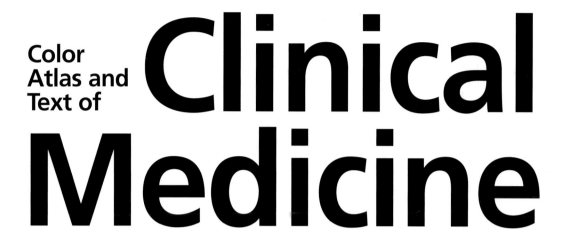

Color Atlas and Text of Clinical Medicine

THIRD EDITION

Charles D Forbes
DSc MD FRCP FRSE
Professor of Medicine
Ninewells Hospital
and Medical School
Dundee, UK

William F Jackson
MA MB BChir FRCP(Glasg)
Medical Writer
Formerly Honorary Consultant
Department of Medicine
Guy's Hospital
London, UK

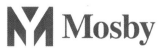 Mosby

EDINBURGH LONDON NEW YORK PHILADELPHIA ST LOUIS
SYDNEY TORONTO 2003

MOSBY
An affiliate of Elsevier Science Limited

First edition 1993
Second edition 1997
Third edition 2003

ISBN 07234 31949
International Student Edition 07234 32953

British Library Cataloguing in Publication Data
A catalogue record for this book is available from the British Library

Library of Congress Cataloging in Publication Data
A catalog record for this book is available from the Library of Congress

Note
Medical knowledge is constantly changing. As new information becomes
available, changes in treatment, procedures, equipment and the use of drugs
become necessary. The authors and the publishers have taken care to ensure
that the information given in this text is accurate and up to date. However,
readers are strongly advised to confirm that the information, especially with
regard to drug usage, complies with the latest legislation and standards of
practice.

your source for books,
journals and multimedia
in the health sciences

www.elsevierhealth.com

Typeset by IMH(Cartrif), Loanhead, Scotland
Printed in Spain

The
publisher's
policy is to use
**paper manufactured
from sustainable forests**

Preface

We have been delighted by the positive reception given to the first two editions of our book, and by its widespread acceptance and adoption around the world. *A Color Atlas and Text of Clinical Medicine* has already been published in English and 14 other languages, and further editions in other languages are in preparation. We are pleased to have had the opportunity to prepare this fully updated third edition, in which the text content has been updated throughout to reflect current knowledge and practice. We have also included a number of new illustrations, especially some representing recent advances in diagnostic imaging.

The style of the book is unchanged and it continues to be aimed at all undergraduate medical students and at those in the early postgraduate years of medical practice. It has also found an important niche in the education of paramedics, especially in the USA, and of students of dentistry, nursing and the other professions allied to medicine world-wide.

Rapid visual identification and interpretation remains a cornerstone of medical practice, but it is increasingly unusual for students to see the full spectrum of clinical presentations of many conditions. This is partly the result of the progressive shift from the investigation and management of patients in a hospital setting, where they may often be seen by large numbers of students, to home and family practice, where direct contact between students and patients is usually much less intensive.

Rapid travel means that most diseases may present anywhere in the world, and we have retained our coverage of all the major traditionally 'tropical' disorders. The inclusion of what may seem rather 'gross' examples of some diseases is also intentional. Advanced disease is far from eradicated on a world-wide basis, and a number of our photographs of severe abnormalities were taken recently. In addition, examples of advanced disease usually carry a powerful educational message, even though most patients in many countries can expect to be diagnosed and treated at an earlier stage.

Our aim in the text has been to match the depth of the shorter medical textbooks, so that this book can be used both as an introduction to clinical medicine and for revision purposes. We also intend that it should be used as a companion to any of the major textbooks of medicine; as such it should provide both a useful visual review of most disorders and a concise summary of their key features.

Most of the illustrations in the book come from our personal collections, but no two individuals could hope to illustrate the broad range of clinical medicine from their own experience alone. We are indebted to the many colleagues listed on pages viii and ix for the full range of pictures we have included, and to other past and present physicians and medical photographers (especially at Guy's Hospital, London, and the Dundee hospitals) for their skilled observations and photography.

The reviewers listed on page viii played a very important role in our task of updating the book for its third edition. We deliberately selected reviewers who had not been involved in the previous edition, and their fresh approach to the book's content was both reassuring and helpful. We also acknowledge the particular help given to us by Dr Leslie Jackson, who has continued his role as reviewer and provider of many of the radiological images in the book.

As with the first edition, we carried out much of our collaborative editorial work within the publisher's office - for this edition mainly in the Edinburgh office of Elsevier Science. We were greatly encouraged by the help and support we received there. We also renew our thanks to Janette Forbes, Barbara Jackson and our families, who have continued to support us despite our many absences from home in the interest of producing this book.

Charles Forbes, Dundee
William Jackson, Oxford

Acknowledgements

REVIEWERS

We are very grateful for the help of a number of colleagues, who reviewed large sections of the book in their specialist fields, and advised us on the content of this third edition. The final selection and drafting of the revised content was entirely our responsibility, but this task was greatly eased by their generous help.

CDF and WFJ

Stuart L Bloom, Consultant Gastroenterologist, The University College London Hospitals, London, UK

Watson Buchanan, Emeritus Professor of Medicine and Consultant Rheumatologist, McMaster University, Hamilton, Ontario, Canada

Rino Cerio, Consultant Dermatologist, Royal London Hospital, London, UK

Stuart M Cobbe, Walton Professor of Medical Cardiology, University of Glasgow, Glasgow, UK

John Dhillon, Consultant Hepatologist, Tayside University Hospitals Trust, Dundee, UK

Tim J Fowler, Consultant Neurologist, Tunbridge Wells and London, UK

David W Gorst, Consultant Haematologist, Royal Lancaster Infirmary, Lancaster, UK

Leslie K Jackson, Consultant Radiologist, Princess Margaret Hospital, Swindon, UK

Robert A MacTier, Consultant Nephrologist, Glasgow Royal Infirmary, Glasgow, UK

Dilip Nathwani, Consultant Physician (Infection) and Senior Lecturer in Medicine, Tayside University Hospitals Trust, Dundee, UK

Paul O'Byrne, Professor of Medicine and Head of the Division of Respiratory Medicine, McMaster University, Hamilton, Ontario, Canada

John A H Wass, Professor of Endocrinology and Consultant Physician, University of Oxford, Oxford, UK

In addition, a number of colleagues in Dundee provided advice on the detailed content of individual sections of the book, and we are very grateful for their valuable contributions:

P G Cachia, (Haematology), **D L W Davidson** (Epilepsy), **A J France** (HIV infection), **A F Ghaly** (Sexually transmitted diseases), **G Leese** (Pituitary disorders), **S M Morley** (Dermatology), **R S McWalter** (Stroke), **A Morris** (Diabetes), **the late C R Pennington** (Gastroenterology), **S D Pringle** (Cardiology), **R C Roberts** (Neurology), **J H Winter** (Respiratory medicine)

vi

PICTURE CONTRIBUTORS

We gratefully acknowledge the generosity of the many colleagues and institutions listed below, who lent us single or, in some cases, multiple pictures.

In all cases, the final responsibility for picture selection, relevance and description rests with us.

CDF and WFJ

G Allan, Glasgow, UK
M C Allison, Newport, UK
J Anderson, Dundee, UK
J Baillie, Durham, NC, USA
M Baraitser, London, UK
D W Beaven, Christchurch, New Zealand
M A Bedford, London, UK
J F Belch, Dundee, UK
C M Black, London, UK
A B Bridges, Stirling, UK
J C Brocklehurst, Manchester, UK
S E Brooks, Christchurch, New Zealand
S E Brown, London, UK
J F Calder, Glasgow, UK
R Cerio, London, UK
G S J Chessell, Aberdeen, UK
S Cobbe, Glasgow, UK
G M Cochrane, London, UK
W B Conolly, Sydney, Australia
N Conway, Southampton, UK
I Cree, London, UK
A Cuschieri, Dundee, UK
D Davidson, Dundee, UK
D R Davies, London, UK
J Dent, Dundee, UK
J Dhillon, Dundee, UK
V Dubowitz, London, UK
K Duguid, Aberdeen, UK
D L Easty, Bristol, UK
C F Farthing, Los Angeles, USA
J Ferguson, Dundee, UK
D C Ferlic, Denver, Colorado, USA
N Finlayson, Edinburgh, UK
R J Flemans, Cambridge, UK
J Forrest, Glasgow, UK
A Forster, Dundee, UK
N J R George, Manchester, UK

H M Gilles, Liverpool, UK
H W Gray, Glasgow, UK
Guy's, King's and St Thomas' School of Medicine, Guy's Campus, London, UK (by courtesy of the Dean)
C A Hart, Liverpool, UK
I Hay, Rochester, MN, USA
P Hayes, Edinburgh, UK
F G J Hayhoe, Cambridge, UK
I S Henderson, Dundee, UK
G Houston, Dundee, UK
L K Jackson, Swindon, UK
M J Jamieson, Aberdeen, UK
D Johnston, Dundee, UK
M Jones, Dundee, UK
R T Jung, Dundee, UK
A Kamal, Lincoln, UK
S Karimjee, London, UK
N Kennedy, Dundee, UK
S Kitamura, Tochigi, Japan
E E Kritzinger, Birmingham, UK
J M Lancer, Sheffield, UK
R E Latchaw, Minneapolis, USA
C Lau, Hong Kong
P Le Souëf, Perth, Australia
M H Lessof, London, UK
D Levinson, Dundee, UK
R W Lloyd-Davies, London, UK
C Lockie, Stratford-upon-Avon, UK
T MacDonald, Dundee, UK
C J McEwan, Dundee, UK
D S McLaren, London, UK
M McMurdo, Dundee, UK
R MacTier, Glasgow, UK
J Mills, Dundee, UK
K L G Mills, Aberdeen, UK
M J Monaghan, London, UK
S Morley, Dundee, UK

R Morton, Chelmsford, UK
A Muir, Dundee, UK
R Newton, Dundee, UK
M Nimmo, Dundee, UK
C O'Callaghan, Leicester, UK
G Page, Aberdeen, UK
A Paton, Oxford, UK
C Paterson, Dundee, UK
J R Pepper, London, UK
W Peters, London, UK
M J Pippard, Dundee, UK
S D Pringle, Dundee, UK
N K Ragge, London, UK
P J Rees, London, UK
R Roberts, Dundee, UK
I S Ross, Aberdeen, UK
M B Rubens, London, UK
M A Sambrook, Manchester, UK
J D Schaller, Boston, USA
K F R Schiller, Oxford, UK
C Schmitt, Durham, NC, USA
J D Shaw, Sheffield, UK
M R Shiu, Coventry, UK
D I H Simpson, Belfast, UK
D J Sinclair, Edinburgh, UK
R Siwek, Aberdeen, UK
L Spitz, London, UK
R C D Staughton, London, UK
P Sweny, London, UK
H M A Towler, Aberdeen, UK
W R Tyldesley, Liverpool, UK
S R Underwood, London, UK
D A Warrell, Oxford, UK
Wellcome Institute Library, London, UK
G Williams, Manchester, UK
J H Winter, Dundee, UK
A Wisdom, London, UK
T Yamaguchi, Hirosaki, Japan

Contents

1 Infections

INTRODUCTION

Infections are the largest cause of morbidity and mortality worldwide. The most common infections are the diarrhoeal diseases, respiratory infection, malaria, measles, hepatitis, schistosomiasis, whooping cough and neonatal tetanus. The course and severity of infection depend on a variety of factors, including the virulence of the strain of infecting organism, the resistance of the population or individual, which may be reduced by famine or intercurrent disease (**1.1**), social factors such as lack of sanitation, poor housing and a contaminated water supply, and the availability of medical facilities providing vaccination or diagnosis and treatment. Ultimately it is always the interaction between the patient (host) and the pathogen that determines the outcome of any infection.

HISTORY

A careful history can often localize the site of a possible infection and may suggest its nature. Viral infections are the most common worldwide. They occur in epidemics, often initially in school-age children, and are passed on to adults. Upper respiratory and diarrhoeal illnesses account for the largest number of cases. Points to be elicited in an assessment of history include:

- recent contact with infected persons (**1.3**), including recent birth (**1.4**).
- previous exposure to infections
- vaccination status
- occupation, social pursuits and hobbies

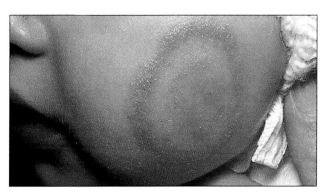

1.2 Tinea (ringworm). Patients with dermatophyte infections act as reservoirs of infection, and ringworm may also sometimes be 'caught' through contact with infected animals. This florid case resulted from infection with *Microsporum canis*.

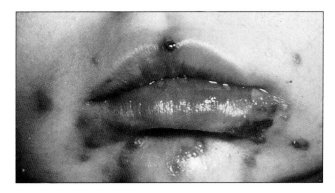

1.3 Primary herpes simplex in and around the mouth. The infection is usually acquired from siblings or parents, and is readily transmitted to other contacts. The infection commonly persists in a dormant phase, but the 'secondary' lesions that occur on reactivation (*see* **p. 19**) are also a common source of infection.

FACTORS THAT MAY AFFECT THE COURSE OF INFECTIONS	
Immune disturbances	**Prosthetic devices and procedures**
HIV infection	Indwelling urinary catheter
Immunosuppression with steroids, cytotoxic drugs	Arterial and venous cannulae
Immune deficiency – hypogamma-globulinaemia and neutropenia	Artificial valves
Leukaemia and lymphoma	Joint prostheses
Various cancers	Vascular grafts
Malnutrition	Chronic ambulatory peritoneal dialysis
Alcoholism and chronic liver disease	Intracranial shunts
Intravenous drug misuse	
Diabetes mellitus	
Splenectomy	

1.1 Factors that may affect the course of infections.

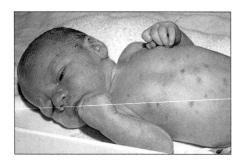

1.4 Mother-to-child transmission is important in a number of infections. This infant has congenital rubella, presenting as a small-for-dates baby with a purpuric rash caused by thrombocytopenia. Children born with congenital rubella are a potential source of infection to others, and it is important that appropriate steps are taken to protect other patients and staff.

- contact with animals (wild or domestic) (**1.2**)
- recent foreign travel, including types of endemic and epidemic diseases and the kind of travel (urban, rural, 'backpacking', etc.)
- migrants should be asked for details of their country and place of origin
- recent dietary history, especially the type/source of food and water
- insect bites

- previous surgery, accidents and the presence of prosthetic devices (**1.5**)
- history of intravenous drug misuse (**1.6**)
- sexual activity and proclivity
- tattooing
- blood transfusion and injections
- recent drug history, including herbal and 'natural' remedies.

CLINICAL EXAMINATION

A careful and complete clinical examination often provides clues to the nature and site of infection. Special attention should be paid to the skin (for nodules, rashes, bites, injection marks (**1.6**)), eyes, lymph nodes (enlargement of which may be local or generalized), the liver and the spleen. With sexually transmitted disease in particular, it is important to examine the genitalia, the perineum, the anus and the mouth. A thorough examination should include taking the patient's temperature and plotting any fever, a general examination for signs of jaundice, dehydration, weight loss, nutritional status, anaemia and oedema, and examination of:

- the mouth, pharynx and throat for ulcers or membranes
- the conjunctiva and retina for petechiae, inflammation and choroidal deposits (**1.7**)
- the tympanic membrane for otitis media (**1.8**)

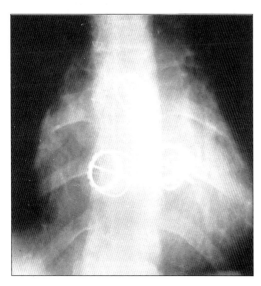

1.5 Prosthetic surgical devices are associated with an increased risk of systemic or local infection. This patient has undergone triple valve replacement with Starr–Edwards' valves, and – like all those who have had heart valve surgery – is at increased risk of contracting infective endocarditis. Similarly, patients who have joint prostheses or other implants are at greater risk of systemic and local infection.

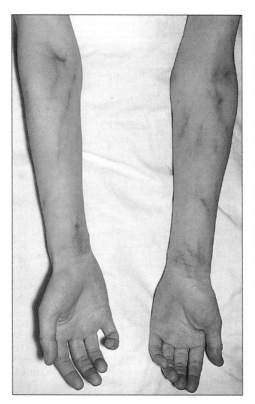

1.6 Intravenous drug misuse typically leads to this appearance, which results from repeated superficial thrombophlebitis of accessible veins in the arm or elsewhere in the body. The sharing and reuse of syringes and needles, together with the lack of aseptic technique, puts these patients at special risk of a wide range of infections, including bacterial septicaemia (sometimes with unusual organisms), systemic fungal infection, hepatitis B, hepatitis C and HIV infection. Right-sided endocarditis is a common complication.

- the skin for rashes (**1.9**), nodules, ulcers or signs of scratching
- nails, for splinter haemorrhages (**3.32**)
- lymph nodes (**1.10**) liver and spleen (**1.11**), which may be enlarged and/or tender to touch
- the heart for evidence of endocarditis or cardiac failure
- the genitalia for ulcers or discharge of pus
- the lungs for the production of sputum and consolidation or cavitation

- the central nervous system for meningism, impairment of conscious level or focal neurological signs
- urine for evidence of infection or bleeding.

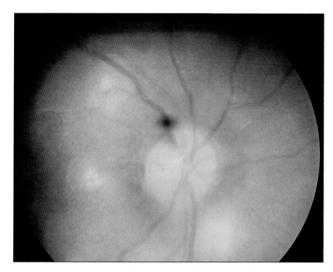

1.7   Choroidal tubercles in acute miliary tuberculosis. This appearance is virtually diagnostic, so it is essential to examine the fundi of any patient in whom miliary tuberculosis is a possibility.

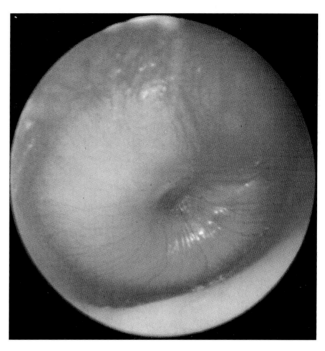

1.8   Severe acute otitis media, with bulging and hyperaemia of the tympanic membrane. The middle ear is filled with purulent fluid. Otitis media is usually symptomatic, but young children may be unable to communicate their earache, so examination with the auriscope is essential.

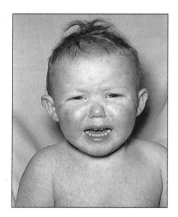

1.9   The face in measles. Rashes may take many forms and have many different distributions in infectious diseases. This miserable child has a characteristic appearance, with a fine, light red maculopapular rash on the skin. Unfortunately, not all rashes are so directly diagnostic.

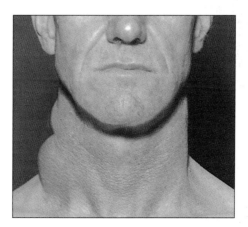

1.10   Enlarged lymph nodes in the posterior triangle on the neck. Lymphadenopathy is a feature of many infectious diseases, and aspiration biopsy of the enlarged nodes is sometimes helpful in diagnosis. This patient presented no other clinical clues to the diagnosis, but histology demonstrated the typical caseating granulomas of tuberculosis (see **pp 32–34**).

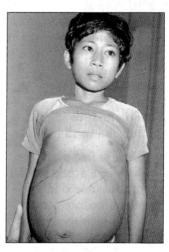

1.11   Gross hepatomegaly and splenomegaly has been marked on the abdomen of this Filipino boy who has schistosomiasis.

INVESTIGATIONS

A number of tests are often needed to give clues to the cause, site and extent of the disease. Many may also be of value in following the progress of the infection and the effects of therapy. Useful investigations include the following:

- a full blood count with a differential count – eosinophilia is an important finding in parasitic infections; lymphocytosis is usually found in viral infections
- erythrocyte sedimentation rate, plasma viscosity or C-reactive protein level (non-specific tests that may be of value in monitoring the course of diseases)
- examination of thick and thin blood films for parasites, especially malaria (**1.148**), trypanosomiasis (**1.12**) and filariasis (**1.157**)
- examination of smears using direct staining (**1.13**), dark-field illumination or fluorescent antibodies
- urinalysis for blood, bile, protein, pus cells and ova of schistosomiasis
- stool microscopy for amoebae, cysts (**1.14**), ova and parasites
- renal and liver function tests
- lumbar puncture for examination of cerebrospinal fluid (CSF) in suspected meningitis

- cultures of blood, urine, stools, throat swab, CSF, pus and so on for viruses, bacteria and fungi
- immunoglobulin levels
- serological tests for specific infections
- rapid diagnostic tests, for example antigen detection and polymerase chain reaction (PCR)
- chest and abdominal X-rays
- stool electron microscopy for rotavirus.

Further specific investigations may be needed to localize the site of the infection, including tomography, ultrasound (**1.139**), isotope scanning (**1.15**), computed tomography (CT) (**1.16, 1.17**) and magnetic resonance imaging (MRI).

Biopsy may be required for a tissue diagnosis. Endoscopy is valuable in obtaining tissue from the lung and alimentary tract, and laparoscopy enables direct inspection and biopsy of the abdominal contents. Tissues that may provide a diagnosis include:

- bone marrow (direct cytology and culture)
- skin (fresh preparations and histology)
- liver (histology and aspiration of abscesses)
- lung – transbronchial biopsy (**1.18**) or aspiration of bronchial washings
- lymph node or spleen
- large and small intestine.

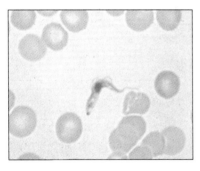

1.12 Blood smear showing *Trypanosoma brucei*, one of the causes of African trypanosomiasis. This finding is diagnostic.

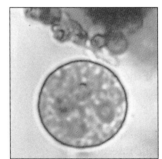

1.14 The mature cyst form of *Entamoeba histolytica*, on stool microscopy, showing the typical appearance with four nuclei. (Iodine, × 1800)

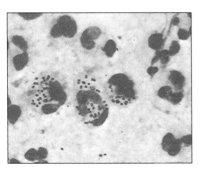

1.13 Intracellular gonococci in a smear of urethral discharge. This appearance is strongly suggestive of gonorrhoea, but definitive diagnosis depends on culture and identification of the organism.

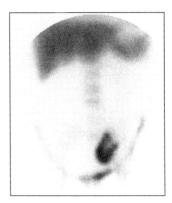

1.15 Isotope scanning, revealing a collection of pus in the left lower quadrant of the abdomen. Here the technique used involved labelling some of the patient's white cells with technetium hexamethyl-propylamine oxime (Tc-HMPAO). This patient had developed a pelvic abscess as a complication of pelvic inflammatory disease (*see* **p. 63**).

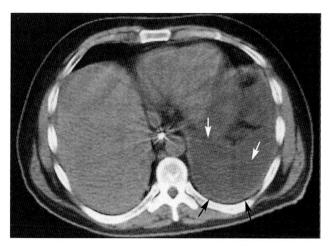

1.16 CT showing a large subphrenic abscess in a patient who developed a persistent fever in association with rather vague pain in his abdomen and shoulder. A large collection of fluid can be seen posteriorly (arrows). Other cuts showed this collection to be between the spleen and the diaphragm.

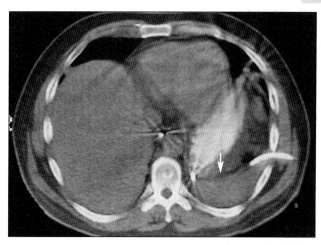

1.17 Percutaneous drainage under CT control yielded 1300 ml of pus, allowing immediate relief of symptoms and culture and sensitivity testing of the contents of the abscess. Part of the drainage catheter can be seen in this view at the same level as 1.16. The spleen (arrow) has moved up on drainage of the abscess, and the contrast-containing stomach is also seen.

Failure to find the cause or type of infection is not uncommon, in which case a 'best guess' trial of appropriate chemotherapy is often used. Indeed, in the very sick patient treatment should be started immediately with supportive measures and 'blind' antimicrobial therapy, which should be continued until the results of investigations dictate a change.

It is important to remember that multiple infections may occur in the same patient. It is common for secondary bacterial infections to occur in patients with primary viral infections, for example; and in patients with gross immunosuppression, such as those with AIDS, several infections often coexist.

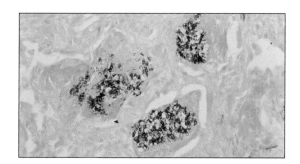

1.18 *Pneumocystis carinii,* dark stained using the Grocott method, in a transbronchial biopsy of the lung. Diagnosis of infections from tissue biopsy is necessary when the organisms are difficult or impossible to culture, as is the case with a number of the secondary infections that occur in AIDS, and with protozoal and helminthic infections. Similar staining of sputum or centrifuged bronchioalveolar lavage fluid may also allow identification of organisms.

IMMUNIZATION

Some infections that previously caused major morbidity and mortality can be prevented through appropriate immunization (vaccination). Immunization in childhood and before international travel is now routine in developed countries. Precise immunization schedules vary from one country to another.

VIRAL INFECTIONS

HIV INFECTION AND AIDS

Infection with the human immunodeficiency virus (HIV) gives rise to a wide range of clinical conditions resulting from progressive immunodeficiency. There is no internationally agreed definition of AIDS (acquired immune deficiency syndrome), but the term is usually used to describe patients with the more serious complications of HIV infection.

HIV infection is most prevalent in sub-Saharan Africa where, in some countries, up to 30% of the adult population have the infection. The infection is now spreading most rapidly in South-East Asia and the Indian subcontinent. The World Health Organization (WHO) estimates that over 33 million people are living with HIV/AIDS worldwide, and that it causes at least 2.3 million deaths per year. The resulting chronic ill health and premature death in the young adult populations of some developing countries will have devastating social and economic consequences. In the developed world, the prevalence is lower and the greater funding and availability of healthcare has also transformed the outlook for many with HIV infection.

Sexual intercourse is the major route of transmission. In the indigenous population of the developed world, unprotected homosexual intercourse remains an important mode of transmission, but heterosexual transmission accounts for the majority of infections worldwide. Coexistent sexually transmitted diseases, especially those causing genital ulceration, enhance the transmission of HIV.

Other important routes of transmission or potential transmission include the transfusion of contaminated blood or blood products, organ transplantation, sharing of syringes by misusers of intravenous drugs, accidental 'needle prick' injury with contaminated needles or surgical instruments, reuse of non-sterile medical equipment and mother-to-child transmission.

VIROLOGY AND IMMUNOPATHOLOGY

HIV is an RNA virus which selectively infects cells that express CD4 on their surface. These include part of the T-lymphocyte population, macrophages and some cells in the central nervous system (CNS). HIV copies its genetic code using reverse transcriptase to produce a double stranded DNA copy which is inserted into the host cell genome and cannot be removed. HIV has its own protease, which helps assemble mature virions in the cell cytoplasm.

HIV antibodies are usually found within 2 weeks of initial infection but can take up to 3 months to reach detectable levels. The HIV antibody test is the preferred method for diagnosing the infection. The rate of growth of HIV in a patient can be estimated by measuring the number of copies of viral RNA in plasma using polymerase chain reaction (PCR) technology (the 'viral load'). The degree of damage to the immune system is best indicated by the CD4 count – the number of CD4 lymphocytes in peripheral blood (normal range $500-1000 \times 10^6$/litre).

The antibody response is not a neutralizing response, so HIV is still able to infect susceptible cells. Some infected cells lie dormant but most are eliminated by cell mediated immunity or cell death from the effects of HIV replication. The loss of CD4 cells is offset by production of new cells from precursors. These new cells are susceptible to HIV infection so the cycle repeats itself. As years go by, the capacity of the immune system to regenerate is lost and manifestations of immunodeficiency become apparent.

CLINICAL FEATURES

Primary HIV infection
Within a few weeks of infection the patient may suffer a glandular fever-like illness and a non-itchy macular rash (**1.19**). During this stage HIV replicates on a huge scale and seeds itself in 'sanctuary sites' in the body (e.g. in the CNS). The symptoms and signs subside over a few days or weeks and the patient returns to normal health.

LATER MANIFESTATIONS OF HIV INFECTION

Later manifestations of HIV infection are determined largely by the degree of immunodeficiency. Some of the common features are listed in **1.20**. Many other opportunistic infections are also seen, and their incidence varies in different parts of the world.

Mild immunodeficiency
Tuberculosis is usually pulmonary, but cavitation is relatively uncommon in HIV infection. Drug resistant strains of tuberculosis are becoming more common, so HIV patients with tuberculosis should be isolated until a response to treatment is apparent or drug sensitivities are known. Standard antituberculous drugs should be used in the first instance (*see* **p. 33**).

Varicella zoster infection commonly presents as shingles (*see also* **p. 20**), often in more than one dermatome (**1.21**). Atypical presentations include recurrent intensely itchy spots with necrotic centres. New lesions of this type may appear over many weeks, mostly on the limbs, but sometimes on the trunk, and they have the appearance of multiple cigarette burns. Like shingles, these lesions respond to aciclovir and related drugs.

Herpes simplex infection in patients with HIV may be mucocutaneous (**1.22**) or disseminated. Aciclovir and other antiviral therapy is often effective in its treatment.

Candidiasis of the oropharynx can be extensive (**1.23**) and may spread to involve the oesophagus (**1.24**), but it usually responds well to appropriate antifungal treatment (*see* **p. 46**).

Kaposi's sarcoma (**1.25–1.28**) is a multifocal tumour initially seen in the skin as purplish brown spots. It later spreads to the gastrointestinal tract and, if untreated, to internal organs. Human herpesvirus 8 infection is thought to be responsible for this neoplasm. It responds well to local radiotherapy and to chemotherapy.

Thrombocytopenia is common in HIV infection. The underlying disorder is excessive destruction of platelets similar to that seen in idiopathic thrombocytopenia. It rarely gives rise to bleeding complications even when the platelet count is less than 10. It responds well to zidovudine.

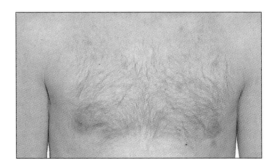

1.19 HIV-related rash in a 22-year-old homosexual man. In addition to this rash, the patient presented with fever, sore throat and headache. HIV serology was negative at this time, but seroconversion was noted 5 weeks later.

COMMON FEATURES OF HIV INFECTION ACCORDING TO DEGREE OF IMMUNODEFICIENCY				
Degree of immunodeficiency	Opportunistic infection	Tumours	Neurological	Other
Mild: CD4 > 200	Tuberculosis Varicella zoster *Candida* Bacterial pneumonia	Kaposi's sarcoma	Peripheral neuropathy	Thrombocytopenia Sweats Arthralgia Persistent generalized lymphadenopathy
Moderate: CD4 200–50	*Pneumocystis carinii* *Toxoplasma* Molluscum contagiosum *Salmonella* Herpes simplex *Cryptosporidium*	Cervical Anal	Myelopathy Dementia	Oral hairy leukoplakia Wasting HIV retinopathy
Severe: CD4 < 50	Cytomegalovirus *Cryptococcus* Atypical mycobacteria	Lymphoma	HIV encephalitis Strokes Venous thrombosis	

1.20   Common features of HIV infection according to degree of immunodeficiency.

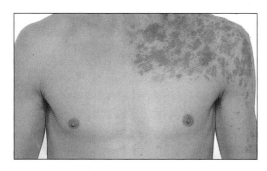

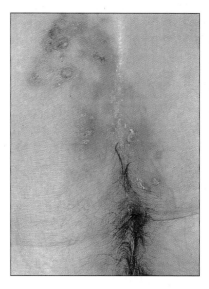

1.22   **Severe perianal herpes simplex** is a common problem in homosexual patients with HIV infection. It may cause great discomfort, but often responds to antiviral treatment.

1.21   Herpes zoster (shingles) is often the first manifestation of immunosuppression in patients with HIV disease. It can also occur in many other patients (*see* p. 20) but multidermatomal involvement is particularly common in HIV infection. In this patient the C4 and C5 dermatomes are affected.

Moderate immunodeficiency

Pneumocystis carinii pneumonia usually presents with a dry cough and breathlessness of several weeks duration. Physical signs of cyanosis and dyspnoea at rest indicate severe disease. The X-ray appearances can be deceptively mild (**1.29**). The diagnosis is made by ELISA tests on sputum (the production of which is induced by the inhalation of nebulized 3% saline) or on bronchoalveolar lavage fluid obtained at bronchoscopy. Treatment is with high dose co-trimoxazole and prednisolone. The steroid protects the patient from acute respiratory failure at the onset of treatment and improves the tolerance to the antimicrobials. Complications of *Pneumocystis* pneumonia include pneumothorax, which can be bilateral and is indicative of severe life-threatening disease.

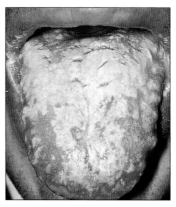

1.23   **Extensive oral infection with *Candida albicans*** in a patient with HIV infection. Note the gross changes in the tongue and the angular cheilitis.

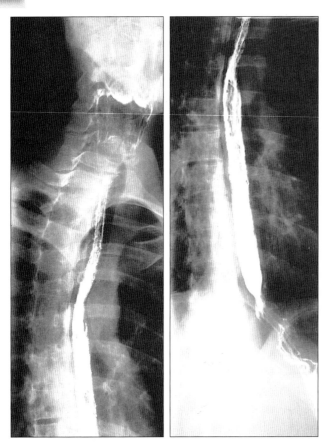

1.24 **Candidiasis of the oesophagus in a patient with HIV infection,** demonstrated by barium swallow. Note the mottled appearance, which results from multiple plaques of candidiasis on the oesophageal mucosa.

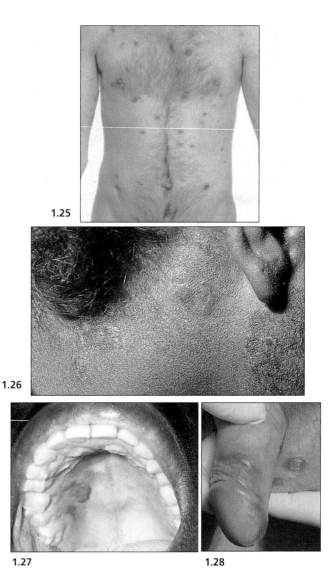

1.25–1.28 **Kaposi's sarcoma** is a common complication of HIV infection. In **1.25** note the multifocal nature of the tumour. **1.26** shows the appearance of similar involvement in a black African patient. Kaposi's sarcoma may also affect mucous membranes, as seen in **1.27**, where there are two obvious plaques of Kaposi's sarcoma on the palate. Similar lesions may be seen throughout the gut and the bronchial tree. Kaposi's sarcoma may occur anywhere on the surface of the body, including the penis and scrotum (**1.28**).

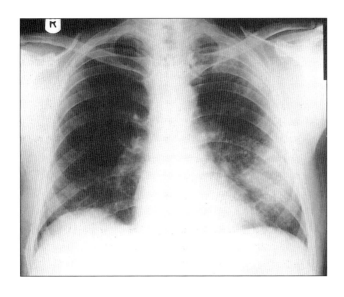

1.29 **Pneumocystis pneumonia** is a common life-threatening opportunistic infection in patients with HIV and in other immunocompromised patients. The area of consolidation in the left lower zone was the only radiological abnormality, but the patient had severe disease, requiring urgent therapy.

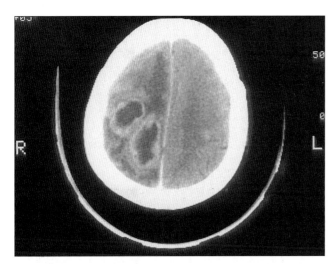

1.30 Cerebral abscesses in the right occipital and parietal areas on a contrast-enhanced CT of a patient with advanced HIV infection. The 'ring enhancement' surrounded by an area of low attenuation (cerebral oedema) is a characteristic finding.

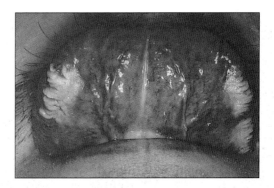

1.31 Hairy leukoplakia in a patient with HIV infection. Note the appearance of ribbed white plaques along the sides of the tongue. The term 'hairy' refers to the histopathological appearance. The cause appears to be proliferation of Epstein–Barr virus in the superficial layers of the squamous epithelium of the tongue.

Cerebral toxoplasmosis presents with headaches, fevers and localizing neurological signs. Cerebral abscesses are characteristic and can be diagnosed by contrast enhanced CT (**1.30**) or MRI of the brain.

Cryptosporidium is the commonest pathogen to be isolated from patients with HIV and diarrhoea, though other protozoa and bacteria may also lead to severe gastrointestinal symptoms, and HIV infection may itself cause enteropathy and malabsorption. Weight loss and wasting may result from prolonged gastrointestinal involvement with any of these organisms.

Carcinomas of the cervix and anus are related to co-infection with human papilloma virus. An annual cervical smear is advisable in women with HIV infection.

Leukoplakia may develop in the mouth (**1.31**)

Myelopathy is heralded by a gradual onset of spastic paresis. Initially it involves the legs but bladder control is also eventually lost. Myelopathy can be arrested by anti-retroviral therapy and some recovery is possible.

Generalized wasting and HIV-induced retinopathy may also begin at this stage.

Severe immunodeficiency

Cytomegalovirus (CMV) retinitis is a painless condition which usually begins with blurred vision in one eye. It is diagnosed by the characteristic features of destructive retinitis and the appearance as shown in **1.32**. The visual loss is progressive and permanent, and it can lead to blindness in a matter of days. Prompt anti-retroviral therapy arrests the disease process.

Mycobacterium avium-intracellulare (MAI) is one of the non-tuberculous mycobacteria which cause significant disease in HIV patients (*see also* **p. 34**). Weight loss, sweats, hepatosplenomegaly, anaemia and abnormal liver function are

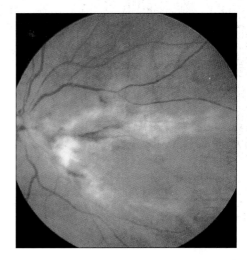

1.32 Cytomegalovirus (CMV) retinitis in a patient with HIV. This destructive retinitis tends to spread along the lines of the vessel and can rapidly progress to irreversible blindness.

among the non-specific features of this systemic infection. Blood culture for mycobacteria or tissue biopsy (liver or bone marrow) reveal the diagnosis. Various treatment regimens have produced temporary improvement but the outlook is usually very poor.

High grade B cell lymphoma (**1.33**; *see also* **p. 435**) is a very serious development with a very poor prognosis. The response to chemotherapy is poor but palliative radiotherapy can be beneficial.

ANTI-RETROVIRAL THERAPY

Initial experience with single drug therapy for HIV infection was disappointing. The benefit was limited due to the development of drug resistance by the virus. Since 1996,

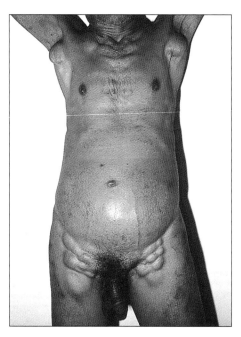

1.33 Non-Hodgkin's lymphoma in a patient with HIV infection. There is massive axillary and inguinal lymphadenopathy. He also had gross hepatosplenomegaly and ascites.

combination therapy – called highly active anti-retroviral therapy (HAART) – has transformed the outlook for HIV patients. Simultaneous use of three or more drugs can circumvent the problem of drug resistance. By reducing viral replication to a minimum, the immune system can regenerate and improve its performance. This immune reconstitution can abolish many of the opportunist infections and produce regression of the tumours. Dramatic improvements in survival and quality of life accompany these treatments.

The aims of HAART are to reduce the viral load to below the minimum level of detection and to raise the CD4 lymphocyte count. Treatment is usually started while the CD4 count is between 350 and 200, and must be seen as lifelong.

COMMONLY USED ANTI-RETROVIRAL DRUGS		
Nucleoside reverse transcriptase inhibitors (NRTI)	**Non-nucleoside reverse transcriptase inhibitors (NNRTI)**	**Protease inhibitors (PI)**
Zidovudine	Nevirapine	Indinavir
Didanosine	Efavirenz	Saquinavir
Lamivudine		Ritonavir
Stavudine		Nelfinavir
Abacavir		Amprenavir

1.34 Commonly used anti-retroviral drugs.

The two targets are reverse transcriptase and HIV protease. The commonly used drugs are listed in **1.34**.

Side-effects of treatment are common. The nucleoside reverse transcriptase inhibitor (NRTI) drugs are toxic to mitochondria and can cause peripheral neuropathy, myopathy, cardiomyopathy, diabetes, pancreatitis and lactic acidosis. These effects are related to duration of therapy. NNRTI (non-nucleoside reverse transcriptase inhibitor) drugs can cause liver function disturbance (nevirapine) and CNS effects (efavirenz). PI drugs (protease inhibitors) often lead to elevated plasma cholesterol and triglycerides.

Mother-to-child transmission can be almost eliminated by treating the mother with HAART during the second half of pregnancy and the child in the first 6 weeks of life. Even single dose nevirapine at the onset of labour reduces the risk of transmission. Breast-feeding is another source of HIV infection for the child and should be avoided if possible.

Post-exposure prophylaxis (for example following a needle stick injury), can prevent transmission but the drugs must be started as soon as possible after the injury.

PROPHYLAXIS AGAINST OPPORTUNISTIC INFECTION

Pneumocystis carinii infection is mostly confined to patients with CD4 counts < 200. Below this level, prophylactic therapy with co-trimoxazole can prevent pneumocystis infection. Other opportunistic infections can also be prevented by appropriate prophylactic therapy.

PREVENTION OF HIV INFECTION

Public health education is the key to prevention. Reducing the number of sexual partners and using condoms during anal and vaginal intercourse are very effective ways to reduce the spread of HIV. Use of HAART in pregnancy can eliminate mother-to-child transmission. Testing of blood donations and organ donors reduces the risk of HIV transmission to the recipients.

THE COMMON COLD

The common cold (acute coryza) is the most common disease caused by infection in the developed world, and the most frequent symptomatic manifestation of upper respiratory tract infection (URTI). These infections may be caused by a range of viruses, including rhinoviruses, respiratory syncytial virus, parainfluenza viruses, coronaviruses and adenoviruses.

Uncomplicated acute coryza leads to nasal congestion (**1.35**), a watery nasal discharge that may become purulent and often a sore throat. Most cases resolve spontaneously, but the common cold may be complicated by secondary bacterial infection,

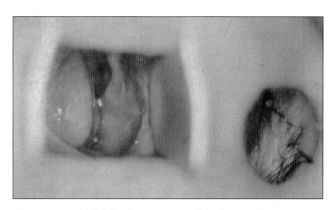

1.35 Acute rhinitis in the common cold. The nasal mucous membrane is oedematous, so the inferior turbinate abuts against the septum causing obstruction, as seen here in a view through a nasal speculum.

leading to sinusitis, otitis media and infection of the lower respiratory tract.

ENTEROVIRUS INFECTIONS

The enteroviruses can be subdivided into three main subgroups: polioviruses, coxsackieviruses and echoviruses (hepatitis A, *see* **p. 386**, is also caused by an enterovirus). All infect man by the faecal–oral route. Initial viral replication takes place in the gut or respiratory mucosa, with subsequent shedding of virus. If host immunity is poor, virus enters the bloodstream and may be disseminated to target organs such as the meninges, nervous tissue, heart and skin.

Enteroviruses can be isolated from stool, pharyngeal secretions, CSF, pericardial fluid and, occasionally, from blood

in severe neonatal infections. Rising antibody titres may be demonstrated to specific enteroviruses. Treatment of enterovirus infections is symptomatic, although trials of antiviral therapy are in progress in severe cases.

Poliomyelitis
Poliomyelitis has an incubation period of up to 14 days and is characterized by an initial flu-like illness followed, if host immunity is poor, by aseptic meningitis. The virus then enters nervous tissue, the main attack being on the anterior horn cells of the spinal cord, causing flaccid paralysis of limb muscles that tends to be asymmetrical and is usually permanent (**1.36, 1.37**). In severe cases, muscles of swallowing and respiration may be involved.

Management is symptomatic, but paralytic poliomyelitis requires skilled physiotherapy. Patients may also need long-term ventilation and, later, the provision of mechanical aids or corrective surgery, or both.

An injectable killed virus vaccine (Salk vaccine) and a live attenuated oral vaccine (Sabin vaccine) are available for prevention of poliomyelitis. This disease is now very rare in the developed world, and a WHO initiative aims to eliminate the disease completely from the rest of the world within the next few years. Nevertheless, the long-term sequelae of the disease will be seen for many years to come.

Coxsackieviruses (groups A and B) and echoviruses
Coxsackieviruses and echoviruses produce a wide variety of clinical syndromes after a short but variable incubation period, including non-specific febrile illness, rashes (**1.38**), myocarditis, pericarditis, meningitis, meningo-encephalitis and, rarely, paralytic disease. Herpangina (ulcerative lesions on the palate and fauces) and hand-foot-and-mouth disease (**1.39, 1.40**) are caused

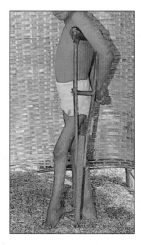

1.36 Paralysis of the left leg as a result of poliomyelitis in an Ethiopian boy. The disease is still a major problem in developing countries.

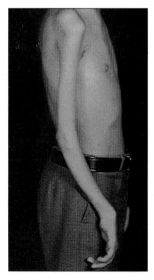

1.37 Flail arm as a result of poliomyelitis in infancy.

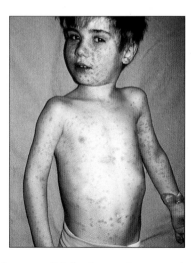

1.38 Echovirus type 19 infection causing a maculopapular rash. Rashes of this kind may be very difficult to distinguish from rubella (*see* **p. 12**), and antibody studies may be required for a firm diagnosis.

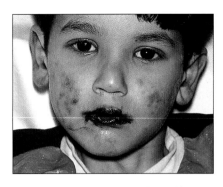

1.39   Hand–foot–mouth disease. This shows the typical rash of bright red macules, with small vesicles on an erythematous base on both cheeks and the lips. Similar lesions occur inside the mouth. This patient has been treated by the topical application of gentian violet.

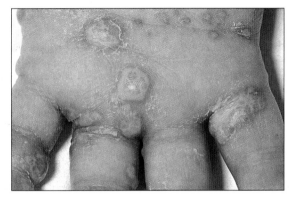

1.40   Hand–foot–mouth disease. Many of the lesions are distributed on the lateral aspects of the fingers, but in this young patient several lesions were also present on the palm.

by group A coxsackieviruses. Epidemic myalgia (Bornholm disease) is a common presentation of infection with group B coxsackieviruses. Both echoviruses and coxsackieviruses can cause severe generalized infection in neonates. The postviral fatigue syndrome may follow coxsackievirus infection.

RUBELLA

The causal agent of rubella is a togavirus that causes a mild illness and is spread by droplets from the respiratory tract. The incubation period is 18–19 days. A pink maculopapular rash appears on the second day of illness (**1.41, 1.42**). On the trunk, the rash becomes confluent and may resemble the rash of scarlet fever. There is usually mild inflammation of the throat and palate, and the posterior cervical lymph nodes become enlarged and tender. The rash fades in about 48 hours and recovery, especially in children, is rapid. Complications include arthralgia (more common in adults), thrombocytopenia and very rarely encephalitis.

The diagnosis is confirmed by the detection of rising titre of IgM antibody in the serum. Treatment is not usually necessary but arthralgia requires relief of pain with analgesics.

Rubella in either childhood or adult life is usually a trivial, self-limiting illness, but the virus can cause serious damage to the developing fetus. Fetal infection can occur at any stage of pregnancy, but the damage tends to be most marked in the first trimester. The sequelae may include signs of infection at birth (**1.4**), microcephaly, deafness, blindness (**1.43**) and congenital cardiac malformations (*see* **p. 225**).

Suspected rubella in early pregnancy should be confirmed serologically; appropriate advice on risk to the fetus and availability of abortion should be given to the parents, if the disease is confirmed. If there is contact with rubella in early pregnancy, it is important to establish the diagnosis in the index case and to check the antibody status of the pregnant contact as soon as possible. A non-immune contact in early pregnancy should be given the option of abortion if rubella

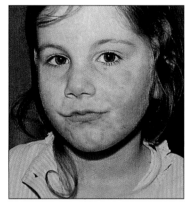

1.41   Rubella, showing the early stage of the rash on the face. Note that the patient shows no signs of catarrh or conjunctival discharge, in contrast to the typical patient with measles.

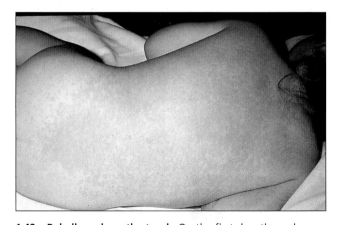

1.42   Rubella rash on the trunk. On the first day, the rash consists of discrete, delicate pink macules. These may coalesce on the second day, as here, but the severity of the rash varies considerably, and it may be missed altogether when the lesions are sparse.

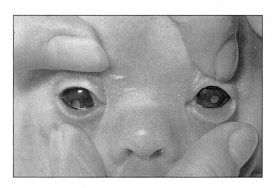

1.43 **Cataracts causing blindness** in this newborn baby with congenital rubella.

develops. If abortion is not performed, hyperimmune globulin can be given and is protective in about 40% of patients.

Prevention may be accomplished by live attenuated vaccine, used on its own or combined with measles and mumps vaccine (MMR). Rubella vaccine should not be given during pregnancy.

YELLOW FEVER

This is an acute mosquito-borne infection caused by a flavivirus which results in a pyrexial illness, with liver and renal involvement and disseminated intravascular coagulation (DIC, *see* **p. 443**). It is found in both Africa and Central and Southern America in a narrow band about the equator, but not in Asia. There are two important cycles of transmission: in the urban type the yellow fever virus is transmitted from an infected person to a non-immune recipient by mosquitoes (*Aedes* sp.); in the sylvan (or jungle) type there is a monkey reservoir and the vector is the *Aedes* sp. in Africa or *Haemagogus* sp. in America.

The spectrum of clinical illness varies from a very mild, transient, pyrexial illness to a rapid, progressively fatal form. The incubation period is short (4–6 days). The appearance of

jaundice (not usually severe), proteinuria and haemorrhage give clues to the diagnosis. Haemorrhage is often apparent initially in the skin but haematemesis may occur and is a poor prognostic sign (**1.44**). In fulminant cases there is progression of liver and renal failure to coma and death. The mortality rate is about 40% in these severe cases.

There is no specific antiviral therapy, and general supportive measures are required for severely ill patients. Yellow fever vaccine gives protection for up to 10 years.

DENGUE FEVER

Dengue fever is a very common disease in many tropical areas, especially South America, sub-Saharan Africa, South-East Asia and India. It is transmitted by *Aedes* sp. mosquitoes which are themselves infected by the dengue virus (or one of four subtypes). The incubation is short (1–2 days). The clinical illness is usually self-limiting, with high fever, arthralgia and a petechial rash.

Dengue haemorrhagic fever is a severe complication of dengue, which usually occurs in second or subsequent attacks in individuals partly immunized by previous infection. The clinical presentation is abrupt with extreme nausea, vomiting and fever. Purpura appears on the second or third day and disseminated intravascular coagulation (DIC) with bleeding from a variety of sites dominates the clinical picture (**1.45, p. 443**). Viraemia and blood loss produce a profound state of shock (dengue shock syndrome, DSS).

There is no specific treatment, but symptomatic treatment with oxygen and blood volume expanders is often essential. Despite this, there is a mortality rate of up to 50% in severe cases. Public health measures for mosquito control are important.

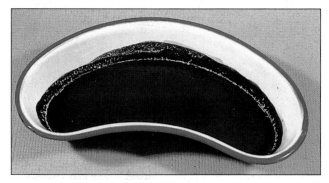

1.44 **'Coffee ground' vomit in yellow fever** has severe implications. As in other conditions, it is a sign of major upper gastrointestinal bleeding.

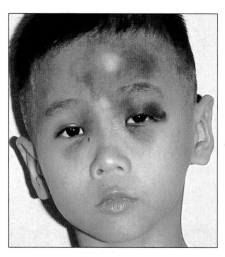

1.45 **Dengue haemorrhagic fever** causing marked ecchymoses associated with DIC in an infected 8-year-old boy in Vietnam.

EPIDEMIC ENCEPHALITIS

Several flaviviruses and togaviruses cause mosquito-transmitted encephalitis in various parts of the world. These include several forms of equine encephalitis in the American continent, Japanese encephalitis (**1.46**) and St Louis encephalitis. Russian spring–summer encephalitis and powassan are similar diseases transmitted by ticks. Encephalitis results rapidly, and the patients present with fever and rigors. There is often rapid deterioration of mental status (*see* **p. 472**). Mortality is high (up to 40%) and there is a high morbidity in the survivors (up to 30%), with residual neurological deficits. There is no specific treatment. Vaccination against Japanese B encephalitis is now available for those travelling to endemic areas.

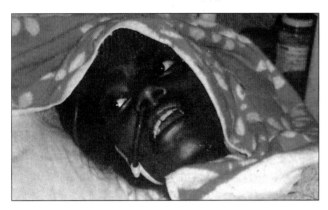

1.46 Encephalitis caused by Japanese B virus can be severe and result in serious sequelae such as mental retardation. Other encephalitis viruses may have similar consequences.

MEASLES

The causal agent for measles is a paramyxovirus, and the disease is highly infectious. It is spread by droplets from the respiratory tract and preschool children are particularly at risk.

The World Health Organization estimates that there are 40 million cases of measles per year, resulting in nearly 1 million deaths – almost exclusively in young children in developing countries.

After an incubation of 10–11 days, the illness starts with fever and coryzal symptoms. Small white spots (Koplik's spots) appear on the buccal mucosa (**1.47**) on the second day. A red, blotchy, maculopapular rash starts on the neck, usually on the fourth day of illness. Thereafter, the rash spreads to the face (**1.9**), trunk and finally to the limbs (**1.48**). As the rash fades, there may be temporary purplish haemorrhagic staining of the skin.

Complications of measles include pneumonia, croup, otitis media, gastroenteritis and, rarely, encephalitis. In developing

countries, these complications lead to a high morbidity and mortality, especially in undernourished children (**1.49, 1.50**). In the developed world, atypical measles may be seen in patients who received early, unsuccessful vaccines.

The diagnosis is usually made on clinical grounds, but if necessary can be confirmed by viral isolation or by serology. Treatment is symptomatic in uncomplicated cases. Appropriate antibiotic therapy is required for bacterial complications such as pneumonia and otitis media. Pneumonia may be rapidly fatal in undernourished children with measles and in immuno-compromised patients.

Active immunization is available; combined with mumps and rubella vaccine (MMR), it should be offered to all children aged between 1 and 2 years, or at 6 months in some developing countries. Passive immunization with normal human immunoglobulin can prevent the disease if given early in the incubation period, but immunity is short-lasting.

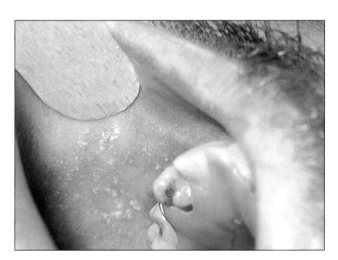

1.47 Koplik's spots in measles are most commonly seen opposite the molars or on the buccal surface of the lips and cheeks. They precede the main rash by several days.

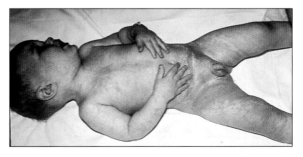

1.48 Measles. The typical maculopapular, morbilliform rash starts on the neck and face and spreads to involve the trunk and the limbs. This infant also had typical catarrh and conjunctivitis.

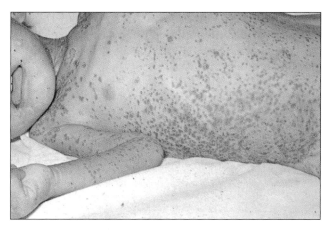

1.49   Measles in an undernourished child in Guatemala. The rash is florid, and is likely to be associated with serious complications, including the development of overt kwashiorkor (*see* **p. 328**).

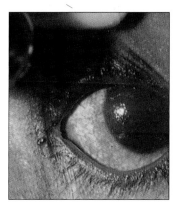

1.50   Measles keratoconjunctivitis and xerophthalmia are common complications of the infection in the malnourished child, especially in those with vitamin A deficiency. The corneal light reflex is distorted, and the preocular tear film is lacking.

No specific therapy is available. If there is salivary gland involvement, attention must be paid to oral hygiene and fluid intake. Diet should be bland. The pain and swelling of orchitis usually responds to a short course of steroid therapy. Antiemetics and intravenous fluids may be required for pancreatitis. Mumps meningitis is a benign illness and needs only bed rest and symptomatic treatment.

Active immunization is available (alone or combined in MMR) and it should be offered to children and adults without a history of the disease.

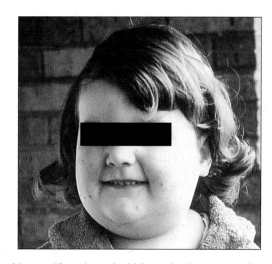

1.51   Mumps. There is marked bilateral enlargement of the parotid glands, which are usually tender, associated with generalized facial oedema. This girl was convalescent when photographed.

MUMPS

The causal organism of mumps is a paramyxovirus which spreads by droplets and saliva. The incubation period is 18–21 days. Most patients with mumps present with swelling of the salivary glands (**1.51**), but other glands may be involved, including the pancreas, the gonads (adults only) and the thyroid gland. The virus may also attack the meninges or the brain, causing aseptic meningitis or encephalitis. Transient deafness can occur during the course of mumps, but permanent nerve deafness is a rare complication.

Salivary gland swelling usually subsides within 2 weeks. About 10–15% of postpubertal males will develop orchitis (**1.52**) which may be unilateral or bilateral. Breasts and ovaries are occasionally involved in females.

The diagnosis can be confirmed if necessary by viral isolation and serology. This is important in patients who present without salivary gland involvement.

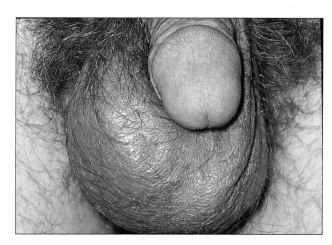

1.52   Mumps orchitis is the most serious complication of the disease in the adult, though it does not usually damage the prepubertal testis. It may be unilateral or bilateral and usually causes severe tenderness.

INFLUENZA

Influenza is an acute viral infection which is spread by droplets from person to person. It is caused by three groups of related myxoviruses which produce fever, prostration, myalgia, headache and anorexia. The viruses undergo frequent antigenic changes, do not produce cross-immunity to each other and give rise to epidemics and pandemics. Five pandemics occurred in the twentieth century with massive mortality: for example, up to 20 million people died in 1918, with millions more having continued morbidity from respiratory and neurological sequelae (postencephalitic parkinsonism, *see* **p. 481**).

Acute infection may present with a spectrum of symptoms ranging from a very mild pyrexia which is rapidly self-limiting to an overwhelming infection with severe myalgia, headache, fever, sore throat, acute tracheitis and even pleurisy. In addition, encephalitis, myositis and myocarditis may supervene, especially in the elderly. Secondary bacterial infection, often with *Streptococcus pneumoniae*, *Staphylococcus aureus* and *Haemophilus influenzae*, is a common complication in the debilitated elderly patient (**1.53**, *see* **p. 175**). Treatment is usually symptomatic, but antiviral drugs may be of value in ameliorating symptoms more rapidly if given early in the course of the disease.

Influenza vaccines are available for people at risk, including the elderly, especially in residential care, asthmatics, those with chronic obstructive pulmonary disease (COPD), the immunocompromised, diabetics and patients with chronic renal disease. Health care workers and others caring for at-risk patients should also be immunized.

The influenza viruses A and B constantly alter their antigenic structure, especially the haemagglutinins and neuraminidases on the surface coat. To be effective in a current epidemic a vaccine must contain these antigens, so the appropriate vaccine varies from year to year. As the vaccines are prepared in chick embryos their use is contraindicated in patients hypersensitive to eggs.

RABIES

Rabies is caused by an RNA virus of the Rhabdoviridae family. Man is infected through bites from a rabid animal, usually a dog or cat, but occasionally a vampire bat, fox, squirrel or rodent. Rarely, the virus may gain entry through a cut, abrasion or area of eczema. The incubation period may be as short as 2 weeks, but in some cases may be as long as 1 year. The virus, once in the body, spreads via peripheral nerves to the CNS causing encephalomyelitis which is almost uniformly fatal. The time from bite to first symptom ranges from about 35 days for bites on the face to 52 days for bites on the limbs.

Initial symptoms include pain and tingling at the inoculation site, extreme restlessness ('furious rabies'), followed by severe spasms of the larynx and pharynx which are brought on by attempts to swallow water, giving rise to the term 'hydrophobia' (**1.54**). Eventually, flaccid paralysis develops and the patient lapses into coma. Some patients, especially those bitten by vampire bats, present initially with flaccid paralysis which often begins in the bitten limb, but which rapidly becomes generalized (dumb rabies). Death results from respiratory paralysis.

If possible, the diagnosis should be confirmed in the animal by histopathological examination of the brain. In humans the virus can be identified by immunofluorescence on skin or

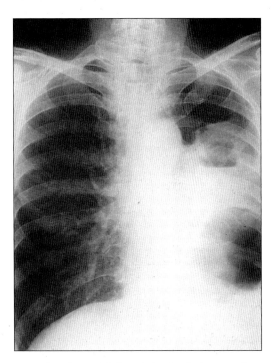

1.53 Secondary bacterial chest infection is the most frequent serious consequence of influenza. In this elderly patient, there is a left mid-zone cavitating pneumonia (note the fluid level in the cavity) and an accompanying left pleural effusion. The causative organism was *Staphylococcus aureus*.

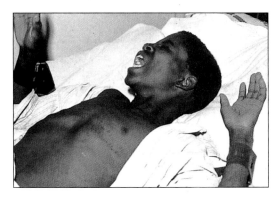

1.54 'Furious rabies' in a 14-year-old Nigerian boy. Inspiratory spasms occur spontaneously or are induced by attempts to swallow. This may lead to fear of water (hydrophobia).

corneal impression smears or by brain biopsy. Serological tests may also be diagnostic, but may be difficult to interpret if vaccination has been given since exposure to the virus.

Management of bitten people includes thorough cleaning of the bite, passive immunization with human rabies immunoglobulin and an immediate course of human diploid cell rabies vaccine. The outlook is poor if treatment is started after the onset of symptoms.

Patients must be nursed in an intensive care unit. Heavy sedation and positive pressure ventilation are required. The disease is usually fatal but there have been several documented cases of recovery.

Prevention includes regular immunization of domestic animals in endemic areas and pre-exposure immunization of people at risk.

LASSA FEVER

Lassa fever is caused by infection with an arenavirus (Lassa fever virus) and is found predominantly in West Africa. Infection with similar viruses causes Argentine and Bolivian haemorrhagic fevers in South America. The vector is the rodent *Mastomys natalensis*. The incubation period is 6–21 days.

Onset of the clinical disease is gradual, with fever, headache and myalgia that particularly affects the legs. In addition there may be conjunctivitis, aphthous ulceration of the mouth, a fine generalized petechial rash and facial oedema (**1.55**). As the platelet count falls, haemorrhage may occur from a variety of sites. A combination of viraemia and haemorrhage produces shock and this may be associated with evidence of viral myocarditis. Encephalitis and permanent cranial nerve impairment may also occur. In severe cases a mortality of up to 20% has been found.

Treatment with ribavirin may be effective when given early in the course of the disease. Symptomatic control of haemorrhage and shock are important. Prevention of spread of the disease depends on public health measures to control contact with rodents and with virus-laden rodent excreta. Hospital outbreaks involve careful handling of all blood and excreta of patients.

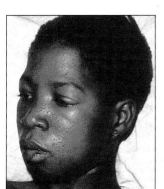

1.55 Facial oedema in Lassa fever is a common feature of severe cases and carries a poor prognosis.

MARBURG AND EBOLA HAEMORRHAGIC FEVERS

These haemorrhagic fevers are characterized by an acute onset fever, papular rash (**1.56**), diarrhoea, proteinuria, hepatitis and haemorrhage. Marburg disease was originally found in people in contact with green monkeys (*Cercopithecus aethiops*) which were obtained from Uganda. Subsequently there was evidence of transmission by needles and directly from person to person. Ebola fever is also found in Uganda and other parts of Central Africa. Both the Marburg and the Ebola virus lead to haemorrhage as a result of platelet dysfunction; profound haemorrhage is the usual cause of death. There is no specific treatment, but patients require intensive circulatory support and control of the disseminated intravascular coagulation (DIC) with heparin; they may benefit from plasma containing virus-specific antibodies. Extensive precautions are needed to prevent the spread of infection.

Haemorrhagic fever occurs widely throughout the world. Other causes include dengue (*see* **p. 13**), yellow fever (*see* **p. 13**), bunyavirus and hantavirus infections. All are potentially fatal conditions.

1.56 African haemorrhagic fever is often accompanied by a widespread papular rash, though this non-specific sign may progress to more serious petechiae and haemorrhage.

HUMAN PARVOVIRUS B 19

Human parvovirus B 19 causes a self-limiting disease known as erythema infectiosum or fifth disease. This common disease occurs in outbreaks, most often in winter and spring . Any age may be affected but it is most common in children aged 6–10 years, in whom the usual presentation is a mild febrile illness followed by marked erythema of the cheeks and the appearance of a pink maculopapular rash (**1.57**). The rash may become confluent and is most marked on the limbs; as it fades, it takes on a lace-like appearance. The rash may come and go over

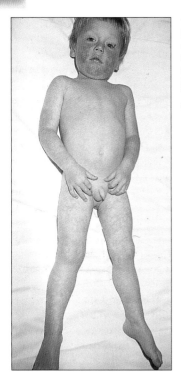

1.57 Erythema infectiosum. This boy's erythematous rash appeared 24 hours after the onset of a mild fever and sore throat. Note the 'slapped cheek' appearance of the face.

multiple painful, shallow ulcers on the tongue, buccal mucosa and lips (**1.3, 1.58**). In genital herpes, ulcers are on the vulva, vagina, cervix or penis (**1.59**). In both instances, the primary lesions are self-limiting and clear in about 10 days. The local eruption may be accompanied by fever and malaise and, in the case of children, refusal to eat or drink. Other sites of primary infection are the fingers (herpetic whitlow) and the cornea (dendritic ulcer, **1.60**). Herpes simplex encephalitis is a rare but very serious presentation (*see* **p. 472**). In the neonate, disseminated herpes simplex is a life-threatening illness.

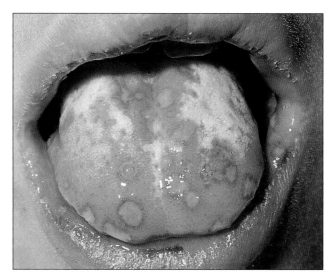

1.58 Severe herpetic gingivostomatitis. This young child was acutely ill with a high fever and had multiple vesicular lesions on the tongue, lips and buccal mucosa. In adult patients, a more common manifestation of herpetic stomatitis is the cold sore; this is usually a reactivation of latent infection.

about 2–3 weeks. Adenopathy, arthralgia and arthritis are common especially in adults infected with the virus. Joints most involved are wrists and knees. The arthritis may, if prolonged, be mistaken for other forms of rheumatism. Transient marrow depression may occur during the course of the illness. In patients with congenital haemolytic anaemia, such as sickle-cell disease, β-thalassaemia or hereditary spherocytosis, an aplastic crisis may be induced (*see* **p. 415**). Maternal infection in the second trimester of pregnancy may result in hydrops fetalis and fetal loss.

The diagnosis can be confirmed by finding a specific IgM antibody in the serum.

As the disease is self-limiting, children require no therapy. Analgesics and anti-inflammatory drugs may be needed for relief of joint pain in adults. If there is an aplastic crisis, blood transfusion is indicated. Intravenous immunoglobulin may ameliorate or terminate bone marrow infection in the immunosuppressed. No vaccine is available for this disease.

HERPES SIMPLEX

The causal agents of herpes simplex are herpes simplex virus types I and II. Type II is usually associated with sexually transmitted genital infection, whereas most other infections are caused by type I. Following the primary infection, the virus remains latent in the tissues and may re-emerge at a later stage to produce local lesions.

Primary infection with type I virus usually occurs in childhood and takes the form of acute gingivostomatitis with

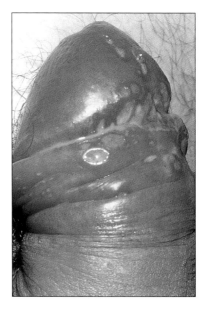

1.59 Primary genital herpes. Note the numerous lesions on the penis and the associated tissue reaction.

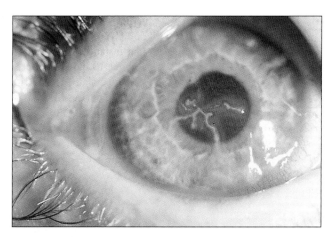

1.60   A primary herpetic dendritic ulcer, stained with fluorescein. Herpes simplex virus proliferates in the epithelial layer of the cornea. Urgent treatment with antiviral drops or ointment is indicated.

Patients with eczema may present with widespread lesions on the eczematous areas (eczema herpeticum, **2.26**).

Reactivation of latent herpes simplex usually occurs in sites related to the primary infection (**1.61**). In the immunocompromised patient, reactivation of the virus may cause very severe local lesions (**1.22**), with generalized viraemia and encephalitis.

Genital herpes has reached epidemic proportions and differs from other sexually transmitted diseases because of the likelihood of spontaneous recurrence. It is extremely contagious, being spread by secretions to partners and to the fetus. There is a causal relationship between genital herpes, cervical cell metaplasia and cervical carcinoma. Herpes simplex virus II is the most common infecting agent in young women.

The primary lesions of genital herpes appear within a day or so of exposure and are thin-walled vesicles which are painful. In women there is usually a vaginal discharge followed by tender lymphadenopathy with generalized fever. Urinary retention may result from extreme pain on micturition or from associated sacral meningomyelitis. Systemic symptoms, including fever,

fatigue and photophobia, occur in 25% of patients; viral meningitis is a rare complication. In men the lesions are found on the glans, foreskin and penile shaft (**1.59**). In addition, lesions may be found in the perineum and perianal regions of homosexual men (**1.22**).

Recurrence of genital herpes is common and may be precipitated by local trauma, menstruation, pregnancy, stress, depression, intercurrent illness or immunosuppression. The recurrence tends to be more localized and not as severe as the first attack. Patients often recognize the prodrome of recurrence with local itching and tingling.

It is important to recognize that both primary and recurrent genital herpes may be asymptomatic (in perhaps 15% of patients).

The virus can be cultured from vesical fluid or from swabs from genital or mouth ulcers. Viral particles can also be identified under the electron microscope. Rising antibody titres may be found in primary herpes simplex.

Most primary lesions are self-limiting and specific therapy is not usually required. Curative therapy is not available. If applied very early, acyclovir cream may abort the development of 'cold sores'. Aciclovir and famciclovir may be used to control both primary genital herpes and recurrences (patients can start treatment at the first prodromal sign of recurrence). Intravenous aciclovir should be used to treat herpes encephalitis and severe infections in the immunocompromised host and in the neonate. An ophthalmological opinion should be sought when there is involvement of the eye.

As with all sexually transmitted diseases, partner tracing, notification and counselling are indicated.

VARICELLA ZOSTER

Varicella zoster causes two distinct diseases – chickenpox (varicella) and shingles (herpes zoster).

Chickenpox

Chickenpox is a highly infectious disease caused by the varicella zoster virus. It is usually mild in children but can be severe in adults and in immunocompromised patients. The incubation period is usually 14–15 days. In adults especially, there may be a short prodromal illness with fever, malaise, headache and occasionally a transient erythematous rash. The true rash is vesicular with a central distribution in the body (**1.62**). The spots are elliptical and come out in crops over a few days. Mucous membranes may also be affected. Scabs form rapidly and most have separated in 10–14 days. The most common complication, especially in children, is skin sepsis, usually due to superinfection with *Staphylococcus aureus* or *Streptococcus pyogenes*, which may lead to a fulminant toxic shock syndrome. Varicella pneumonia, which can be life-threatening, occurs mainly in adults who smoke and in the immunocompromised (**1.63**, **10.65**, **10.91**). Other rare complications include encephalitis, cerebral ataxia and haemorrhagic chickenpox.

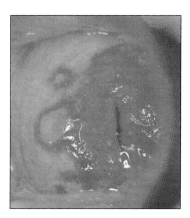

1.61   Recurrent herpes simplex on the cervix. The ulcers have recurred in a common primary site for genital infection. Other common sites include the external genitalia and the lips.

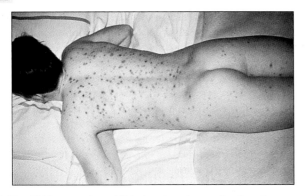

1.62 Chickenpox in a child, showing the predominantly central distribution of the rash (which used to be of great importance in differentiating chickenpox from the now-eradicated smallpox, in which the rash is predominantly peripheral).

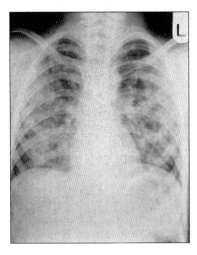

1.63 Chickenpox pneumonia affects mainly adults, and produces a severe illness with the characteristics of acute inflammatory pulmonary oedema. Chest X-ray shows widespread soft, nodular opacities throughout both lungs. The complication varies in severity from mild to life-threatening.

which is always unilateral, appears along the line of one or two dermatomes (**1.64**). The lesions are vesicular on an erythematous base. In ophthalmic herpes (**1.65**), especially if the nasociliary branch of the nerve is affected, there may be corneal ulceration (as in herpes simplex, **1.60**) and iridocyclitis. Ophthalmic herpes zoster is a medical emergency: corneal scarring and other serious complications may occur. Dissemination of virus in the bloodstream may result in the appearance of scattered chickenpox lesions elsewhere on the body. Viraemia may be overwhelming in immunocompromised patients. Pain may precede the skin rash, and postherpetic neuralgia can be prolonged and severe, especially in the elderly.

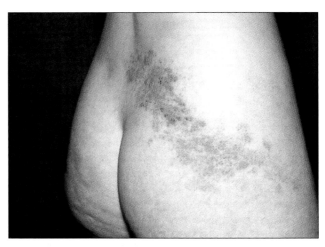

1.64 Herpes zoster affecting the L2 dermatome. The rash shows the characteristic 'band' distribution, starting from the midline, where some vesicles can be seen.

The diagnosis is usually made on clinical grounds but electron microscopy, viral culture and serology may be required in difficult cases.

Children should, if possible, be prevented from scratching the spots to prevent scarring and secondary infection. In adults, and children at greatest risk of complications, aciclovir can reduce the duration of symptoms if administered within 24 hours of rash onset. If the disease is severe, especially in the immunocompromised patient, aciclovir may be used parenterally.

There is no active vaccine. Varicella zoster immune globulin may modify or prevent the disease if given within 1 week of contact.

Shingles

Shingles is caused by reactivation of latent varicella virus in sensory root ganglia in patients previously infected with chickenpox. Reactivation is common in the elderly and in immunocompromised patients (**1.21**). The skin eruption,

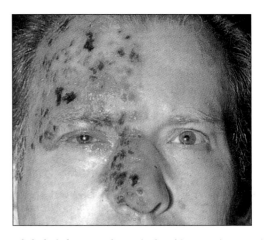

1.65 Ophthalmic herpes. The vesicular skin eruptions are in the distribution of the ophthalmic division of the fifth cranial nerve. Serious opthalmic complications are a real threat, especially when the tip of the nose is affected (this indicates involvement of the nasociliary nerve, which also supplies the cornea).

The most common complications are bacterial superinfection of the skin lesions and postherpetic neuralgia. Occasionally there may be motor nerve involvement, as in the Ramsay Hunt syndrome when seventh nerve paresis occurs (**1.66, 1.67**). Meningo-encephalitis is a more serious but rarer complication.

Aciclovir, famciclovir or valaciclovir given orally within 72 hours, or in severe cases intravenously, along with local applications of aciclovir skin cream, may hasten healing and reduce viral shedding, and there is some evidence that the new antiviral agents may prevent or reduce postherpetic neuralgia. Analgesics and amitriptyline are almost always required for pain control. If there is involvement of the eye, an antiviral should be given and an ophthalmological opinion should be sought.

thrombocytopenia. Intrauterine infection may cause fetal death. Severe neonatal cytomegalovirus infection causes jaundice, hepatosplenomegaly (**1.69**), purpura, neurological damage and chorioretinitis. The infected infant may, however, appear normal at birth, and develop symptoms later.

The finding of specific IgM in serum is diagnostic of acute infection. Isolation of virus from urine or sputum may simply indicate prolonged excretion after past infection.

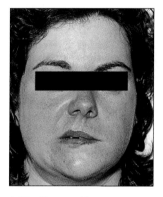

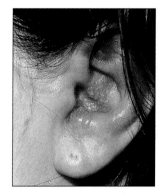

1.66 Ramsay Hunt syndrome (geniculate zoster). The patient has a left seventh nerve paresis. Full recovery occurs in about 50% of cases.

1.67 Ramsay Hunt syndrome (geniculate zoster). The left ear of the patient shown in 1.66 showing the presence of herpetic vesicles in the external auditory mentus, which receives a small sensory branch from the facial nerve.

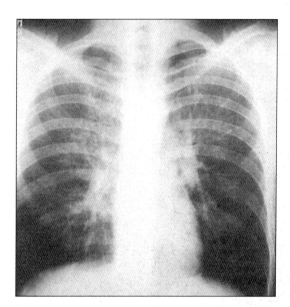

1.68 Cytomegalovirus (CMV) pneumonia is often known as CMV pneumonitis, as the infection is generalized, and consolidation may not be seen on X-ray. CMV is second only to *Pneumocystis* as a cause of pulmonary disease in patients with HIV infection, and it is also seen in other immunocompromised patients, including those on anticancer therapy, systemic steroids, and drugs such as azathioprine and cyclophosphamide used to prevent organ transplant rejection. CMV pneumonia cannot be diagnosed on clinical grounds or X-ray appearances alone.

CYTOMEGALOVIRUS

Like other herpesviruses, cytomegalovirus remains latent in the body after primary infection and may only reactivate if the patient is stressed or becomes immunocompromised. The virus may be transmitted by respiratory secretions, sexually, by blood transfusion or by organ transplantation. Maternal infection spreads transplacentally or perinatally to the fetus.

Most cytomegalovirus infections in the immunocompetent are subclinical, but there may be a glandular fever-like syndrome with fever, generalized lymphadenopathy, abnormal liver function tests and atypical mononuclear cells in the blood. Primary infection or reactivation of latent infection in the immunocompromised patient may cause serious illness with pneumonia (**1.68**), chorioretinitis (**1.32**), gastroenteritis, involvement of the CNS, haemolytic anaemia and

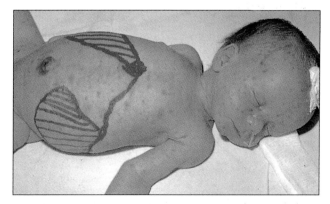

1.69 Congenital cytomegalovirus infection. This infant has massive splenomegaly, hepatomegaly and a purpuric rash. A similar picture may be caused by a number of prenatal virus infections.

Cytomegalovirus inclusion bodies in biopsy specimens from the lung or gastrointestinal tract are diagnostic, so biopsy provides definitive diagnosis in the immunocompromised patient.

Most acquired infections are self-limiting but severe disease, especially in the immunocompromised, should be treated with intravenous ganciclovir or phosphonoformate. Treatment may have to be prolonged; relapses are common unless maintenance therapy is continued on a long-term basis. In post-transplant patients, cytomegalovirus infection may be prevented by antiviral prophylaxis.

EPSTEIN–BARR VIRUS INFECTIONS

Infectious mononucleosis

The Epstein–Barr virus (EBV) is the causal agent of infectious mononucleosis. Primary infection with EBV is often subclinical, especially in young children. Older children and young adults usually present with symptoms of glandular fever.

In the most common form of the disease, there is enlargement of glands both in the anterior and posterior triangles of the neck, and usually in the axillae and groins. The fauces and palate become inflamed and oedematous. There may be palatal haemorrhages and a whitish or yellow pseudomembrane appears on the tonsils (**1.70**). There is usually marked nasopharyngitis and often puffiness of the face.

In the more generalized form of the disease, throat involvement is less marked. Presenting features are fever, generalized adenitis, splenomegaly and occasionally jaundice (**9.35**). There may also be a pink, maculopapular rash on the trunk and limbs (**1.71**). A rash is more often seen in patients who have been given ampicillin or related drugs (**1.72**).

Complications of infectious mononucleosis include myocarditis, autoimmune haemolytic anaemia, thrombocytopenia and

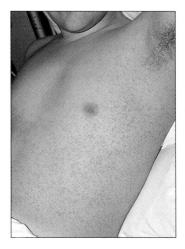

1.71 Rash in infectious mononucleosis may be the result of the infection itself, as here. The maculopapular rash usually emerges during the second week of illness, and it is often indistinguishable from that of rubella (**1.42**).

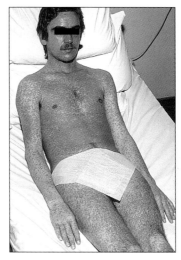

1.72 Rashes in infectious mononucleosis are most commonly caused by the administration of ampicillin or related penicillin compounds (these are often administered early in the disease on the presumption that the patient has bacterial pharyngitis). Ampicillin rashes occur more commonly in patients with infectious mononucleosis than in other patients, so the appearance of this kind of rash in a patient with typical symptoms points strongly to the diagnosis of infectious mononucleosis.

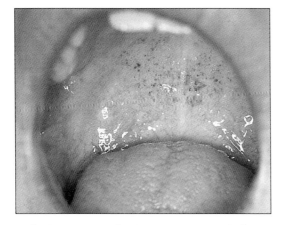

1.70 Infectious mononucleosis. Numerous petechial haemorrhages are seen in the hard palate. In many patients there is also a tonsillitis, indistinguishable from that seen in acute streptococcal pharyngitis (**1.82**).

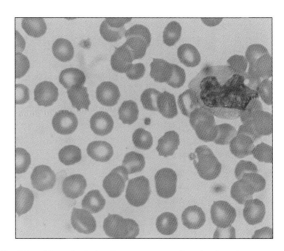

1.73 Blood film in infectious mononucleosis showing an atypical mononuclear cell. There is a wide variation in cell size and shape and mitotic activity is greatly enhanced, but the cellular structure is not fundamentally deranged.

meningo-encephalitis. Splenic rupture is a rare complication which is usually associated with trauma. A chronic fatigue syndrome may follow EBV infection.

The diagnosis is aided by the identification of atypical mononuclear cells in peripheral blood (**1.73**). The Paul–Bunnell test for heterophil antibodies usually becomes positive in the second or third week of the illness. In children under about 7 years, the Paul–Bunnell or Monospot test is rarely positive, and diagnosis should be confirmed by EBV serology (EBV IgM).

Treatment is symptomatic. Antibiotics are not indicated and ampicillin and related drugs should not be prescribed because of the high incidence of allergic reactions. Steroid therapy may be indicated if there is respiratory obstruction or autoimmune manifestations.

Burkitt's lymphoma and nasopharyngeal carcinoma

EBV has been implicated in the aetiology of Burkitt's lymphoma, a transmissible neoplastic tumour particularly involving the head and neck (**1.74**) that is found in tropical Africa. The disease has a similar range of distribution to malaria, and it is thought that the virus may be transmitted via mosquitoes.

EBV has also been implicated in some nasopharyngeal carcinomas, and it may play a role in the genesis of hairy leukoplakia (**1.31**) and in other premalignant and malignant disease.

ROSEOLA (SIXTH DISEASE)

Roseola infantum is a common, benign exanthematous disease of young children. After a rapid onset high fever, which lasts for a few days and then resolves, a generalized rubelliform rash appears (**1.75**). There may be cervical node enlargement and febrile convulsions may complicate the acute stage. The rash fades after 24–48 hours, and the patient usually makes a complete and uncomplicated recovery.

The disease is caused by human herpes 6 virus (and the disease is also known as sixth disease).

ORF

Orf (contagious pustular dermatitis) is a paravaccinia virus infection of sheep and goats, which causes an eruption on the animals' lips. It is sometimes contracted by those who work with these animals, and in humans it usually causes a single papule on the skin of the hand, which develops from a flat vesicle to a haemorrhagic bulla. Occasionally, more than one papule may occur (**1.76**). The lesions are usually self-limiting, but may ulcerate and may act as a trigger for the onset of erythema multiforme (*see* **p. 76**). Regional lymph node enlargement is common. Milkers' nodules are similar lesions, caused by cowpox virus and seen in farm workers dealing with cattle. Other differential diagnoses include anthrax, vaccinial infection and infection with *Erysipelothrix rhusiopathiae*.

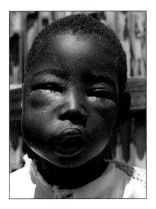

1.74 Burkitt's lymphoma, causing gross facial swelling in an African child.

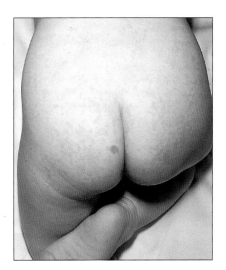

1.75   Roseola infantum. An erythematous macular or rubelliform rash appears. It is often particularly prominent on the buttocks and fades within 2 days. If the child has been treated with an antibiotic for the fever, the rash may be mistaken for drug sensitivity.

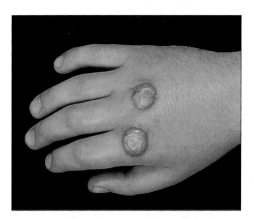

1.76   Orf. Around 3–7 days after inoculation from an infected sheep or goat, one or more firm, painless, dark papules may appear on the finger or hand. These develop into pustules, but the condition is self-limiting, usually clearing within 4–8 weeks.

BACTERIAL INFECTIONS

STAPHYLOCOCCAL INFECTIONS

Staphylococcus aureus, a Gram-positive coccus, causes a wide variety of community-acquired and nosocomial infections. *S. aureus* is found in the nose in 15% of adults in the community and is also commonly carried on the skin. Carriage rates are higher in hospital personnel. Organisms are transmitted by direct contact, by fomites and by aerosol (sneezing). They survive for long periods on dry surfaces but are easily killed by disinfectants and antiseptic solutions. In hospitals, patients with a higher risk of carriage include those taking steroids, those with diabetes mellitus, intravenous drug misusers and those on haemodialysis. The emergence of strains of the organism with multiple resistance to antibiotics is causing major problems of management and infection control.

Certain areas of the body, especially the nasal mucosa and the skin of the axilla, groin and perineum, may become colonized by staphylococci; given favourable circumstances, the organisms may invade the skin and subcutaneous tissue. Tissue breakdown and abscess formation are characteristic of staphylococcal lesions (**1.77**). Staphylococcal infection is a common cause of exacerbations in patients with atopic dermatitis (*see* **p. 71**). Staphylococci may also enter the blood with subsequent involvement of other organs such as bone (**p. 144**), joints, lungs (**1.53, 1.78, 4.28, 4.29**), heart valves (**p. 231**), brain or meninges.

In addition to causing local sepsis, *S. aureus* produces a number of toxins. Epidermolytic (exfoliative) toxin is responsible for the syndrome of toxic epidermal necrolysis (Lyell's disease, scalded skin syndrome). In this, there is sudden onset of fever and marked generalized erythema of the skin, followed by loss of large areas of the superficial layers of the epidermis, which produces an appearance resembling severe scalding. This condition occurs mainly in children (**1.79**). Ritter's disease is a neonatal form of the same condition.

Staphylococcal toxic shock syndrome is a relatively rare condition (about 40 cases in 58 million people in the UK per year). It is due to the production of an exotoxin (TSST-1) by *S. aureus*. Sufferers present with an acute onset influenza-like illness with sudden high fever (> 39°C), vomiting, diarrhoea, muscle aches and a sunburn-like rash resembling that of scarlet fever (*see* **1.83**). The patients often become rapidly disorientated. There is a mortality rate of about 5–10%. Many of the initial cases were in young women using superabsorbent tampons. This group now accounts for one-half of the cases;

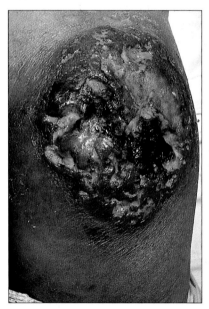

1.77 **A massive staphylococcal carbuncle,** in which the infection has caused tissue breakdown and multiple interconnected abscesses. Lesions of this kind are found most commonly in diabetic patients.

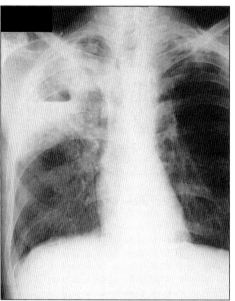

1.78 **Staphylococcal pneumonia** in a 20-year-old intravenous drug misuser. The organisms were introduced by a contaminated intravenous injection, but a similar picture may occur in debilitated or immunocompromised patients secondary to staphylococcal skin infection. Note the presence of a large cavity (septic infarct) in the right upper zone. The possibility of right-sided endocarditis should always be considered when this picture is seen in an injecting drug misuser.

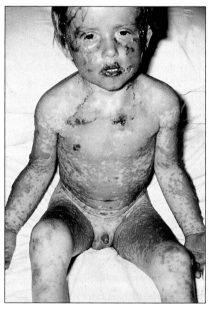

1.79 **Toxic epidermal necrolysis** (scalded skin syndrome), in which the skin is extremely painful, and large patches of necrotic epidermis slide off the underlying layers at the slightest pressure, leaving extensive raw areas. The condition occurs mainly in children, but a similar syndrome may occur at any age as a consequence of drug hypersensitivity (**2.149**).

others include patients after surgery and those with burns, boils and insect bites. Men, women and children may be affected. The diagnosis may be confirmed by culture of swabs from the lesion or from a tampon. Blood cultures are usually negative. Patients usually have a high white cell count, lowered platelets (from DIC), renal impairment and elevated creatine phosphokinase (CPK) from muscle injury.

Most *S. aureus* organisms are resistant to penicillin and ampicillin, so the drugs of choice for most infections are penicillinase-resistant antibiotics. In patients with an allergy to the penicillins, and especially if the organisms have multiple resistance to antibiotics, choice of appropriate antibiotic therapy must depend on sensitivity testing; therefore, close cooperation with microbiologists is essential, and treatment should be in accordance with locally agreed antimicrobial policy. Methicillin-resistant *S. aureus* (MRSA) is resistant to methicillin, flucloxacillin and gentamicin and severe infections require treatment with a glycopeptide antibiotic such as vancomycin.

Epidemics of infections with MRSA have now occurred in many countries. These organisms, like other *S. aureus*, are carried in the nose and skin, particularly of patients or staff with eczema. MRSA accounts for between 10 and 15% of nosocomial infections. Admission of such a patient to a ward requires rigorous measures to control infection, which may involve closing wards or hospitals. Staphylococcal abscesses should be drained (**1.80, 1.81**), and full supportive measures are required for all serious infections including toxic epidermal necrolysis and toxic shock syndrome.

S. epidermidis and related coagulase-negative staphylococci are important causes of infection in patients with prosthetic devices (especially heart valves (**1.5**), joints, shunts and vascular grafts), in patients undergoing chronic peritoneal dialysis and in those with indwelling vascular or urinary catheters. They are the most common cause of hospital-acquired bacteraemia, and are increasingly penicillin resistant. Specialist advice should be sought on treatment, which may need to be protracted.

Infection can also occur on heart valves that have been damaged as a result of acute rheumatism or are congenitally abnormal (**p. 231**).

STREPTOCOCCAL INFECTIONS

Streptococcus pyogenes is carried harmlessly by up to 15% of the population, but causes a wide variety of infections including tonsillitis, scarlet fever, skin lesions (impetigo, erysipelas and cellulitis), puerperal sepsis and septicaemia. The organisms are transmitted by direct contact, by droplets from the respiratory tract or indirectly through food, dust or fomites. Late complications of *S. pyogenes* infections include acute rheumatic fever, post-streptococcal glomerulonephritis, Henoch–Schönlein purpura, toxic shock and erythema nodosum.

Streptococcal tonsillitis is an acute illness with fever, marked general malaise and pain on swallowing. There is inflammation and oedema of the palate and fauces with spotty exudate on the tonsils (**1.82**). The anterior cervical lymph nodes are enlarged and tender. Local complications include otitis media, streptococcal rhinitis, sinusitis and peritonsillar abscess (quinsy). As with all streptococcal infections, late complications may appear about 10 days after the onset of the illness, especially in patients not treated with antibiotics. The diagnosis of streptococcal tonsillitis can be confirmed by culture of throat swabs. There is usually a marked polymorph leucocytosis in peripheral blood. The diagnosis may be confirmed in retrospect, by the finding of a raised antistreptolysin O titre (ASOT).

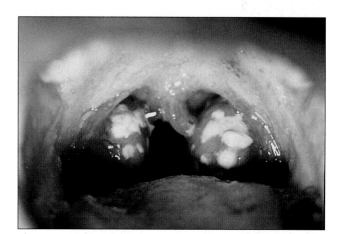

1.82   Acute streptococcal pharyngitis. There is pus in the tonsillar crypts, and some palatal petechiae are also seen. The patient acts as a reservoir of *Streptococcus pyogenes*: the organisms multiply in the pharynx and may be disseminated to others by coughing, sneezing or by direct contact with oral secretions. A similar appearance may be seen in patients with infectious mononucleosis. Treatment with a penicillin is indicated for streptococcal pharyngitis, but ampicillin and related drugs may cause a drug rash if the true diagnosis is infectious mononucleosis.

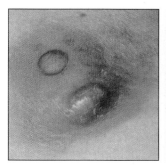 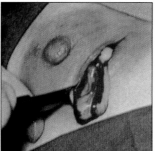

1.80   1.81

1.80, 1.81   Staphylococcal abscesses should be drained, as they are very unlikely to respond to antibiotic treatment alone. On the surface, this breast abscess did not appear large, but a large volume of pus was released when it was incised. After evacuation of the pus, the wound should be packed and left open.

Scarlet fever is a streptococcal infection characterized by the appearance of an erythematous rash (**1.83**). The disease is seen mainly in children, who are susceptible to streptococcal erythrogenic toxin. Scarlet fever is usually associated with streptococcal tonsillitis but it may also follow infection of wounds or burns (streptococcal toxic shock syndrome). The rash is a generalized punctate erythema which affects the trunk and limbs. As the rash fades, there may be desquamation of skin. Other characteristics of the disease are circumoral pallor (**1.83**) and white strawberry tongue (**1.84**). Complications of scarlet fever are similar to those of streptococcal tonsillitis.

Streptococcal infections of skin and tissues

Erysipelas and cellulitis are skin and tissue infections with *S. pyogenes* which are usually found in middle aged and elderly patients. Sites most often involved are the face (**1.85**), legs, hands and arms (**1.86**). General symptoms include fever, malaise, rigors and sometimes delirium. The local lesion consists of an area of spreading erythema with a well demarcated edge. Regional lymph nodes become tender and enlarged. There is a tendency for erysipelas to recur in a previously affected area.

A similar clinical picture, erysipeloid, may be produced by infection with *Erysipelothrix rhusiopathiae* (**1.87**), though systemic symptoms are rare. This is an occupationally acquired infection in farmers, meat and fish processors and veterinary surgeons.

Necrotizing fasciitis is due to subcutaneous infection usually with β-haemolytic streptococci but sometimes with *S. aureus* or other anaerobic organisms. Patients who have diabetes mellitus

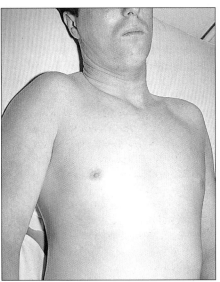

1.83 Scarlet fever showing a typical erythematous rash on the trunk and a hint of the classic circumoral pallor, with some oedema of the face.

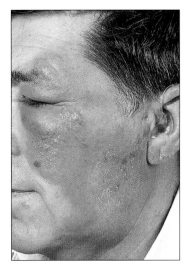

1.85 Erysipelas of the face. During the acute stage, the eyelids may become so swollen that they cannot be opened. The entire face may become erythematous, and this appearance is accompanied by an unpleasant sensation of tightness and burning.

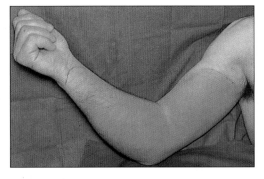

1.86 Cellulitis caused by streptococcal infection which entered through an apparently trivial knuckle injury. Other common sites of entry for the bacteria are areas of infected eczema and fungal infections of the toe-web with fissuring.

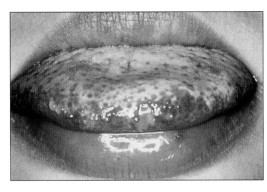

1.84 White strawberry tongue in scarlet fever. The oedematous red papillae protrude through a thick, white, furry membrane. This appearance is typical of the first 2 days, but later the white fur peels off, to leave a deep red strawberry tongue.

1.87 Erysipeloid (fish handler's disease) produces a similar clinical picture to erysipelas, although the systemic reaction is usually relatively slight.

or are on steroids are more likely to be affected. The organisms may be introduced by penetrating trauma or after surgery. The patients are usually febrile and shocked with local tenderness, occasionally with crepitus over the affected area and with a dusky red–blue appearance of the skin. Gas may be found on X-ray (as in gas gangrene, **1.94**). The organism may be identified by blood culture, culture of the affected tissue or Gram staining of the tissue. Treatment consists of urgent surgical intervention with debridement of the affected area and fasciotomy where appropriate (**1.88**).

Impetigo is most commonly seen in children and is a superficial infection of skin, usually caused by either *Streptococcus pyogenes* or *Staphylococcus aureus*. It may occur *de novo* or as a secondary infection in areas of eczema or in pediculosis of the scalp. The lesions, which are often on the face, start as thin-walled vesicles that rupture and form yellowish crusts (**1.89**). Infection is often spread by scratching.

Penicillin is the drug of choice for infections with *S. pyogenes*. In necrotizing fasciitis high dose I.V. clindamycin must be added to high dose I.V benzylpenicillin. Antibiotic therapy for all streptococcal infections should be continued for 10 days in order to lessen the risk of rheumatic fever. In cases of allergy to penicillin, erythromycin is the second choice drug. Impetigo usually responds to topical antibiotic therapy.

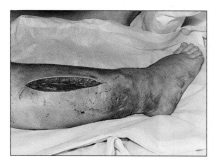

1.88 Necrotizing fasciitis, treated by fasciotomy. Note the extensive cellulitis and erysipelas, with some blistering of the skin. Subcutanenous infection was extensive in this patient, and was accompanied by gas formation and crepitus.

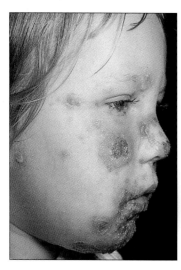

1.89 Impetigo of the face. The superficial nature of the infection and the characteristic honey-coloured serous crusting are typical.

STREPTOCOCCUS PNEUMONIAE INFECTION

Streptococcus pneumoniae ('pneumoccoccus') is an important cause of human disease at the extremes of age and in those with underlying disorders including diabetes mellitus, alcoholism, asplenism and immunosuppression. *S. pneumoniae* infection is the principal cause of community acquired pneumonia (**4.107** *see also* **p. 175**) and otitis media (**1.8**), and causes 30-50% of bacterial meningitis in adults (*see* **p. 471**). Bacteraemia occurs in 25-30% of cases of pneumonia and 80% of cases of meningitis.

The case fatality rate from pneumococcal pneumonia is 5–7% and from meningitis 15–20%, despite antimicrobial therapy. Prompt treatment with benzylpenicillin is required, but resistant strains are emerging worldwide.

The currently available polysaccharide vaccine contains 23 serotypes and is 70% effective in preventing pneumonia and bacteraemia. The vaccine is less effective in infants and the immunosuppressed. New conjugate vaccines should be more effective.

MENINGOCOCCAL INFECTION

The causal agent of meningococcal infection is *Neisseria meningitidis*, a Gram-negative diplococcus with nine serogroups of which groups A, B and C are the commonest cause of epidemics. Infection results from inhalation of droplets. Meningococci colonize the pharynx, often giving rise to a carrier state (in 5–20% of the normal population); they may, however, spread from the pharynx to the blood and meninges. No age is exempt from meningococcal disease but young children and young adults are most at risk, especially those in a closed environment such as a school or camp. Epidemics occur in winter and spring in temperate climates and in the dry season in the tropics.

The incubation period is usually 2–10 days. Infection produces a wide spectrum of illness from fulminating septicaemia, which can kill in a few hours, to a subacute illness with intermittent fever and a 'flea-bite' type rash. The most common presentation is meningitis (*see* **p. 471**) with or without septicaemia – the main features of which are high fever, severe headache, signs of acute meningeal irritation, often a purpuric rash and rapid deterioration of consciousness. The case fatality rate is 10% in meningococcal meningitis and 20% in meningococcal septicaemia. Fulminating septicaemia (Waterhouse–Friderichsen syndrome) is a devastating illness with extensive skin haemorrhage (**1.90**, **1.91**), disseminated intravascular coagulation (DIC, **10.109**, **10.114**) and circulatory failure due to adrenal haemorrhage. These patients usually do not live long enough to develop meningitis.

Meningococci can be cultured from blood, pharynx, skin lesions and CSF, and rapid diagnosis by polymerase chain reaction (PCR) is now possible. If examined, the CSF is found to be purulent with a marked polymorph leucocytosis. Lumbar puncture may, however, be hazardous because 'coning' of the

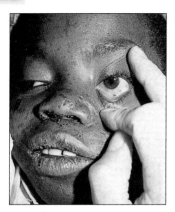

1.90 Meningococcal septicaemia in a Nigerian boy with meningitis, associated with repeated nosebleeds and petechial haemorrhages in the conjunctivae and skin.

brainstem may occur with disastrous consequences. Prior CT scan is recommended, especially if the clinical features suggest raised intracranial pressure. If the clinical diagnosis is not in doubt, therapy can be started without CSF examination.

The clinical state and laboratory findings are a poor guide to prognosis, and meningococcal infection should always be treated urgently. Intravenous benzylpenicillin is still a drug of choice and should be given for 5–7 days. In most developed countries a third generation cephalosporin, such as ceftriaxone, is now used instead of benzylpenicillin. Intensive care nursing with full supportive therapy is required, especially for fulminating septicaemia with multiple organ dysfunction.

Close contacts of the index case should receive prophylactic therapy – usually with rifampicin or ciprofloxacin. Vaccines may be used to contain epidemics. These include the group A + C bivalent vaccine and the A + C + Y + W–135 tetravalent vaccine. These produce immunity for 2–3 years in patients over the age of 2 years, but do not alter the rate of nasal carriage. Vaccines are not yet available against group B – the most common cause of meningococcaemia in the UK and some other countries.

ANTHRAX

The causal agent of anthrax is *Bacillus anthracis*, a spore-bearing organism. Most human infections result from contact with animals or animal products, such as hides, wool or bones, and therefore most cases occur in farmers, vets and abattoir workers. Anthrax has an unfortunate potential for use in germ warfare and biological terrorism, and anthrax spores may persist in the environment for many years.

The spores of *B. anthracis* may enter human skin through cuts or abrasions, or they may be ingested or inhaled. Human to human transmission of anthrax does not occur. The spores are phagocytosed by macrophages and the vegetative form of the bacillus is produced. Clinical features of cutaneous anthrax appear with 3–4 days of infection. The cutaneous lesions are usually single and are most common on exposed sites, especially hands, arms, head or neck. The classic anthrax lesion is the malignant pustule (**1.92**). This starts as a red papular lesion that vesiculates and becomes necrotic in the central area and finally dries up to form a thick, blackish scab which may take several weeks to separate. There is usually marked erythema and oedema of the surrounding tissues. Fever, headache and malaise accompany most lesions. Anthrax septicaemia is much less frequent in humans than in animals, and the untreated mortality of cutaneous anthrax can be as high as 20 per cent.

Gastrointestinal anthrax is less common than cutaneous infection. It usually presents about 7 days after the ingestion of spores, with fever, abdominal pain and gastrointestinal bleeding. The mortality is up to 50 per cent.

Inhalation anthrax has an incubation period of 4–6 days from the inhalation of spores. There is a prodromal illness with fever, malaise, nausea, cough and vomiting with rapid progression to respiratory failure, coma and death. Mortality is about 95 per cent.

Anthrax bacilli can be identified in stained smears from the lesion. Confirmation is by culture or animal inoculation, although rapid diagnostic tests (ELISA and PCR) are available in some centres. Treatment requires the early use of combinations of antibiotics (penicillins and rifampicin or doxycycline). Erythromycin can be used if patients have

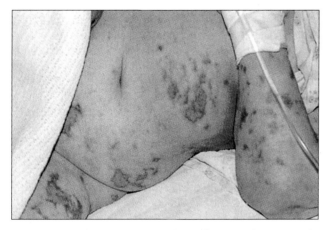

1.91 Fulminating meningococcal septicaemia is characterized by extensive purpuric lesions, a high fever, shock and evidence of disseminated intravascular coagulation (DIC).

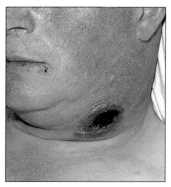

1.92 Anthrax. A single malignant pustule in a typical position on the neck. The patient was a porter who carried animal hides over his shoulders.

penicillin allergy. Post-exposure prophylaxis and initial treatment (before confirmation of the diagnosis) with ciprofloxacin is effective and this may be combined with immunization with an inactivated vaccine. The vaccine is also suitable for people in high-risk occupations. Other preventive measures include improvement of working practices, animal vaccination, proper disposal of animal carcasses and sterilization of animal products such as bone meal.

As a result of an accidental release of 1 gram of aerolised material (approximately 890 million spores) from a biological weapons plant in Russia in 1979, approximately 70 people died and up to 60 000 required treatment. Most of those who died had inhalational anthrax, contracted within 4 km of the point of release. The use of anthrax in major warfare would be complicated by difficulties in its mode of delivery and by its lack of specificity for the target group. Nevertheless, as seen recently in the USA, its use in biological terrorism can cause illness and death, while also inducing great fear in the general population.

CLOSTRIDIAL TISSUE INFECTIONS

Deep, penetrating wounds, including those produced by subcutaneous or intramuscular drug abuse are often contaminated by a range of *Clostridium* spp. (including *C. tetani*, *perfringens*, *septicum* and *novyi*). These organisms may produce two main syndromes:

- clostridial cellulitis
- clostridial myonecrosis with the release of gas into the tissues (gas gangrene).

Clostridial cellulitis may be superficial and of relatively minor consequence, but it may lead to rapidly progressive tissue destruction. In anaerobic conditions, associated with large amounts of devitalized tissue, clostridia may produce extensive myonecrosis and release gas, which tracks along the tissue planes. Gas gangrene has also been recorded at the site of intramuscular injections.

The clinical features of myonecrosis occur within a few days of injury, especially in wounds with muscle damage, fractures, retained foreign bodies and impairment of the arterial supply. Patients present with severe pain in the proximity of the wound, which rapidly becomes swollen with 'woody hard' oedema (**1.93**). A thin, watery, sweet-smelling discharge is often noted, and this becomes brown or frankly bloody later. Gas in the tissue planes may be apparent on X-ray before it can be felt (**1.94**). If a limb is involved, the part distal to the infection rapidly becomes cold, oedematous and pulseless before frank gangrene appears. The patient remains conscious during this time and has few other features, the clinical state being dominated by great pain at the site. There may be a slight fever. Progression of the condition leads to anorexia, profuse diarrhoea, circulatory collapse and renal and hepatic failure. There may be massive haemolysis.

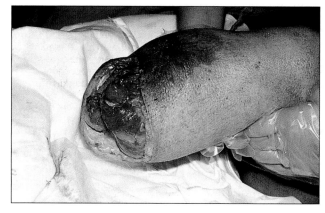

1.93 Clostridial cellulitis after amputation in a 45-year-old man who had been injured in a railway accident. The necrosis of skin and muscle is clearly seen.

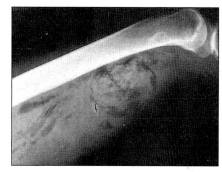

1.94 Gas gangrene in the soft tissues of the thigh after a penetrating injury. The combination of myonecrosis and gas results in swelling and impaired distal circulation.

Treatment consists of extensive early surgical debridement of the affected part under penicillin cover. The use of specific antitoxins and hyperbaric oxygen is controversial. Circulatory support is necessary to prevent renal failure. Death is inevitable if treatment is not available, and may also occur suddenly and unexpectedly during surgery.

TETANUS

Clostridium tetani is a spore-bearing organism that produces a powerful exotoxin that acts on the CNS, preventing feedback inhibition of neural discharges. Spores are present in the soil, and humans may be infected by inoculation of spores, usually into a deep wound, but sometimes even through minor breaks in the skin. Agricultural workers, athletes, road traffic accident casualties and the elderly (with waning immunity) are particularly at risk. Neonates are also at risk (**1.95**), especially if the umbilicus is handled in an unclean manner (for example, the use of dung dressings in parts of the developing world).

After an incubation period ranging from a few days to about 3 weeks, muscle rigidity develops. This is often first noted as

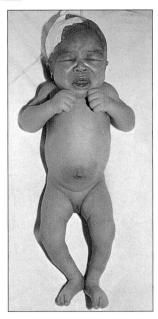

1.95   Neonatal tetanus. All the key diagnostic features are seen. Tetanus has resulted from unclean handling of the umbilical cord; note the inflammation around the umbilicus. The classic features of tetanus – trismus, risus sardonicus and muscle spasms of the arms and legs – are all present.

jaw stiffness (trismus), but later becomes generalized, producing opisthotonos. Painful muscle spasms occur and these are often triggered by sensory stimuli such as loud noises. There may also be involvement of the autonomic nervous system. The severity of the disease is inversely proportional to the length of the incubation period.

The diagnosis is made on the history and clinical features of the disease. Patients with tetanus require intensive care nursing. Obvious wounds should be cleaned and debrided. Human tetanus immunoglobulin and penicillin should be administered as soon as possible. Moderate spasms can be controlled by diazepam, but severe tetanus may require full muscle relaxation and intermittent positive pressure ventilation.

Primary immunization should be achieved in early childhood with three doses of diphtheria, pertussis and tetanus (DPT) vaccine. Booster doses of tetanus toxoid are required every 10 years to maintain immunity, especially before pregnancy. After a penetrating injury an additional booster dose of toxoid should be given unless the previous booster dose was within 5 years. If the history of previous immunization is uncertain and if wounds are heavily contaminated, antitetanus human immunoglobulin should be given and a course of tetanus toxoid started.

BOTULISM

Botulism results from ingestion of the endotoxin of *Clostridium botulinum* or, in some cases, from the release of endotoxin by surviving ingested organisms in the gut. This is usually caused by bacterial or spore contamination of improperly canned or preserved meat and meat products, which allows growth of the organism and toxin production. Rarely, wounds may be infected with *C. botulinum*. The toxin interferes with the release of acetylcholine at the neuromuscular junction and, as a result

progressive descending muscle paralysis dominates the clinical picture with diplopia, laryngeal and pharyngeal palsy and generalized symmetrical paralysis of muscles, especially those of the cranial and respiratory systems. Loss of the pupillary reflex is an early sign.

Botulinum toxin is the most toxic material known to man, and it is estimated that 1 gram has the potential to kill one million people. The toxin has potential uses in biological warfare and terrorism, and its distribution as an aerosol or in deliberately contaminated food are the most likely methods, as it is rapidly inactivated by standard water treatment processes.

The diagnosis of botulism is confirmed by finding toxin in the food, gastric contents or faeces by specialised laboratory testing, which takes days to complete; so clinical diagnosis on the basis of symptoms and signs is necessary. Airway support with assisted ventilation is the keystone of treatment. Antitoxin is of value and antibiotics may have a role if organisms survive in the gut. Mortality is about 50%. Public health measures are aimed at prevention during food preparation for preservation, especially when this is done at home. A trivalent antitoxin is available for prophylaxis after exposure and also for those presenting with early symptoms. It neutralizes the toxins of *C. botulinum* types A, B and E. Contraindications to its use are a history of hay fever, asthma or other allergy.

DIPHTHERIA

Diphtheria is now rare in the developed world as a result of effective immunization campaigns, but is still relatively common in some countries, including Russia and other countries in the CIS. It may be found in travellers returning from endemic areas. The causal agent is *Corynebacterium diphtheriae*. The most common type of diphtheria is faucial–pharyngeal in which the local lesion takes the form of a greyish-white translucent membrane, which may start on the tonsils (**1.96**), but which tends to spread to the palate, uvula

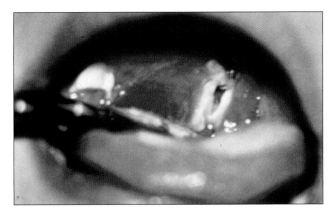

1.96   Diphtheria membrane in the pharynx. The membrane is usually white or greyish-yellow in colour, and the child may have relatively few symptoms at this stage.

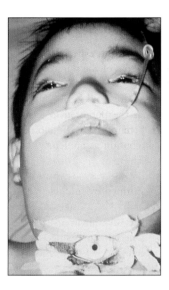

1.97 Respiratory obstruction is a life-threatening complication of diphtheria, and the need for urgent tracheostomy was the reason that most doctors carried a small penknife before the advent of effective immunization. This child has a palatal palsy (hence the nasogastric tube), and a 'bull neck' (a characteristic appearance of cervical oedema).

- cervicofacial actinomycosis, in which the presentation is a reddish indurated subcutaneous mass in the anterior triangle of the neck or submandibular region; there may be slight tenderness with low-grade fever and general symptoms of malaise
- pulmonary actinomycosis usually involves previously damaged lungs, for example cavitation after pulmonary tuberculosis (*see* **p. 178**)
- abdominal actinomycosis usually involves the appendix and caecum and presents with lower abdominal pain, low-grade fever and a slow-growing abdominal mass; it may occasionally be seen in association with an intrauterine device.

In all these sites, the infection may ultimately discharge through the skin, forming sinuses (**1.98**). Classically, these sinuses discharge typical 'sulphur granules'.

A prolonged course of high-dose penicillin is the treatment of choice.

and pharynx. Other sites of the local lesion include the anterior nares, larynx and skin. The organisms multiplying in the local lesion produce a powerful exotoxin which especially affects the heart and the CNS.

Toxic complications include cardiogenic shock, cardiac arrhythmias and sudden cardiac arrest. Nervous system damage is due to demyelination of motor nerves. This may lead to paralysis of extraocular muscles, palate and pharynx and, more rarely, to paralysis of limbs and respiratory muscles. Obstruction of the airway by a membrane is a life-threatening complication of laryngeal diphtheria, in which exhaustion due to respiratory muscular effort may be rapidly followed by death (**1.97**).

The diagnosis is confirmed by culture of the organism from the local lesion. Diphtheria antitoxin should be given with penicillin or erythromycin, but antitoxin is prepared from horse serum and allergic reactions are common; it should only be given when the index of suspicion for diphtheria is high. Bed rest is important, especially in the presence of cardiac involvement. Laryngeal obstruction may require intubation or tracheotomy.

Infants should be immunized against the disease with combined diphtheria, pertussis and tetanus vaccine. The Schick test can determine immune status, but is now rarely used. Low-dose diphtheria vaccine should be given to adults whose immunity is uncertain if there is a chance of exposure (for example travellers to an endemic area or workers in infectious disease units).

ACTINOMYCOSIS

Infection with *Actinomyces israelii*, an anaerobic filamentous bacterium, is uncommon in the West. The organism can be found as a commensal in the mouth and intestine, and it may invade any part of the body when immunity is suppressed. Three sites are commonly involved:

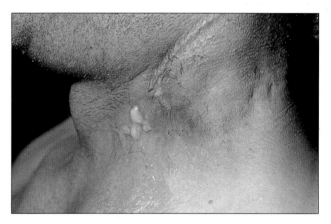

1.98 Cervical actinomycosis. The patient presented originally with an indurated subcutaneous mass in the anterior triangle of the neck. The chronic nature of the condition is demonstrated by the signs of a previous sinus higher up in the neck, which has healed, and an actively discharging sinus below it.

NOCARDIASIS

Nocardiasis can be an acute, subacute or chronic infection by a family of Gram-positive filamentous 'higher' bacteria. These are usually inhaled, but occasionally may enter via penetrating wounds of the skin (usually the foot). The organisms have a worldwide distribution and are soil saprophytes. Most infections occur in people who have pre-existing immunosuppression resulting from cancer, cancer therapy, steroid therapy, alcoholism or HIV infection. Pulmonary nocardiasis appears similar to any other pneumonia, with fever, productive cough and progressive signs of lung consolidation. Despite antibiotics, the disease progresses to cavitation, and there may be direct spread to the pleural cavity with empyema formation. Bloodborne spread to the brain and other organs occurs. Surgical drainage of the abscesses is required, along with prolonged antimicrobial therapy.

TUBERCULOSIS

After a period of decline lasting for most of the twentieth century, the incidence of tuberculosis (TB) is now increasing again in much of the developed world. TB has always been endemic in poorer countries, and the incidence there is also on the increase, particularly in young adults and in refugee groups. The World Health Organization (WHO) estimates that one-third of the world's population is already infected with TB, that TB kills more that 2 million people per year, and that a further 300 million people worldwide will become infected over the next decade.

The twentieth century reduction in the incidence of TB in the developed world was probably encouraged by improved social conditions, mass miniature radiography, good contact tracing, BCG (Bacille Calmette–Guérin) vaccination of schoolchildren and the use of effective antituberculous therapy. Cases continued to occur in the elderly, the debilitated, alcoholics, diabetics, immunocompromised patients, refugees and other recent migrants from unstable or developing countries. Tuberculosis is a frequent (and treatable) complication of HIV infection, but patients with HIV account for only a minority of new cases in the developed world. The most potent risk factor for TB in the developed world seems to be socioeconomic deprivation.

In the developing world, socioeconomic deprivation is of great importance, as is interaction with HIV infection, especially in sub-Saharan Africa and many parts of Asia.

Mycobacterium tuberculosis is spread mainly by droplets, and relatively casual contact may be sufficient to ensure spread. The organisms gain entry to the body by inhalation, ingestion or occasionally by inoculation through the skin. Primary infection usually involves the lungs (**1.99**, **1.100**), but parts of the gastrointestinal tract may also be affected, and there is usually lymph node involvement. The organisms provoke granuloma formation, often with caseation and cavitation.

Occasionally, primary infection may lead directly to more widespread disease – usually by haematogenous spread that may occur at any stage of the disease. More commonly, the primary focus of infection in the lung heals, but the healed granuloma continues to contain viable organisms. If host resistance is lowered in later life, TB may be reactivated, spreading locally and, via the bloodstream, throughout the

1.99

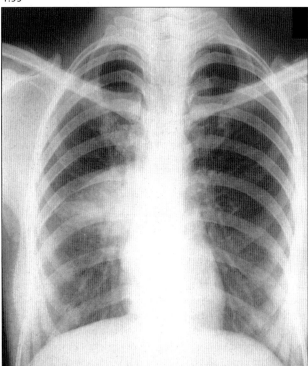

1.100

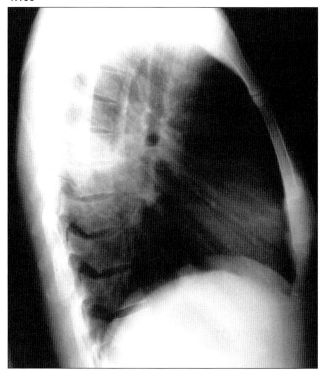

1.99, 1.100 Primary tuberculosis in the apical segment of the right lower lobe. The PA film shows the primary focus, and its position, just below the fissure, is confirmed by the lateral film. The PA film also shows slight hilar enlargement. In most cases, the primary focus heals with extensive calcification, but viable organisms remain within the healed focus. This patient was a 23-year-old Indian woman who had recently come to the UK, and the infection responded to combined antituberculous chemotherapy.

body and producing many possible manifestations. Major complications include the following:

- miliary TB – diffuse haematogenous spread throughout the body, often visible as miliary mottling in the chest X-ray (**1.101**)
- pulmonary TB (*see* **p. 178**)
- gastrointestinal TB in the ileocaecal area (*see* **p. 367**)
- genitourinary TB affecting the kidneys and other parts of the genitourinary tract (*see* **p. 286**)
- tuberculous meningitis and space-occupying tuberculomas of the brain (*see* **p. 471**)
- tuberculous osteomyelitis (*see* **p. 144**)
- tuberculous arthritis (*see* **p. 118**)
- skin manifestations, including lupus vulgaris (**2.51**) and erythema nodosum (**2.45**)

- eye involvement (**1.7**)
- constrictive pericarditis (*see* **p. 237**)
- adrenal involvement leading to Addison's disease (*see* **p. 302**)
- lymph node enlargement (**1.102–1.103**).

TB in people in or from the developing world is often extrapulmonary and investigation of any such patient with unexplained pyrexia should include chest X-ray, tuberculin skin test, culture of sputum and Ziehl–Neelsen (Z–N) staining (**4.14**) of sputum, and culture of urine and stool, and, if indicated, gland or marrow biopsy or CSF examination with Z–N staining and culture. TB in the immunocompromised patient, including patients with HIV infection, may be a primary infection or a reactivation of a previously inactive infection. By the time of diagnosis, the disease may be widely disseminated and careful investigation and management is required.

Treatment of infection with typical *M. tuberculosis* requires combination drug therapy to prevent the emergence of resistant strains of the organism. Drugs available for use include isoniazid, rifampicin, ethambutol, pyrazinamide, thiacetazone and streptomycin. Conventional drug therapy, as used in the developed world, lasts for 6–9 months or more, depending upon the combination of drugs used. WHO's strategy for curing patients with TB is to use 'directly observed treatment, short-course' (DOTS), a regimen lasting no more than 6 months. In DOTS, patients are observed taking each dose of treatment by a member of the medical team. Patients who have not attended for therapy can then be followed up, with the aim of controlling TB in the individual and the population.

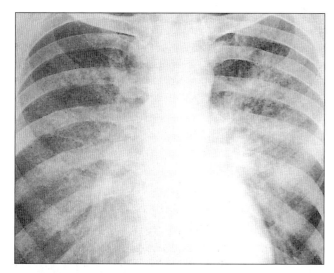

1.101   Miliary tuberculosis. The appearance of miliary mottling on the chest X-ray is characteristic, but not diagnostic, of miliary TB; similar appearances may be found in other forms of pneumonia, in sarcoidosis and in some occupational lung diseases.

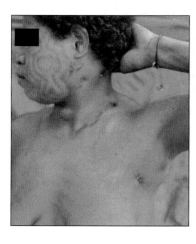

1.102   Enlarged tuberculous lymph nodes in the neck and axilla of a Fijian woman with widespread TB. Discharging sinuses are visible in the axilla and at the angle of the jaw.

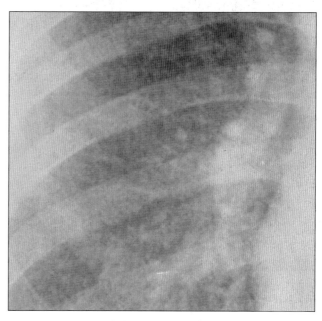

1.103   Hilar node enlargement is a common finding in tuberculosis, usually in association with pulmonary involvement. The right hilar nodes are seen to be enlarged in this close-up view.

The general level of mycobacterial resistance is low, and correctly treated TB is curable in at least 98% of cases. However, there has recently been much concern about the development of multiple drug-resistant tuberculosis (MDRTB). Outbreaks of MDRTB have been reported in HIV care facilities and prisons in the USA, and elsewhere, including the UK, mainly in HIV-positive patients. Spread of MDRTB is best prevented by early diagnosis, culture and sensitivity testing of tubercle bacilli, careful monitoring of therapy and its effects and appropriate precautions against cross-infection.

Cell-mediated delayed hypersensitivity to TB can be demonstrated by the use of tuberculin tests, including the Mantoux, Heaf and tine skin tests (**1.104**). Patients who have latent TB infection usually react positively to these tests; however, their main value is in conjunction with vaccination programmes. Those found to be 'tuberculin negative' can be immunized. BCG is a live vaccine prepared from an attenuated strain of *M. bovis*. This stimulates a hypersensitivity reaction to *M. tuberculosis*. A papule or benign ulceration develops within a few weeks and this slowly heals; delayed healing, extensive ulceration (> 10 mm), subcutaneous abscess formation or regional lymph node enlargement are recognized complications.

BCG vaccination may offer up to 80% protection against TB infection and is recommended for the following groups if they are negative on tuberculin testing:

- contacts of patients with open TB
- healthcare workers who have direct patient contact (especially those working with immunocompromised patients)
- children aged between 10 and 14 years
- handlers of animal species liable to develop tuberculosis
- travellers to countries where TB is endemic.

In some parts of the world, for example Malawi and southern India, BCG has been shown to offer no protection against *M. tuberculosis* infection. The reasons for this difference in efficacy are unclear.

NON-TUBERCULOUS MYCOBACTERIAL (NTM) INFECTIONS

Young adults and the elderly, together with those of any age with HIV infection and other immunosuppressed patients, are susceptible not only to infection with *M. tuberculosis* but also to infection with other mycobacteria. *M. scrofulaceum* is particularly likely to produce lymph node infections (**1.102**), whereas other organisms such as *M. avium-intracellulare* (MAI) and *M. kansasii* may produce almost any of the manifestations of typical tuberculosis. MAI is a particularly important cause of disseminated disease in patients with HIV infection (it may also occasionally produce a low-grade pneumonia in otherwise normal individuals). The organisms may be found on blood culture, acid-fast staining of stool smears, or culture or histology of bone marrow. Infections with these organisms are often very difficult to treat because of multiple drug resistance, but can usually be managed with a cocktail of drugs (rifabutin, clarithromycin and ethambutol).

Mycobacterium bovis, formerly a common cause of tuberculosis in the West, is now a rare cause of the disease in man, as a result of the careful control of the infection in cattle. *M. marinum* and related mycobacteria may cause fish tank or swimming pool granulomas (**1.105**). *M. marinum* and *M. ulcerans* grow preferentially at cooler temperatures and usually affect the skin where they produce nodular lesions locally and along the line of draining lymphatics. The nodules slowly break down to produce ulcers. Antimicrobial drugs may be necessary.

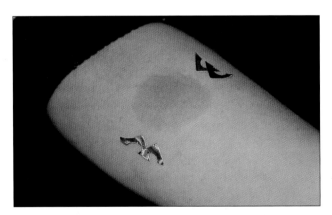

1.104 Mantoux test – positive reaction. The test is carried out with purified old tuberculin, which is injected intradermally. In those who have had previous exposure to tubercle bacilli, a positive reaction appears within 48 hours. This consists of erythema and induration, and may be graded by intensity and size. The distance between the tips of the skin markers on each side is 1 cm.

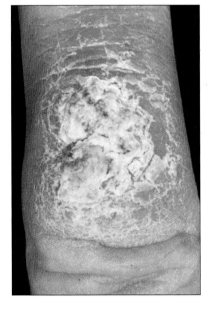

1.105 Fish tank granuloma. This middle-aged woman, who kept tropical fish, had a 6-month history of painless nodules on the dorsum of her right index finger. The single lesion resulted from infection with *Mycobacterium marinum* (*balnei*), an organism that infects fish.

LEPROSY

Leprosy, which is caused by *Mycobacterium leprae*, remains an important disease in tropical and subtropical countries. Infection is spread by droplets from infected nasal mucosa, but prolonged close contact is required. The incubation period is usually between 3 and 15 years. The spectrum of disease activity in leprosy depends upon the host's immune response to the infection.

Lepromatous leprosy develops when the response is poor. In this form, there are widespread lesions which contain enormous numbers of bacilli. There is involvement of nasal mucosa, skin (**1.106**), testicular tissue and later of nerves. Marked destructive lesions of the face and palate may result, and neurotrophic atrophy may lead to loss of the extremities (**1.107–1.109**).

In tuberculoid leprosy host immunity is good and bacilli are rarely seen in lesions. Patients present with erythematous or hypopigmented skin lesions (**1.110**) and with asymmetrical thickening of nerves (**1.111**).

The term 'borderline leprosy' is used when there are features of both lepromatous and tuberculoid disease. This may eventually evolve into one or other form of the disease.

The diagnosis is easily made when bacilli are demonstrated in smears from nasal mucosa or skin in lepromatous disease. Biopsy of skin or affected nerve is required for diagnosis of tuberculoid disease.

Multiple drug therapy with rifampicin, dapsone and clofazimine is now recommended. Good supportive measures, including surgical correction of deformities, are also important.

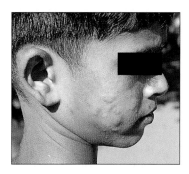

1.106 Lepromatous leprosy. There is infiltration and oedema of the cheek and thickening of the ear.

35

1.107

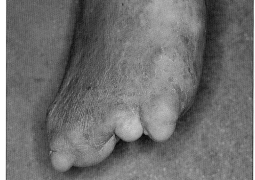

1.108

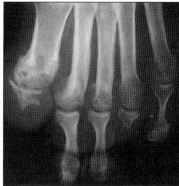

1.107, 1.108 Neurotrophic atrophy in lepromatous leprosy eventually leads to erosion of the extremities (left). In these patients, the terminal phalanges were all eroded to a variable extent (right).

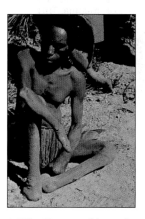

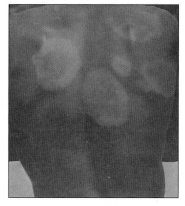

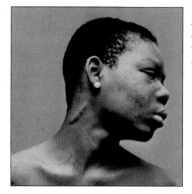

1.111 Nerve thickening in tuberculoid leprosy. Thickening of the great auricular nerve is common.

1.109 Near total loss of the hands and feet in late stage leprosy, as a result of long-standing neurotrophic atrophy.

1.110 Tuberculoid leprosy. The early tuberculoid lesion is characterized by macules showing loss of sensation and hypopigmentation.

No specific vaccine is available at present but the BCG vaccine may have a useful role in stimulating immunity.

LISTERIOSIS

The bacterium *Listeria monocytogenes* has a worldwide distribution and is found in nature in rotting vegetation, unpasteurized milk and cheeses, water and 5% of human faeces. Despite this, human disease is uncommon, affecting principally pregnant women and patients who are immunocompromised. Transplacental transmission results in fetal infection that often overwhelms and kills the fetus, which is then aborted. Occasionally, the child is born with severe malformations. Infection acquired at term delivery usually presents with meningitis at 4–6 weeks, but these babies have disseminated disease with cardiorespiratory failure, diarrhoea and shock. The mortality in this condition is high, despite modern therapy. About one-half the infections occur in adults, especially in the presence of lymphoreticular neoplasia, diabetes mellitus alcoholism or drug treatment with systemic steroids, anti-cancer therapy or immunosuppresion following organ transplantation. Infection presents acutely with fever, vomiting, diarrhoea and often signs of meningism. There may also be a purulent conjunctivitis that can produce corneal ulceration and the regional lymph nodes may be involved. Listeria is a very important cause of bacterial meningitis in the elderly and in patients receiving anti-cancer therapy. The mortality is high, despite the use of antibiotics. High dose I.V. ampicillin and gentamicin are the drugs of choice.

ESCHERICHIA COLI INFECTIONS

Escherichia coli serotypes are a common cause of infection in most organs of the body. In particular, *E. coli* is a common cause of urinary tract infection (**p. 284**), gastroenteritis (**p. 367**), pneumonia (**p. 175**), meningitis (**p. 471**) and septicaemia.

Verocytotoxin-producing *E. coli* (VTEC) is an epidemic disease with a high incidence in summer and early autumn. The most common VTEC implicated in human infection is *E. coli* 0157, which produces a range of illnesses that include a mild self-limiting gastroenteritis and haemorrhagic colitis with severe fever, colic and bloody diarrhoea. The main reservoirs are cattle, and meat products such as beefburgers are often implicated, together with milk products, raw vegetables and drinking water. A small number of severe cases develop haemolytic uraemic syndrome (HUS). In HUS-induced renal failure there is a very significant morbidity with long-term renal impairment and a mortality of about 10%. The condition is more likely to occur in young children and the elderly. In adults, disseminated intravascular coagulation (DIC, *see* **p. 443**) may develop.

The diagnosis depends on culture of *E. coli* 0157 from faeces. DNA probes can detect verocytotoxin in faecal samples and serology can be used to detect a rising antibody titre and the 0157 antigen.

SALMONELLOSIS

Salmonella organisms cause a range of clinical syndromes:

- enteric fever (typhoid or paratyphoid fever)
- focal infections (e.g. osteomyelitis, *see* **p. 143**)
- enterocolitis (food poisoning) (*see* **p. 367**)
- asymptomatic carrier state.

Enteric fever

The causal serotypes of enteric fever are *S. typhi* and *S. paratyphi* A, B and C. These organisms are species-specific to man, and transmission is by the faecal–oral route, either by direct contact or indirectly through contamination of water or food. Most cases diagnosed in developed countries are imported.

Enteric fever is primarily a septicaemic illness that starts after an incubation period of 7–14 days, with non-specific flu-like symptoms that increase in severity during the first 2 weeks of the illness. The temperature rises in a step-like fashion, reaching its highest level in the second week, by which time there is marked toxaemia. There may be diarrhoea, but many patients remain constipated throughout the illness. Signs include furred tongue, rose spots on the trunk (**1.112**), abdominal distension and splenomegaly. During the third week, the temperature declines, but at this stage a number of potentially fatal complications may occur, including intestinal haemorrhage and perforation, pneumonia, cholecystitis, meningitis and osteomyelitis. Osteomyelitis is especially common in patients who have sickle-cell anaemia (**3.153, 10.46**). Death earlier in the illness is usually related to septicaemia and toxaemia. Paratyphoid is similar to but less severe than typhoid.

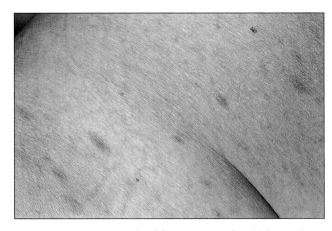

1.112 Rose spots in typhoid fever consist of pinkish macules or maculopapules, measuring 2–4 mm in diameter. The spots blanch on pressure.

Diagnosis is by blood, stool and urine culture. The Widal test measures agglutinating antibody titres but may be difficult to interpret in immunized patients and for this reason is now rarely used. Chloramphenicol has been widely used in treatment despite the associated (low) risk of aplastic anaemia, but drug resistance is now common and ciprofloxacin is the usual treatment of choice. Approximately 3% of patients will become long-term carriers, usually harbouring the organisms in the biliary tract.

Prophylaxis against typhoid is by the use of one of two injectable vaccines, or by a live-attenuated oral vaccine, but the maximum efficacy of prophylaxis is probably about 70%. These vaccines have no activity against paratyphoid.

PLAGUE

Focal epidemics of plague still occur in some countries (including the USA) despite public health measures. The organism responsible is *Yersinia pestis* which is retained in a reservoir of woodland rodents (sylvatic plague) and the domestic rat (murine plague). The vector from rat to man (and occasionally cats and dogs) is usually the rat flea, but cases of infection have been reported by direct transmission from an infected animal and by aerosol from infected patients. The possible development of plague as an agent of biological warfare or terrorism is another potential source of infection in the future.

The most common type is bubonic plague in which, after an incubation period of 2–4 days, the patient develops a fulminant illness with fever, headache and enlarged matted inguinal or axillary lymph nodes (buboes) (**1.113**) that may suppurate and discharge. DIC is common and results in bleeding from many sites, especially from the nose, and alimentary, respiratory and urinary tracts. The diagnosis can be made at this time by blood culture and by direct aspiration of the nodes. A fluorescent antibody test is also available.

When the organism is inhaled, there is rapid onset of an overwhelming pneumonia with severe toxaemia and rapid death (pneumonic plague). In biological warfare or terrorism, aerosolised plague would cause fever, cough, chest pain and haemoptysis with signs consistent with severe pneumonia 1 to 6 days after exposure. These features would be rapidly followed by septic shock, with a very high mortality rate. Early treatment and prophylaxis with streptomycin or gentamicin, or with tetracycline or fluoroquinolone classes of antimicrobials is most likely to be effective in reducing the morbidity and mortality of plague of natural or malicious origin.

Public health measures to control the rat population in urban situations and the migration of rats are important, as there are no reasonable methods available to control the potential sylvan reservoir. Control of the flea population is possible with insecticides, but these may be environmentally dangerous. Vaccination is possible in selected individuals at risk.

CHOLERA

Cholera is an acute diarrhoeal illness that results from colonization of the small intestine with the organism *Vibrio cholerae*, which produces a specific exotoxin that interferes with the sodium and water homeostasis of the lining cells of the intestine. The result is massive secretion of isotonic fluid into the gut and severe extracellular fluid loss with hypovolaemic shock, potassium depletion and acid–base disturbance.

The disease is usually transmitted by the faecal–oral route, often in contaminated food and water. The incubation period may vary from a few hours to a few days before the abrupt onset of profuse watery painless diarrhoea (rice water stools). Muscle cramps may appear as the levels of electrolytes fall. Circulatory shock rapidly supervenes if treatment is not available. The patient has a typical appearance with extreme dehydration – sunken eyes (**1.114**), poor skin turgor, tachycardia, thready pulse and hypotension. Acute tubular necrosis causes renal failure and this, together with severe hypovolaemic shock, is the common cause of death.

The diagnosis is made clinically and prompt replacement of water and electrolytes is the key to success. The widespread use of oral rehydration with a solution of water, sugar and salt can greatly increase survival rates in cholera epidemics. Hydration status can be monitored clinically (determination of eyeball pressure or skin turgor, or by assessment of jugular venous pressure). Biochemical control of acid–base balance and sodium and potassium levels is helpful if available. Administration of

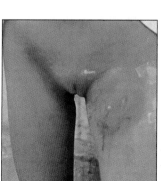

1.113 Bubonic plague. One of the most characteristic clinical features is lymphadenopathy with suppuration, especially in the inguinal and axillary regions.

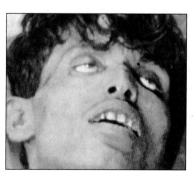

1.114 Choleraic facies. Extreme dehydration has led to the typical appearance of deeply sunken cheeks and eyes. Despite the moribund appearance of the patient with cholera, rehydration can lead to complete recovery if started before the onset of renal failure.

oral broad-spectrum antibiotics halves the duration of the illness and the stool volumes and also shortens the duration of excretion of the organism. Public health measures to improve sanitation and provide a source of fresh water are of paramount importance. Current cholera vaccine provides little protection against acquiring the disease and does not alter its spread. More effective vaccines are in development.

HAEMOPHILUS INFLUENZAE INFECTIONS

Haemophilus influenzae, a Gram-negative coccobacillus, may be a commensal in the upper respiratory tract. It may, however, also be involved in lower respiratory tract infections, especially infective exacerbations of chronic obstructive pulmonary disease (COPD, *see* **pp. 169, 175**). It is also an important cause of bacterial meningitis, especially in children under the age of 2 years and, occasionally, the elderly. Meningitis is often caused by the type b strain. Vaccination is now available against type b (Hib) and is usually given at the same time as diphtheria, pertussis and tetanus (DPT) and polio vaccinations.

LEGIONELLOSIS

The Legionellaceae are aerobic Gram-negative bacilli which have been found worldwide and are associated with outbreaks of pneumonia and lesser pyrexial illnesses. An increased risk of *Legionella* infection is associated with old age, male sex, cigarette smokers, alcohol excess, chronic chest disease or immunosuppression and a recent history of travel. The airborne route of transmission has been proven in many outbreaks, usually by water aerosols from air-conditioning systems, humidifiers, shower heads and taps. Direct person-to-person transmission has not been shown, nor has infection from drinking contaminated water. The incubation period is 2–10 days.

Two distinct diseases may occur after infection with *L. pneumophila*: Pontiac fever and legionnaires' disease.

- Pontiac fever, named after the city in which it was first described, is an acute pyrexial illness with fever, headache and myalgia. The disease is self-limiting over the course of 1 week.
- Legionnaires' disease has a spectrum of clinical severity. The features range from trivial to an acute-onset multisystem infection with pneumonia (**1.115**), encephalitis and liver and renal impairment. The dominant feature is the progressive nature of the pneumonia, which is associated with a 20% mortality (*see* **p. 175**). Diagnosis depends on sputum culture, detection of urinary antigen (the most rapid investigation) and serology. Treatment may require respiratory and renal support. Erythromycin with or without rifampicin, plus ciprofloxacin in severe cases, are the drugs of choice. Public health measures include the addition of biocides to the water used in air-conditioning plants.

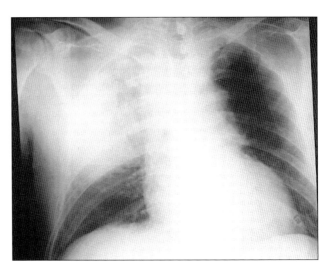

1.115 **Chest X-ray in legionnaires' disease,** showing extensive pneumonic shadowing in the right upper zone. The patient was severely ill, with a high fever and delirium.

BACTEROIDES INFECTION

The most common and most important of the *Bacteroides* spp. is *B. fragilis*, an anaerobic Gram-negative bacillus that is a commensal of the human bowel. It may become pathogenic in the presence of tissue injury and anoxia. It is frequently found in pus from abdominal wounds, after pelvic surgery, in liver abscesses, in empyema after aspiration, and in brain abscesses. The pus is particularly foul smelling. *B. fragilis* infection is also found in spreading gangrene of skin and muscle, for example in Fournier's gangrene (**1.116**). Treatment is with metronidazole.

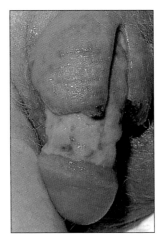

1.116 **Fournier's gangrene of the penis and scrotum.** The causative organism was *Bacteroides fragilis*. Good wound care and split skin grafting resulted in complete healing.

BRUCELLOSIS

Brucellosis in humans is caused by infection with one of six species of *Brucella*, depending on the animal source of infection: the most important are *B. melitensis* (goats), *B.*

abortus (cattle) and *B. suis* (pigs). The organism infects the genitourinary tracts of animals and may be ingested in milk and milk products or meat, or directly through cuts in the skin. The disease occurs occasionally in workers in contact with animals, for example farmers, abattoir workers, veterinary surgeons and butchers. Epidemics may occur from the ingestion of unpasteurized milk and milk products.

The incubation period is usually up to 3 weeks, but the first symptoms may not appear for many months and are usually low-grade 'undulant' fever, headache, myalgia, anorexia, pains in the joints and over the spine, orchitis and general debility. A more acute presentation may be high swinging fever, lymphadenopathy and tender hepatosplenomegaly. Almost every organ of the body may be involved in the acute process, which gradually subsides to be replaced by a chronic disease characterized by progressive asthenia, depression, loss of weight associated with intermittent fever, chronic bone and joint degeneration and hepatosplenomegaly.

The diagnosis is made by blood culture during the acute phase or a rising titre of agglutinins. Specific immunoglobin (IgM) tests are now available. Treatment is with tetracycline plus rifampicin for 6 weeks or co-trimoxazole in children. Public health measures include testing cattle with the brucellin skin test, certification of disease-free stock and pasteurization of milk.

PERTUSSIS

Pertussis (whooping cough) is a serious illness that mainly affects young children but is increasingly also seen in adults who were not immunized in childhood or whose immunity has lessened with age. The causal agent is *Bordetella pertussis*, and spread is by droplets from the respiratory tract.

Catarrhal symptoms and cough appear after an incubation period of 7–10 days. By about the tenth day of illness, the cough has usually become spasmodic and may be followed by a whoop. At the end of a spasm of coughing, mucus is expectorated and there is frequently vomiting. In severe cases there may be 20–30 spasms of coughing per day, and frequent vomiting may lead to weight loss and dehydration. The illness usually lasts about 4–6 weeks, but in some patients coughing may persist for several months.

Pneumonia and otitis media may occur as a result of bacterial superinfection. There may be mechanical complications, such as subconjunctival haemorrhage (**1.117**), epistaxis, haemoptysis or ulcers of the tongue. Hernias may develop and there may be rectal prolapse. Atelectasis results from mucous plugging of bronchi or bronchioles. Convulsions, either anoxic or caused by encephalopathy, can be life-threatening.

The causal organism can be identified in pernasal swabs, by culture or by immunofluorescence. The white blood cell count is usually raised with marked lymphocytosis.

Physiotherapy during spasms aids mucus expectoration. Small, frequent meals and attention to fluid intake prevent weight loss and dehydration. Antibiotics are of little benefit in the established case. Erythromycin given very early in the disease may have some effect and it has a place in prophylaxis in child contacts. Cough suppressants are contraindicated and sedation should be reserved for patients with convulsions.

Prophylaxis is available with combined diphtheria, pertussis and tetanus (DPT) vaccine.

TULARAEMIA

Tularaemia is a zoonosis caused by the Gram-negative rod *Francisella tularensis*. It is acquired from an animal reservoir (usually a rodent) directly, by contaminated food or water, by inhalation, by handling an infected carcase or indirectly by ticks. Tularaemia may occur in most parts of the world. The use of aerosolized preparations of *F. tularensis* in biological warfare or terrorism is also a future possibility.

The clinical presentation of 'natural' tularaemia is often with a febrile illness with a skin ulcer and enlargement of the regional lymph nodes. There may be a secondary necrotizing pneumonia from the primary lesion, or inhalation of the organism may produce a primary pneumonia. Pericarditis and meningitis are rare but serious complications with a high mortality. Intentional tularaemia would probably present with pneumonia, pleurisy and hilar lymphadenopathy 3 to 5 days after inhalation. Without treatment, the usual clinical course would progress to respiratory failure, shock and death. The organisms are usually sensitive to streptomycin, gentamicin, doxycycline and ciprofloxacin. Prophylactic use of doxycycline or ciprofloxacin may be useful in the early post-exposure period, but vaccination offers only limited protection against inhalational tularaemia and it not recommended at this stage. However, routine vaccination is appropriate for those who are at high risk of exposure to the organism, for example some laboratory workers, forest rangers and hunters.

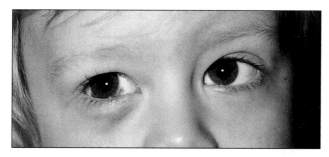

1.117 Subconjunctival haemorrhage in pertussis occurs because the intrathoracic pressure rises sharply during violent paroxysms of coughing and leads to sudden surges in capillary pressure. In this child, the subconjunctival haemorrhage is accompanied by bleeding into the lower lid – a rarer complication. No permanent harm results, and these complications resolve rapidly.

NON-VENEREAL TREPONEMATOSES

For venereally transmitted treponemal disease (syphilis) *see* **p. 58**.

Yaws

Yaws is a chronic infection with *Treponema pertenue* that has a worldwide tropical distribution. Children are often infected through pre-existing skin lesions when in contact with a person with infectious yaws, but congenital infection does not occur. There is an incubation period of 4–6 weeks and the primary lesion is a papule that grows and discharges ('mother yaw'). There is usually inguinal lymphadenopathy. This primary lesion heals over a period of 4–8 months. A crop of secondary lesions occurs over a period of 6 months – these often involve the skin (**1.118**) and long bones. Longer-term infection results in multiple destructive lesions of bones (**1.119**), joints and skin.

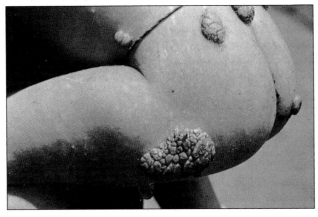

1.118 Secondary framboesiform yaws, occurring in a Papuan child. These classic lesions are often accompanied by secondary lesions at mucocutaneous junctions.

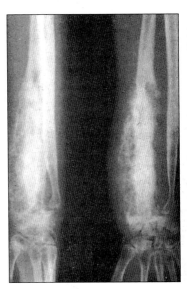

1.119 Yaws osteitis. This X-ray of the forearms shows focal cortical rarefaction and periosteal new bone formation. Similar appearances may be seen elsewhere in the body, especially in the tibia ('sabre tibia'), as in tertiary syphilis.

Diagnosis is made by demonstration of the treponemes and by serology. Treatment of the early lesions is with penicillin. Public health measures include improvements in personal hygiene, dressing of open wounds and community prophylaxis with antibiotics.

Pinta

Pinta is a chronic skin infection with *T. carateum* found in South America, which causes a generalized multicoloured rash. The lesions start slate blue and become brown and eventually white, leaving the skin mottled and blotchy (**1.120**). There is no general hazard to health and the effects are cosmetic and psychological. Penicillin controls the progress of the disease.

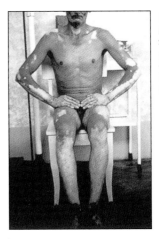

1.120 Depigmented lesions of pinta. These 'pintids' start as small papules and develop into plaques with actively growing edges which become confluent. In the late stages the 'pintids' become depigmented.

Bejel

Bejel is a chronic inflammatory disease of skin and mucous membranes caused by a non-venereal treponeme that eventually produces chronic granulomas of skin and bone. It occurs in childhood, and is found particularly in the dry regions of Africa, the Balkans and Australia. The secondary features include a maculopapular rash (**1.121**) with regional lymphadenopathy. Transmission is by direct person-to-person

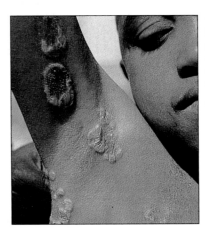

1.121 Secondary rash in bejel or 'endemic syphilis'. A florid maculopapular eruption with associated adenitis is usually the first sign of this nonvenereal infection.

contact or by fomites. Widespread use of penicillin has led to a decline in incidence with eradication in some countries.

CANCRUM ORIS

Cancrum oris is caused by infection with a mixed flora of anaerobic organisms, including *Borrelia vincentii*. The condition is seen in malnourished, deprived children who have become immunosuppressed or who are debilitated with another disease such as measles or acute leukaemia. The infection usually starts as gingivitis and rapidly spreads to involve the buccal mucosa, the cheek, the mandible and the maxilla. If the gangrenous areas heal, they leave major disfigurement. The mortality is very high despite antibiotic treatment.

LYME DISEASE

Lyme disease was originally diagnosed in the village of Old Lyme, Connecticut, USA and the infecting spirochaete, *Borrelia burgdorferi*, identified and isolated. The organisms infect the skin, nervous system, heart and joints. Most cases in North America have rheumatological features but in Europe there is a preponderance of dermatological and neurological features. The organism is transmitted by the bite of infected ticks (*Ixodes ricinus* in Europe and Asia and *I. scapularis* in North America) which are to be found on sheep, deer, horses, game-birds and other animals. The populations most likely to be affected are those working in forest and moorland areas, for example wood-cutters and shepherds, and those passing through, such as climbers and hikers.

There are three clinical signs:

- The first stage is local skin infection spreading from the tick bite. This is erythema chronicum migrans – a chronic indurated rash with a characteristic red margin and central clearing (**1.122**, **5.89**). This is associated with generalized

fever and systemic upset. Multiple skin lesions may appear at different stages of development and there may be regional lymphadenopathy, myalgia and arthralgia. There may be early clinical evidence of involvement of the CNS.

- The second stage reflects early disseminated infection and is found some weeks to months later. There may be clear evidence of CNS involvement, with neuritis (the seventh nerve is often affected), encephalitis, myelitis and cerebral vasculitis, and optic neuropathy. Carditis is often present with rhythm disturbances, transient atrioventricular block, pericarditis and heart failure. Arthralgia and myalgia represent early features of involvement of the musculoskeletal system. Frank arthritis and myositis is commonly seen in North American patients, whereas neurological involvement is more common in European patients.

- The third stage represents chronic organ involvement, months to years after the initial infection. In North America the joints are particularly targeted, especially the knee joints, and 10–20% of patients have chronic disease (**1.123**). Chronic infection of the brain may appear as spastic paresis with ataxia. Chronic polyneuropathy may be associated with acrodermatitis chronica atrophicans; this mainly affects the extensor surfaces of the extremities which become bluish-red. The skin may also become atrophic and wrinkly and fibrous nodules may appear adjacent to the joints.

The diagnosis is made on clinical grounds as culture of *B. burgdorferi* is difficult from body fluids. Serological tests are available but must be interpreted with care.

A wide range of antibiotics have been used singly and in combination. Despite this, a significant number of patients have disease progression and may require a change of therapy. Therapy should be given in high dosage for a prolonged period.

41

1.122 Erythema chronicum migrans. This characteristic rash should raise a strong clinical suspicion of the diagnosis of Lyme disease. Unless this is noted, the diagnosis may often be missed. Note the chronic induration, with a characteristic red margin (arrows) and central clearing. Sometimes (not in this patient) an eschar from the tick bite may be seen near the centre of the lesion.

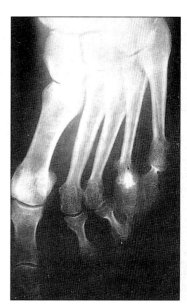

1.123 Chronic arthritis in Lyme disease. These severe arthritic changes in the foot occurred in a patient who had first noted the characteristic skin rash more than 10 years earlier.

Of major importance is the prevention of tick bites by protective clothing and prompt removal of ticks. There is no evidence that prophylactic antibiotics are of any value, but a vaccine for high-risk individuals is being evaluated.

LEPTOSPIROSIS

Humans acquire leptospirosis from direct or indirect contact with animals, especially cattle and rodents. The most common rodent carrier is the brown rat, *Rattus norvegicus*. Farm workers, vets, sewer workers and fish-farm workers are particularly at risk and account for 50% of reported cases, and other at-risk groups include people in contact with rat-infested water, for example canoeists, swimmers and wind surfers on inland waterways. The causal organisms are members of the species *Leptospira interrogans* of which there are 202 serovars. *L. hardjo* (cattle) and *L. icterohaemorrhagiae* (rats) are the serovars most often associated with human diseases.

Leptospires can penetrate the mucous membranes of the eyes and nasopharynx or may enter from skin cuts or abrasions; within 24 hours most tissues of the body are infected. The disease course is then biphasic.

In the first week of illness there are influenza-like symptoms, with fever, shivering, headache, myalgia and conjunctival suffusion (**1.124**).

The second phase of the illness is characterized by multisystem involvement, by the disappearance of the organism from the blood and the appearance of antibodies. In classic Weil's disease (*L. icterohaemorrhagiae*) the patient becomes jaundiced and haemorrhages appear on skin and mucous membranes. There are signs of meningitis, renal failure, adult respiratory distress syndrome, uveitis and DIC.

Death may occur in the second or third week from cardiac or renal failure in 10–20% of patients.

There is usually a polymorph leucocytosis in leptospiral infection. Early in the illness, organisms can be identified in the blood, CSF and urine by culture or dark-ground microscopy. Diagnosis is confirmed by the finding of rising titres of specific IgG and IgM antibodies in paired sera.

In severe infection the patient usually requires intensive care facilities. Dialysis may be required for renal failure. Antibiotics are effective if given early in the illness. High-dose benzylpenicillin is the drug of choice, but tetracycline and erythromycin may also be used.

Prevention methods include rodent control in farms and industrial areas, avoidance of rat-infested waters and wearing protective clothes.

TRACHOMA

Trachoma is a type of chronic conjunctivitis caused by infection with *Chlamydia trachomatis*, which has a worldwide distribution. In endemic areas it is transmitted from eye to eye by hands or flies, and in non-endemic areas it may be transmitted from the genital tract to the eye, especially in the newborn. A patient with trachoma presents with the features of conjunctivitis; minute lymphoid follicles in the conjunctiva are typical of early infection (**1.125**). Chronic inflammation leads to scarring and formation of a pannus. Further scarring leads to distortion of the eyelid, with turning-in of the eyelashes (entropion), which abrades the cornea further (trichiasis). Destruction of the goblet cells leads to a 'dry eye', which in turn exacerbates the corneal injury and rapidly results in blindness (**1.126**). The diagnosis is made from the clinical picture and the therapeutic response to tetracycline. Public health measures are of paramount importance. Corneal grafting is of value in selected patients.

C. trachomatis is also a common cause of non-gonococcal urethritis and pelvic inflammatory disease (*see* **p. 63**); and a strain of *C. trachomatis* is the cause of lymphogranuloma venereum (*see* **p. 63**).

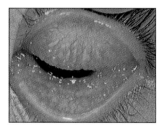

1.125 Early trachoma. Small pinhead-sized, pale follicles are present in the epithelium over the tarsal plates, as can be seen especially in the everted upper lid.

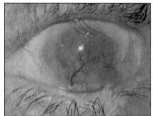

1.126 Blindness resulting from late stage corneal scarring in trachoma.

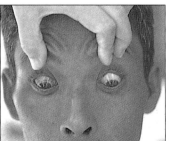

1.124 Leptospirosis causing conjunctival suffusion. This patient washed regularly in rat-infested water.

PSITTACOSIS

Psittacosis is an infection caused by *Chlamydia psittaci*, which infects parrots, parakeets, turkeys, pigeons, ducks, chickens and other birds. Infection is acquired by inhalation of dried infected bird faeces and more rarely by handling the feathers or the carcase, by a bird bite or by other close contact. The disease is found in people working with birds, such as pet shop employees, pigeon handlers and poultry workers. The incubation period is about 7–10 days followed by a mild influenza-like illness. More severe infections are associated with fever, malaise, anorexia, myalgia and headache. Chest features predominate with cough, mucoid sputum that may be blood-stained and, rarely, pleuritic pain from pneumonia. Splenomegaly in a patient with pneumonia is an important diagnostic sign. Spontaneous recovery usually occurs over several weeks, but neurological signs, liver or renal failure indicate a poor prognosis. The diagnosis of pneumonia is confirmed by a chest X-ray (*see* **p. 176**); there may be some elevation in white cell count and erythrocyte sedimentation rate (ESR); the diagnosis is made by isolation of the organism or, usually, by serology. Tetracyclines remain the drugs of choice.

CHLAMYDIA PNEUMONIAE INFECTION

Infection with *Chlamydia pneumoniae* is common (20% of blood donors in the UK have the antibody). Usually the clinical result is a relatively mild respiratory tract infection. Hoarseness as a result of pharyngitis is the most common problem followed by a fever, cough and general malaise from a mild form of pneumonia. Chest X-ray may show changes, usually confined to a single lobe of the lung. Elderly patients may develop more severe pneumonia.

The diagnosis depends on the serological testing and a rising antibody titre on serotype specific immunofluorescence. The route of transmission is from person to person by way of droplets of respiratory secretions.

The treatment of choice is tetracycline or erythromycin.

MYCOPLASMA INFECTION

Mycoplasmas are the smallest free-living organisms, and differ from other bacteria in that they lack a cell wall. The most important mycoplasmas infecting man are *Mycoplasma pneumoniae*, *M. hominis* and *Ureaplasma urealyticum*. *M. pneumoniae* is a frequent cause of respiratory infections in children and young adults, being spread by airborne droplets. The other mycoplasma organisms are associated with infections of the urogenital tract (*see* **p. 64**).

Epidemics of infection with *M. pneumoniae* last for about 2 years, occurring in cycles of 4 years. The incubation period is 14–21 days. The spectrum of illness caused by *M. pneumoniae* ranges from mild upper respiratory infection to severe atypical pneumonia. There may also be involvement of other organs with acute myocarditis, pancreatitis, aseptic meningitis and encephalitis, ear infection (bullous) and skin involvement (erythema multiforme, *see* **p. 76**) and Stevens–Johnson syndrome (*see* **p. 77**). Patients with atypical pneumonia present with fever, lassitude, malaise and a non-productive cough. Chest pain is not usually prominent. Physical signs on

examination of the chest are often less impressive than the X-ray findings, which may be unilateral or bilateral (**4.108**). Segmental lobular consolidation is frequently seen, but there may be changes suggesting bronchopneumonia or simply a general haziness fanning out from the hilum.

Laboratory findings include a high ESR and relatively low white blood cell count. Cold agglutinins appear in the blood in about 50% of patients and, if present, may be associated with haemolytic anaemia. The diagnosis is confirmed by demonstration of a specific IgM antibody to *M. pneumoniae*. Mild infection usually resolves spontaneously. Moderate or severe infections should respond to a course of erythromycin or tetracycline.

TYPHUS AND RELATED INFECTIONS

A range of diseases caused by the family Rickettsiaceae are harboured in the intestines of a range of arthropods (lice, fleas, ticks). They infect animals and man, often in epidemic form. Such infections are found worldwide and all have similar clinical presentations as the rickettsia invades the endothelium of blood vessels to produce vasculitis and local thrombosis followed by tissue necrosis.

The most important disease historically is typhus, which is caused by infection with *Rickettsia prowazekii*, carried by the human louse. Epidemics of infection are usually associated with disasters such as war or earthquakes. After a short incubation period (up to 7 days) there is rapid onset of fever, headache, myalgia and prostration.

A rash appears soon afterwards (**1.127**), which is petechial initially before becoming confluent. Gangrene of the feet and hands (**1.128**) may then appear with areas of skin necrosis, renal failure and coma. Diagnosis is serological because culture exposes laboratory personnel to an unnecessary hazard. Tetracycline is the drug of choice and vaccination is available. Public health measures to control lice are mandatory.

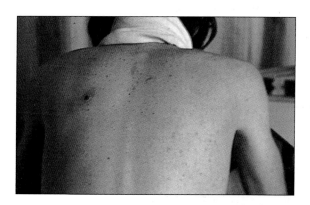

1.127 The rash in tick typhus. An 'eschar' forms at the site of the infective tick bite, and this is followed by a more generally distributed rash.

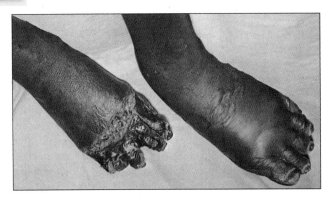

1.128 Peripheral gangrene in severe typhus. This serious complication follows the vasculitis and thrombosis associated with the disease.

Related disorders include Rocky Mountain spotted fever, murine typhus, scrub typhus and trench fever all of which are caused by different rickettsiae carried by different vectors.

Q FEVER

Q fever is an acute pyrexial illness that is caused by infection by a rickettsial-like organism, *Coxiella burnetii*. Infection is usually acquired from an animal source by inhalation of dust, from infected milk, or by direct handling. The usual animal sources are cows, sheep and goats and the organism is spread between them by ticks. After exposure, the incubation period is about 2–3 weeks before the onset of fever, myalgia, petechial rash, headache followed by cough and pleuritic chest pain caused by pneumonia (**1.129** and *see* **p. 175**). Most patients recover rapidly, but occasionally progression occurs with hepatitis (*see* **p. 385**), endocarditis (*see* **p. 231**), uveitis and orchitis. The diagnosis is dependent on serology and treatment is with tetracycline. Rifampicin is added in endocarditis.

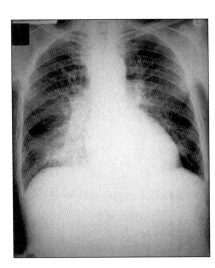

1.129 Right lower lobe pneumonia in a patient with Q fever. The patient had a cough and pleuritic chest pain after a febrile illness of several days. The chest X-ray also shows evidence of a pericardial effusion. Q fever was diagnosed.

FUNGAL INFECTIONS

HISTOPLASMOSIS

Histoplasmosis occurs in many areas of the world and is particularly common in parts of the American Midwest. It is caused by a fungus, *Histoplasma capsulatum*, which is found in the soil, and transmitted by inhalation of fungal spores. The incubation period is usually 5–20 days.

In several respects, the clinical picture of histoplasmosis resembles that of tuberculosis:

- Primary pulmonary histoplasmosis – which is often asymptomatic – is the first manifestation. It produces radiological features identical to those of the primary focus in tuberculosis (**1.99, 1.100**) and heals in a similar way. The radiological appearance may sometimes resemble miliary tuberculosis (**1.130**), and calcification may eventually occur (**1.131**). Complications at this stage may include pneumonia, pleural effusions, erythema nodosum (**2.45**) or erythema multiforme (**2.47, 2.48**).
- Chronic pulmonary histoplasmosis is usually clinically indistinguishable from pulmonary tuberculosis, producing a similar range of complications (*see* **p. 33**).

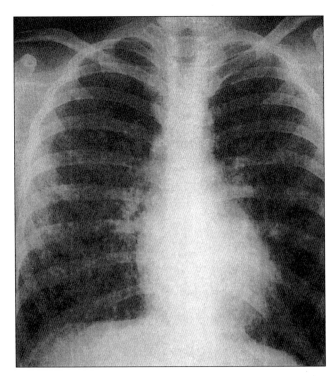

1.130 Primary pulmonary histoplasmosis may be asymptomatic, or it may result in a transient symptomatic respiratory infection. In this patient, the appearance of miliary mottling could represent miliary tuberculosis, pneumoconiosis or pulmonary metastases, and other tests are necessary to confirm the diagnosis.

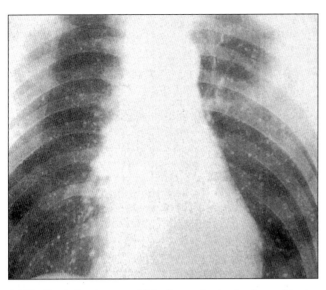

1.131 Healed pulmonary histoplasmosis. Again, the residual fibrosis and calcification are reminiscent of TB, or of healed chickenpox pneumonia.

- Disseminated histoplasmosis may occur at any stage of the disease, leading to complications that include chronic pericarditis, granulomatous hepatitis, chronic meningitis and destructive lesions of skin and bone.

Definitive diagnosis is made by culture or histology, and serology and histoplasmin skin testing are also useful. In endemic areas, over 90% of the population have serological evidence of previous infection.

Only severe histoplasmosis requires treatment with anti-fungal therapy (amphotericin B).

African histoplasmosis is caused by *H. duboisii*. It does not cause pulmonary lesions, but skin lesions (**1.132**), lymph node involvement and lytic bone lesions are common.

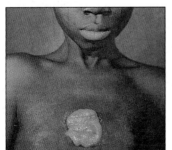

1.132 African histoplasmosis producing a large destructive skin lesion. Similar appearances may occur in disseminated infection with *Histoplasma capsulatum*, especially in immunosuppressed patients.

ASPERGILLOSIS

Inhalation of the spores of the ubiquitous fungus *Aspergillus fumigatus* (occasionally *A. flavus* and *A. niger*) may produce three forms of disease in the lung:

- In normal people, inhalation of spores may give rise to an acute pneumonia, which is usually self-limiting over several weeks. In patients who are immunosuppressed, blood-borne dissemination may take place to orbit, brain and skin.
- In patients with pre-existing lung disease, especially in those with bronchiectasis or cavities, *Aspergillus* can form large colonies. Balls of hyphae may reach several inches in diameter (aspergilloma) (**1.133**, **4.41**, **4.42**). These are usually found on routine X-ray, but may occur with haemoptysis.
- In allergic bronchopulmonary aspergillosis (ABPA), which usually occurs in previously asthmatic patients, infection is followed by intermittent episodes of asthma and pneumonia, with eosinophilia and bronchial plugging with mucus. Repeated episodes of pneumonia may produce progressive bronchiectasis or pulmonary fibrosis, or both (**1.134**, *see* **pp. 173, 185**).

45

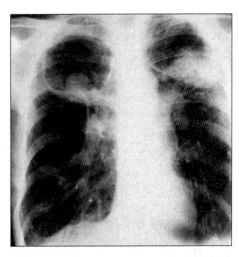

1.133 Bilateral aspergillomas, occurring in upper lobe cavities caused by old tuberculosis. If left untreated, the balls of fungus might ultimately grow to fill the cavities completely.

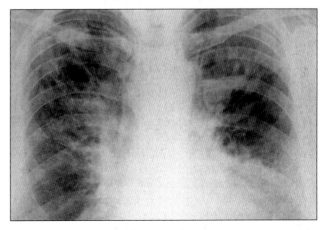

1.134 Allergic bronchopulmonary aspergillosis, showing widespread changes of bronchiectasis, predominantly central in distribution, with associated fibrotic scarring.

Systemic aspergillosis is an important form of nosocomial infection that occurs mainly in patients with neutropenia or immune deficiency (most commonly in those with acute leukaemia, or after renal or cardiac transplantation). It is commonly fatal unless diagnosed early and treated aggressively. It may present as pneumonia.

The diagnosis of aspergillosis depends on the demonstration of hyphae in the sputum, positive serology, positive skin prick test (in ABPA; *see* **p. 151**) or typical radiological appearances. Corticosteroids are of value in treating allergic pneumonitis. Amphotericin B and itroconazole are used in invasive disease. Surgery may be required to remove the cavity that contains an aspergilloma.

CRYPTOCOCCOSIS

Cryptococcus neoformans is a fungus with a worldwide distribution and is thought to be spread in bird droppings. Inhalation of the spores of this and related fungi gives rise to a low-grade granulomatous pneumonia. This may heal spontaneously, but it is occasionally complicated by cavitation, bilateral hilar lymphadenopathy and pulmonary fibrosis.

The most serious complication is meningo-encephalitis, a particularly common problem in patients with AIDS who have opportunistic cryptococcal infection. In addition, chronic infection of skin, bone, liver, heart and kidney may occur.

Cryptococcal infection cannot be diagnosed on clinical grounds. The detection of cryptococcal antigen in the CSF by polymerase chain reaction is the 'gold standard' for the diagnosis of cryptococcal meningitis In other sites, biopsy is usually necessary.

CNS infection is still potentially fatal, but treatment with amphotericin B, fluconazole or flucytosine has reduced the mortality rate.

COCCIDIOIDOMYCOSIS

Coccidioidomycosis is a common disease in South America and the southern USA that results from the inhalation of the fungal spores of *Coccidioides immitis*, which are widely disseminated in soil. Most infections are asymptomatic and the presence of the organism is detected by skin testing. In a small number of patients there is an acute pneumonia, often associated with arthralgia and erythema nodosum (**2.45**) or erythema multiforme (**2.47, 2.48**). The disease may be severe in pregnancy and in patients who are immunosuppressed. Chronic lung infection may follow (**1.135**) and there may be evidence of general dissemination to bones, joints, brain and skin. Diagnosis depends on the identification of mycelia and on serology. Treatment is with amphotericin B or ketoconazole. Surgery may be indicated for chronic pulmonary or bone lesions.

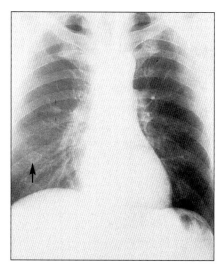

1.135 Chronic coccidioidomycosis. The nature of the coin lesion (arrow) seen in the right lower zone (a coccidioidoma) was confirmed by aspiration needle biopsy.

Paracoccidioidomycosis and blastomycosis are broadly similar diseases that are caused by inhalation of the fungi *Paracoccidioides brasiliensis* and *Blastomyces dermatitidis*, respectively. They are found mainly in the American continent. The diseases tend to be milder than coccidioidomycosis, but skin lesions are prominent in blastomycosis and occasional dissemination of both conditions has been reported.

CANDIDIASIS

Candidiasis results from infection by *Candida albicans*, a budding yeast-like organism that can infect the skin and the mucosa of the mouth, intestine and genital tract. Young infants, pregnant women, diabetics, people with prosthetic heart valves, patients on broad-spectrum antibiotics and people immunocompromised by drugs or disease are especially susceptible to *Candida* infections. *Candida* is an important and common cause of nosocomial infections. In immunocompromised patients, particularly those with neutropenia and underlying haematological malignancy, dissemination of infection via the bloodstream may be life-threatening. Oral or genital candidiasis is often the first opportunistic infection to appear in HIV infection; if mucocutaneous candidiasis occurs in an adult patient who is neither diabetic nor taking an oral contraceptive preparation HIV infection is a likely underlying cause.

On mucous membranes, candidiasis appears as curd-like spots or plaques ('thrush') on a red base (**1.23, 1.136, 1.137, 10.66**). Vaginal (**1.138**) or penile candidiasis is usually accompanied by irritation and itching of the region. Oesophageal candidiasis (**1.24, 8.39**) causes retrosternal pain and dysphagia. Moist areas of skin are susceptible to infection (**2.61**) and the nails may be infected (**2.62**). Infants with oral candidiasis often have involvement of the skin of the groin and perineum. Almost any organ of the body may be involved in systemic candidiasis.

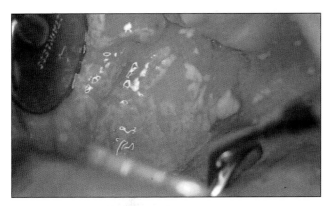

1.136 Oral thrush showing the characteristic curdy white patches of acute *Candida* infection. In all but newborn babies this infection implies underlying disease or debility, and further investigation of the patient may be necessary. It is important not to confuse thrush with other causes of white oral mucosal lesions (e.g. lichen planus, **2.70**).

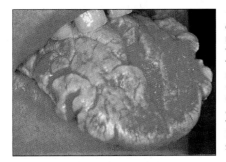

1.137 Chronic candidiasis of the mouth. The deep fissuring of the tongue is the end result of long-term *Candida* infection (compare this appearance with the acutely infected tongue seen in **1.21**).

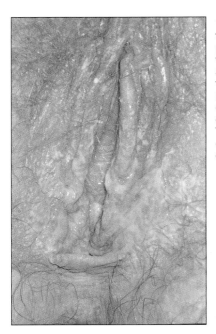

1.138 Vaginal thrush is a common problem in adult women during or after antibiotic treatment, in pregnancy and during oral contraceptive use. The curdy white discharge is characteristic.

Candida organisms can easily be identified in smears made from skin or mucosal lesions and stained with methylene blue. Confirmation of infection is by culture from the local lesions or from the blood in systemic candidiasis.

Mucocutaneous candidiasis usually responds to local therapy with antifungal agents in preparations suitable for the site of infection. Oral fluconazole may be required for severe gastrointestinal or genital candidiasis. Systemic candidiasis requires intravenous therapy with fluconazole or amphotericin B alone, or combined with flucytosine. Predisposing factors such as diabetes and HIV infection should be sought and treated.

PROTOZOAL INFECTIONS

AMOEBIASIS

Amoebiasis is endemic in many tropical areas where sanitation is poor. Spread of infection is by the faecal–oral route, usually through ingestion of amoebic cysts in contaminated water or food. The causal agent is *Entamoeba histolytica* and the time from ingestion of cysts to the appearance of symptoms may be up to 1 year.

Patients infected with *E. histolytica* may present in several ways:

- with acute dysenteric symptoms: malaise, fever, abdominal pain and the passage of frequent loose stools containing blood and mucus (amoebic colitis, *see* **p. 368**)
- with less severe relapsing diarrhoea over a period of weeks or months
- with symptoms mimicking those of an intestinal tumour, caused by granulomatous masses (amoebomata) in the bowel wall (**8.115**, *see also* **p. 368**)
- carrier states exist without obvious clinical illness
- liver abscess may occur without evidence of concurrent or previous bowel infection (*see* **p. 388**)
- pleura, lung and pericardium may be involved in spread from the liver
- skin may be involved by abscess formation or directly as a result of sexual contact.

Vegetative forms of amoebae should be sought in fresh (hot) stools or in scrapings from bowel ulcers seen at sigmoidoscopy. Suspected liver abscess is diagnosed by ultrasound (**1.139**), isotope scanning, CT (**9.40**), or by diagnostic aspiration (**1.140**). Antibody levels to amoebae are raised in most cases of liver abscess, but are of less value in dysenteric illness.

Both amoebic dysentery and amoebic liver abscess respond to metronidazole. Chloroquine may be used as additional therapy in liver abscess. Therapeutic aspiration of the abscess is now rarely required but progress towards healing should be monitored by ultrasound scanning. Diloxanide furoate is effective in clearing amoebic cysts from the gut in the carrier state.

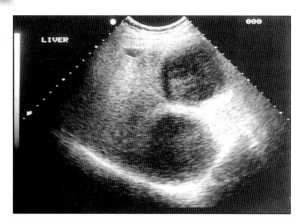

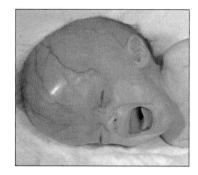

1.141 Hydrocephalus is a major complication of congenital toxoplasmosis and is usually associated with substantial cerebral damage.

1.139 Amoebic liver abscesses seen on a ultrasound in a patient who presented with right upper quadrant pain and fever. The patient had recently returned to the UK from extensive travels in Africa.

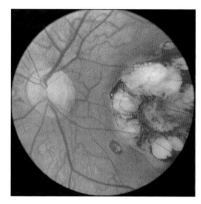

1.142 Necrotizing choroidoretinitis is an invariable complication of congenital toxoplasmosis, and it also occurs in about 1% of patients with the acquired disease. Note the pigmented atrophic scar in the fundus. Ultimately, progression of the untreated disease may result in blindness.

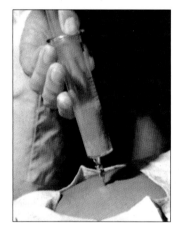

1.140 Aspiration of an amoebic liver abscess is useful for diagnostic purposes and may still have occasional therapeutic value in patients with large abscesses. Note the characteristic chocolate-coloured pus.

TOXOPLASMOSIS

The causal organism of toxoplasmosis is *Toxoplasma gondii*, a protozoan parasite. The organism has many vertebrate hosts but the sexual cycle occurs only in cats, which pass the infective oocysts in their faeces. Man is infected by eating meat containing tissue cysts or by the ingestion of oocytes from cat faeces.

Women infected during pregnancy may transmit the organism transplacentally to the fetus. Abortion is likely if the fetus is infected in early pregnancy. Congenital toxoplasmosis may be a severe life-threatening illness with fever, hepatosplenomegaly, rash, hydrocephalus (**1.141**), brain damage and choroidoretinitis (**1.142**). Infants may, however, appear normal at birth or may have only minor clinical abnormalities.

Toxoplasmosis acquired in childhood or adult life is often subclinical but it may cause a glandular fever-like syndrome with fever, malaise and swelling of one or more glands. Occasionally the disease is more widespread with involvement of liver, spleen, heart, meninges, brain and eyes (**1.142**). Primary infection or reactivation of latent infection in immunocompromised patients, including those with HIV infection, is likely to cause particularly severe illness, including cerebral abscesses (**1.30**). *Toxoplasma* is the most common cause of CNS infection in patients with AIDS.

The diagnosis is confirmed by serology. In cerebral toxoplasmosis CT or MRI may aid diagnosis and lymph node biopsy may also be helpful.

Acquired toxoplasmosis in immunocompetent patients usually requires no treatment. Congenital toxoplasmosis and severe illness should be treated with pyrimethamine plus sulphonamide or pyrimethamine plus clindamycin. Therapy may have to be prolonged and in the immunocompromised patient maintenance therapy may be required for life. Spiramycin is advised for use in pregnancy.

Prevention includes thorough cooking of meat and meat products and the avoidance of areas, such as children's sand pits, likely to be contaminated with cat faeces.

MALARIA

Malaria is the major cause of morbidity and mortality in many tropical and subtropical countries. The World Health Organization estimates that there are 300 million cases and

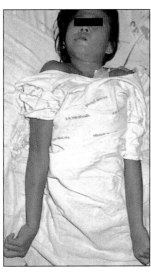

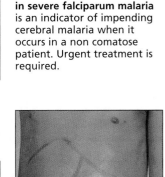

1.144 Retinal haemorrhage in severe falciparum malaria is an indicator of impending cerebral malaria when it occurs in a non comatose patient. Urgent treatment is required.

1.143 Classic decerebrate rigidity in a Thai woman with cerebral malaria.

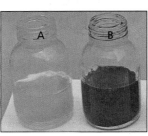

1.145 'Blackwater' (B) compared with normal urine (A). Acute haemolytic crises resulting in haemoglobinuria occur in severe attacks of falciparum malaria (blackwater fever).

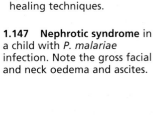

1.146 Tropical splenomegaly syndrome (TSS) is associated with chronic malaria infection and is thought to result from an abnormal immunological response. Note the outline of the massive spleen. The scars result from the local application of traditional healing techniques.

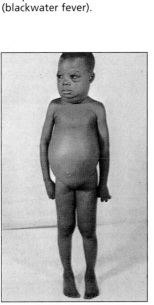

1.147 Nephrotic syndrome in a child with *P. malariae* infection. Note the gross facial and neck oedema and ascites.

1.1 million deaths per year worldwide. Over 90% of the deaths are in Africa, two-thirds among children. The number of cases imported into non-endemic areas grows each year as a result of increasing world travel.

Four species of the genus *Plasmodium* cause human malaria:

- *P. falciparum* – malignant tertian
- *P. vivax* – benign tertian
- *P. ovale* – ovale tertian
- *P. malariae* – quartan.

The insect vector is the female *Anopheles* mosquito. Infection with *P. falciparum* causes the most severe illness. Increasing geographic spread of resistance of this organism to chloroquine and other antimalarial drugs is causing major problems in the management and control of the disease.

Presenting features of an acute malarial attack are protean and may include fever, rigors, sweating, headache, myalgia, gastrointestinal upset and respiratory symptoms. The initial presentation may be with mild influenza-like symptoms, for example, so it is essential to consider the possibility of malaria in any patient in or returning from an endemic area, and even in those who live near or work in international airports. In severe falciparum malaria there may be collapse, convulsions and coma (cerebral malaria, **1.143**). The presence of retinal haemorrhage (**1.144**) in the non-comatose patient heralds the rapid onset of cerebral symptoms. Splenomegaly and anaemia are usual in the acute attack. Acute haemolytic crises may be associated with haemoglobinuria (blackwater fever, **1.145**).

Chronic infection may be associated with massive splenomegaly (tropical splenomegaly syndrome (TSS), **1.146**) or with the nephrotic syndrome (**1.147**).

The diagnosis is confirmed by examination of thick and thin blood films and the identification of parasites in red cells (**1.148**). Thrombocytopenia is common.

Chloroquine is the treatment of choice for benign tertian or quartan malaria. Chloroquine resistance is spreading and up-to-date advice is required before falciparum malaria is treated.

49

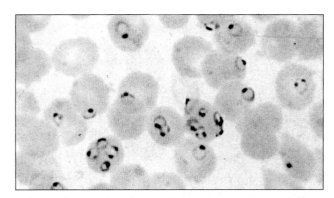

1.148 Blood film in *P. falciparum* infection showing ring form trophozoites in red cells. All blood stages in the life cycle of the parasite may be seen in films taken at different times, and blood film examination remains the cornerstone of diagnosis.

Quinine is now used to treat falciparum malaria from most regions because of the worry of potential resistance to chloroquine. A course of primaquine should also be given to patients with benign tertian or ovale tertian malaria to prevent recurrence (unless the patient has glucose-6-phosphate dehydrogenase deficiency, where primaquine may induce haemolysis).

Preventive measures include mosquito control, personal measures to avoid mosquito bites and, often, prophylactic therapy for people entering or living in a malarious area. Advice given to travellers should be up to date and should take account of the relative risk of acquiring infection, the degree of resistance of parasites in the area and the potential side-effects of drugs used in prophylaxis. As malaria in most regions is now chloroquine resistant, prophylaxis usually involves the use of mefloquine, chloroquine with proguanil or sometimes doxycycline. Global control of malaria may be achieved if a reliable vaccine becomes available.

LEISHMANIASIS

Leishmaniasis is a common tropical disorder caused by infection with protozoa of the genus *Leishmania*, which is transmitted between people or from animals by the bite of the infected female sandfly. The protozoa may cause visceral, mucosal or cutaneous infection. WHO estimates that at least 12 million people are infected worldwide, and that 350 million are at risk of infection.

In the visceral form, the organism (*L. donovani*) multiplies in macrophages. After an incubation period of 2–6 months there is extensive reticulo-endothelial proliferation (kala-azar, literally 'black sickness', so called because deepening pigmentation of the skin is commonly seen). Clinically these patients present with recurrent fever, lymphadenopathy, firm, non-tender massive splenomegaly (**1.149**) and bone marrow suppression. Leucopenia with a relative lymphocytosis is often present. In light-skinned patients there may be hyperpigmentation of the skin, especially on the hands, feet and abdomen. The death rate in untreated patients is high from intercurrent infections, marrow suppression or bleeding. Treatment is with organic pentavalent antimony – I.V. sodium stibogluconate. After successful treatment of visceral leishmaniasis, dermal lesions may reappear (post kala-azar dermal leishmaniasis, PKDL, **1.150**).

The various cutaneous forms of leishmaniasis present with single or multiple chronic but localized skin ulcers (**1.151**), and, with some species, chronic mucocutaneous lesions. They are subdivided into 'Old World' and 'New World' cutaneous leishmaniasis and are known by a wide range of local names in different countries. Transmission occurs via sandflies or directly by contact with open lesions. The diagnosis is made by finding parasites in smears of skin adjacent to the sores or by a positive leishmanin skin test. Specific antibody tests and DNA probes are now also available. Treatment of these local lesions is often

unsatisfactory, but they may respond to direct heating to 40ºC, to sodium stibogluconate or to levamisole.

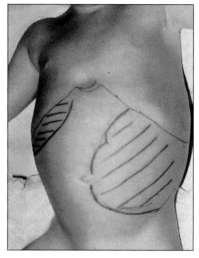

1.149 Massive splenomegaly in an 18-month-old boy with visceral leishmaniasis. For other causes of splenomegaly see **10.63**.

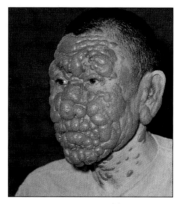

1.150 Post kala-azar dermal leishmaniasis (PKDL) in a patient who had been treated for visceral leishmaniasis 2 years earlier. The patient was completely cured by further chemotherapy.

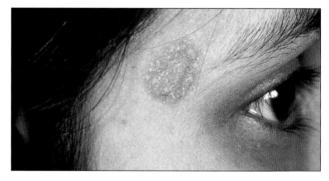

1.151 Cutaneous leishmaniasis. This lesion on the face of a woman from western India resulted from infection with *Leishmania tropica*. This parasite often produces dry, single lesions, which represent a granulomatous response to the initial infection. The lesions may heal spontaneously, and may sometimes be treated by cryotherapy, but systemic therapy with sodium stibogluconate is often required for definitive treatment.

TRYPANOSOMIASIS

There are two major types of trypanosome infection: African trypanosomiasis, including sleeping sickness, and American Chagas' disease.

African trypanosomiasis is caused by subspecies of *Trypanosoma brucei* and the natural vector is the tsetse fly. About 8–12 days after a bite by an infected tsetse fly, a trypanosomal chancre may develop at the site (**1.152**). After a period that may vary from months to years, a systemic reaction occurs, associated with fever and lymphadenopathy (**1.153**). After an indeterminate time, the infection involves the CNS starting with mild behavioural changes and rapidly progressing to coma and death.

American trypanosomiasis (Chagas' disease) is a result of infection by *T. cruzi* and is found in Central and South America. The disease is transmitted by the faeces of blood-sucking triatomid bugs (*Triatoma infestans*). In the acute infection, there may be a mild pyrexia and skin rash with patients occasionally developing myocarditis. The initial local skin lesion is the chagoma which is painful and swollen (**1.154**). Most patients present with chronic disease many years after the infection. The common presentations are chronic cardiomyopathy, and dilatation of the oesophagus (*see* **p. 350**) or colon. Dysrhythmias of various types and degrees are common in Chagas' disease, and death may result from Stokes–Adams attacks. The disease may be diagnosed on blood or lymph node films, by animal culture or by serology.

WORM INFESTATIONS

LYMPHATIC FILARIASIS

The infecting nematodes *Wuchereria bancrofti*, *Brugia malayi* and *B. timori* are found in the tropics worldwide and produce disease in man by lymphatic obstruction. WHO estimates suggest that over 120 million people worldwide are affected. Mosquitoes of the species *Culex*, *Anopheles* and *Aedes* transmit the larvae of *W. bancrofti*, and *Mansonia* and *Anopheles* mosquitoes transmit *B. malayi* and *B. timori*. The larvae enter the regional lymphatics and mature. They may live in this situation for many years.

Within 3 months of infection there is intermittent fever and sweats, with photophobia, myalgia and lymphangitis in most areas of the body. Localized areas of swelling follow, for example leg oedema (**1.155**), ascites, hydrocele, pleural effusion. Local abscess formation and chronic sinuses may form. Massive chronic oedema of the legs produces elephantiasis (**1.156**). The diagnosis is made by demonstration of the microfilariae in blood films (**1.157**). Treatment is with diethylcarbamazine or albendazole and a 20-year WHO global elimination programme, utilizing albendazole, is now in progress.

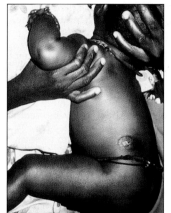

1.152 African trypanosomiasis – the trypanosomal 'chancre'. The lesion marks the site at which the tsetse fly inoculated the patient with the trypanosome. Chancres are rare in indigenous patients, but common in visitors.

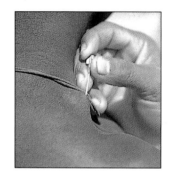

1.153 Puncture of an enlarged supraclavicular lymph node and examination of the aspirate is a valuable aid to diagnosis in African trypanosomiasis, especially in the Gambian form of the disease.

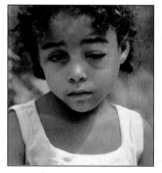

1.154 'Chagoma' in American trypanosomiasis. In this case, the inoculation occurred within the conjunctival sac, and the chagoma has caused marked local oedema with lid swelling and chemosis. This is a common site of inoculation, and this unilateral appearance is termed Romana's sign.

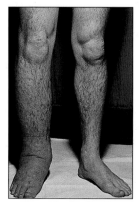

1.155 Chronic lymphatic oedema in the right leg as a result of long-standing lymphatic filariasis. The patient was a seaman who had been working in the Far East coastal trade for 15 years.

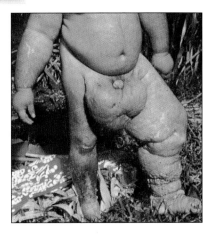

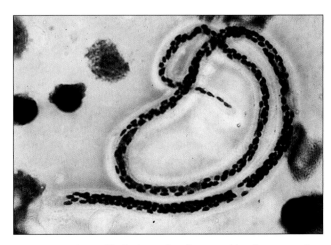

1.156 Gross elephantiasis of the leg, scrotum and hand caused by *W. bancrofti* in a patient in Tahiti. Elephantiasis on this scale may cause incapacitating deformity and radical surgery may be required to remove surplus tissue.

1.157 Lymphatic filariasis can be diagnosed by demonstrating the parasite (in this case *W. bancrofti*) in a blood film.

LOIASIS

Loiasis is filarial infection with *Loa loa* and is found in western Central Africa. The disease is transmitted by the bite of tabanid flies of the genus *Chrysops*, which live in tropical rain forests (*C. dimidiata* and *C. silacea*). Larvae enter the human skin, where they mature. The adult females migrate continuously throughout the subcutaneous tissues and may pass in front of the eyes, under the conjunctivae, where they produce severe discomfort (**1.158**). The intense subcutaneous inflammatory reaction involved in the passage of the adult worms produces skin nodules (Calabar swellings, **1.159**). In the heart, the microfilariae may cause endomyocardial fibrosis. The diagnosis may be confirmed by finding sheathed microfilariae in biopsy samples of the swellings. The migrating worms may be removed under local anaesthesia (**1.160**). Treatment is with diethylcarbamazine.

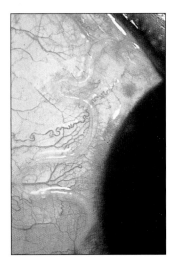

1.158 Adult *Loa loa* in the eye. The movement of the adult worm under the conjunctiva causes congestion and considerable irritation.

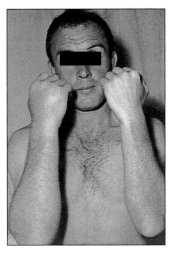

1.159 Calabar swelling in the right hand and arm caused by loiasis. Recurrent large swellings lasting about 3 days are characteristic and are most frequently seen in the hand, wrist and forearm. They indicate the tracks of the migrating adults in the connective tissue. A marked eosinophilia (60–90%) accompanies this phase of the infection.

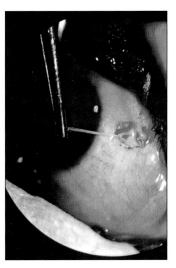

1.160 Extraction of *Loa loa* worm from the eye. The adult worm can be extracted with fine forceps after anaesthetizing the conjunctiva.

ONCHOCERCIASIS

Onchocerciasis is a variety of cutaneous filariasis caused by infection by the tissue-dwelling *Onchocerca volvulus*. It is found predominantly in Africa (where it is known as 'river blindness'), Yemen and South America. Larvae enter the skin via the bite of the blackfly vector of the genus *Simulium* and then migrate to the subcutaneous tissues where they mature into adults. The adult worms may live in the body for 10–15 years. Larvae develop from the female worms to form unsheathed microfilariae which migrate in the subcutaneous tissues and the eye. The major symptoms result from a hypersensitivity reaction to dead microfilariae. In the skin, this produces nodules which, if very large, may give an appearance called 'hanging groins'.

The eye lesions can be catastrophic for affected individuals and populations. They include keratitis (**1.161**) and choroiditis with eventual optic atrophy and blindness. The diagnosis is made by demonstrating motile microfilariae in a skin biopsy preparation (skin snip). Removal of the adult worms in the nodules by nodulectomy prevents the continued production of microfilariae.

Therapy is with ivermectin, which has fewer adverse effects than previous treatments. A successful current WHO campaign aims to eliminate onchocerciasis.

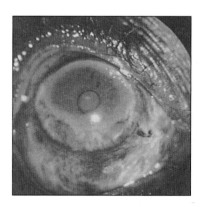

1.161 Severe keratitis in a patient with onchocerciasis.

DRACUNCULOSIS

Dracunculus medinensis (Guinea worm) is a nematode that migrates within the body tissues. Active foci of this disease are now found only in sub-Saharan Africa and in Yemen. Humans are infected by drinking water containing the microcrustacean *Cyclops*, which is infected with the larval form of *D. medinensis*. The larvae are liberated in the human stomach and migrate through the connective tissue planes of the body, a process that can take up to 1 year. Once fertilized, the female migrates to a limb where she produces a painful vesicle which ulcerates. This allows the female worm to protrude a loop of her uterus through the ulcerated skin. On contact with water, larvae are

released and in fresh water wells the cycle continues. Patients usually present at the painful stage of vesiculation when the worms can be removed mechanically (**1.162**). If the worms die, they may be found in calcified subcutaneous nodules (**1.163**). Public health measures and education of the population are necessary for prevention. Surgery is possible for local lesions and a range of anthelmintics is available. A current WHO programme aims to eliminate this parasite.

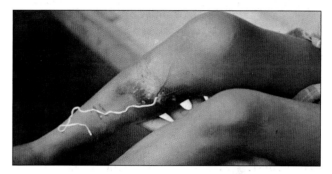

1.162 Dracunculosis in the region of the right knee joint. The infestation can cause arthritis and considerable disability, but the physical removal of some worms may be possible at this stage.

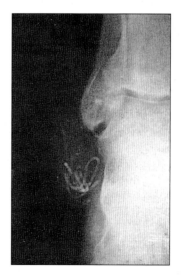

1.163 Dracunculosis. Dead, calcified worms in the region of the ankle joint, where they formed a large, palpable subcutaneous nodule.

TOXOCARIASIS (VISCERAL LARVA MIGRANS)

The eggs of the ascarid worms, *Toxocara canis* and *T. cati*, are to be found in soil contaminated by dog and cat faeces. Infection occurs when they are accidentally ingested, usually by young children. The eggs hatch in the intestine and migrate in the bloodstream to the liver and lungs but do not develop beyond the larval form. Migration of the larval worm (visceral larva migrans) may produce haemorrhage and granuloma formation. Eosinophilia is a common finding and there may also be intermittent fever, cough, asthmatic attacks, dermatitis,

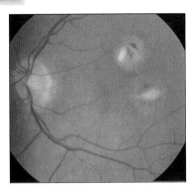

1.164 Toxocariasis. End-stage scarring of the retina in a child with otherwise subclinical toxocara infection. Sometimes the retinal appearances may suggest a melanoma or other tumour, and the eye may even be enucleated in error.

occasionally hepatosplenomegaly and retinitis (**1.164**). Usually, the acute attack remains undiagnosed and the healed lesions may be found coincidentally in the eye where they must be differentiated from neoplasms. The diagnosis can be confirmed serologically. Prevention is possible if pet owners worm their animals regularly and stop the fouling of children's play areas. Occasionally, treatment is necessary and the drug of choice is diethylcarbamazine.

CUTANEOUS LARVA MIGRANS

Cutaneous larva migrans, also known as 'ground itch' or 'creeping eruption', is the result of intact skin penetration by the larvae of a range of hookworms whose normal host is non-human, for example *Ancylostoma braziliense*, *A. caninum*, *A. duodenale*, *Necator americanus* and *Strongyloides stercoralis* (*see also* **p. 368**). The larvae cannot develop further in humans, but migrate in the subcutaneous tissues where they provoke a severe erythematous and vesicular reaction, with pruritus at the point of entry (**1.165**). These lesions are often complicated by a secondary bacterial infection. The feet and lower limbs are often involved and the condition is most common in children. The diagnosis is confirmed by finding larvae in biopsy material. Treatment is with topical thiabendazole ointment.

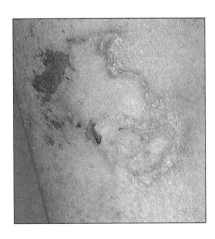

1.165 Cutaneous larva migrans on the shin. The skin lesion was erythematous and itchy, and the patient had a marked eosinophilia.

TRICHINOSIS

Trichinosis is a worldwide disease that results from the ingestion of pig, bear or wolf meat containing the encysted larvae of *Trichinella spiralis*. The larvae develop into adults in the small intestine and penetrate the wall to enter the bloodstream where they move to all body tissues, especially muscle and brain. Migrating larvae are associated with eosinophilia, fever, diarrhoea, myalgia and periorbital oedema (**1.166**). In severe infection, there may be evidence of meningo-encephalitis, psychiatric syndromes, myocarditis and pneumonia. The disease may be suspected on clinical grounds, as it may occur as a localized outbreak, and the larvae can be found in muscle biopsies. Serology is also valuable. Thiabendazole is of value in the intestinal phase and systemic steroids may be required in severe encephalitis or myocarditis. Education in the need for thorough cooking of meat products is important in prevention and the deep freezing of pork has significantly reduced transmission.

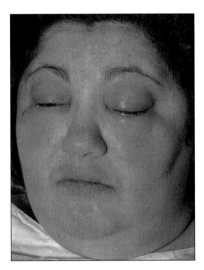

1.166 Gross periorbital and facial oedema are a common feature in trichinosis and are usually associated with malaise and eosinophilia.

SCHISTOSOMIASIS (BILHARZIAS)

Schistosomiasis is an infection with a wide distribution caused by five types of blood flukes of the genus *Schistosoma*. Humans are infected by the cercarial stage of the parasites released from freshwater snails in ponds, canals, lake edges and streams. Penetration of intact skin occurs rapidly and the schistosomes migrate into the portal system to mate and then to a part of the venous system to lay eggs. *S. haematobium* is found in the bladder and pelvic organs, whereas the others (*S. mansoni*, *S. intercalatum*, *S. japonicum*, *S. mekongi*) are usually found in the rectal venous plexus. Eggs laid in these venous plexuses are shed into the bladder or rectum and returned to the local water supply to complete the cycle through the snail population. Cercarial penetration of the skin may produce an itchy papular eruption (**1.167**) and this may be followed by myalgia, headache and abdominal pain.

In intestinal schistosomiasis the late manifestations of the disease include abdominal pain, diarrhoea, malabsorption and, occasionally, intestinal obstruction and rectal prolapse. Cirrhosis of the liver is also frequently found with associated portal hypertension, splenomegaly (**1.168**) and oesophageal varices (**1.169**). In *S. haematobium* infection the major signs are in the urinary tract, with recurrent haematuria (**1.170**) and

eventually bladder calcification, obstructive uropathy (**1.171**) and renal failure. Migration of eggs to the lungs may cause massive chronic fibrosis.

Diagnosis is by detection of the characteristic ova in the stools, urine or on biopsy (**1.172**) or with an ELISA test. Public health measures may inhibit the cycle of the parasite. Treatment of patients is with praziquantel given as a once-daily dose, depending on the patient's weight.

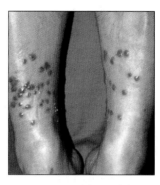

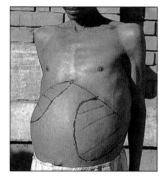

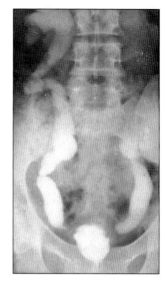

1.167   Dermatitis resulting from the penetration of the skin by cercariae. In this case, the reaction is to avian schistosomes, which are otherwise non-pathogenic to humans, but a similar, though often less marked, reaction may occur to the invasion of pathogenic schistosomes.

1.168   Schistosomiasis causing massive hepatosplenomegaly. The greatly enlarged spleen is accompanied by an enlarged, irregularly fibrosed liver. The appearance is typical of advanced intestinal schistomsomiasis.

1.171   Intravenous urogram (IVU) in advanced *S. haematobium* infection, showing a severely contracted and irregular bladder, associated with severe constriction of the lower end of both ureters, and gross dilatation and tortuosity of the rest of the ureters with bilateral hydronephrosis.

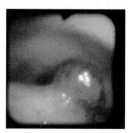

1.172   A schistosomal polyp in the descending colon, as seen through a colonoscope. Biopsy provided diagnostic information. It is not necessary to find a polyp to achieve the diagnosis. 'Blind' biopsy of the rectum through a proctoscope will often yield positive results.

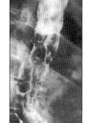

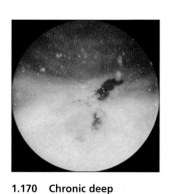

1.170   Chronic deep ulceration of the bladder, seen through a cystoscope in a patient with *S. haematobium* infection. Note the bilharzial tubercles at the top of the picture, and the 'ground glass' appearance of the mucosa below.

1.169   Oesophageal varices are a common accompaniment of portal hypertension (*see* **p. 383**). Massive varices, like those outlined on this barium swallow, occur commonly in advanced schistosomiasis; they may lead to death from haematemesis.

PARAGONIMIASIS

Infection in humans occurs from eating uncooked freshwater crabs and crayfish, which harbour the metacercarial form of *Paragonimus westermani* (lung fluke). The disease is found worldwide, but especially in South-East Asia. The larval worm hatches in the human stomach and migrates through the gastric wall into the peritoneal cavity, and through the diaphragm into the pleural cavity and lung. The mature adult worms produce local necrosis in the lungs (**1.173**) and the patient presents with haemoptysis, cough and fever. Cavitation with massive haemoptysis, pneumonia, pleurisy and empyema are also found. Healing takes place, with eventual pulmonary fibrosis. The liver and brain may also be infected. The diagnosis can be made from sputum and faecal examination. Eosinophilia is common and should trigger a search for ova. Radiography of the chest

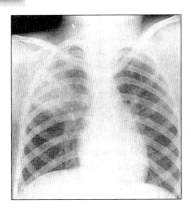

1.173 Paragonimiasis. A necrotic area is seen in the right lung field. The symptoms and signs of paragonimiasis in the lungs are often confused with those of tuberculosis.

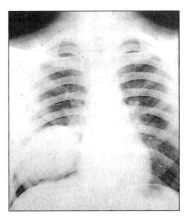

1.174 Hydatid cyst in the right lung.

may show infiltration, cyst formation, effusion and empyema. Public health measures include proper sanitation, and education about adequate cooking of shellfish. Drug treatment is with praziquantel or bithionol.

HYDATID DISEASE

Human infection with *Echinococcus granulosus* is found worldwide, especially in countries with a large sheep industry. Accidental ingestion of the eggs results from contamination of food with canine faeces (usually dog). Hatching of the eggs in the intestine produces a six-hooked oncosphere which migrates through the intestinal wall and is carried to all body tissues by the circulation, especially to the liver and lungs, and more rarely to the CNS and bone, where cyst formation occurs. In humans that is the end of the cycle, but if the eggs were ingested by a herbivore (sheep, cattle, pig, deer) which was subsequently eaten by a dog, the cysts would form adult tapeworms in the canine intestine and new egg production would be initiated.

In humans, the cysts may grow to a large size and produce daughter cysts and pressure on surrounding tissues. The clinical presentation depends on the organ(s) most affected.

Cysts are contained by a definite membrane; the fluid within, if liberated into the body cavities, may produce anaphylactic shock and death, and it will lead to dissemination of tapeworm heads (protoscolices) that then form further cysts. Over the course of time, cysts may become calcified.

Cysts are demonstrated by conventional X-rays (**1.174**), ultrasound and CT (**1.175**). Serological diagnosis (ELISA test) is also helpful and may be used as a screening test.

Surgery may be required to remove cysts that are causing pressure symptoms. The fluid must be aspirated and the cyst cavity filled with formalin to kill the potentially infective protoscolices and to detoxify the residual fluid. The cyst lining should then be marsupialized. Public health measures involve public education in endemic areas about transmission, personal hygiene and the prevention of feeding offal to dogs.

A more serious disease is caused by *E. multilocularis* which is found in foxes, wolves, farm dogs and cats. Humans are infected in a similar fashion and the oncospheres migrate to

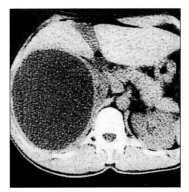

1.175 Massive hydatid cyst (*Echinococcus granulosus*) in the liver of a 14-year-old Kuwaiti boy, demonstrated by CT.

lung, liver and brain. The developing cyst is not covered by a membrane and tends to grow progressively in size. It may be mistaken for a cancer and may embolize to other tissues. It has an untreated mortality rate of about 80%.

Control of the disease requires at least a 10-year cycle of eradication in sheepdogs, in which the dogs are wormed every 6 weeks using praziquantel.

SPARGANOSIS

Sparganosis is mainly seen in the Far East. Infection in humans is acquired by drinking water or eating raw frog or snake contaminated by copepods (crustacea) that carry a larval tapeworm (*Diphyllobothrium mansoni*). Migration of the larvae to the skin, eyes and other tissues produces an acute inflammatory reaction; for example in the eye, severe periorbital oedema may be found. The adult worm may be removed from its subcutaneous or conjunctival site (**1.176**). Education and public health measures are important.

OTHER INFECTIONS

The range of agents known to cause human infections is frequently extended. Thus, cat-scratch fever, until recently of

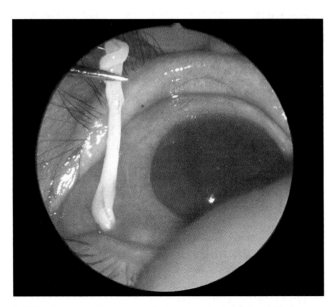

1.176 Sparganosis. Removal of a mature larva from the conjunctival site to which it has migrated.

unknown cause, is now known to be the result of infection with the bacterium *Bartonella henselae*, and other members of this genus have been shown to be responsible for Oroya fever, trench fever and bacillary angiomatosis-peliosis.

In addition, a large number of viruses, bacteria, fungi and protozoa not discussed elsewhere in this book may produce infections, especially in debilitated or immunocompromised patients.

Many of these organisms may exist as harmless commensals in healthy individuals. Others may be acquired from the environment (especially in a hospital setting), but are of danger only to those with impaired defence mechanisms.

The possibility of the use of biological agents as weapons in war or terrorism is unfortunately important. This has already been discussed in relation to anthrax (**p. 29**), botulism (**p. 30**), plague (**p. 37**) and tularaemia (**p. 39**). Other human pathogens, including Venezuelan equine encephalitis, are known to have been investigated for this purpose, and it is unfortunately possible that smallpox (eradicated from the world by 1977 following an intensive WHO campaign) could be deliberately reintroduced as a biological weapon. As smallpox is frequently fatal and highly contagious, and as routine vaccination of the world population ceased by 1980, this could have a major impact on any target population.

OTHER PROBABLE INFECTIONS

A number of other disorders are believed to be of infective origin. The association between *Helicobacter pylori* infection and peptic ulceration is clear (**p. 350**), and many believe that as yet unidentified infections may account for granulomatous conditions such as sarcoidosis, Crohn's disease and temporal arteritis. Much research has focused on the possible role of infectious agents in rheumatoid arthritis and the connective tissue disorders, and underlying infective agents such as *Chlamydia pneumoniae* may even prove to play a role in coronary heart disease and other thrombotic disorders.

KAWASAKI DISEASE (MUCOCUTANEOUS LYMPH NODE SYNDROME)

Kawasaki disease is an acute febrile disease in which mucocutaneous inflammation is associated with lymph node enlargement and systemic vasculitis. Its cause remains unknown but is presumed to be an infection because of the occurrence of epidemics, clusters and seasonal peaks. It most commonly affects children under 5 years; in the UK there is an incidence of about four per year per 100 000 children in this age-group. There are major differences in countries round the world, for example in Japan it is at least 30 times more common than in the UK.

The usual presentation is fever with conjunctivitis (**1.177**). The most common vasculitic complication is coronary arteritis, associated with coronary microaneurysms in about one-third of patients. The result may be death from myocardial infarction, arrhythmias or ruptured aneurysms. Most children recover, but they are at long-term risk of morbidity from accelerated atherosclerosis.

In addition to the dominant cardiac features, there may be arthritis, pneumonitis, hepatitis, splenomegaly, gastroenteritis, aseptic meningitis and nephritis.

As there is no recognized diagnostic test, the syndrome is diagnosed according to American Heart Association diagnostic guidelines, which require the presence of fever of 5 or more days' duration and four of the following five features: bilateral conjunctivitis; inflammation of mucous membranes of the upper respiratory tract; rash; tender cervical lymphadenopathy; and peripheral oedema, erythema or desquamation.

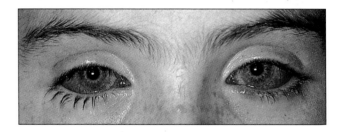

1.177 Bilateral conjunctivitis in a child with Kawasaki disease. The marked conjunctival injection is typical, though not diagnostic, of Kawasaki disease – a condition that is presumed to be infective in origin. Prompt diagnosis and treatment are essential to reduce the risk of coronary artery damage.

Treatment consists of the use of aspirin and high-dose intravenous gammaglobulin, which are believed to reduce the risk of coronary artery damage.

PRION DISEASES

A number of chronic progressive fatal neurological disorders of man and animals have now been shown to result from the transmission of a modified cell membrane protein called prion protein (PrP). Prion proteins are resistant to heat and chemical sterilization. Sensitivity to infection with prions seems to have a strong genetic basis, though it is possible that genetics influence the speed of development of the resulting pathological changes rather than the onset of infection. The most important prion diseases in man are Creutzfeldt–Jakob disease (CJD), variant Creutzfeldt–Jakob disease (vCJD), kuru and Gerstmann–Sträussler–Schienker syndrome (GSS). The underlying pathology in all these diseases is a spongiform encephalopathy.

Creutzfeldt–Jakob disease (CJD)

CJD is a rare but rapidly progressing dementing illness that is invariably fatal. About one in 10 cases are familial. Most cases are sporadic and are found worldwide with an annual incidence of about one case per million of the population. Case-to-case transmission by innoculation has also been well documented and recently highlighted in people who have had organ transplants and processed pituitary extracts of growth hormone.

The clinical presentations of classic CJD include focal neurological signs, dementia, myoclonus, akinetic mutism and cortical blindness. Death usually occurs within three months to one year of onset.

The diagnosis is made on clinical grounds. The EEG may show pseudoperiodic triphasic waves late in the disease. MRI and CT may be normal or show a degree of cerebral atrophy (**11.36**). Single photon emission tomography may show cerebral and cerebellar impairment of uptake of the tracer, hexamethyl-propylenamine labelled with ^{99m}Tc.

There is no specific treatment and management is directed at patient and family support.

Variant Creutzfeld–Jakob disease (vCJD)

It is now considered that bovine spongiform encephalopathy (BSE), a prion-induced disease of cattle, is transmissible to man by the ingestion of prion-containing bovine nervous or lymphatic tissue, and that such transmission can lead to a dementing illness broadly similar to CJD. This new entity is defined as variant CJD (vCJD), as it differs from classic CJD in several ways. It appears to occur predominantly in younger patients, has a more prolonged clinical course than classic CJD, and shows consistent florid amyloid plaques in the cerebral and cerebellar cortex.

The usual clinical presentation is with non-specific behavioural and psychiatric disturbances, including depression, anxiety and withdrawal. Sensory abnormalities may also occur early. After some months most patients develop a progressive cerebellar syndrome, myoclonus, dementia and akinetic mutism. The clinical course from onset to death so far ranges from 9 months to 3 years.

It is possible that the incubation period of vCJD may vary, and that some patients may not develop symptoms for many years after ingestion of infected material. For this reason, the size of the anticipated epidemic of vCJD in the UK (and elsewhere) is impossible to predict.

Unlike other prion diseases, the PrP in clinically evident vCJD is detectable in tonsillar biopsies, but it is not yet clear whether a negative tonsillar biopsy can be used to exclude the diagnosis. The EEG is abnormal in vCJD, but does not show the specific changes seen in classic CJD.

As with classic CJD, there is no specific treatment for vCJD. Attention is focused on early recognition of cases (a difficult task) and appropriate medical, nursing and social support as the illness progresses to death.

Kuru

Kuru is localized to one tribe who live in the Papua New Guinea highlands and is related to cannibalism of dead relatives, especially the brains and viscera. Women and children are most susceptible: they prepare the bodies for eating and the prion may enter via skin cuts and abrasions, via the conjunctiva or by ingestion. Affected individuals develop progressive cerebellar ataxia, dysarthria, dystonia and myoclonus ('kuru' means shivering or trembling). Dementia occurs late in the disease. Kuru has many similarities to vCJD. There are no specific changes on EEG or CT scan. Since the apparent cessation of cannibalism the disease is rare.

Gerstmann–Sträussler–Scheinker syndrome (GSS)

GSS is an extremely rare disease that may occur sporadically but is mainly transmitted as an autosomal dominant. It often presents in the early twenties and thirties with progressive cerebellar ataxia and loss of short-term memory. Dementia and bradykinesia are late features. Progression is much slower than CJD or kuru and life expectancy can be up to 10 years.

SEXUALLY TRANSMITTED DISEASES

The WHO estimates that at least 333 million new cases of curable sexually transmitted disease (STD) occur annually worldwide. These new cases comprise *Trichomonas* (170 million), *Chlamydia* (89 million), gonorrhoea (62 million) and syphilis (12 million). These diseases are all preventable and curable, but they currently represent a major cause of morbidity in both the developing and the developed world (though the incidence of syphilis and gonorrhoea in the developed world has declined in recent years).

HIV infection (**p. 5**) is a major incurable STD, and a number of other infectious diseases can be sexually transmitted. There is now good evidence that the presence of genital ulceration or inflammation resulting from curable STD may greatly increase the risk of transmission of HIV infection. The presentation, progression and treatment of all other STDs may also be significantly altered in the presence of HIV infection.

Some STDs can also be transmitted by other routes. For example, HIV infection and hepatitis B and C can be transmitted by needle-sharing among drug misusers and in therapeutic blood products. Syphilis can be transmitted by unscreened blood transfusion; it is closely related to non-sexually transmitted endemic treponemal diseases (bejel, yaws and pinta, *see* **pp. 40–41**).

In this section we cover most of those diseases that are predominantly or exclusively sexually transmitted (the STDs). HIV infection is covered on **page 5**, genital herpes infection on **page 18** and hepatitis B and C on **page 386**.

It is important to consider the health of a patient's sexual partners whenever a sexually transmitted disease is diagnosed, and to instigate appropriate tracing, investigation, counselling and treatment.

GENITAL WARTS

Genital warts are sexually transmitted and are caused by DNA viruses, the human papillomaviruses (*see also* **p. 78**). They affect the genitalia and the perianal region and are found most commonly in men on the corona and frenum of the penis (**1.178**), and in women on the labial folds of the vulva (**1.179**), in the lower third of the vagina and on the cervix. The time from sexual contact to the appearance of the lesion is about 2–3 months. The warts are usually multiple and they often grow together and spread to involve the whole perineum and anal

region (condylomata acuminata, **8.11**). The rate of spread is increased in patients who are immunocompromised.

Infection with human papillomavirus is probably a causative factor in cervical neoplasia. It is strongly associated with premalignant changes in the cervical epithelium, which may progress to invasive carcinoma of the cervix. Similar epithelial changes may occur on the penis, vulva and anus, though their significance is less clear.

Spontaneous healing of warts may take place and this can sometimes be accelerated with topical applications such as podophyllin.

GONORRHOEA

Gonorrhoea is caused by *Neisseria gonorrhoeae* (the 'gonococcus') and the disease is transmitted by sexual contact. Neonatal infection may also occur during passage of the infant through the birth canal.

The incubation period is less than 1 week. In men there is purulent urethral discharge (**1.180**) and dysuria, sometimes with associated epididymitis and inflammation of regional lymph nodes. Proctitis occurs in homosexual men (**1.181**). Many women are asymptomatic, but there may be dysuria and vaginal discharge if there is cervicitis (**1.182**). Infection may spread to Bartholin's glands, the uterus, the fallopian tubes and the pelvic peritoneum, where it is one cause of chronic pelvic inflammatory disease. Blood spread may occur causing fever, skin rash and painful arthritis (**3.8**). Lesions may be seen in the mouth and pharynx after oral sex. Infants infected during birth usually develop ophthalmia neonatorum (**1.183**).

The diagnosis is by microscopy (**1.13**) and culture of pus from the urethra, cervix, rectum, mouth or, in the case of

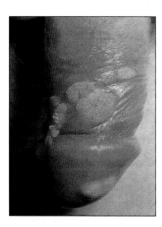

1.178 Plane warts of the prepuce and glans penis. Genital warts vary greatly in appearance. They may be sessile, filiform or hyperplastic.

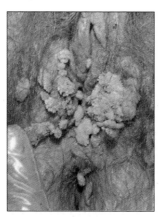

1.179 Florid labial, perineal and perianal warts. Associated cervical lesions may put this patient at increased risk of carcinoma of the cervix.

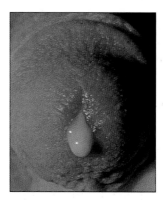

1.180 Gonorrhoea. The typical purulent urethral discharge can often be demonstrated during examination by 'milking' the urethra. The patient also has associated meatitis.

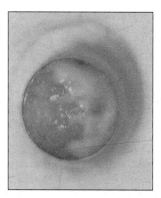

1.181 Gonococcal proctitis as seen through a proctoscope. Note the erythematous mucosa and the profuse purulent exudate.

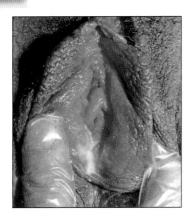

1.182 Gonorrhoea in a symptomatic woman. Note the purulent discharge, which usually indicates the presence of cervicitis.

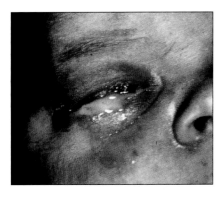

1.183 Ophthalmia neonatorum. Purulent conjunctivitis follows 2–5 days after birth in the infected infant, and may be associated with septicaemia.

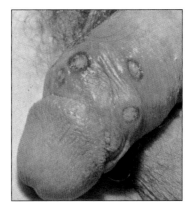

1.184 Chancroid of the prepuce, showing typical multiple ulcerating lesions.

neonates, the conjunctivae. Alternatively, nucleic acid probe, ELISA and polymerase chain reaction may be used.

Single-dose therapy with procaine benzylpenicillin (procaine penicillin) or amoxicillin, each given with probenecid, is often effective, but penicillin-resistant strains are now common in some parts of the world (e.g. South-East Asia and Africa). Longer treatment may be required if there is spread of infection. If the organisms are resistant to penicillin, alternative drugs include spectinomycin, the cephalosporins and ciprofloxacin. Concomitant infection with *Chlamydia trachomatis* (**p. 63**) is common and may require additional treatment. Tracing and treatment of contacts is important to prevent spread of infection.

CHANCROID

Chancroid is characterized by painful genital ulceration followed by tender inguinal lymphadenopathy. The organism responsible is *Haemophilus ducreyi*, a Gram-negative bacterium with a worldwide distribution (though infection in developed countries is now rare). It is most common in men, but this suggests significant underdiagnosis in women. The incubation period is usually 2–5 days. The first lesion is a tender, painful macule which becomes pustular and, on bursting, forms a painful ulcer which has a necrotic grey membrane. Lesions are usually found on the glans or shaft of the penis (**1.184**) or

around the anus. In women, they may appear on the cervix, vagina, vulva or perianal region. They may also be found occasionally on other skin surfaces and in the mouth. Regional lymphadenopathy (buboes) is invariable and may occasionally suppurate and leave chronic fistulae.

The diagnosis can be made in most cases by culture of exudate or pus, or by polymerase chain reaction. Treatment is with co-trimoxazole or tetracycline. Sexual partners should be identified and screened if possible.

GRANULOMA INGUINALE

Granuloma inguinale is an infectious disease resulting from *Calymmatobacterium granulomatis*, a Gram-negative bacterium. It is usually transmitted sexually and is found predominantly in Africa, Papua New Guinea, India and the Caribbean but some cases have been reported in homosexual men in the USA and Europe. The clinical signs develop 1–10 weeks after exposure. An indurated papule usually forms on the penis, labia or anal margin but extragenital lesions are common on the face, lips and neck. These primary lesions may be tender and produce a foul-smelling discharge. Regional lymphadenopathy is usual (**1.185**) and suppuration and secondary infection are common. Extensive scarring may be found in the healing phase (**1.186**).

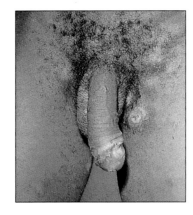

1.185 Granuloma inguinale, showing a typical ulcer on the inner thigh. The ulcerated lesion is deep and its floor is covered by a thick, offensive, purulent exudate. Bilateral inguinal lymphadenopathy is present.

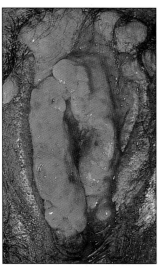

1.186 Granuloma inguinale of the vulva. The disease often runs a chronic course and is associated with mutilating ulceration, chronic swelling and ultimately extensive scarring.

Diagnosis is by finding the typical Donovan bodies in Gram-stained exudate. Exclusion of the other venereal infections is essential.

SYPHILIS

Syphilis is an STD characterized by an initial illness followed by a long latent period before late manifestations of the disease appear. The causative organism is the spirochaete *Treponema pallidum*. Congenital syphilis results from transplacental infection of the fetus.

Syphilis is still a common disease (12 million new cases per year), mainly in the developing world where many patients have advanced disease before they come to medical attention. This makes transmission to sexual partners and children more likely.

In the developed world, syphilis is relatively rare, but it is now seen more frequently in patients with HIV infection, in whom the disease progresses more rapidly.

Three stages of the disease are recognized:

- The primary stage occurs after an incubation period of about 3 weeks; a painless ulcerated lesion (chancre) develops at the

site of inoculation. In men, the lesion is usually on the penis (**1.187**) or anus (in homosexuals). In women the lesion may be on the vulva (**1.188**), but if it is in the vagina or on the cervix it may be missed. Chancres are highly infective, but are self-limiting and heal in about 4–6 weeks.
- The secondary stage represents systemic spread of infection and follows about 2 months after the primary lesion. Features of this stage include fever, widespread macular rash, wart-like lesions (condylomata lata) in the genital area (**1.189**), snail-track ulcers on the buccal mucosa (**1.190**), generalized lymphadenopathy and occasionally aseptic

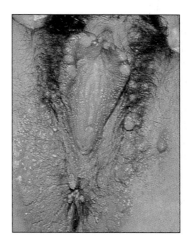

1.188 Syphilis – typical chancre of the labium majus.

61

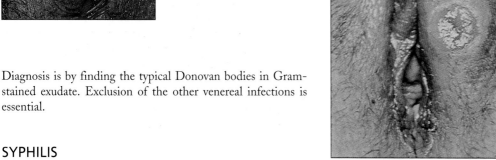

1.189 Secondary syphilis. Gross condylomata lata of the vulva and anus. Note the resemblance to warts (condylomata acuminata).

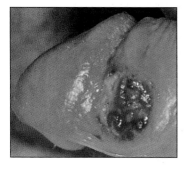

1.187 Syphilis – typical primary chancre in the coronal sulcus. A small red macule enlarges and develops through a papular stage, becoming eroded to form a typical round, painless ulcer. If untreated, the ulcer usually heals after 4–8 weeks.

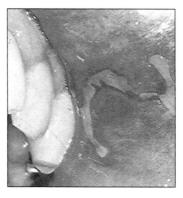

1.190 Secondary syphilis – classic 'snail-track' ulcer of the buccal mucosa. Other mucosal lesions at this stage may be round or oval in shape.

meningitis. This stage is also self-limiting and is followed by a latent period of 2–20 years, before symptoms of the tertiary stage appear.

- Features of the tertiary stage include the development of chronic granulomatous lesions (gummata) in skin (**1.191**), mucosa and bone, vascular lesions (aortic aneurysm – **1.192**) and lesions of the CNS (meningovascular syphilis (**11.6**), general paralysis of the insane, tabes dorsalis) which may also lead to destructive joint disease (**1.193, 1.194**). Neurosyphilis progresses rapidly and aggressively in patients who also have HIV infection. Adequate therapy in the early stages of syphilis should prevent the tertiary stage developing.
- Congenital syphilis may result in abortion or stillbirth. Infants may be severely affected at birth or may appear normal and develop manifestations of disease in later childhood (**1.195, 1.196**).

The diagnosis is confirmed by finding spirochaetes in the primary lesion or in exudates during the secondary stage. Serological tests include non-specific antigen tests (e.g. VDRL) or specific antitreponemal tests (TPI, TPHA, FTA).

1.193 1.194

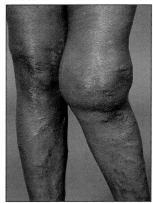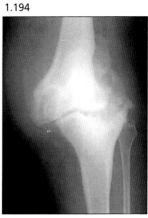

1.193, 1.194 **Tertiary syphilis** – Charcot joints. In tabes dorsalis, impaired pain and position sensation, combined with muscular hypotonia, often lead to the destruction of joints and inappropriate new bone formation, as seen in these clinical and radiological examples. Charcot joints may also occur in patients with diabetes, leprosy and syringomyelia.

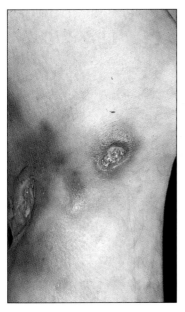

1.191 **Tertiary syphilis – gummata of the skin.** The lesions start as subcutaneous masses, which increase in size before breaking down to form typical gummatous ulcers. The ulcers are painless, and have sharply defined 'punched out' edges and an indurated base that is occupied at this stage by a slough of necrotic tissue. In contrast to the ulcerating lesions in primary and secondary syphilis, *Treponema pallidum* organisms cannot be found.

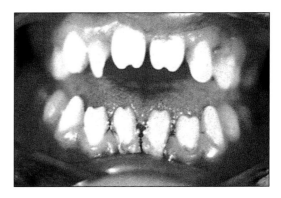

1.195 **Congenital syphilis (Hutchinson's teeth).** The incisors have a typical appearance with a 'peg' or 'screwdriver' shape and marginal notching.

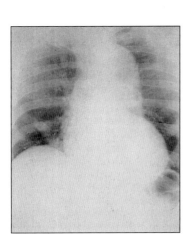

1.192 **Tertiary syphilis** – a large aortic aneurysm on chest X-ray. The aneurysm results from vasculitis affecting the vasa vasorum of the aorta.

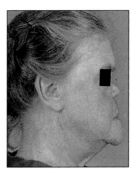

1.196 **Congenital syphilis.** Treponemal infection of bone leads to epiphysitis, retardation of bone formation and separation of the epiphyses, with resulting interference with growth. In the nasal bones, the infection results in destruction of the nasal septum and the classic 'saddle nose', giving the characteristic facies of congenital syphilis.

CSF examination should be carried out if neurosyphilis is suspected.

Parenteral penicillin is the drug of choice. Steroid cover should be used in the first few days of therapy to prevent a Jarisch–Herxheimer reaction (caused by toxins released by the dying spirochaetes). Alternative drugs for patients with penicillin allergy include erythromycin and tetracycline.

LYMPHOGRANULOMA VENEREUM

Lymphogranuloma venereum is an STD caused by a strain of *Chlamydia trachomatis* (serovar L) that is found in many tropical countries. The primary lesion appears, within a few days of sexual contact, on the genitalia, in the anus or in the mouth as a small indurated papule, and heals rapidly without leaving a scar. Lymph node enlargement develops in 2–8 weeks and the nodes undergo suppuration and may discharge though the skin (**1.197**). There may be systemic upset with fever, arthralgia, splenomegaly, generalized lymphadenopathy and meningism. Healing may be associated with extensive scarring and local oedema resulting from lymphatic obstruction; strictures of the vagina, urethra or rectum may form.

The diagnosis is made by finding the organism in the local lesions or by serology. Treatment is with tetracycline, and suppurating lymph nodes should be aspirated via normal skin to prevent fistulae forming.

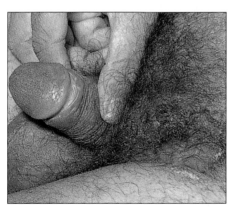

1.197 Lymphogranuloma venereum showing superficial ulceration and enlarged lymph nodes (buboes) in the left inguinal region.

OTHER *CHLAMYDIA TRACHOMATIS* INFECTIONS

Eight serovars of *C. trachomatis* (D–K) are spread by sexual contact and cause genital infections (serovars A–C cause trachoma, **p. 42**; serovar L causes lymphogranuloma venereum, *see above*).

Infection with this organism in men accounts for about one-half the cases of non-gonococcal urethritis and about one-third of cases of acute epididymitis. In women, it accounts for about 60% of cases of pelvic inflammatory disease and 50% of cases of cervicitis.

The usual symptoms in men are dysuria, urethral discharge and epididymitis (painful swollen scrotum). In women pelvic infection is accompanied by lower abdominal pain, fever and tenderness of the uterus on vaginal examination (pelvic inflammatory disease). About 30% of babies born to mothers with *C. trachomatis* in the vagina develop conjunctivitis and 20% develop chlamydial pneumonia. In addition, they may develop a reactive arthritis.

The diagnosis is made by enzyme immunoassay of infected urethral, cervical samples or of 'first-catch' urine samples, or alternatively using nucleic acid probes or polymerase chain reaction techniques. Contact tracing and screening is important.

63

NON-GONOCOCCAL URETHRITIS

Chlamydia trachomatis is one of the most common causes of sexually transmitted non-gonococcal urethritis. The incubation period is short (5–10 days) and is usually followed by a urethral (**1.198**) or vaginal discharge and severe dysuria. A variety of complications may occur including cervicitis, salpingitis and urethral stricture.

Mycoplasma hominis, M. genitalium and *Ureaplasma urealyticum* are other recognized causes of non-gonococcal urethritis.

Diagnosis is usually made by the finding of a leucocytic urethral exudate and excluding gonorrhoea, but *C. trachomatis* may be identified by other techniques (*see above*).

Treatment is with tetracycline for the patient and sexual partners.

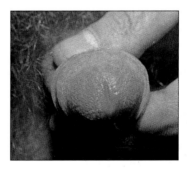

1.198 Typical non-gonococcal urethritis, with mucopurulent discharge. Although the discharge is often more watery than that in gonorrhoea (**1.180**), gonorrhoea must always be excluded by Gram stain and culture.

PELVIC INFLAMMATORY DISEASE

Pelvic inflammatory disease (PID) is a general term for a range of infections of the female organs of reproduction. It is most commonly found in sexually active women in the 15–25 years age-group. The socioeconomic factors that predispose to pelvic inflammatory disease are early age of onset of sexual activity, multiple sexual partners, recent change of partner, previous STD, use of an IUCD, recent gynaecological procedure or recent pregnancy, and failure to use a condom. The results of long-term infection include recurrent pelvic pain, vaginal discharge, dysuria, infertility due to fibrosis, a high incidence of ectopic pregnancies and the risk of pelvic abscess (**1.15**).

Pelvic inflammatory disease is usually caused by ascending infection with the patient's own vaginal organisms or with sexually transmitted organisms. *Chlamydia trachomatis* is the most common infection in the developed world, followed by *Neisseria gonorrhoea*, but *Bacteroides* sp., *Mycoplasma hominis* and *M. genitalium* may all cause pelvic inflammatory disease.

The diagnosis may require laparoscopy with direct viewing of the anatomical changes, followed by bacterial cultures and serology. Ultrasound is of value in excluding ectopic pregnancy or other major contributing pathology, such as fibroids of the uterus or ovarian cysts.

Treatment, for example with tetracycline and metronidazole, should be aimed at the likely infecting organisms.

Counselling and treatment should be offered to all partners. In addition, the possibility of concurrent HIV infection should always be remembered.

TRICHOMONIASIS

Trichomoniasis is an STD caused by the protozoan *Trichomonas vaginalis*. The incubation period is 3-21 days. In women, it presents as an acute or recurring vaginitis characterized by an extremely irritant, foul-smelling vaginal discharge that is often frothy and yellow (**1.199**). The symptoms may subside, but the patient continues to carry the trichomonads and is infectious to her sexual partners. In men, the organism may cause recurrent urethritis and prostatitis. The diagnosis is made by the finding of numerous motile organisms in a wet mount of vaginal, prostatic or urethral secretions or a spun sample of urine, or by culture.

Treatment of all sexual partners with metronidazole is important.

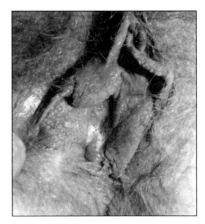

1.199
Trichomoniasis. Typical vulvovaginitis, with profuse, foul-smelling purulent frothy discharge.

ANAEROBIC BACTERIAL VAGINOSIS

Anaerobic bacterial vaginosis is accompanied by a profuse fishy-smelling vaginal discharge that is associated with vulvar itch and dysuria. There is usually a profuse white vaginal discharge and vulval or vaginal erythema, oedema or fissuring. The pH of the vaginal fluid is usually > 5. The 'amine' test can be performed on a drop of vaginal secretion on a slide by adding a drop of potassium hydroxide. If the test is positive there is a transient ammonia-like odour (positive sniff test). It is important to exclude the possibility of *Candida* infection (*see* **p. 46**).

Gram staining of the vaginal fluid shows epithelial cells, the surface of which are studded with bacteria (so-called 'clue' cells).

Culture usually grows anaerobes *Gardnerella vaginalis* and *Mycoplasma hominis*. Treatment involves local or systemic metronidazole or other antimicrobial agents, or both. The role of sexual transmission and whether there is a need to treat sexual partners is still unclear.

2 Skin

HISTORY AND EXAMINATION

A careful history and full examination of the dermatological patient is essential. First, establish the duration and evolution of a skin lesion or eruption as this will provide the basis for further questions and investigations. For example, a lesion may have been present from birth, or it may have developed in the past few days or weeks. Dermatoses may precede or coincide with other events such as intercurrent illnesses, a course of drugs, contact with animals, chemicals or plants or perhaps travel abroad. There may have been a previous episode of a similar dermatosis or someone else in the family may recently have had a similar problem.

The appearance and distribution of skin lesions are characteristic in many conditions. Often a dermatosis will start with a typical lesion and then spread in a particular pattern, as for example the herald patch of pityriasis rosea. Lesions may be confined to one body site, such as the face in acne rosacea, or to light-exposed sites or to a group of sites such as scalp, eyelid and eyelashes, face and chest in seborrhoeic dermatitis. Psoriasis characteristically affects the extensor surfaces of limbs, whereas atopic dermatitis affects the flexor surfaces. Some dermatoses, for example erythema multiforme, tend to have peripheral lesions first, affecting hands and feet before moving centrally. Skin eruptions may be symmetrical, more suggestive of an endogenous cause, or asymmetrical, when exogenous factors may be relevant. If a dermatosis settles during a vacation, only to recur on return to work, a factor at the work site may be important.

An accurate description of the skin lesion is essential. The morphology of a lesion should be defined carefully as macular, papular, pustular or nodular. The presence of scale or crust, the colour of both recent and fading lesions, the presence of background sun damage in the form of wrinkles and skin thinning, abnormal pigmentation, changes in colour and distribution of hair all combine to make a characteristic picture that can often provide more information than subsequent investigations.

Finally, the dermatosis may be symptomatic: pain or pruritus are the most common symptoms. Painful lesions suggest active inflammation or infection; pruritus is very common and subjective, but can be useful in making a diagnosis. For example, the sudden onset of an itchy dermatosis, worse at night, in a person with no previous skin problems is highly suggestive of scabies – but look for the characteristic lesions before making a diagnosis. Itch can be distressing, causing embarrassment and loss of sleep, and should be acknowledged sympathetically. Pain can precede the development of either herpes simplex or zoster lesions.

General health is also important. Many skin conditions are a reflection of underlying systemic conditions, so attention to a history of other illnesses, a brief systemic inquiry and recognition of other factors, such as arthritis, anaemia, weight gain or loss, thyroid enlargement, lymphadenopathy, all form part of the examination of the skin.

INVESTIGATIONS

SKIN BIOPSY

Skin biopsy is a useful and common investigation, as the histology of a lesion will establish, confirm or refute the clinical diagnosis in most cases. The biopsy should be well planned; early lesions are more informative as secondary infection or excoriation in mature lesions may mask underlying changes. A representative lesion should be selected, with attention to local anatomy, healing and potential scar formation. Although a punch biopsy is adequate for some conditions, an ellipse of skin, including normal and abnormal skin, is usually preferable (**2.1**). The size and depth of biopsy depend on the nature of the

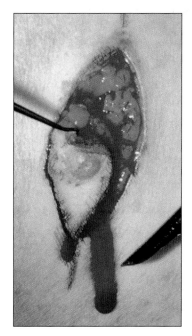

2.1 Excision biopsy of a lesion on the leg. The ellipse for excision is placed in the direction of the skin-crease line, and a small margin of normal skin is removed with the lesion.

lesion and the investigations required, but most biopsies should include dermis down to subcutaneous fat. Tissue should be sent for bacterial or viral culture, for routine histology (**2.2**) or for immunofluorescence staining (**2.3**, **2.75**, **2.79**, **3.11**). Special stains, for example for fungal elements, should also be requested.

SAMPLES FOR MICROBIOLOGICAL INVESTIGATIONS

Swabs can be taken from lesions with exudate or pus; blister fluid can be aspirated for culture or microscopy for bacterial or viral infection. Interpreting results requires some knowledge of commensal organisms and potential pathogens (**2.4**).

Blood samples may be needed for culture, ASO titres, fluorescent treponema antibody-absorption (FTA-ABS) tests, paired samples for viral titres or serology for other infections such as viral hepatitis or HIV infection.

Fungal elements are found in keratin from nail clippings, hairs and skin scrapings. Examination under Wood's lamp is occasionally helpful in identifying infections. For example, *Microsporum* species fluoresce blue–green, (**2.5**, **2.6**), and erythrasma (infection with *Corynebacterium minutissimum*) fluoresces pink. The affected skin should be scraped firmly, using a scalpel blade held at 45° to the skin surface. Scrapings are collected in a fold of black paper or on microscope slides; adequate quantities are required for both microscopy and culture. Direct microscopy of skin scrapings treated with potassium hydroxide may reveal fungal hyphae and spores

2.2

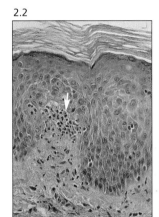

2.3

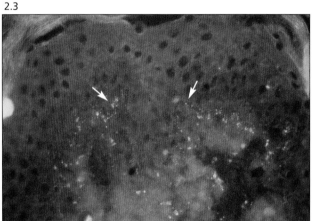

2.2, 2.3 Skin biopsy yields valuable information in many dermatological disorders. This patient has dermatitis herpetiformis (DH). A formalin-fixed perilesional biopsy (H&E stain) shows a papillary tip microabscess (arrow), which is typical of DH (**2.2**). Immunofluorescence on an unfixed section (**2.3**) shows IgA deposition in the papillary tips (arrows). These abnormalities occur at the level at which the subepithelial split subsequently develops in this blistering condition.

2.4 Skin commensals and common pathogens.

SKIN COMMENSALS AND COMMON PATHOGENS		
COMMENSALS	*Corynebacterium*	'Diphtheroids' (Gram-positive rods) aerobic or anaerobic, for example *C. acnes*
	Micrococcacea	Gram-positive cocci, for example *Staphylococcus albus* (*Staphylococcus aureus* in 10%)
	Gram-negative bacilli	e.g. *Proteus* (5–15%)
	Pityrosporum ovale	Yeast in sebaceous glands or scalp
	Candida	Varying species, including *C. albicans*
	Demodex folliculorum	A mite on face or scalp
PATHOGENS	*Corynebacterium*	*C. minutissimum* (erythrasma) *C. acnes* (acne vulgaris)
	Micrococcacae	*Staphylococcus aureus*
	Streptococci	Beta haemolytic group A (C, D and G may be pathogens)
	Gram-negative bacilli	*Pseudomonas, Klebsiella, Escherichia coli*
	Yeasts	*Candida albicans* (opportunistic) *Pityrosporum orbiculare*
	Fungi	Dermatophytes: *Trichophyton, Epidermophyton* and *Microsporum*

2.5

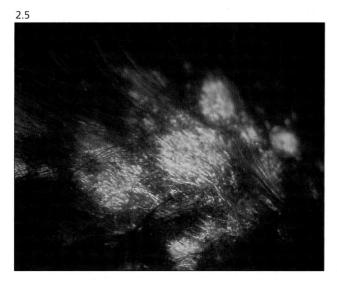

2.6

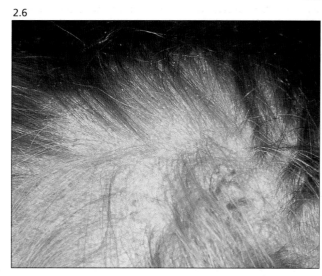

2.5 & 2.6   Wood's light is a long-wave ultraviolet light (UVA), which is useful in evaluating a range of skin conditions. In this patient, a superficial fungal infection of the scalp fluoresces blue–green (**2.5**). The appearance of the scalp of the same patient in normal light is shown in **2.6**. The patient has ringworm (*see* **p. 79**).

(**2.7**), and culture allows identification of the dermatophyte species. Scabies infestation may be confirmed by looking for adult mites in skin scrapings (**2.8**).

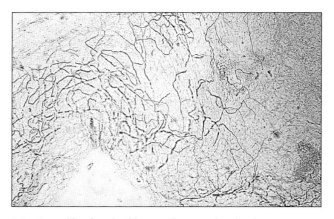

2.7   Fungal hyphae in skin scrapings can be clearly seen microscopically after treatment of the scrapings with KOH.

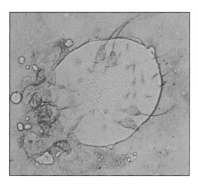

2.8   Scabies mite. The discovery of even a single mite or egg seen microscopically in skin scrapings confirms the diagnosis.

PATCH TESTING

Patch testing is designed to detect delayed hypersensitivity, or cell-mediated immune reactions, which may be the basis of an inflammatory rash. A careful history is very important for this investigation to be worthwhile. The patient may need to supply materials from suspect cosmetics, footwear or industrial processes. A visit to the work site of patients with suspected industrial dermatitis can be helpful. For this test, the suspect allergens are applied to the skin surface, using defined concentrations mixed in a paraffin ointment, under a special chamber (**2.9**, **2.10**). After 72 hours a positive test shows erythema and blistering at the contact site (**2.11**, **2.12**). A vast range of potential allergens exists; choosing the correct 'battery'

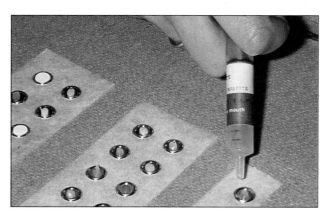

2.9   Preparation for patch testing. Common sensitizers are dissolved in water or soft paraffin ointment and applied in sequence to special aluminium chambers (Finn chambers).

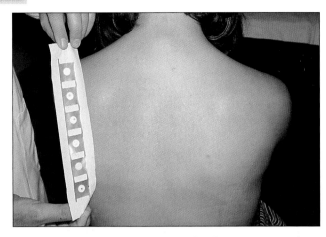

2.10 **Patch testing.** The aluminium chambers are mounted on hypoallergenic tape and applied to the back.

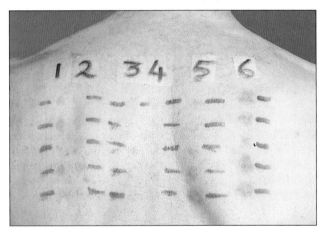

2.11 **Positive patch test results** in a gardener who became sensitized to chrysanthemums and other plants and developed contact dermatitis.

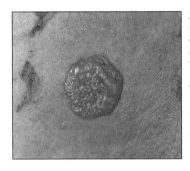

2.12 **An extreme positive patch test reaction in close-up.** There is extensive erythema and vesiculation. Ulceration may subsequently occur at the site. This patient reacted to rubber additives; she was a dental surgeon who developed severe contact dermatitis after wearing latex gloves.

COMMON CAUSES OF CONTACT DERMATITIS	
Allergen	**Component of**
Nickel	Coins, buckles, jewellery
Formaldehyde Ethylene diamine	Preservatives, stabilizers or bases for cream and ointments
Parabens	
Wool alcohols	
Chlorocresol	
Chinoform	Topical antiseptics
Neomycin	Topical antibiotic
Paraphenylene diamine (PPD)	Hair and textile dye
Thiuram mix	Rubber additives
Mercapto-mix	
Carba-mix	
PPD mix	

2.13 **Common causes of contact dermatitis.**

of test substances depends on the history, nature of the dermatosis and knowledge of potential sensitizers (**2.13**). A standard battery of common sensitizers is available, together with extra lists, for example for patients with leg ulcers or chronic otitis externa, or for hairdressers; a range of common facial sensitizers, plant allergens or medicaments and bases of common topical therapies may be indicated. Contact dermatitis to topical steroids should be considered in patients who have used a wide range of preparations, usually over many months. Immediate contact patch tests for allergens suspected of causing urticarial reactions are occasionally helpful. The suspect allergen is applied directly to the skin and left on, unoccluded, for 30 minutes. An urticarial weal developing at the site of the allergen indicates a positive reaction. Photopatch testing involves the application of a suspected topical allergen together with ultraviolet irradiation. A range of wavelengths of ultraviolet may be used and non-irradiated control tests are included.

IGE AND RADIOALLERGOSORBENT TESTS

IgE is often but not always raised in atopic dermatitis, but does not reflect the severity of the dermatosis or response to treatment. More often a raised level reflects associated asthma. Radioallergosorbent tests (RASTs) demonstrate levels of specific IgE, indicating potential sensitizers such as animal dander, house-dust mites and a range of other potential inhaled or ingested allergens.

OTHER DIAGNOSTIC SKIN TESTS

Skin-prick tests with allergen extracts result in immediate (type I) skin reactions; in atopic dermatitis frequent false-positives occur and skin-prick tests are more useful for hayfever or asthma sufferers (*see* **p. 151**).

Tuberculin tests (*see* **p. 34**) require intradermal antigen injection, with readings at appropriate intervals.

FURTHER INVESTIGATIONS

Haematological and biochemical tests are frequently used in primary skin disorders and the dermatological manifestations of systemic disease, and for monitoring drug therapy, for example methotrexate, retinoids, dapsone or cyclosporin. Immunological investigations, including antinuclear antibody, immune complexes, complement levels and autoantibodies, may be required. Underlying medical or surgical problems should be investigated appropriately.

PSORIASIS

Psoriasis is a common disorder affecting about 2% of the population. The onset may be at any age, with peaks around 20 and 60 years. Men and women are affected equally. A positive family history is found in 30% of patients; in those developing the disease at an earlier age there is an increased association

with HLA CW6. The disease is characterized histologically by abnormal keratinocyte differentiation and hyperproliferation with inflammation, involving both lymphocytes and polymorphonuclear leucocytes and an associated vasodilatation of superficial dermal vessels. Investigations into the inherited basis of this disorder are complicated by genetic heterogeneity and to date no gene has been characterized. Environmental factors such as infection are also important.

Clinically, psoriasis is characterized by variability and unpredictability. The rash may be intermittent, undergo spontaneous remission or be lifelong. In general a chronic condition, it may flare acutely and, rarely, be life-threatening. Patients generally feel well but they can experience considerable emotional distress and social isolation. There is an association between the severity of psoriasis and alcohol intake.

The most common presentation is **chronic plaque psoriasis**, generally affecting extensor surfaces in a symmetrical pattern (**2.14**, **2.15**, **3.52**). Lesions are clearly demarcated erythematous plaques covered with coarse scales that may be removed by gentle scraping (**2.16**). Involvement of flexures, especially inframammary or groin areas (**2.17**), is also common. In these sites the rash is not usually scaly and is often confused with fungal or yeast infections. The scalp may be involved alone or with other lesions; psoriasis in the scalp may be both 'felt' and seen. The hairline (**2.18**) and behind the ears are common sites.

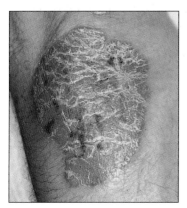

2.14 Psoriasis affecting the extensor surfaces of the arms. Other plaques are visible on the trunk.

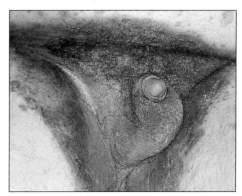

2.16 Psoriasis. Typical small plaques, showing typical silvery scales. These can be removed by gentle scraping with a spatula or fingernail.

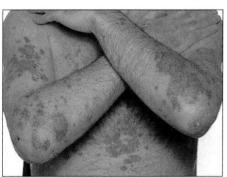

2.15 Psoriasis on the extensor surface of the elbow.

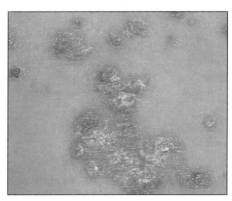

2.17 Psoriasis caused severe pruritus in this man. The discoloration of the lesions results largely from tar therapy.

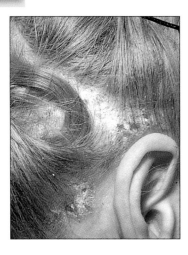

2.18 Psoriasis of the scalp and hair margin. The patchy nature of scalp involvement helps to distinguish psoriasis from other conditions, such as dandruff and seborrhoeic dermatitis.

A resistant plaque in the sacral area is also very common. Involvement of nails include coarse 'pitting', as on a thimble (**3.5**), onycholysis (**2.19**) or gross thickening of the nail with underlying hyperkeratosis.

Guttate psoriasis is an abrupt onset of psoriasis with droplet shaped erythematous scaly lesions scattered widely over trunk and limbs with no predilection for extensor surfaces (**2.20**). It may be triggered by a preceding streptococcal throat infection, and is more common in children and young adults. It usually clears completely but classic psoriasis may appear in later life.

Erythrodermic psoriasis (**2.21**) can be a life-threatening condition. The rash starts as common psoriasis but spreads to become confluent and often indistinguishable from other forms of erythroderma.

Arthropathy occurs in 10–15% of psoriatic patients. Classically, distal interphalangeal joints (**3.53**) and large joints such as ankles and knees are involved and the rheumatoid factor is negative. Rarely, the arthritis can be severe, producing 'arthritis mutilans' of the hands and feet with resultant severe disability (**3.54**, **3.55**).

Localized chronic **pustular psoriasis** may occur without other evidence of psoriasis (**2.22**, **3.56**). Generalized pustular psoriasis is a rare presentation that may be fatal. It may be precipitated by topical or systemic steroid use, drug reactions or infections. Crops of sterile pustules occur, with fever and systemic upset.

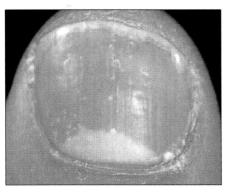

2.19 Psoriasis affecting the nail, causing pitting, onycholysis, discoloration and thickening.

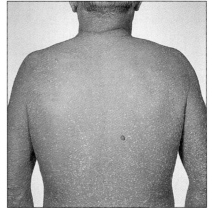

2.21 Erythrodermic psoriasis is potentially life-threatening, and it closely resembles other forms of erythroderma in which the whole skin surface is involved. The management of patients with severe erythroderma is as urgent as that of a patient with severe burns.

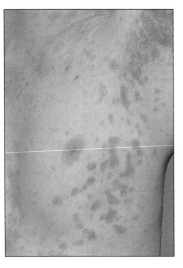

2.20 Guttate psoriasis in a 17-year-old. The condition resolved completely within a few months.

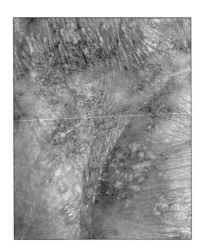

2.22 Pustular psoriasis of the palms. The palms and soles are the most common areas for this localized form of psoriasis. The pus is usually sterile, and the hands are not tender or oedematous.

The treatment of psoriasis depends upon its location and severity but may involve topical emollients, dithranol, tar or steroids. Ultraviolet B radiation alone, and ultraviolet A radiation combined with an oral psoralens (PUVA) are often effective for widespread disease, but systemic treatment with retinoids, methotrexate, cyclosporin A or other drugs may be necessary for stubborn disease.

DERMATITIS

'Dermatitis' and 'eczema' are synonyms; in practice, the term 'eczema' is usually restricted to dermatitis seen in atopic individuals. 'Dermatitis' means inflammation in the skin. It may be acute with weeping, crusting and vesicle formation, subacute, or chronic with dryness, scaling and fissuring and lichenification (especially in atopic individuals; **2.23**). The skin eruption is almost always itchy and secondary infection is common. Dermatitis may be exogenous (contact, irritant, infective or photodermatitis) or endogenous (e.g. atopic, seborrhoeic, discoid). Most often the diagnosis can be established by the distribution pattern and morphology of the skin eruption together with a detailed history.

Atopic dermatitis begins in childhood, between 2 and 6 months of age, affecting about 2% of the population, although the prevalence does appear to be increasing. A family history of atopy is present in 70% of cases. Hayfever and/or asthma may develop as the child gets older. Over 90% of children are free from dermatitis by the age of 12 years, but predicting this for an individual child is difficult. Few patients with the classic features are seen beyond the age of 30 years. In infants the face, neck and trunk are involved (**2.24**), with sparing of the napkin

area. Flexural involvement appears later, behind knees, elbows, wrists and ankles (**2.25**) and lichenification may result from repeated scratching (**2.23**, **2.91**). Hand dermatitis is common in later years. Secondary infection is common (**2.26**) and staphylococcal infection is often responsible for exacerbations of dermatitis. Itch can be severe and causes much distress to patients and families. Food allergy, especially to eggs, fish and dairy products, may be relevant in some patients, especially infants and young children.

A number of abnormalities may be detected in the skin in atopic dermatitis, but the underlying mechanisms are still unclear. Immunological abnormalities include a tendency to increased IgE levels, a predisposition to anaphylactic reactions, increased reactivity to skin-prick tests and a reduction in local

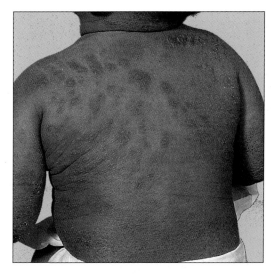

2.24 Infantile eczema in a dark-skinned child, affecting the face, neck and trunk. In a Caucasian child, the lesions are red rather than violaceous in colour.

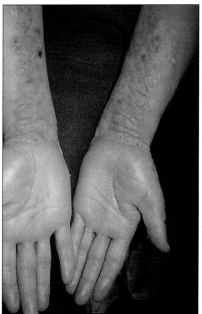

2.23 Lichenified eczema results from repeated scratching of lesions in eczematous patients.

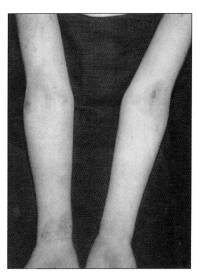

2.25 Flexural atopic dermatitis. This girl shows the typical childhood distribution. As the lesions are itchy, they are usually scratched repeatedly and become excoriated. In the long term, lichenification results (*see* **2.23**). Even non-flexural skin is dry and may be itchy.

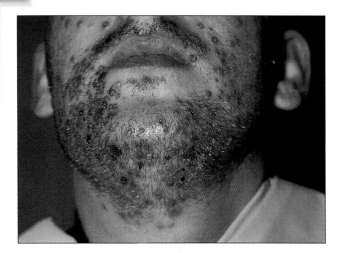

2.26 **Secondary infection in eczema.** Patients with atopic dermatitis have defective cell-mediated immunity, and are more susceptible to bacterial, viral and fungal infections. This man has a herpes simplex infection (eczema herpeticum), which has prevented him from shaving (*see* **p. 18**).

cell-mediated immunity; the latter leads to an increased tendency to viral infections such as molluscum contagiosum, viral warts and herpes simplex, and a reduced incidence of contact dermatitis. Changes in essential fatty acid metabolism have been described and some patients benefit from gammalinoleic acid supplements in the diet. Minor degrees of ichthyosis and keratosis pilaris are commonly seen; the skin is generally dry, with increased transepidermal water loss and a reduced resistance to irritant substances.

Neurodermatitis or lichen simplex is a localized chronic dermatitis, perpetuated by the itch–scratch cycle. Common sites are the nape of neck or lower leg (**2.27**). The pruritus is

often disproportionate to the rash and lichenification is common. The initial cause of the rash is often not established and the condition can be difficult to treat. There may be clinical overlap between this condition and chronic nodular prurigo, which is characterized by multiple small irritable patches widely scattered over the body (**2.28**).

Discoid dermatitis is characterized by discrete circular or oval patches of dermatitis in a symmetrical pattern often on extensor surfaces, almost always in adults. Exogenous causes should be excluded but often no cause is found (**2.29**).

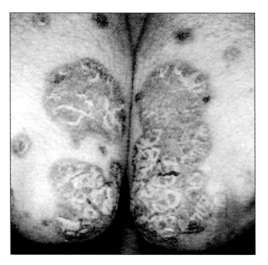

2.28 **Chronic nodular prurigo.** This condition usually affects middle-aged and elderly women who present with pruritic nodules on the legs and arms. A few cases may have an underlying iron deficiency, but the majority are a form of neurodermatitis.

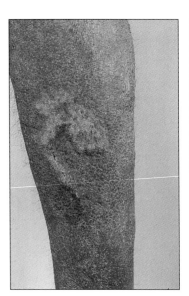

2.27 **Neurodermatitis,** or lichen simplex chronicus, usually presents with a single, flexed, lichenified plaque, which is perpetuated by repeated rubbing or scratching, either as a habit or as a response to stress. In this Asian patient, the end result was post-inflammatory hypopigmentation.

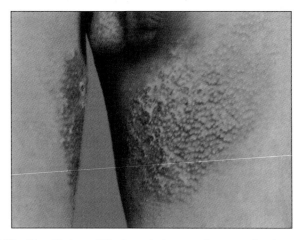

2.29 **Discoid dermatitis.** Round plaques of eczema develop, usually on the extensor surfaces of the limbs. The condition often occurs in patients who have no previous history of atopic dermatitis. The lesions are subacute, with erythema, mild oedema and some vesiculation.

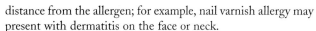

Pompholyx is a variant of eczema in which recurrent vesicles or bullae affect the palms (**2.30**) and fingers, or soles, or both. It is characterized by remissions and relapses, which are sometimes provoked by heat, emotional stress, or an active fungal infection of the feet. There have been reports that the ingestion of small amounts of nickel in susceptible patients may trigger an attack.

Contact dermatitis is an allergy (type IV, delayed hypersensitivity) to a substance present on the skin surface. The relevant factor may be immediately obvious – for example nickel, perfume, shoe rubber or plants (**2.31–2.33**). A wide range of potential allergens exists in domestic and industrial life; a careful history and relevant patch tests should establish the diagnosis. The rash can be chronic, patchy and some

distance from the allergen; for example, nail varnish allergy may present with dermatitis on the face or neck.

Stasis dermatitis is associated with venous insufficiency. It is often complicated by oedema, infection, ulceration and contact dermatitis to topical medicaments or bandages (**2.34**). A secondary, widespread symmetrical dermatitis may develop.

Seborrhoeic dermatitis occurs in infancy as cradle cap, with scattered erythematous patches on the head and neck and an associated napkin rash. In adults, scaling in the scalp, blepharitis, red scaly patches in nasolabial folds (**2.35**), around the ears and on the presternal area are characteristic; intertrigo may occur. It occurs in 3–5% of young adults; extensive seborrhoeic dermatitis may occur in early HIV infection. The yeast *Pityrosporum ovale* is increased in the scaly epidermis in this condition and is now implicated in its pathogenesis.

In **irritant dermatitis** the rash is caused by physical or chemical irritation and damage of the skin; allergy is not usually implicated. Soaps, detergents, foods and building materials can

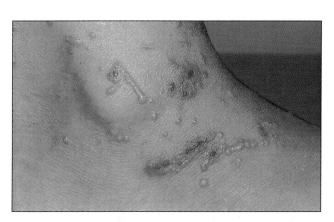

2.30 Pompholyx, or pustular eczema, of the hand. This form of atopic eczema may be provoked by external factors, including a fungal infection elsewhere on the skin (an 'id reaction') or possibly the ingestion of small amounts of nickel by a patient with contact sensitivity to the metal. Secondary infection of the vesicles is common, and both topical corticosteroid and systemic antibiotic treatment are often required.

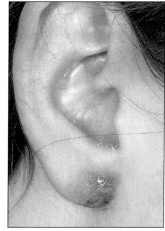

2.32 Contact dermatitis to nickel affects 10% of European women. Nickel is a common component of jewellery such as rings, necklaces and earrings and of fasteners in clothing. Nickel in earrings gave rise to earlobe eczema in this young woman.

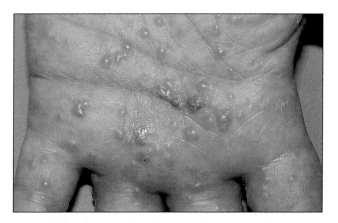

2.31 Contact dermatitis to poison ivy is a common problem in North America. This 15-year-old boy presented with linear eczematous lesions on his ankle.

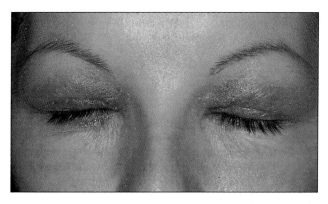

2.33 Contact blepharitis. Characterized by redness and swelling of the eyelid margins, this can result from contact dermatitis caused by eye make-up, as in this 22-year-old woman.

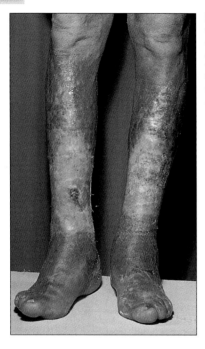

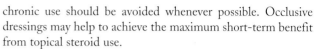

2.34 **Stasis eczema** is commonly seen in elderly women, in association with venous insufficiency or frank ulceration. Often, as here, there is also marked pigmentation as a result of haemosiderin deposition.

chronic use should be avoided whenever possible. Occlusive dressings may help to achieve the maximum short-term benefit from topical steroid use.

In the long term, patients with dermatitis of any cause should avoid soap and use lubricants liberally. Other therapy, as outlined in **2.37**, is indicated in selected patients.

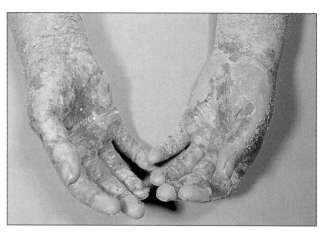

2.36 **Irritant dermatitis** on the hands of a 39-year-old man. It resulted from exposure to irritant chemicals at work.

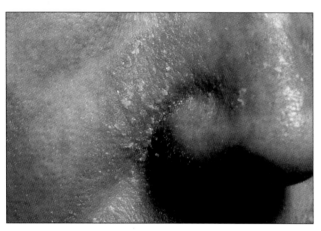

2.35 **Florid seborrhoeic dermatitis** in close-up, showing typical red, scaly lesions. This patient was HIV positive (*see* **p. 5**); however, although this is a common problem in HIV-infected patients, most patients with seborrhoeic dermatitis do not have HIV infection.

all produce this pattern. Hand dermatitis is the most common form (**2.36**). Asteatotic dermatitis is common in elderly and hospitalized patients.

The principles of management in dermatitis are similar, whether the diagnosis is atopic eczema or contact dermatitis (**2.37**). Allergen or irritant avoidance is particularly important in contact dermatitis and if there is hand involvement.

Most eczema responds best to topical corticosteroids, but it is important to avoid the local (**2.38**, **2.91**) and systemic side-effects associated with excessive steroid use. In general, topical steroids should be used intensively for short periods, and

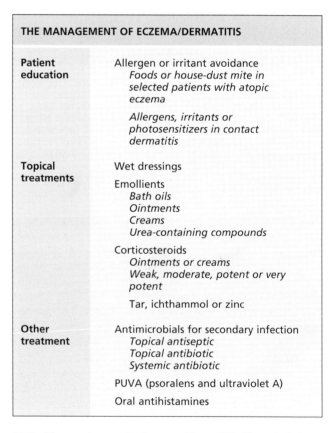

THE MANAGEMENT OF ECZEMA/DERMATITIS

Patient education	Allergen or irritant avoidance *Foods or house-dust mite in selected patients with atopic eczema*
	Allergens, irritants or photosensitizers in contact dermatitis
Topical treatments	Wet dressings
	Emollients *Bath oils Ointments Creams Urea-containing compounds*
	Corticosteroids *Ointments or creams Weak, moderate, potent or very potent*
	Tar, ichthammol or zinc
Other treatment	Antimicrobials for secondary infection *Topical antiseptic Topical antibiotic Systemic antibiotic*
	PUVA (psoralens and ultraviolet A)
	Oral antihistamines

2.37 **The management of eczema/dermatitis.** The principles of management are similar, whatever the cause.

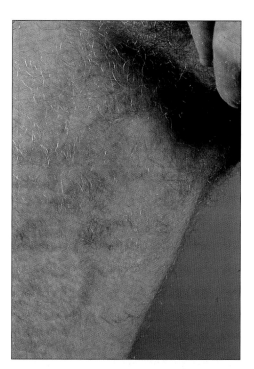

2.38 Topical corticosteroid-induced striae on the thigh of a patient with atopic eczema. These were caused by overuse of potent steroid therapy. It is essential to avoid the inappropriate and/or excessive use of topical steroids in such treatment for all dermatological conditions. Additional complications of excessive steroid therapy include other skin changes as seen in Cushing's syndrome (**7.23–7.25**), delayed healing of wounds, masking of fungal and bacterial infections, and exacerbation of pustular acne.

URTICARIA

Urticaria is common and usually patients present with acute, transient but recurrent, pruritic, erythematous swellings, resulting from localized oedema within the skin. Each weal usually lasts a few minutes to hours and clears leaving no residual marks. The number of lesions varies from one or two to a widespread rash (**2.39**). Patients may exhibit dermographism (which also occurs in 10% of the normal population; **2.40**). The itch of urticaria can be severe. Rarely, urticaria is associated with angioedema of the face or lips and in a more life-threatening pattern with swelling of the tongue and respiratory tract (**2.41**, **2.42**) and an anaphylactic reaction (*see* **p. 168**). Similar reactions can occur in other organs including the gastrointestinal tract or the joints.

The aetiology of urticaria is either obvious – as when associated with specific foods, for example strawberries or seafood – or, more commonly, unknown. Both immunological and non-immunological factors may be involved, and many distinct types of urticaria have been described (**2.43**).

Most patients require treatment with antihistamines and the eruption generally settles quickly. In some cases it can

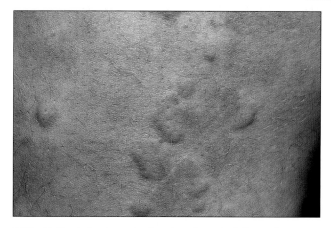

2.39 Urticaria in close-up, showing characteristic weals, surrounded by an erythematous flare.

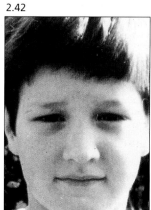

2.40 Dermographism is a skin reaction pattern in which the patient responds to anything more than a very light touch with a weal and flare reaction. This can be simply tested with firm finger pressure, as shown in this patient from a well-known London teaching hospital.

2.41 2.42

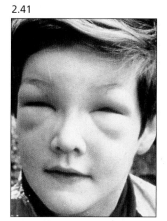

2.41 & 2.42 Severe angioedema in a 9-year-old boy after a bee sting. The patient required immediate treatment with adrenalin (epinephrine) to overcome a generalized anaphylactic response, and showed gross facial swelling. **2.42** shows the same patient without angioedema.

CLASSIFICATION OF URTICARIA

Type	Aetiology
IgE-dependent	Atopic
	Specific antigen sensitivity, e.g. food, intestinal worms, penicillins
Physical	Dermographism, pressure, heat, cold, water, sunlight, cholingeric
Complement-mediated	Hereditary angioedema, e.g. C_1-esterase inhibitor deficiency
	Acquired, e.g. lymphoma
	Autoimmune
Substances which directly stimulate mast cell degranulation	Drugs, e.g. opiates, quinine, chlortetracycline, aspirin
	Chemicals, e.g. dextran, azo-dyes, benzoates
	Food, e.g. egg white, strawberries and shellfish
Histamine-containing foods	For example, some cheeses, mackerel and tuna fish
Contact urticaria	IgE-mediated, pharmacological, idiopathic
Idiopathic	Unknown

2.43 Classification of urticaria.

become chronic, recurring for many months or years. Food diaries can be kept and exclusion diets may help in some cases. Some patients respond to the avoidance of aspirin and foods containing high amounts of azo dyes such as tartrazine, which can potentiate urticaria (*see* **p. 371**). Urticarial lesions that persist for some days and leave bruising marks in the skin are suggestive of underlying vasculitis and need to be investigated more thoroughly.

REACTIVE ERYTHEMAS

Reactive erythema without urticaria may occur in response to many known or unknown stimuli and may take a number of different forms.

Erythema nodosum is primarily an inflammation of the subcutaneous fat (panniculitis), with involvement of the adjacent vasculature. It is an immunological reaction provoked by various infections, drugs and a variety of other causes (**2.44**).

The characteristic lesions are tender red nodules occurring on the lower legs and sometimes the forearms (**2.45**). Some patients also have painful joints and fever. The lesions resolve in 6–8 weeks, often leaving a bruise-like appearance. Management depends on the identification and elimination of the underlying cause.

SOME CAUSES OF ERYTHEMA NODOSUM

Infections

Bacterial (e.g. streptococcal, tuberculosis, brucellosis, leprosy)

Mycoplasma

Rickettsia

Chlamydia

Viral

Fungal (e.g coccidioidomycosis, histoplasmosis)

Drugs

e.g. sulphonamides, contraceptive pill

Systemic disease

e.g. sarcoidosis, inflammatory bowel disease, Behçet's disease

2.44   Some causes of erythema nodosum.

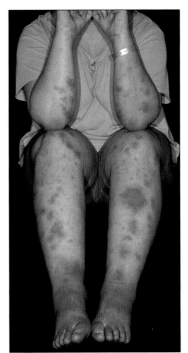

2.45   Erythema nodosum occurring in a classic distribution over the front of the legs and forearms. The appearance reflects the patchy inflammation of subcutaneous fat and small vessels, probably as the result of a type III (immune complex) allergic mechanism. Erythema nodosum has many causes (**2.44**), of which the most common in the developed world is now drug therapy – especially with sulphonamides. This patient also had arthralgia and a mild fever, and further investigation revealed an underlying diagnosis of sarcoidosis.

Erythema multiforme is also immunologically mediated. It usually follows an infection or drug therapy, but other factors have occasionally been implicated, and no cause is apparent in up to 50% of cases (**2.46**). The eruption typically takes the form of annular plaques over the palms, soles, limbs and sometimes over the trunk (**2.47**). Characteristic 'target' lesions made up of two concentric plaques may blister in the centre (**2.48**). When combined with mucous membrane involvement, erythema

SOME CAUSES OF ERYTHEMA MULTIFORME

Viral infection, e.g. herpes simplex, hepatitis, orf

Mycoplasma infection

Bacterial infections

Fungal infections, e.g. coccidioidomycosis

Parasitic infections

Drugs

Pregnancy

Malignancy and its treatment with radiotherapy

Idiopathic (50%)

2.46 Some causes of erythema multiforme.

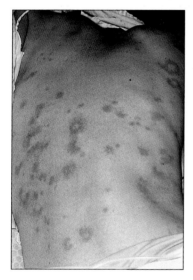

2.47 Erythema multiforme is a form of reactive erythema that probably involves both type III and type IV immunological mechanisms. Typically, it starts with a symmetrical eruption of target-like lesions on the hands and feet. These may blister centrally and they spread proximally, the extent depending on the severity of involvement. The cause of the lesions in this patient was unknown, but they were preceded by a pyrexial illness and antibiotic treatment.

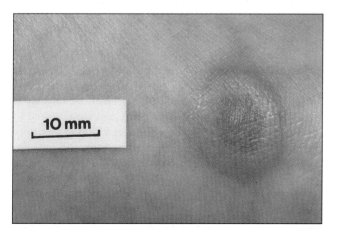

2.48 Erythema multiforme. A close-up view of a typical lesion on the palm. The centre of the target is beginning to blister.

multiforme is called the **Stevens–Johnson syndrome** (**2.49**). Lesions in the tracheobronchial tree in such patients may lead to asphyxia, and conjunctival and corneal involvement may result in blindness. Genital ulcers may cause urinary retention and phimosis or vaginal stricture after they have healed. Severe Stevens–Johnson syndrome may progress to become indistinguishable from toxic epidermal necrolysis, a condition that may also be provoked directly by staphylococcal infection or drug therapy (**1.79, 2.149**).

Erythema chronicum migrans is another form of reactive erythema, which may be associated with Lyme disease (**1.122**) or rheumatic fever (**5.89**).

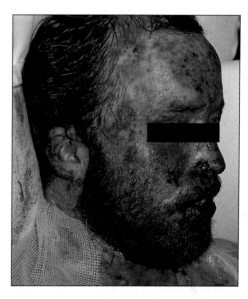

2.49 Stevens–Johnson syndrome, in its severe form, is a widespread erythema multiforme with oral, genital and conjunctival involvement, and widespread skin lesions, as on this patient's face. This form of the disease is most common in patients with *Mycoplasma pneumoniae* infection.

INFECTIONS AND INFESTATIONS

BACTERIAL INFECTIONS

Surface commensals include diphtheroids and micrococci – mainly *Staphylococcus epidermidis*. A minority of people carry *Staphylococcus aureus* in the nose, perineum or axillae (**2.4**). Damaged epidermis predisposes to secondary infection.

Staphylococcccal infections include impetigo (**1.89**), which is highly contagious (impetigo can also be caused by *Streptococcus pyogenes*). Furuncules (**2.50**) are boils that may occur singly or in crops; multiple or large lesions suggest underlying diabetes mellitus (**1.77**). Staphylococci may cause toxic epidermal necrolysis in children (**1.79**).

Erysipelas (**1.85**) is a **streptococcal infection** usually associated with systemic upset. Recurrent attacks may occur,

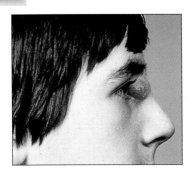

2.50 A boil (furuncle) is caused by a staphylococcal infection of a hair follicle with the accumulation of pus. This results in severe pain, and is usually followed by the spontaneous discharge of yellow pus. A boil in this location carries the risk of septicaemia and cavernous sinus thrombosis (*see* **p. 480**).

leading to chronic lymphoedema. Necrotizing fasciitis, a rapidly progressive often fatal condition, may also be due to a group A β-haemolytic streptococcal infection.

Syphilis should be remembered as a cause of skin eruptions (*see* **p. 61**). The primary chancre is typically a painless ulcer. Secondary syphilis must be distinguished from pityriasis rosea, measles, drug eruptions, guttate psoriasis and lichen planus. Tertiary syphilis (**1.191**) resembles granulomatous conditions such as sarcoid.

Patients with **tuberculosis** (*see* **p. 32**) may present with lupus vulgaris, a chronic nodular scarring rash (**2.51**). Warty

resolution occurs (30% in 6 months) but painful or multiple lesions may need treatment (**2.52**, **2.53**, **8.11**, *see also* **p. 59**).

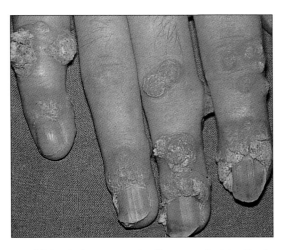

2.52 Multiple viral warts on the fingers. A florid collection of warts like this should raise the suspicion of a possible underlying impairment in cell-mediated immunity.

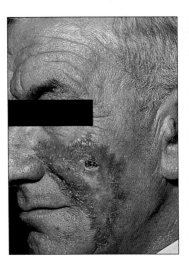

2.51 Lupus vulgaris on the cheek. This is a rare presentation of tuberculosis in the developed world, but it still occurs in developing countries and in immunosuppressed patients. The slowly extending lesion is hyperpigmented at its margin, and depigmented in the healing central zone. Ulceration has also occurred. This patient is generally pigmented as a result of Addison's disease, after tuberculous infection of the adrenals (*see* **p. 302**).

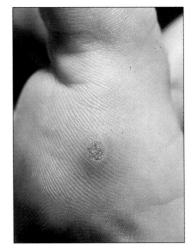

2.53 A plantar viral wart, popularly known as a 'verruca'. Single and multiple plantar warts are common, especially in schoolchildren who may acquire them from swimming-bath floors. They are characteristically flat with a callus on the surface, but may extend subcutaneously. They are often painful, and should be treated to relieve symptoms and prevent transmission to others.

tuberculosis or scrofuloderma occur less commonly. Erythema nodosum (**2.45**) or induratum may be associated with tuberculosis.

Skin lesions in **leprosy** reflect the patient's immune response (*see* **p. 35**)

VIRAL INFECTIONS

Viral warts are caused by the human papilloma virus (more than 50 subtypes exist). Warts are common; their morphology varies with anatomical site and viral subtype. Spontaneous

Herpes simplex types I and II cause primary (sometimes asymptomatic) and recurrent infections on extragenital and genital sites. Recurrent lesions are preceeded by tingling or pain, usually appear in the same place, and are triggered by various factors such as infection or sun exposure. Grouped vesicles on an erythematous base persist for a few days (*see* **p. 18**). Secondary bacterial infection may occur. Infection may complicate atopic dermatitis (Kaposi's varicelliform eruption).

Herpes zoster (shingles) is caused by the varicella zoster virus, reactivated in a sensory nerve root (where it persists after chicken pox). Pain in the affected dermatome precedes the rash of scattered blisters and erythema (*see* **p. 20**). Haemorrhagic lesions and scattered lesions elsewhere on the body suggest underlying neoplasia or immunosuppression. Corneal ulcers and scarring may follow involvement of the ophthalmic branch of the trigeminal nerve. Postherpetic pain is common (*see also* **p. 20**).

Molluscum contagiosum is caused by a pox virus. The umbilicated pearly lesions (**2.54**), often multiple, are more common in childhood and resolve spontaneously after becoming inflamed. Residual marks may persist for some months.

Pityriasis rosea occurs in children and young adults (a viral aetiology is suspected but unproven). A herald patch (**2.55**) precedes subsequent lesions, which tend to be distributed along the rib lines (**2.56**). The lesions are usually asymptomatic but may be itchy. They persist for 4–6 weeks.

FUNGAL AND YEAST INFECTIONS

Dermatophyte fungi (genera *Trichophyton*, *Microsporum* and *Epidermophyton*) live on keratin and evoke a variable amount of inflammation. Clinical lesions are termed tinea or ringworm. Presentation depends on body site, but it is usually as plaques of scaling erythema, with variable itch (**1.2**, **2.5**, **2.6**, **2.7**, **2.57**, **2.58**). Nail involvement causes onycholysis and

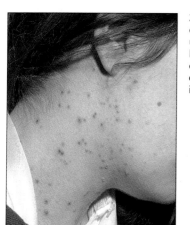

2.54 Molluscum contagiosum. Note the umbilicated, pearly lesions. The condition occurs most commonly in childhood and is also seen in adults.

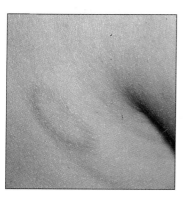

2.55 The herald patch in pityriasis rosea commonly precedes the later multiple lesions by several days. It is usually oval, and has a surrounding collar of fine white scales.

2.56 Pityriasis rosea. The herald patch can still be seen, but there is now a widespread itchy skin eruption, largely following the lines of the ribs.

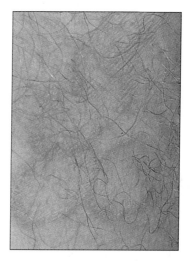

2.57 Tinea corporis. These annular lesions ('ringworm') are on the thigh. Note the scaly margins, which can be scraped and examined for fungal hyphae and spores (**2.7**).

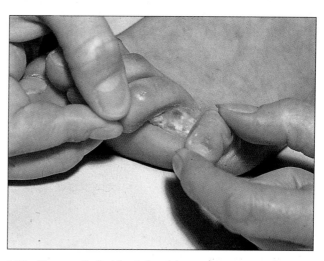

2.58 Tinea pedis ('athlete's foot') is a very common infection between the fourth and fifth toes, especially in those who wear tight or poorly ventilated footwear.

dystrophy (**2.59**) and scalp infection patchy hair loss (**2.60**, *see also* **p. 89**).

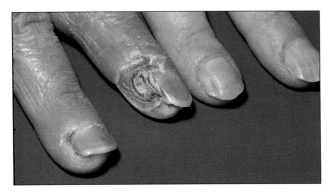

2.59 Chronic dermatophyte infection of the nails and the surrounding soft tissue of the index fingers of the right hand. For comparison, the corresponding fingers of the left hand are shown. The patient was a heavy smoker, and tar staining is evident in the right hand fingers. Finger clubbing is obvious in the fingers of the left hand. This was associated with carcinoma of the bronchus.

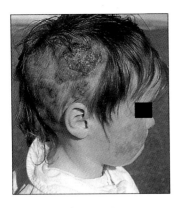

2.60   Fungal infection of the scalp, which has resulted in severe pustular inflammation (kerion) and hair loss in an infant from a deprived background.

Candida infections caused by *Candida albicans* yeast commonly occur in moist, flexural sites (**2.61**). Predisposing factors include diabetes mellitus, pregnancy, broad-spectrum antibiotics and obesity (*see also* **p. 46**). Chronic candida

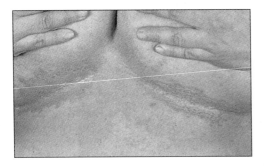

2.61   Candidiasis of the skin (intertriginous candidiasis) below both breasts in an obese diabetic.

paronychia may be complicated by additional bacterial infection; wet work or poor circulation are predisposing factors. Chronic mucocutaneous candidiasis is associated with widespread candida infection of the skin, mucous membranes and nails (**2.62**).

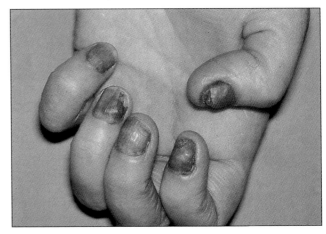

2.62   Nail changes in a patient with chronic mucocutaneous candidiasis. There is onycholysis, a yellow-brownish pigmentation, with pitting and ridging, and the nails are soft, friable and easily split. Chronic mucocutaneous candidiasis normally begins in childhood, is associated with a defect in cell-mediated immunity and may be associated with autoimmune endocrine disorders including hypoadrenalism, hypothyroidism or diabetes mellitus. In adults the condition may occur in the presence of a thymoma. Lengthy, intensive treatment is required to eliminate this fungal nail infection.

Pityriasis versicolor is caused by yeasts (*Pityrosporum orbiculare*) producing widespread scaly lesions on the upper trunk and back (**2.63**), pale in dark skins and darker in fair skins. Recurrent attacks are common.

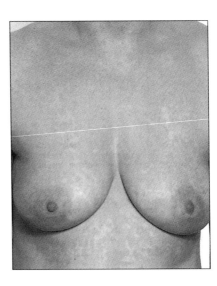

2.63   Pityriasis versicolor. Typical lesions in a 28-year-old woman.

INFESTATIONS

Infestations result from invasion of the body by arthropods, including insects, mites and ticks. Only a few are discussed here.

Insect bites are reactions to injected antigens, causing weals, persisting papules and sometimes blisters (**2.64**). Lesions may occur in recurrent crops (papular urticaria), and are often secondarily infected.

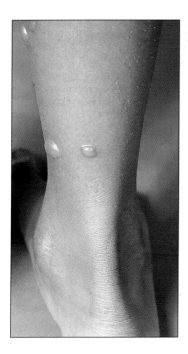

2.64 Insect bites producing a bullous reaction in an 8-year-old child.

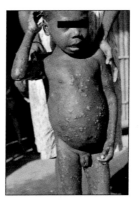

2.66 Scabies with secondary infected eczema in a boy from Papua.

Lice infestations are caused by *Pediculus humanus* (var. *capitis* and *corporis*) and *Pthirus pubis*. The lice suck blood, causing pruritus, scratching and secondary infection. Their eggs, known as nits, are attached to hairs (or clothing with body lice; **2.67**). Head lice occur irrespective of cleanliness, whereas body lice are mainly found on vagrants and those who wash themselves or their clothes only rarely. Pubic lice are commonly sexually transmitted.

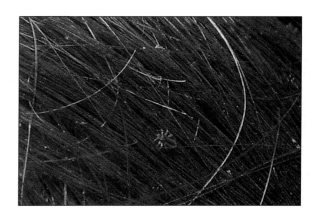

2.67 Head louse infestation (pediculosis capitis). This close-up picture shows a single louse clearly enough to count its six legs, and a number of egg capsules (nits) attached to the hairs.

Scabies is caused by the mite *Sarcoptes scabiei* var. *hominis* (**2.8**). Transmission occurs through close body contact. The adult mite lays eggs in burrows in the skin (**2.65**). Sensitization to the mites results in a widespread secondary eczema (**2.66**) and severe pruritus, worse at night. Household contacts must be treated to prevent recurrences.

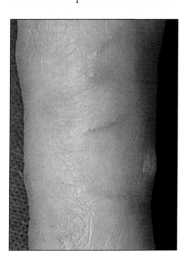

2.65 Scabies. Typical burrows on the finger.

LICHEN PLANUS

Lichen planus accounts for only 1–2% of new referrals to the dermatology clinic. It affects both sexes equally and usually occurs in those aged 30–60 years.

The classic presentation is easy to diagnose with 'purple, pruritic, polygonal papules'. These commonly occur on the wrists, low back, ankles (where they may be chronic and hypertrophic) and feet (**2.68**) but lesions may be widespread. If severe, lesions may blister. The Koebner phenomenon may be seen (**2.69**).

Mucosal lesions are common and may present before or without those on other affected sites. Mouth lesions are

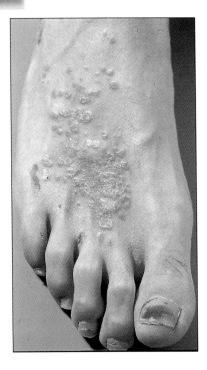

2.68 **Lichen planus.** The polygonal papules on the dorsum of the foot are typical of the chronic form of the disorder, and the lesions are commonly itchy. Dystrophic nail changes are common in lichen planus.

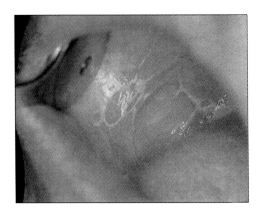

2.70 **Oral lesions are relatively common in lichen planus.** The classic appearance is of white reticulations on the buccal mucosa, as here, but the disease may also take an erosive form and similar lesions may occur on the tongue. Biopsy is usually advisable to confirm the diagnosis.

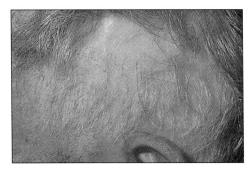

2.71 **Lichen planus in the scalp** of a 68-year-old man. There is depigmentation and scarring caused by biopsy-proven lichen planus that was active for over 30 years.

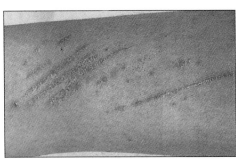

2.69 **Koebner's phenomenon in lichen planus.** Typical lesions may occur in a scratch when the disease is active, as here along the lines of bramble scratches.

diagnostic, with lacy white striae on the buccal mucosa (**2.70**). Ulceration may occur. Genital lesions especially affect the vulva or the glans and shaft of the penis.

Hair loss may occur, sometimes with irreversible scarring alopecia (**2.71**). Nail changes include irregular coarse pits or linear streaks, or adhesions between the skin and the nail plate, causing pterygium formation.

The histology is characteristic and should confirm the diagnosis if required.

Most cases settle within 1–2 years, but the rash may recur or become chronic. Post-inflammatory hyperpigmentation may persist. Topical or systemic steroid treatment may be required in severe cases.

The aetiology is unknown. Similarities between lichen planus and the skin lesions of chronic graft-versus-host disease suggest an autoimmune aetiology. An association with primary

biliary cirrhosis and other autoimmune diseases has also been reported.

Lichenoid reactions, mimicking lichen planus, may result from therapy with drugs such as gold, chloroquine and thiazide diuretics, or after contact with colour photograph developer.

BULLOUS DISORDERS

Blisters develop when fluid collects between layers of the epidermis, or between the epidermis and dermis, as a result of inflammation (external or internal) or shearing forces. They are a feature of many conditions, for example dermatitis (**p. 71**), herpes simplex (**p. 18**) and insect bites (**p. 80**). The bullous disorders are distinguished by characteristic immunofluorescent staining either within the epidermis or at the dermoepidermal junction, in conjunction with the appropriate clinical features.

Dermatitis herpetiformis is an uncommon disorder in which groups of intensely itchy blisters appear on elbows (**2.72**), shoulders, buttocks (**2.73**) and knees. There may be an associated gluten enteropathy (*see* **p. 356**). Skin biopsy

characteristically shows subepidermal microabscesses or blisters (**2.2**) and immunofluorescence shows granular IgA deposits in dermal papillae (**2.3**). Patients with this disorder have a high prevalence of tissue types HLA B8 (85–90%) and DRw3. Although the disease is well controlled with dapsone and a gluten-free diet, treatment may need to be long term as the condition persists for many years, and there is some evidence to suggest a risk of small bowel lymphoma, as in coeliac disease.

Bullous pemphigoid is a condition predominantly affecting elderly patients in which large tense itchy blisters appear on any body site (**2.74**). The blisters may be preceded by pruritus alone or with an urticarial type rash. Skin biopsy shows subepidermal blisters and immunofluorescence shows linear IgG (occasionally IgA) and C3 at the dermoepidermal junction (**2.75**). The pemphigoid antigen is located within the hemidesmosomes but there is no evidence that the antibody is directly pathogenic; it may have a role in activating

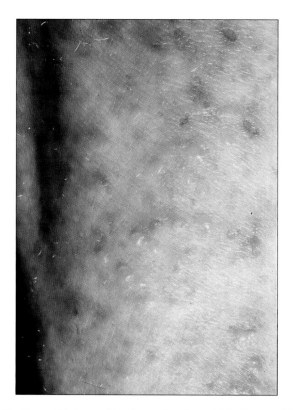

2.72   Dermatitis herpetiformis on the elbow. This 65-year-old man had a history of a recurrent eruption of vesicles and crusts on his elbows, head, neck and lower back. The lesions are intensely itchy, and the vesicles are easily ruptured by scratching.

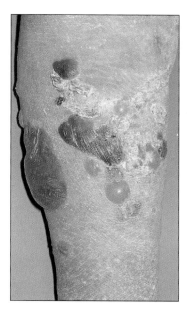

2.74   Pemphigoid. Some of the blisters have become haemorrhagic, as often occurs.

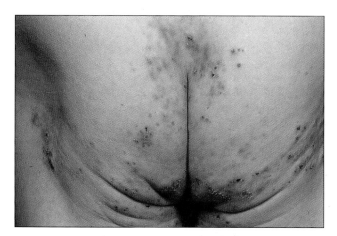

2.73   Dermatitis herpetiformis in the sacral and buttock areas. The vesicles have been ruptured by scratching, and are healing, leaving pigmented scars.

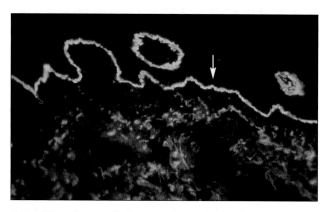

2.75   Direct immunofluorescence in pemphigoid reveals IgG deposition in the basement membrane (arrow) in perilesional skin biopsies. Granular deposition of C3 is often observed.

complement pathways that then cause local inflammation. Circulating anti-basement membrane antibodies are present in up to 75% of patients, but the titre does not reflect disease activity. Oral lesions are uncommon. The disease runs a chronic, often self-remitting course over months to years. Treatment with prednisolone and azathioprine can be helpful.

Pemphigus gestationis (formerly known as herpes gestationis) is a rare dermatosis of pregnancy resembling pemphigoid clinically and histologically (**2.76**). It remits post partum, but tends to recur with subsequent pregnancies.

Pemphigus vulgaris is a severe, chronic disorder affecting middle-aged to elderly patients. Many patients present with oral lesions before developing the skin lesions, which are predominantly erosions as the blisters are flaccid and easily ruptured (**2.77**, **2.78**). Lesions occur predominantly on the trunk, face or pressure points, but all body sites can be affected. Skin biopsy shows intraepidermal blisters and immunofluorescence shows diffuse staining between epidermal cells, with IgG and C3 (**2.79**). Circulating autoantibodies are generally present and the titre reflects disease activity. The course of this disease is prolonged, often with serious complications despite therapy. The condition can be caused by drugs, such as penicillamine, captopril and rifampicin.

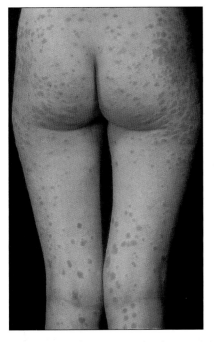

2.76 Pemphigus gestationis. This rare disorder presents with vesicles and bullae during pregnancy or the puerperium. It resembles bullous pemphigoid, but can sometimes be distinguished from it by immunofluorescence techniques. The condition tends to recur in subsequent pregnancies.

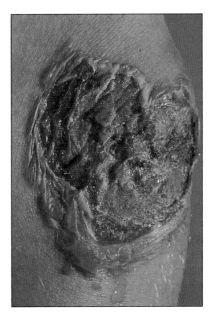

2.78 Pemphigus vulgaris blisters are thin and painful, with an intraepidermal split. They often become secondarily infected.

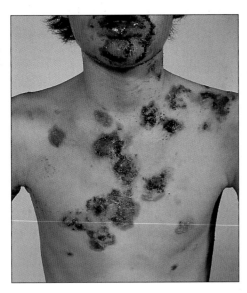

2.77 Pemphigus vulgaris in a 13-year-old boy. The blisters rupture easily, and are often associated with similar lesions on mucous membranes, especially in the mouth.

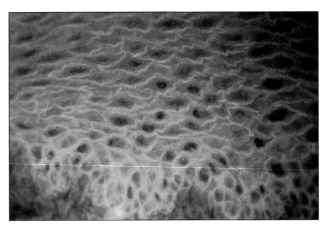

2.79 Direct immunofluorescence in pemphigus vulgaris, showing intercellular epidermal deposition of IgG. C3 and occasionally IgM may also be deposited.

Blisters are a common feature of **porphyrias** (*see* **p. 332**).

Inherited blistering diseases are an uncommon group of disorders occurring in infancy or childhood. Recent advances in molecular biological techniques have enabled the cause of many of these conditions to be determined. **Epidermolysis bullosa simplex** is a group of disorders characterized by splitting of the basal cells of the epidermis, above the dermoepidermal junction. Many of these disorders have been shown to be caused by point mutations in the cytoskeletal proteins, the keratins, in particular keratins K5 and K14, which provide resilience to the basal epidermal cells. These conditions are inherited as autosomal dominant disorders, although many cases are sporadic. In the more severe, and less common, inherited blistering diseases known as **dystrophic epidermolysis bullosa**, the blister forms at or below the dermoepidermal junction (**2.80**). These disorders are due to point mutations in either laminin V, a protein integral to the basement membrane, or collagen VII, which connects the basement membrane to the underlying dermal structures. These variants of epidermolysis bullosa may be either dominantly or recessively inherited.

levels of androgen hormones may account for hormonal influences; acne may be associated with hirsutism and obesity in the polycystic ovary syndrome (*see* **p. 308**). Duct abnormalities and obstruction at the epidermal opening of the pilosebaceous unit also have a role. The face (**2.81**), back (**2.82**) and chest are affected with a range of lesions from small papules and pustules to comedones and deeper, painful cysts, on a

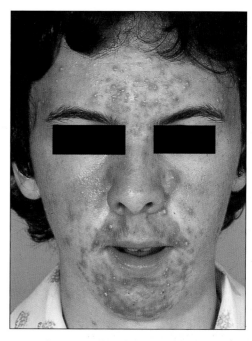

2.81   Acne vulgaris usually involves the face. This 17-year-old shows the typical features of moderately severe acne. He has many papular and pustular lesions at different stages of evolution, and the older lesions are healing with scarring.

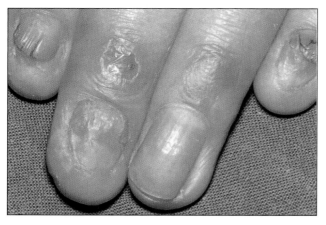

2.80   Epidermolysis bullosa (dystrophic form). From early childhood, minor trauma has caused blistering in this patient. The blisters heal with scarring, as shown here. Note also the dystrophic nail changes.

ACNE

Acne vulgaris is a very common chronic inflammatory disorder of the pilosebaceous unit. It occurs in adolescence, usually earlier in girls, and may persist for some years (infantile acne may also occur rarely). It results from a combination of factors: there is increased sebum production (this alone does not cause acne), together with infection and inflammation due to *Propionibacterium acnes* within the sebaceous glands, where breakdown of fatty acids triggers inflammation. Increased endorgan sensitivity within the sebaceous gland to normal

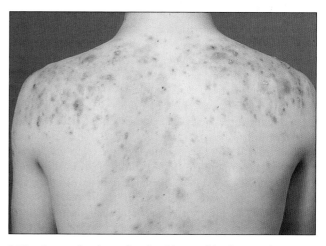

2.82   Acne vulgaris on the shoulders and back – another common site. Again, a wide range of lesions are seen, including some large pustules, and scarring is occurring on healing.

background of seborrhoea. Subsequent scars may be depressed (**2.83**) or hypertrophic, but adequate treatment should prevent scar formation.

Less commonly, drug-induced acne may follow treatment with corticosteroids, androgenic hormones, oral contraceptives or anticonvulsant drugs.

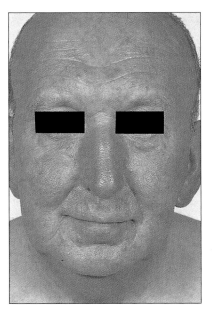

2.84 Acne rosacea. This patient shows typical papules and pustules, superimposed on a generally erythematous facial skin. His eyes were normal, but conjuctivitis and keratitis may occur.

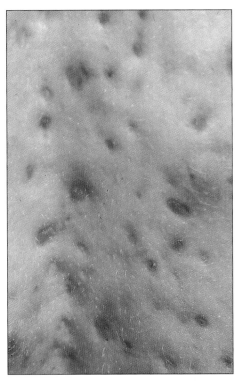

2.83 Acne scars – a close-up view. In this patient, the scars are depressed, but hypertrophic scars may also occur.

Acne rosacea occurs in an older age group than acne vulgaris and has a vascular component to it. Flushing, often precipitated by hot foods, warm environment or sunlight, occurs in association with small papules and pustules over the forehead, cheeks and chin in a symmetrical pattern (**2.84, 9.45**). Seborrhoea is not necessarily present. Despite the obvious improvement with antibiotic therapy (topical or systemic) no infective cause has been demonstrated; skin microflora are often normal and an association with the mite *Demodex folliculorum* (a skin commensal) has not been substantiated. Rosacea lymphoedema may develop and become persistent and **rhinophyma** (**2.85**) may develop. Inflammatory ocular conditions – most commonly conjuctivitis but also rosacea keratitis, a more serious complication – may occur in up to 50% of patients and may precede the skin manifestations. The rash is exacerbated by topical steroids and sometimes aggravated by sunlight. Rosacea must be distinguished from seborrhoeic dermatitis, perioral dermatitis, sarcoidosis and the facial rash of systemic lupus erythematosus.

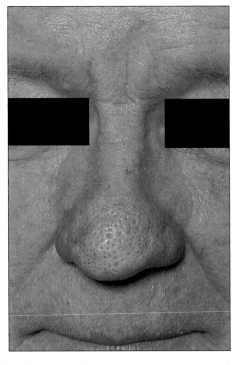

2.85 Rhinophyma usually occurs as a long-term complication of acne rosacea. The nose is characteristically red and bulbous. The 'strawberry' appearance results from hyperplasia of the sebaceous glands and connective tissue. The follicle openings become prominent.

DISORDERS OF PIGMENTATION

Most disorders of pigmentation result from excess or insufficient melanin, the dominant pigment in the skin. Other pigments include haemosiderin, bilirubin and carotene.

Congenital disorders of pigmentation include freckles, simple lentigines and café-au-lait patches in neurofibromatosis (**2.86**). Less common conditions include oculocutaneous albinism (defective melanin production that affects hair, eyes and skin, sparing pigmented naevi, **2.87**), incontinentia pigmenti (initial blisters leave whorled pigmentary lesions in adult life) and lentigines round the mouth in Peutz–Jeghers syndrome (**2.88**). Xeroderma pigmentosum patients show excessive freckling in light-exposed areas (*see* **p. 100**). Urticaria pigmentosa occurs in childhood as scattered brownish-pink macules that urticate on rubbing.

Vitiligo (**2.89**) develops in 1% of the population. The white patches show total loss of melanocytes. A personal or family history of other autoimmune disorders may be present.

Hyperpigmentation may be a sign of underlying endocrine disease, such as Addison's disease, acromegaly, Cushing's syndrome or hyperthyroidism. Patchy facial pigmentation (chloasma or melasma) is common in pregnancy or with oral contraceptives. Tumours may cause diffuse pigmentation through ectopic adrenocorticotrophic hormone (ACTH) production or localized pigment changes such as acanthosis nigricans (**2.90**).

Hyperpigmentation is seen in cirrhosis, renal failure, haemochromatosis (slate-grey colour; **9.52**) and porphyria (**7.139**).

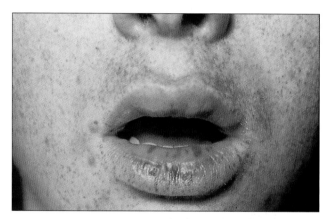

2.88 Peutz–Jeghers syndrome. Dark brown pigmentation is found particularly on the lips and around the mouth, but also on the hard and soft palate, buccal mucosa and, occasionally, on the feet and hands. There is an association with multiple intestinal polyps, some of which undergo malignant transformation.

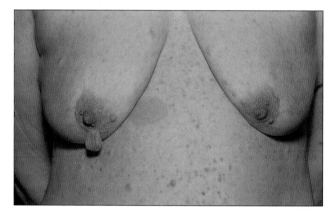

2.86 Neurofibromatosis (von Recklinghausen's disease, type I, *see* **p. 490**). Note the subcutaneous nodular tumours arising in the sheaths of peripheral nerves, the pigmented pedunculated tumours on the skin surface and the brown (café-au-lait) patches.

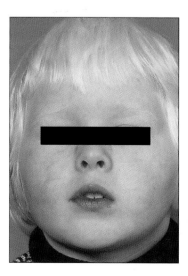

2.87 Albinism. This child has typical white skin and hair. His eyes were also affected; he had pink irises and photophobia.

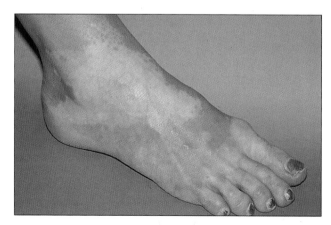

2.89 Vitiligo is often first noticed in the hands, but may be found throughout the body. It is characterized by multiple, well-demarcated areas of hypopigmentation that progressively enlarge. It is often associated with other autoimmune disorders, and – in about one-third of cases – there is a family history.

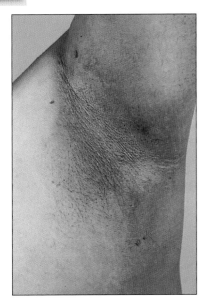

2.90 **Acanthosis nigricans** in an Asian patient. Patchy velvety brown hyperpigmentation and thickening of flexures develops. In older patients, this is often a marker of underlying malignant disease, but the condition may occur in diabetes and other endocrine disorders and as an isolated abnormality.

DISORDERS OF KERATINIZATION

Keratinization disorders result from abnormalities of epidermal maturation, with scaling and thickening of the skin, with or without inflammation. Gene defects have now been identified in several of these conditions, and study of these disorders has helped to clarify the mechanisms of differentiation in the normal epidermis and in other disorders of keratinization.

Ichthyosis vulgaris is a common (1:300) autosomal dominant condition of scaly skin that appears in early childhood (**2.92**). The scales are small and spare the flexural areas, and the condition improves with age. There is an association with keratosis pilaris. X-linked ichthyosis occurs in early infancy, with larger, darker scales and flexural involvement and persists in adult life. The gene defect is located on the X chromosome and affected individuals have a defect in the enzyme steroid sulphatase.

Other rare forms of ichthyosis also occur. These conditions result from mutations in the genes for keratins K1, K10, or K2e, proteins present in the upper layers of the epidermis.

Acquired ichthyosis is usually associated with underlying conditions such as Hodgkin's disease, other lymphomata, sarcoid or malabsorption.

Keratoderma of palms and soles may be inherited or acquired. Various patterns such as punctate, striate or diffuse thickening occur. Diffuse keratoderma (tylosis) may be familial (**2.93**) and has rarely been associated with underlying neoplasia. Some forms of keratoderma are due to mutations in keratin genes K6 and K9 (this protein is only found in palm or sole skin).

Connective tissue disorders such as systemic lupus erythematosus, dermatomyositis or morphoea may cause local or diffuse pigment changes.

Drugs causing pigmentation include antimalarials, phenothiazines, minocycline, busulfan, cyclophosphamide, bleomycin and arsenic. Psoralens, used for photochemotherapy, produce a deep tan.

Exogenous causes of pigmentation include carotene (carotenaemia) and compounds containing silver (argyria). Tattoos are a common form of exogenous pigmentation.

Post-inflammatory hypopigmentation or hyperpigmentation may result from inflammatory conditions such as lichen planus, dermatitis (**2.91**), or discoid lupus erythematosus, especially in darker-skinned people.

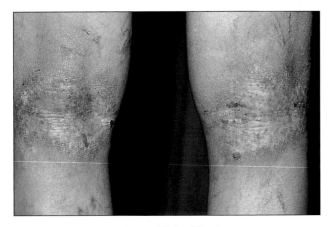

2.91 **Hyperpigmentation and lichenification** are common complications of chronic atopic dermatitis. Note the thinning of the skin around the gross lesions, which results from inappropriate use of topical corticosteroid therapy.

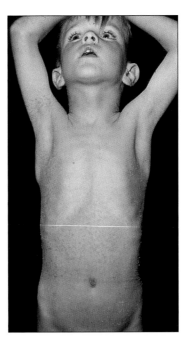

2.92 **Ichthyosis vulgaris** is a dominant condition that causes scaly skin from early childhood onwards. Its name reflects the resemblance of the skin to scaly fish skin.

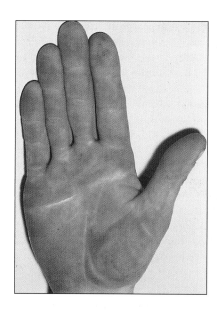

2.93 Keratoderma of the palm in a girl with familial tylosis.

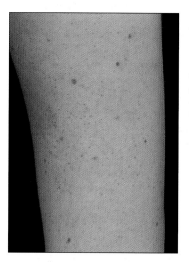

2.94 Keratosis pilaris on the outer surface of the upper arm. In this common disorder, the hair follicles are plugged with keratin, giving the skin a rough texture. The disorder is only of cosmetic importance.

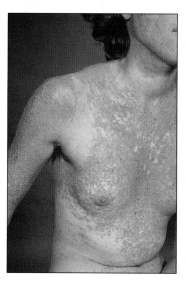

2.95 Darier's disease. In this dominant familial disorder there are large numbers of hard reddish papules, which may coalesce.

Keratosis pilaris is a common abnormality of keratinization at the hair follicle ducts that presents in childhood as roughened areas on upper outer arms and legs (**2.94**). The face and eyebrows may be affected.

Darier's disease (keratosis follicularis) is a rare autosomal dominant condition that appears in the mid-teens as small scaly reddish-brown papules on chest, back, scalp or flexures (**2.95**). Histology is diagnostic. Nail abnormalities include linear streaks and notching, and punctate lesions may be seen on hands or feet. The gene defect has been located but the candidate protein has yet to be identified.

HAIR DISORDERS

HAIR LOSS (ALOPECIA)

Hair loss can be diffuse or focal and may not be associated with any underlying inflammation or scarring. Androgenic alopecia is common in men (in whom the incidence approaches 100% in Caucasians) but also occurs in women. The pattern of hair loss includes frontal recession and thinning over the vertex, with more diffuse loss commoner in women. The extent and rate of hair loss are related to undefined genetic and hormonal factors.

Alopecia areata is a common cause of focal hair loss (**2.96**), characterized by many short exclamation mark hairs at the edges of the lesion. The underlying pathogenesis is a chronic inflammatory process triggered by a variety of environmental factors (e.g. infection) and probably represents a type of organ-specific autoimmune disease. Regrowth usually occurs within

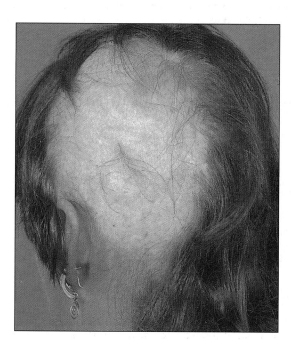

2.96 Severe alopecia areata in a 24-year-old woman. There are no features to suggest infection of the scalp.

weeks or months, but further episodes may occur. Alopecia totalis (**2.97**) and loss of all body hair (alopecia universalis) can occur, and associated fine pitting of the nails may be seen. A family history of alopecia areata occurs in up to 20% of cases and a family or personal history of atopy or other autoimmune disorders may also be present.

Fungal infection of the scalp causes patchy hair loss. If significantly inflamed, the lesion is called a kerion (**2.60**). Regrowth is usually good but permanent scarring may result from extensive inflammation.

Traction alopecia results from repeated tension on the hairs, as in some Afro-Caribbean and Asian hair styles (**2.98**).

Trichotillomania is patchy hair loss due to rubbing or pulling, commonly in childhood; hairs are broken off close to the surface.

Scarring alopecia may result from inflammatory dermatoses, such as lichen planus (**2.71**), discoid lupus erythematosus or scleroderma, and from trauma, burns or irradiation.

Diffuse hair loss after pregnancy, severe febrile illnesses or operations is termed **telogen effluvium** (loss in telogen growth phase). Cytotoxic drugs such as cyclophosphamide cause anagen effluvium. Iron-deficiency anaemia, hypothyroidism or hyperthyroidism, systemic lupus erythematosus and drugs such as heparin, vitamin A derivatives (retinoids) and oral contraceptives may cause hair loss.

EXCESSIVE HAIR

Hirsuties (hirsutism) is an excess of terminal hair growth in a male pattern distribution in women (**2.99**, **7.52**, **7.53**). Mild facial hirsuties is common, increasing after the menopause. In younger women, especially when hirsuties is associated with menstrual irregularity or with other signs of virilization, investigations to exclude conditions such as polycystic ovaries, ovarian tumours, virilizing adrenal tumours or Cushing's syndrome and congenital adrenal hyperplasia (heterozygote form) should be considered.

Hypertrichosis, a localized or overall increase in hair, may be drug induced, as with minoxidil, corticosteroids, diazoxide (**2.100**) or phenytoin, or associated with gross malnutrition, anorexia nervosa (**7.123**) or some variants of porphyria. Localized hypertrichosis occurs with some pigmented naevi and in the lumbosacral region in association with diastematomyelia (**11.106**).

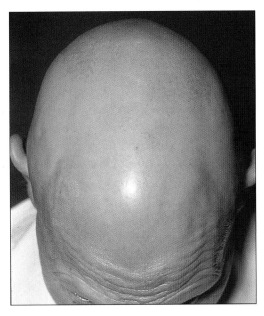

2.97 Alopecia totalis developed from severe alopecia areata in this patient. A similar appearance may result from the use of some cytotoxic chemotherapy for malignant disease.

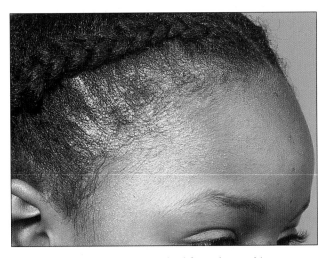

2.98 Traction alopecia has resulted from the combing involved in maintaining a traditional hairstyle in this patient.

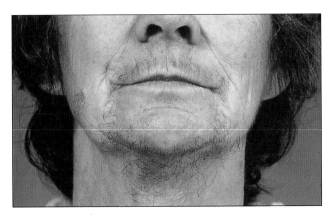

2.99 Hirsuties was the presenting symptom in this woman who was found to have an arrhenoblastoma.

in renal disease, and changes with some drugs such as antimalarials or tetracyclines.

Koilonychia is seen in iron-deficiency anaemia (**2.103, 10.6, 10.18**). **Clubbing of nails** (**2.59, 2.104, 2.105, 4.2, 4.95**) is

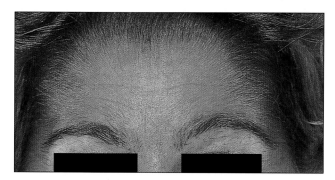

2.100   Gross hypertrichosis in a 32-year-old woman who was being treated with minoxidil for severe renal hypertension. Topical minoxidil is now used as a treatment for baldness in some countries.

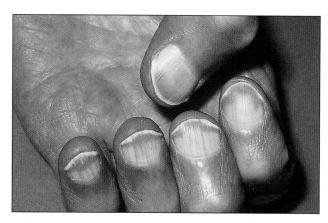

2.102   Leuconychia (opaque white nails) may occur in chronic liver disease and other conditions in which the serum albumin is low, such as nephrotic syndrome. In this patient, marked ridging of the nails is also present.

NAIL DISORDERS

Inherited abnormalities of nails are present in some genodermatoses, such as nail–patella syndrome, pachyonychia congenita (caused by a mutation in keratin K6, K16 or K17 genes) and ectodermal dysplasias. In these conditions often all finger nails and toe nails are affected (20-nail dystrophy). Scarring of nails occurs in some forms of epidermolysis bullosa dystrophica (**2.80**). Subungual exostoses cause overlying nail dystrophy.

Acute or chronic trauma may cause subungual splinter haemorrhages (**3.32**) or haematomas, gross thickening of the nail (onychogryphosis) or onycholysis of individual nails. Habit tic nail dystrophy of thumb nails and bitten nails, with damaged cuticles are common.

Yellow nails (**2.101**) are seen with chronic lymphoedema and in some chronic lung diseases. Other colour changes include leuconychia in liver disease (**2.102**), half-and-half nails

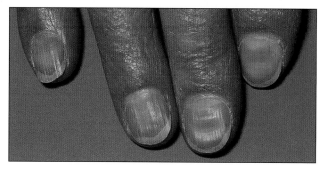

2.103   Koilonychia is usually a marker of underlying iron deficiency. The nails are brittle and spoon-shaped, as is particularly evident here in the thumb and index finger. This middle-aged woman had long-standing menorrhagia.

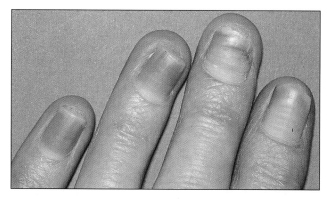

2.101   Yellow nail syndrome is a disorder in which there is progressive yellowing and thickening of the nails with absence of the lunula and a degree of onycholysis. There is often an association with chronic lung disease and peripheral lymphoedema.

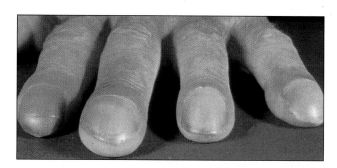

2.104   Gross clubbing of the nails in a 72-year-old man with carcinoma of the bronchus. Note the so-called 'nicotine sign' – staining of the index and middle finger by tar from his heavy cigarette smoking.

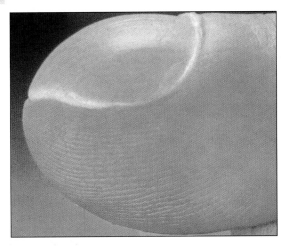

2.105 Gross clubbing of the nail. Note the filling-in of the nail fold, the increased curvature of the nail in both directions, giving a 'beaked' appearance, and the increased volume of the finger pulp.

associated with cyanotic heart disease, carcinoma of the bronchus, some chronic lung diseases and some chronic gastrointestinal diseases; alternatively it may be congenital.

Beau's lines are horizontal grooves that appear on all nails after severe illness. Splinter haemorrhages may be seen in vasculitis in association with connective tissue diseases (**3.32**) or in bacterial endocarditis. **Onycholysis** (**2.19**, **2.59**, **2.62**) may be due to fungal infection or psoriasis, drug induced, or associated with hyperthyroidism. Median nail dystrophy occurs without skin changes and the cause is unknown. Peripheral vascular disease predisposes to chronic paronychia.

Changes occur in dermatological conditions such as psoriasis (**2.19**), dermatitis, lichen planus, fungal (**2.59**) and yeast (**2.62**) infections and alopecia areata. Tumours may develop under or around the nail base, including malignant melanoma (**2.106**), glomus tumours and myxoid cysts.

SKIN TUMOURS

Skin tumours are common and may originate from the epidermis, melanocytes or any of the dermal components. Early detection of malignant tumours is vital.

COMMON BENIGN TUMOURS

Seborrhoeic keratoses or **basal cell papillomas** occur in the middle years, mainly on the trunk and face, with a roughened, warty, greasy surface and a superficial, stuck-on appearance (**2.107**). Lesions may be multiple, sometimes heavily pigmented, and they can be traumatized. They are commonly misdiagnosed as malignant melamonas.

Skin tags are simple papillomas that occur round the neck and in body folds (**2.108**). They are often familial.

Milia are common on the face or at the site of healed blisters (**2.109**). They are superficial cysts of sweat ducts.

Keratoacanthoma (**2.110**) is a rapidly growing ulcerating tumour, more common in middle-aged or elderly subjects. It should resolve spontaneously, within 9 months. Clinical distinction from a squamous cell carcinoma can be impossible. If the history is uncertain, biopsy is essential.

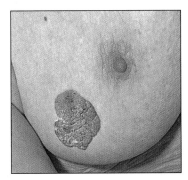

2.107 Seborrhoeic keratosis (seborrhoeic wart). These benign lesions are increasingly common with age, and they appear predominantly on unexposed Caucasian skin.

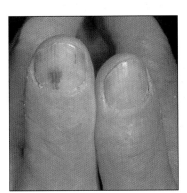

2.106 Subungual melanoma. A persistent dark lesion below a nail should be biopsied, as this is a common site for malignant melanoma. Pigmentation of the nail fold is particularly sinister.

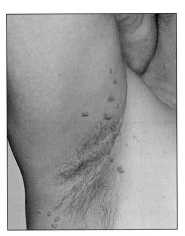

2.108 Skin tags in the axilla. These are small benign papillomas.

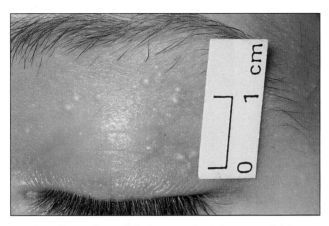

2.109 **Milia on the eyelid.** These are harmless, superficial, keratin-filled cysts, which are usually found on the face. In this location, it is important not to confuse these with xanthelasmas (see **p. 325**).

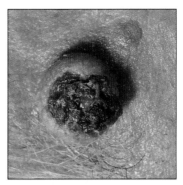

2.110 **Keratoacanthoma on the neck.** This ulcerating tumour, with a central keratin plug, grows rapidly but resolves spontaneously. Biopsy may be necessary to exclude a malignant lesion.

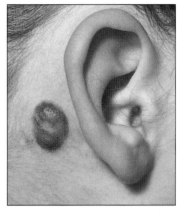

2.111 **Cavernous haemangioma.** 'Strawberry naevi' appear early in life and enlarge progressively. Parents can be reassured that most will resolve spontaneously before puberty.

93

Cavernous haemangiomata (**2.111**) appear at or soon after birth. Single or multiple lesions, of varying size, occur at any site. Ulceration and trauma with haemorrhage can occur but lesions are best left to regress spontaneously unless causing obstruction to vision.

Capillary haemangiomata (port-wine stains) are present at birth and do not fade with age. Cosmetic camouflage or laser treatment may be needed. Unilateral facial haemangioma may be associated with cerebral haemangiomata in the Sturge–Weber syndrome (**11.118**).

Pyogenic granulomas grow rapidly, tend to occur at sites of trauma, may be single or multiple and can recur.

Dermatofibromas (**2.112**) are more common in women, often pigmented, may be multiple and generally occur on limbs.

Keloids are persisting areas of exuberant scar tissue. Certain body sites, individuals and races are predisposed to this reaction.

Neurofibromata may be solitary or multiple and associated with café-au-lait patches in type I neurofibromatosis (**2.86** and see **p. 490**). Adenoma sebaceum is associated with tuberous sclerosis (**11.121**).

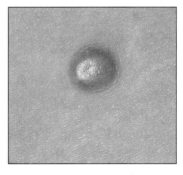

2.112 **Dermatofibroma on the thigh.** The lesion is raised, pink and firm, and is surrounded by a halo of hyperpigmentation. These benign lesions are often multiple on the legs and thighs in middle-aged women.

MELANOCYTIC TUMOURS

Congenital melanocytic naevi (moles) appear during the first few years of life. Most people have between 20 and 30; some have many more. The common mole should be uniformly pigmented, with a regular margin (**2.113–2.115**). A halo of pale skin around a mole may be seen in adolescence. Occasionally congenital moles are large (greater than 1 cm; **2.116**), multiple or confluent (bathing trunk pattern). These lesions carry a risk of malignant transformation. Moles deeper in the dermis appear blue in colour (**2.117**). Moles tend to regress in old age.

If moles change in size, become irregular in shape or pigmentation, itch or bleed they should be regarded as unstable and potentially malignant. Sunburn can irritate and activate moles. During pregnancy, moles tend to increase in size and darken.

Malignant melanomas (**2.106, 2.118, 2.119**) usually arise de novo but may develop from pre-existing moles. The incidence of this tumour is increasing, especially in fair-skinned people with high sun-exposure. The prognosis is much better if tumours are detected early. Melanoma may develop after some years in a lentigo (**2.120**). Amelanotic melanomas may be missed, especially in periungual sites. Malignant melanomas may occur in the eye (**2.121**).

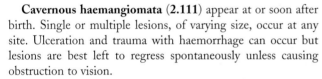

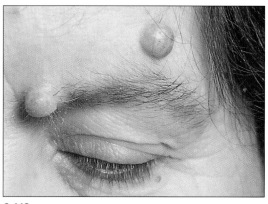

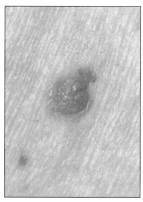

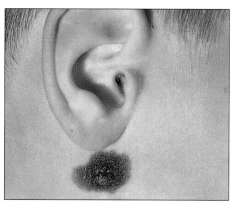

2.113   2.114   2.115

2.113–2.115 Benign melanocytic naevi (moles), showing a range of normal appearances. Pigmentation is even, but may vary from pale (**2.113**) to dark brown (**2.115**). There is no hint of malignant change in **2.113**. The irregular margin in the lesion seen in **2.114** aroused sufficient suspicion for the lesion to be biopsied. Despite the slightly irregular margin, the mole in **2.115** is probably congenital and almost certainly benign; but, if it were to change in shape, pigmentation or size, or if it were to bleed, biopsy would be necessary.

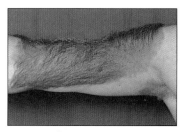

2.116   A large congenital pigmented melanocytic naevus. Note that hairs can grow in melanomas. Large lesions like this should be carefully observed for malignant change.

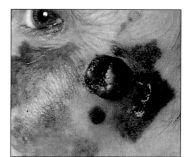

2.119   Malignant melanoma on the hand. The centre of the tumour is now amelanotic, but the local invasion remains pigmented and the patient had widespread secondary deposits.

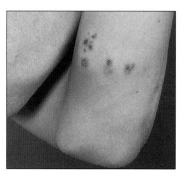

2.117   A group of blue naevi on the arm. These lesions are usually benign.

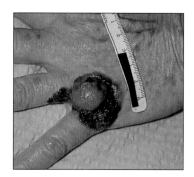

2.120 Lentigo malignant melanoma. Lentigo is a flat, dark brown lesion on the cheek of an elderly person. It should be regarded as a melanoma-*in-situ*, and may become frankly malignant, as here.

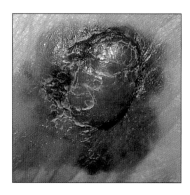

2.118   Malignant melanoma. Note the superficial spread in the skin and the varying level of pigmentation. The lesion had also bled. Prognosis depends on the depth of invasion of the tumour in the skin.

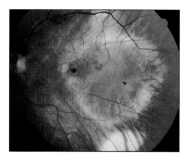

2.121   A large choroidal malignant melanoma, revealed by ophthalmoscopy. Malignant melanomas may also occur in the iris and conjunctiva. This tumour was treated by enucleation of the eye.

NONEPITHELIAL MALIGNANT TUMOURS

Secondary tumour deposits may occur in the skin. Common tumours that metastasize to the skin include breast (in addition to Paget's disease of the nipple), stomach, bronchus (**2.122**, **4.166**) and kidney. Hodgkin's disease and B-cell lymphomas may have skin lesions (**10.83**).

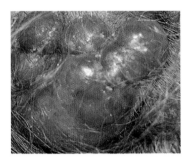

2.122   Skin secondaries, in this case in the scalp from a primary carcinoma of the bronchus. Such lesions are relatively uncommon.

Mycosis fungoides is a cutaneous T-cell lymphoma. It commonly manifests itself as a patchy superficial dermatitis (**2.123**) that evolves slowly into plaques and tumours.

Kaposi's sarcoma is another important skin tumour. Formerly rare outside Africa, it has now become a common complication of HIV infection, especially in homosexual men (*see* **p. 8**).

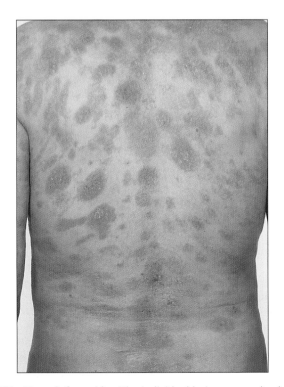

2.123   Mycosis fungoides. The individual lesions grow slowly over a period of years. They are red, thickened plaques, often with fine scales, which are itchy and may later ulcerate.

PREMALIGNANT AND MALIGNANT EPITHELIAL TUMOURS

Solar keratoses (**2.124**, **2.125**) occur on sun-exposed sites as patches of erythema and scale that gradually thicken. The adjacent skin shows signs of sun damage with wrinkling and loss of elasticity. Common sites are the face, ears and backs of hands. Malignant change occurs in a minority of lesions. Keratoses on the ears must be distinguished from chondrodermatitis nodularis helicis chronica, which is characteristically painful on pressure and almost always unilateral.

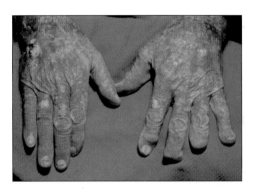

2.124   Solar keratoses – small, firm and scaly plaques – are commonly found on the extensor aspects of the hands and other exposed areas of skin in elderly people and in individuals on long-term immunosuppressive treatment (e.g. renal transplant recipients).

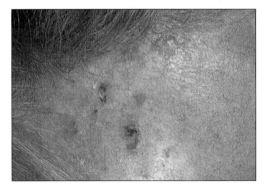

2.125   Solar keratosis. These lesions occur after long exposure to sunlight and are potentially malignant, with a latent period of at least 10 years.

Bowen's disease is an *in situ* squamous cell carcinoma that appears as persistent erythematous slightly scaly patches, which gradually enlarge. The surface is usually flattened and occasionally ulcerates. Patches may be multiple and occur anywhere on the body, especially on lower legs. An invasive carcinoma may develop (**2.126**).

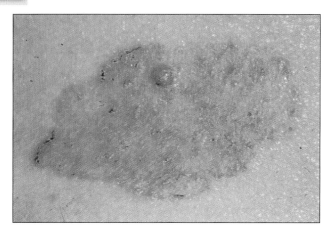

2.126 Bowen's disease – a persistent brownish *in situ* squamous cell carcinoma that slowly enlarges. An invasive carcinoma may develop under the crust or as a nodule, as here.

Leukoplakia (2.127) occurs as persistent white patches on mucous membranes, in the mouth or vulva, and may be an indication of underlying dysplasia.

Basal cell carcinomas are slow growing, locally invasive malignant tumours (**2.128, 2.129**). A pearly margin, telangiectatic vessels and central recurrent ulceration are typical, but variations such as multifocal, pigmented and morphoeic lesions may occur. Basal cell carcinomas are

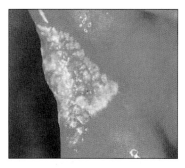

2.127 Leukoplakia may take several forms, all involving white patches on mucous membranes. In speckled leukoplakia, white areas alternate with areas of atrophic red epithelium. The risk of malignant transformation is high.

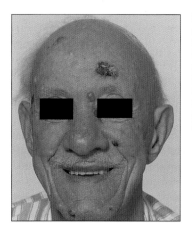

2.128 Multiple basal cell carcinomas. The lesion on the bridge of the nose is typical of the common presentation as a slowly enlarging nodule. The other lesions demonstrate various stages of progression to ulcerated lesions (rodent ulcers).

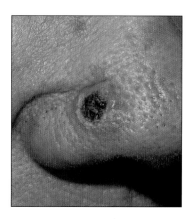

2.129 Basal cell carcinoma ulcerates at a later stage, usually with a shallow ulcer, with a very narrow indurated edge and a smooth shallow base.

especially common on the head and neck, but can occur anywhere on the body.

Squamous cell carcinomas occur especially on sun-exposed sites (**2.130**), but also in areas of chronic scarring or inflammation. Metastases occur more frequently from lesions at mucous membrane junctions such as on the lip.

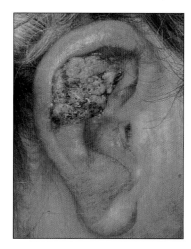

2.130 Squamous cell carcinoma begins as a small nodule, but slowly grows to produce the typical lesion seen here. The ulcer has thick edges and an irregular granular base; and it usually produces a serous discharge.

VASCULITIS AND AUTOIMMUNE CONNECTIVE TISSUE DISORDERS

Vasculitis implies the presence of inflammation within blood vessel walls, with resultant vessel damage, haemorrhage or infarction. The clinical expression of this process depends on the size of vessel involved, from capillaries to small muscular or larger arteries. Circulating factors may initiate the inflammation (immune complexes, cryoglobulins); the vessel damage ranges from endothelial cell swelling to fibrinoid necrosis of the vessel wall or a granulomatous response (as in Wegener's granuloma). The inflammatory infiltrate may involve polymorphonuclear leucocytes or lymphocytes. Skin lesions of vasculitis tend to be purpuric and palpable, may ulcerate and are painful (**2.131, 2.132**).

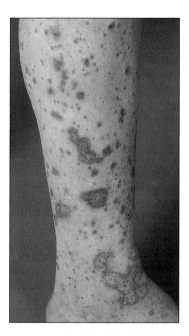

2.131 Leucocytoclastic vasculitis. This 57-year-old woman with rheumatoid arthritis developed widespread, painful, palpable purpura on both legs. Initially, the lesions were scattered and discrete, but in this picture some have coalesced and become necrotic in the centre. Leucocytoclastic vasculitis is also known as allergic or hypersensitivity vasculitis or anaphylactoid purpura and it has many possible causes. The lesions result from the deposition of immune complexes in the postcapillary venules.

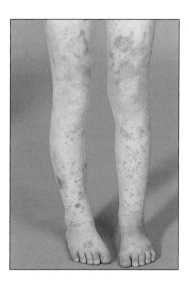

2.133 Henoch–Schönlein purpura, associated with swelling of the left knee and renal involvement in a child aged 4 years. The rash was also present on the back of the legs and the buttocks.

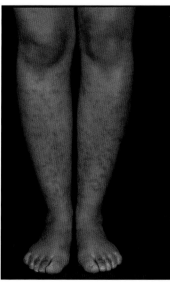

2.132 Livedo vasculitis in a 23-year-old Asian woman with systemic lupus erythematosus. The characteristic livedo or reticular appearance reflects the occurrence of small vessel vasculitis at a deeper level of the skin than in leucocytoclastic vasculitis.

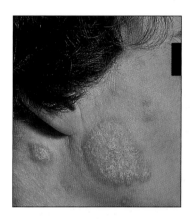

2.134 Discoid lupus erythematosus. Slowly enlarging recalcitrant pink scaly plaques are seen on the face, ears and scalp. The lesions are aggravated by sunlight, and they clear centrally with atrophy and scarring.

Conditions in which vasculitis is the predominant feature include Henoch–Schönlein purpura (**2.133**; small vessel vasculitis, with purpura, arthritis and glomerulonephritis;, *see also* **pp. 275, 439**) and polyarteritis nodosa (*see* **pp. 127, 275**). Vasculitis may be a feature of other connective tissue disorders, such as systemic lupus erythematosus, drug reactions, malignant disease or infections.

Discoid lupus erythematosus (DLE) manifests itself as chronic plaques, commonly on face, scalp or ears (**2.134**), with erythema, scaling and follicular plugging. Lesions persist, with scarring and depigmentation, but systemic features are absent.

Systemic lupus erythematosus (SLE) may present with an acute facial rash of butterfly distribution (**3.73, 3.74**), often

photoaggravated (**3.75**). Vasculitis may occur (**2.132**). Other features of systemic lupus erythematosus are described on **page 121**.

Rheumatoid arthritis (*see also* **p. 107**) may be associated with vasculitis (**2.131**) and subcutaneous nodules (**3.29**). It may also be accompanied by pyoderma gangrenosum, a destructive, necrotic ulcerative process that may destroy large areas of skin (**2.135**). Pyoderma gangrenosum may also complicate other diseases, especially ulcerative colitis, Crohn's disease, myelofibrosis and multiple myeloma.

Systemic sclerosis has several skin manifestations (*see* **p. 123**).

Morphoea is localized plaques of dermal sclerosis, often pigmented, that appear without other underlying disease. Scarring occurs in the skin (**2.136**) and may affect adjacent bone, but the condition usually clears spontaneously.

Dermatomyositis commonly involves the skin (**3.85, 3.86**), as may other connective tissue disorders, including relapsing polychondritis (**3.93**), Reiter's syndrome (**3.56–3.58**) and Behçet's syndrome (**3.100–3.103**).

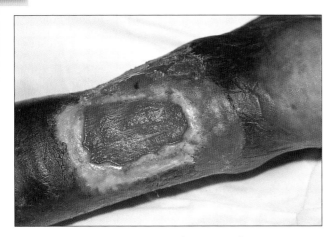

2.135 Pyoderma gangrenosum. This West Indian man developed a pustule over the lower leg that progressed to a tender, superficial necrotic ulcer. Note the typical purple undermined edge. The lesion persisted for months and partially responded to topical corticosteroids and minocycline. Eventually, it responded to systemic corticosteroids. Pyoderma gangrenosum is usually suggestive of underlying systemic disease, but none was found in this patient.

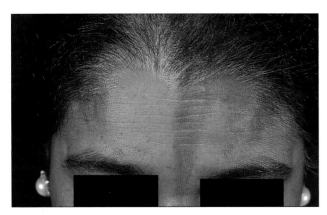

2.136 Morphoea 'en coup de sabre' (resembling the scar from a sabre cut). This form of localized morphoea can involve subcutaneous tissues and even bone. It is a variant of linear morphoea and, if the scalp is involved, can be associated with scarring and subsequent hair loss. Despite the severe local involvement, systemic sclerosis is not seen in this condition.

THE SKIN IN OTHER MULTISYSTEM DISORDERS

A number of other multisystem disorders have cutaneous manifestations or complications. These can be important clues to the diagnosis and should be sought carefully.

Many **systemic infections** have skin manifestations (*see* **Ch. 1**), and a broad range of skin complications has been noted in HIV infection.

Diabetes may be associated with a number of skin conditions, including acanthosis nigricans (**2.90**), staphylococcal (**1.77, 2.50**)

and candidal infection (**2.61, 2.62**), gangrene (**7.92**) and trophic changes, such as ulcers, especially in the skin of the legs. Two specific, and probably related, conditions are seen in diabetics, though they may also occur in non-diabetic patients.

- **Granuloma annulare** occurs as groups of flesh-coloured papules in rings or crescents, most commonly on the extensor surfaces of the hands and fingers (**2.137**).
- **Necrobiosis lipoidica** occurs as erythematous plaques over the shins (**2.138**). These gradually develop a waxy appearance and brown pigmentation. Care is needed to prevent skin breakdown and ulceration.

Xanthomas may be the first indication of underlying hyperlipidaemia, either primary or secondary to underlying disorders such as diabetes or renal disease (*see* **p. 324**).

Sarcoidosis has several skin manifestations, some of which, such as lupus pernio, are diagnostic of the condition (*see* **p. 179**).

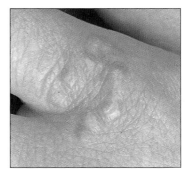

2.137 Granuloma annulare on the finger. Note the ring of flesh-coloured papules. This condition may occur in otherwise healthy individuals or in patients with diabetes.

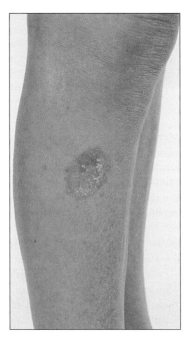

2.138 Necrobiosis lipoidica in a 50-year-old woman with diabetes. Note the surface scaling and atrophy. Ulceration may occur in more advanced and extensive lesions. Necrobiosis lipoidica is usually a complication of diabetes.

CLASSIFICATION OF PHOTODERMATOSES

Acute	Idiopathic	Photoaggravated dermatosis	Exogenous chemical	Degenerative or neoplastic	Genetic or metabolic
Sunburn	Polymorphic light eruption	Acne rosacea	Phototoxic and photoallergic reactions (drugs, plants or chemicals)	Solar keratoses (squamous cell carcinoma)	Porphyrias
	Solar urticaria	Systematic lupus erythematosus		Basal cell carcinoma	Albinism
	Chronic actinic dermatitis (photodermatitis; actinic reticuloid)	Dermatomyositis		Melanoma	Xeroderma pigmentosum
		Darier's disease		Photoageing	Rothmund–Thomson syndrome
	Actinic prurigo	Herpes simplex			Cockayne's syndrome
	Hydroa vacciniforme	Vitiligo			Bloom's syndrome
		Lichen planus			Hartnup disease
		Psoriasis (some patients)			
		Atopic dermatitis (some patients)			

2.139   Classification of photodermatoses.

Generalized pruritus is a common presentation to the dermatologist. There may be a dermatological explanation for the itch, such as dermatitis or scabies, but, more often, especially in the elderly, no abnormality is detected in the skin, except scratch marks. Pruritus may be the first presentation of a wide range of conditions – including drug reactions, liver disease such as primary biliary cirrhosis (**9.49**), chronic renal failure, haematological conditions such as anaemia or polycythaemia, hyperthyroidism or hypothyroidism, diabetes or malignant disease such as Hodgkin's disease – and needs careful investigation.

Cutaneous signs of many other conditions are illustrated throughout this book.

PHOTODERMATOSES

Many skin conditions are affected by ultraviolet radiation, either positively, as when it is used as a therapeutic agent, or adversely, as the cause or an exacerbating factor of a dermatosis. Within the ultraviolet radiation spectrum, the ultraviolet A and ultraviolet B wavebands are the most significant, as ultraviolet C is mainly absorbed within the atmosphere. Although most ultraviolet radiation comes from the sun, the use of sunbeds as artificial sunlight has resulted in a rising incidence of ultraviolet-induced disorders.

The wide range of photodermatoses is summarized in **2.139**.

Idiopathic photodermatoses should be distinguished from other dermatoses aggravated by ultraviolet radiation or the reactions of normal skin to ultraviolet radiation damage (such as inflammation, tanning, thickening of the epidermis and suppression of local cell-mediated immunity).

Polymorphic light eruption is a common disorder affecting 10–20% of the population, predominantly females. It is generally worse in spring and early summer. The rash develops within a few hours of sun exposure as itchy erythematous papules, plaques or vesicles on exposed sites (**2.140**).

Chronic actinic dermatitis (also known as photodermatitis or actinic reticuloid) is a rare disorder that usually presents in older men, as a severe chronic dermatitis of exposed sites (**2.141**), often in association with multiple contact allergies. Other rare photodermatoses include solar urticaria, in which

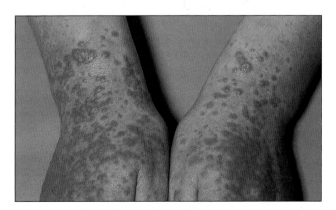

2.140   **Polymorphic light eruption.** This female patient has typical itchy erythematous papules over the forearms and hands. The mechanism of this reaction – the most common form of 'sun allergy' – is not known, but it is provoked by ultraviolet B light in the sunburn range. The reaction commonly occurs on the face and arms, but may also appear in other sun-exposed areas. It may develop at any time from 2 hours to 5 days after sun exposure – most commonly it appears within 24 hours.

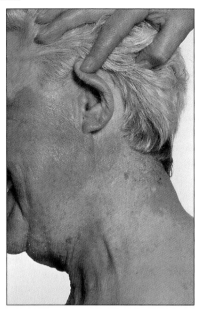

2.141 Chronic actinic dermatitis (photodermatitis) is a severe eczematous reaction which is limited to light-exposed areas. Note the typical distribution of a photodermatosis, with sparing behind the ears, under the chin and below the collar line. In this case, the cause was unknown and prevention of exposure to light was the major preventive measure. In many cases, however, a similar reaction may result from photosensitizing drug therapy.

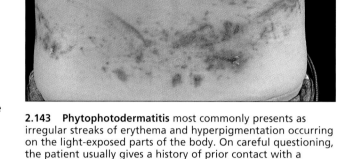

2.143 Phytophotodermatitis most commonly presents as irregular streaks of erythema and hyperpigmentation occurring on the light-exposed parts of the body. On careful questioning, the patient usually gives a history of prior contact with a sensitizing plant. This gardener's skin had been exposed to giant hogweed.

urticarial weals appear within minutes of sun exposure and resolve within 1–2 hours, hydroa vacciniforme, a painful vesicular rash on the face, and actinic prurigo, a persistent itchy papular or nodular eruption on exposed sites; the last two are more common in children.

Many dermatoses can be **photoaggravated** including acne rosacea, systemic lupus erythematosus (**3.75**), lichen planus, psoriasis and atopic dermatitis in some patients.

Photosensitive drug eruptions may be induced by ultraviolet radiation exposure with, for example, phenothiazines, thiazide diuretics, sulphonamides, or tetracyclines. These reactions may present as either an acute phototoxic reaction (**2.142**) or as a more chronic photodermatitis (**2.141**). Several plant families also contain substances that may induce photosensitivity (phytophotodermatitis) in the skin, including cow parsley, hogweed, rue, and bergamot. The sensitivity results from contact with psoralen compounds within the plants (**2.143**). Bergapten (the active ingredient in oil of bergamot) and other furocoumarins are also found in some perfumes.

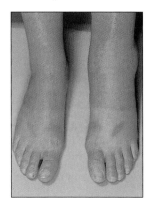

2.142 A phototoxic drug eruption, occurring in exposed skin not covered by footwear. This woman had been treated with doxycycline.

Photosensitivity is a common problem in patients with several variants of porphyria (*see* **p. 332**), whereas patients with vitiligo or albinism lack the melanin protection in the skin and are liable to both acute and chronic ultraviolet radiation damage.

Patients with the rare inherited disorder **xeroderma pigmentosum**, who have inherited defects in DNA repair after ultraviolet exposure, are abnormally sensitive to the tumorogenic effects of ultraviolet B.

DRUG REACTIONS IN THE SKIN

Skin eruptions (rashes) are the most common sign of adverse reactions to drug therapy, although any organ system can be involved. Many drug reactions are not truly allergic in their nature and it is important to distinguish between the characteristics of non-allergic and allergic reactions (**2.144**). Drugs that have been frequently implicated in allergic reactions are listed in **2.145**.

Drug therapy may lead to a wide range of skin pathologies, but some features are especially suggestive of drug eruptions. The skin eruption is usually widespread and symmetrical. Typically, it develops within 10–14 days of the start of therapy, but it may develop sooner if there has been previous exposure to the same or a similar drug. Reactions may develop rapidly, within minutes, if a type I hypersensitivity reaction of anaphylaxis, angioedema or urticaria is present. Alternatively, drug eruptions can develop when a patient has been on treatment for some time, perhaps triggered by some additional, intercurrent factor. When a patient is on multiple drug therapy, drugs commonly associated with eruptions should be identified (e.g. **2.150**), together with those that have been introduced recently, and withdrawal or substitution of alternative therapy carefully planned. It is important to

DIFFERENCES BETWEEN NON-ALLERGIC AND ALLERGIC DRUG REACTIONS		
Difference	**Non-allergic**	**Allergic**
Quantities required to provoke reaction	Large	Minute
Cumulative effect	Often necessary	Usually none
Relationship between allergic effect and pharmacological action	Often present	No connection
Same effect reproduced by pharmacologically different chemicals	Rare	Common
Clinical picture	Uniform	Varied

2.144   Differences between non-allergic and allergic drug reactions.

DRUGS FREQUENTLY IMPLICATED IN ALLERGIC DRUG REACTIONS	
Aspirin	Muscle relaxants
NSAIDs	Tranquillizers
Penicillins	Anti-hypertensives
Sulphonamides	Anti-arrhythmics
Anti-tuberculous drugs	Iodinated contrast media
Nitrofurans	Antisera and vaccines
Antimalarials	Organ extracts, e.g. insulin, ACTH
Griseofulvin	Heavy metals
Hypnotics	Allopurinol
Anticonvulsants	Penicillamine
Anaesthetic agents	Antithyroid drugs

2.145   Drugs frequently implicated in allergic drug reactions.

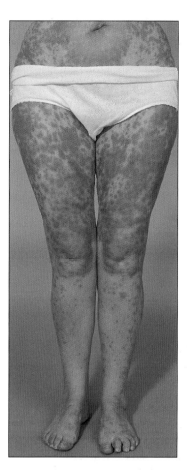

2.146   **Ampicillin rash often presents as a symmetrical erythematous maculopapular eruption.** This patient had a history of previous penicillin rashes, which had not been taken into account when the ampicillin was prescribed.

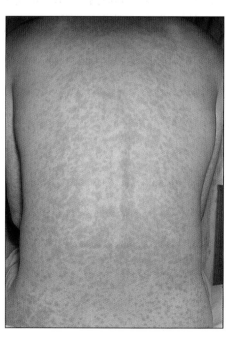

2.147   **A morbilliform eruption in a patient treated with co-trimoxazole.** The offending agent here is usually the sulphonamide component, and similar rashes may occur when other sulphonamides are administered.

recognize that an allergic reaction may not be caused by the active drug itself; it may be due to a preservative, colouring agent or bulking agent in the tablet or syrup. Factors such as infection may modify the development of a drug reaction, as with the ampicillin rash seen in patients with infectious mononucleosis (**1.72**).

Morbilliform and maculopapular eruptions are common (**2.146, 2.147**) and may develop into severe erythroderma (exfoliative dermatitis), clinically indistinguishable from that found in other conditions such as psoriasis (**2.21**).

True immediate-type hypersensitivity to penicillin and many other drugs may lead to **urticaria** (**2.39**), **angioedema**

(**2.41**) and life-threatening anaphylaxis (*see* **p. 168**). Similar reactions may develop as a result of idiosyncratic direct release of inflammatory mediators such as histamine by nonallergic mechanisms, as in aspirin-sensitive individuals.

Fixed drug eruptions are rashes or solitary skin lesions that recur at the same site each time the causative drug is taken (**2.148**). Sulphonamides, barbiturates and the laxative phenolphthalein are common causes.

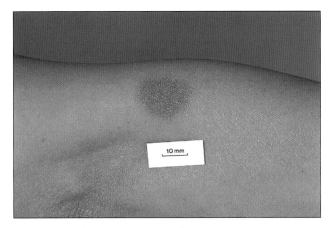

2.148   Fixed drug eruption, so-called because the lesion recurs at the same site after each administration of the causative drug. A common cause, as here, is phenolphthalein, found in various proprietary laxative preparations. The lesion is intensely itchy.

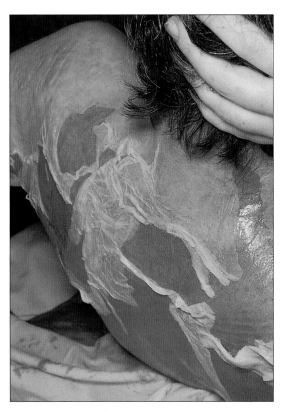

2.149   Toxic epidermal necrolysis, the 'scalded skin syndrome' in an adult. The most common cause is drug allergy, but in children it is more commonly the result of infection (*see* **1.79**).

Erythema multiforme may be evoked by drug therapy (*see* **p. 76**). It is a component of, and may develop into, the life-threatening Stevens-Johnson syndrome (*see* **p. 77**).

Erythema nodosum (**2.45**) may be provoked by drug therapy; so too may vasculitic and purpuric reactions. Another major drug reaction is **toxic epidermal necrolysis**, the 'scalded skin syndrome' (**2.149**). Drug allergy is the most common cause of this syndrome in adults.

Some drugs are used despite a known high frequency of rashes. Gold therapy may be used for its powerful effect in severe rheumatoid arthritis, for example, but it often provokes a psoriasiform eruption, which may persist despite withdrawal of the drug (**2.150**).

A number of drugs may produce **phototoxic or photoallergic reactions**, in which the rash appears on light-exposed areas (**2.141**, **2.142**). These patients must be distinguished from those with underlying photosensitivity caused by conditions such as systemic lupus erythematosus or porphyria.

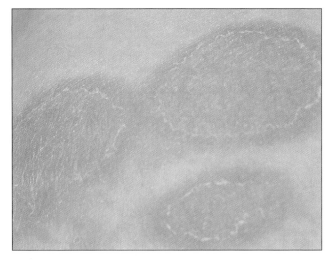

2.150   Gold sensitivity is most commonly manifest as a psoriasiform eruption. Gold rashes are not uncommon in rheumatoid patients, and they may persist despite withdrawal of gold therapy.

3 Joints and bones

HISTORY

In a patient with joint disease, a detailed clinical history and examination is essential to determine the severity of the disease and the nature and extent of subsequent investigations.

The most common symptoms are pain and stiffness. In inflammatory arthritis, these are worse in the morning and are relieved by movement of the joint or joints; there is redness, swelling and an increase in skin temperature over the joint. These features are uncommon in mechanical joint diseases and pain is worse on use of the joint and towards the end of the day. It is relieved by rest.

Information regarding the number and the distribution of joints affected is important; for example:

- gouty and septic arthritis tend to present with acute onset monoarthritis (one joint) (**3.1**, **3.2**)
- the peripheral joint involvement in ankylosing spondylitis and enteropathic arthritis is oligoarticular (four joints or fewer)

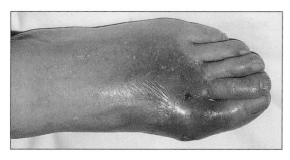

3.1 Monoarthritis. The acute onset of a hot, red, very tender metacarpophalangeal joint of the big toe is a classic presentation of gout (*see* **p. 120**). In this patient, acute gout was complicated by secondary infection; but even in the absence of infection acute arthritis may produce such intense inflammation that it is confused with cellulitis (*see* **3.68**, **3.69**).

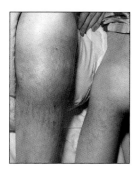

3.2 Acute arthritis of the right knee. The knee is swollen, tender to touch, warm on palpation and is held in flexion. A patellar tap can be demonstrated, and the effusion can be confirmed by aspiration.

- rheumatoid arthritis (RA) and systemic lupus erythematosus (SLE) are polyarticular (five or more joints) (**3.3**)
- a proximal and broadly symmetrical distribution is suggestive of RA
- an asymmetrical presentation favours seronegative arthritis
- in seronegative arthritis, there may also be axial joint involvement with spinal and lower back pain.

The variation of the symptomatology over time also provides useful diagnostic information; for example:

- osteoarthritis (OA) is usually persistent and may be insidiously progressive
- RA may be relapsing and remitting
- recurrent episodes of severe monoarthritis suggest gout or pseudogout.

Although most forms of arthritis are spontaneous in their onset, in some patients specific factors of aetiological importance can be identified. For example, trauma may precipitate an attack of gout and aggravate OA, and infection may cause non-specific polyarthralgia (e.g. parvovirus), Reiter's syndrome (genital or intestinal infection) or a septic arthritis (gonorrhoea).

Extra-articular features are also important:

- skin psoriasis suggests psoriatic arthritis
- nodules occur in RA and tophi in gouty arthritis
- ocular symptoms may occur in many forms of arthritis
- the seronegative arthropathies are often complicated by mucocutaneous lesions.

Joint function can be assessed by asking patients simple questions about difficulty in dressing and washing unaided, working in the kitchen, climbing up and down stairs, getting in and out of a car, etc.

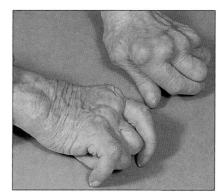

3.3 Polyarthritis in chronic rheumatoid arthritis. The finger joints are not acutely inflamed, but there is major residual deformity of the hand. End-stage arthritis of this severity should now be rare when arthritis is well managed.

EXAMINATION

Simple general observation will provide much information. The patient may have difficulty sitting on, or rising from, a chair, have an abnormal gait and show reluctance to shake hands in fear of pain. Distribution of joint involvement should be noted. On inspection of the individual joints look for erythema, swelling, deformity and muscular atrophy resulting from disuse (**3.4**):

- deformities are classified as either fixed or reducible, and in accordance with their deviation from the normal anatomical position (valgus, varus, ulnar, radial, flexion, etc.)
- the range of active movement should be assessed, so that limitation of joint movement is noted before palpation
- on palpation, joint tenderness should be noted; an increase in skin temperature indicates active inflammation; the type

of swelling may be appreciated (thickened synovium has a boggy feeling; osteophytes or tophi feel hard and irregular)
- joint effusion may be demonstrated (**3.2**) and crepitation can be felt (fine crepitation caused by bone and cartilage irregularities)
- grip strength can be assessed by asking the patient to squeeze the examiner's second and third fingers.

A comprehensive and systematic examination should also be carried out to reveal extra-articular features such as episcleritis, nodules (**3.29**) and vasculitis in RA; skin psoriasis and nail lesions in psoriatic arthropathy (**2.19**, **3.5**); iritis (**3.48**), mucocutaneous lesions and cardiac complications in ankylosing spondylitis; conjunctivitis (**3.6**) and urethritis in Reiter's syndrome; tophus deposition in gouty arthritis (**3.7**); and septic vesicular lesions in gonococcal arthritis (**3.8**)

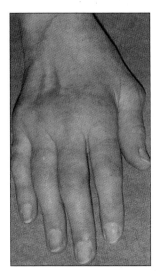

3.4 Rheumatoid arthritis. There is swelling of the metacarpophalangeal and the proximal interphalangeal joints, subluxation with ulnar deformity, and a fixed flexion deformity in the first metacarpophalangeal joint. Note also the disuse atrophy of the intrinsic muscles of the hands.

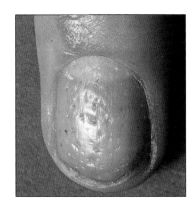

3.5 Pitting of the nails may be a clue to the diagnosis of psoriatic arthropathy. This patient also has a small psoriatic plaque on the finger. More severe nail changes may occur (see **2.16**).

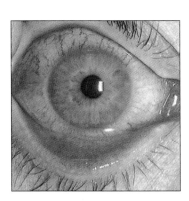

3.6 Conjunctivitis is a frequent extra-articular feature in many rheumatic disorders.

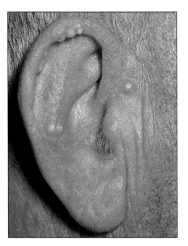

3.7 Tophaceous deposits in the ear and elsewhere may occur in chronic gout. They may discharge a thick toothpaste-like material, which can be shown on polarized light microscopy to be urate crystals (see **3.13**).

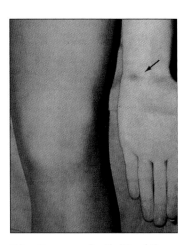

3.8 Gonococcal arthritis of the knee. The association of extra-articular skin lesions, such as the vesicular lesion seen here on the volar surface of the wrist (arrowed), with the arthritis points to a systemic infection.

INVESTIGATIONS

An investigative programme for the rheumatological patient may include haematology, immunopathology, blood biochemistry, joint fluid analysis and radiography.

HAEMATOLOGY

Full blood count
- leucocytosis and thrombocytosis suggest an inflammatory process
- thrombocytopenia may occur in SLE
- a normochromic, normocytic anaemia may indicate a chronic disease such as RA
- a microcytic anaemia (**3.9**) may indicate chronic gastrointestinal blood loss caused by the use of non-steroidal anti-inflammatory drugs (NSAIDs).

Erythrocyte sedimentation rate (ESR)
- a raised erythrocyte sedimentation rate (ESR) or plasma viscosity suggests an inflammatory condition.

C-reactive protein (CRP)
- C-reactive protein (CRP) is a more sensitive indicator of inflammatory activity than ESR or plasma viscosity, but the result is not available for at least 24 hours as it is measured by radioimmunodiffusion.

IMMUNOPATHOLOGY

Rheumatoid factor
- positive in 80% of patients with RA; high titres indicate aggressive disease
- may also be found in other connective tissue disorders such as Sjögren's syndrome, SLE and systemic sclerosis
- may also be found in infectious disease, B-cell lymphoproliferative disorders and in healthy elderly people.

Antinuclear antibody (ANA)
- antinuclear antibody (ANA) (**3.10**, **3.11**) is common in connective tissue disorders, but relatively non-specific and may be found in normal individuals.

Other antibodies
- for example anti-DNA antibodies in SLE, anti-nRNP in mixed connective tissue disorder, anti-neutrophil cytoplasmic antibodies (ANCA) in Wegener's granulomatosis.

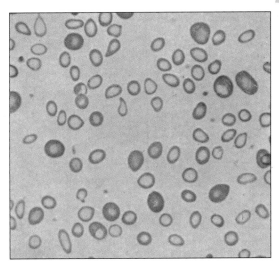

3.9 Microcytic anaemia in a patient with chronic rheumatoid arthritis. Most red cells have a central pallor (hypochromia) and a small diameter (microcytosis). The anaemia resulted from long-term gastrointestinal blood loss as a side-effect of non-steroidal anti-inflammatory drug use.

105

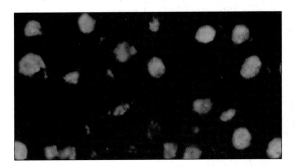

3.10 Antinuclear antibody as revealed by indirect immunofluorescence. The test serum came from a patient with systemic lupus erythematosus (*see* **p. 121**).

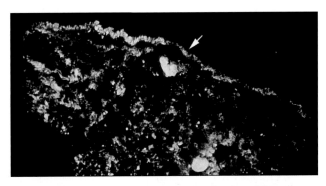

3.11 The lupus band test demonstrates the deposition of complement C3b and immunoglobulin in the skin at the dermo-epidermal junction, shown here as a continuous band of IgM (arrow) by direct immunofluorescence (the background fluorescence in the dermis is not significant). Non-lesional skin that has not been exposed to the sun should be used for this test. A positive result is strongly suggestive of a diagnosis of systemic lupus erythematosus.

BLOOD BIOCHEMISTRY

Renal and liver function
- abnormal function may indicate extra-articular complications and provide guidance to diagnosis and treatment.

Uric acid level
- high level may suggest gouty arthritis.

Calcium level
- hypercalcaemia in sarcoidosis (uncommon).

JOINT FLUID ANALYSIS

Naked eye appearance on aspiration (3.12)
- colour, viscosity and turbidity; active synovial inflammation gives a thin turbid appearance.

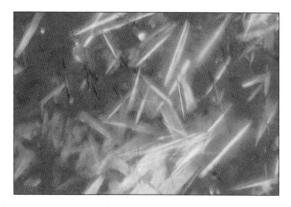

3.12   Joint aspiration may yield valuable information and may relieve symptoms. It must be performed using sterile techniques to prevent the risk of introduction of infection into the joint. In this case, over 40 ml effusion was aspirated from the knee. The effusion was not purulent, and the presence of large numbers of mononuclear cells on microscopy was consistent with the diagnosis of OA.

Microscopy
- white cell count with differential count: polymorphonuclear cells predominant in RA, gouty arthritis and septic arthritis; mononuclear cells predominant in OA
- under polarized light urate crystals are negatively birefringent (**3.13**); calcium pyrophosphate dihydrate crystals are weakly positively birefringent (**3.14**).

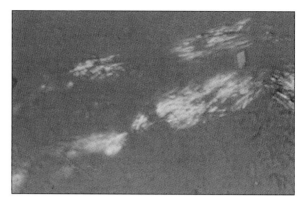

3.14   Polarized light microscopy reveals weakly positive birefringence in the rhomboidal crystals of calcium pyrophosphate dihydrate ingested by leucocytes, which are found in joint aspirates from patients with pseudogout.

RADIOGRAPHY

Plain radiographs
- useful in assessing soft-tissue swelling, joint space loss, erosions, sclerosis, calcification, etc. (**3.15**).

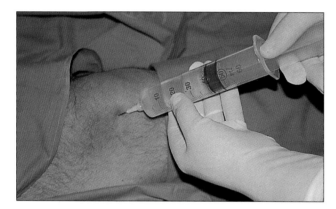

3.13   Polarized light microscopy reveals strongly negative birefringence in the needle-shaped urate crystals found in a joint aspirate from a patient with acute gout.

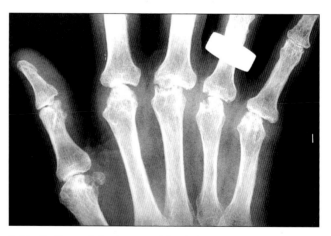

3.15   Radiograph in rheumatoid arthritis. Note the multiple erosions of the metacarpals, the loss of joint spaces, the presence of bone cysts and the subluxation of the metacarpophalangeal joint of the thumb.

OTHER INVESTIGATIONS

These are less often requested and include:

- ultrasound (**3.27**)
- CT scanning
- MRI scanning (**3.16**)
- arthrography (**3.28**)
- arthroscopy and synovial tissue biopsy (**3.17**)
- scintigraphy (**3.18**)
- thermography
- HLA tissue typing.

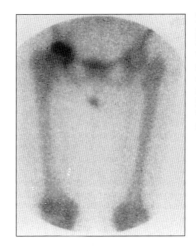

3.18 Acute monoarthritis of the right hip revealed by technetium bone scanning. The increased count over the right hip is a reflection of the increased blood flow to the joint associated with acute arthritis.

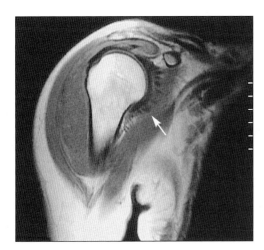

3.16 MRI has an evolving role in the imaging of bones and joints. The patient has synovial chondromatosis, a condition in which multiple cartilaginous bodies are present in the synovium. These were not visible on plain X-ray but are clearly seen on the scan (arrow). Calcification is also seen (to the left of the arrow). The gap between the two synovial layers reflects the presence of an effusion in the joint.

THE ARTHROPATHIES

RHEUMATOID ARTHRITIS (RA)

Rheumatoid arthritis (RA) is a common condition with a worldwide distribution, more prevalent in temperate climates. In Western communities the prevalence is 1–3%, with women more commonly affected than men (3:1), and the peak age of onset is 30–50 years. The aetiology is unknown, but is most probably multifactorial. The high risk conferred by HLA-DR4 suggests a genetic component. Environmental factors such as viral infections have been suggested. The initial pathology is synovitis with oedema, vascular dilatation and polymorphonuclear cell infiltrate. This is followed by lymphocyte and plasma cell infiltration and proliferation of the synovial lining cells. As the disease progresses, the synovial tissue becomes fibrosed and granulation tissue (pannus) develops and erodes the cartilage (**3.19**).

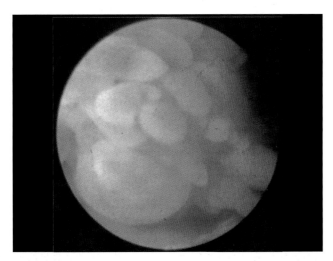

3.17 Arthroscopy can be performed in many joints. The procedure sometimes allows a visual diagnosis, permits confirmatory biopsy and may also allow corrective surgery. Arthroscopy of the knee in this patient with rheumatoid arthritis revealed multiple synovial villi.

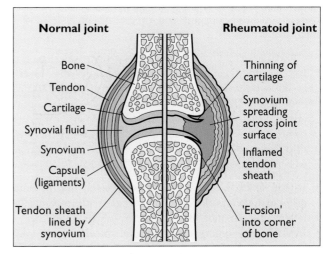

3.19 A diagramatic cross-section of a normal synovial joint (left) and a joint affected by rheumatoid arthritis (right).

Over 70% of patients present with a bilateral and symmetrical polyarthritis, usually of insidious onset. All synovial joints may be affected, but certain joints more commonly so (**3.20**). Patients complain of joint pain, stiffness and swelling that are worse in the early morning. There may also be constitutional symptoms with general malaise and anorexia. The clinical course is that of relapse and remission.

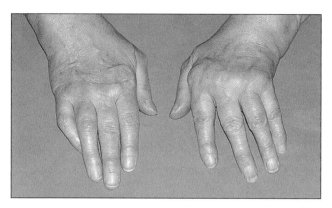

3.21 Advanced rheumatoid arthritis affecting the metacarpophalangeal and proximal interphalangeal joints of the hands. There is also wasting of the small muscles of the hands. Ulnar deviation and other deformities have occurred as a result of subluxation.

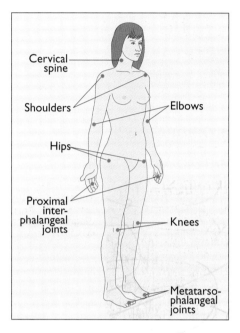

3.20 Joints commonly affected by rheumatoid arthritis.

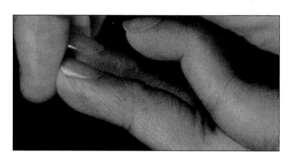

3.22 Swan-neck deformity is common in advanced rheumatoid arthritis. It is brought about by disruption of the volar plate of the proximal inter-phalangeal joint, sometimes with associated rupture of the insertion of the flexor sublimis.

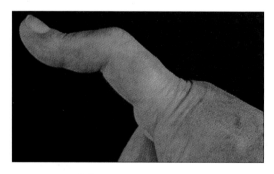

3.23 Boutonnière deformity. This common deformity in advanced rheumatoid arthritis results from the rupture of the central slip of the extensor tendon over the proximal interphalangeal joint. The lateral slips of the extensor tendon mechanism are displaced to the sides and maintain the deformity.

Early changes include fusiform swelling of the proximal interphalangeal joints, soft-tissue enlargement around the metacarpophalangeal joints and progressive wasting of the interosseous muscles.

Later, characteristic deformities of the joints develop:

- In the hands, there is subluxation and ulnar deviation (**3.21**) at the metacarpophalangeal joints; swan-neck (**3.22**) and boutonnière (**3.23**) deformities occur at the interphalangeal joints; dorsal subluxation of the ulnar styloid at the wrist is common, and may contribute to rupture of the fourth and fifth extensor tendons when there is also inflammation within the extensor tendon sheaths (**3.3, 3.24**).

- In the forefoot, the metatarsophalangeal joints become dislocated; there is clawing of the toes and patients complain of a painful sensation like 'walking on pebbles' (**3.25**).

- In the knees, swelling may result from synovial hypertrophy (**3.17**) and effusion; varus and fixed flexion deformities of the knees are common and popliteal (Baker's) cysts are sometimes felt; rupture of these cysts causes sudden calf pain

with swelling that can mimic deep vein thrombosis (**3.26, 3.27, 3.28**).

- The disease also commonly affects the elbows and in more advanced cases the hips and neck.

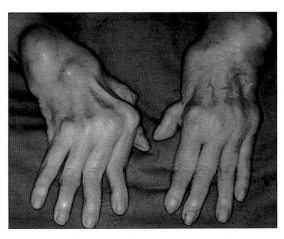

3.24 Severe advanced rheumatoid arthritis of the hands. There is massive tendon swelling over the dorsal surfaces of both wrists, severe muscle wasting, ulnar deviation of the metacarpophalangeal joints and swan-neck deformity of the fingers.

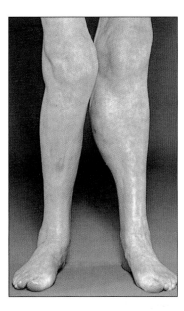

3.26 Advanced rheumatoid arthritis has resulted in a valgus deformity of the right knee and swelling of the left calf caused by the rupture of a Baker's cyst.

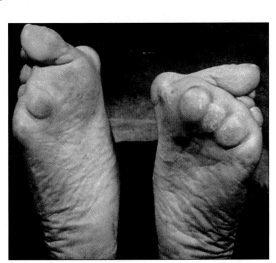

3.25 Rheumatoid arthritis of the feet. Gross destructive changes with multiple subluxations cause painful deformity that severely limits mobility.

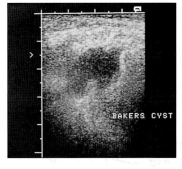

3.27 Baker's cyst of the knee, demonstrated by ultrasound, the usual diagnostic method. This cyst has not ruptured.

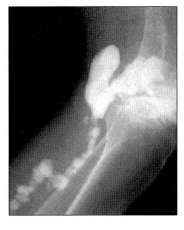

3.28 Arthrogram showing a ruptured Baker's cyst. Contrast has leaked from the Baker's cyst producing the clinical picture shown in **3.26**.

Patients may present with extra-articular features, most of which are associated with vasculitis. These patients tend to have a poorer prognosis:

- Skin manifestations include:
  - rheumatoid nodules (**3.29**)
  - skin rashes, often purpuric
  - ulceration (**3.30**)
  - nail-fold and finger-pulp infarcts (**3.31, 3.32**)
  - pyoderma gangrenosum (**2.135**).
- Raynaud's phenomenon may occur; it is characterized by finger blanching (vasospasm) and usually precipitated by cold or emotion (*see* **p. 243**).

- Keratoconjunctivitis sicca (dry eyes, either alone or as part of Sjögren's syndrome (*see* **p. 125**) and episcleritis are common ocular manifestions (**3.33**); scleritis (with blue sclerae, *see* **3.118**) and scleromalacia are rare but serious, as they can lead to eyeball perforation (**3.34**); steroid-induced cataracts and chloroquine-induced retinopathy may occur when these agents are used in treatment.

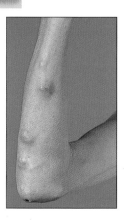

3.29 Rheumatoid nodules. The upper forearm and elbow are the most common sites for skin nodules in rheumatoid arthritis. These nodules result from vasculitis, and they may ulcerate or become necrotic, as has occurred at the elbow in this patient. Such nodules are often painless and cause no symptoms, but surgery is occasionally indicated for cosmetic reasons.

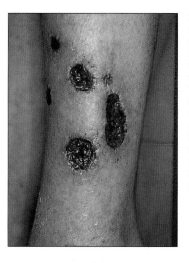

3.30 Deep arterial ulceration of the legs in rheumatoid arthritis. Such ulcers result from vasculitis and are often very difficult to treat. They may respond to a combination of aggressive therapy for rheumatoid arthritis and meticulous local care, but amputation is sometimes necessary when such ulceration is severe and progressive.

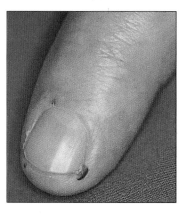

3.31 Nail-fold infarction caused by vasculitis may occur in rheumatoid arthritis and some connective tissue diseases, but a very similar appearance may result from nail trauma in normal individuals.

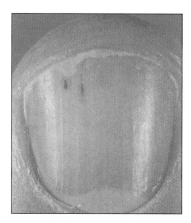

3.32 Splinter haemorrhages may be another result of vasculitis in rheumatoid arthritis, but they are a rather non-specific sign; they may be caused simply by trauma and have little value in diagnosis.

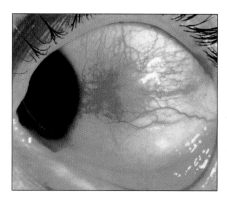

3.33 Rheumatoid episcleritis may present acutely as a localized area of inflammation. It is a common ocular complication of rheumatoid arthritis but does not carry the same poor prognosis as scleritis.

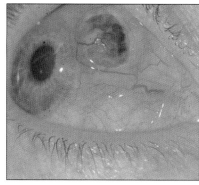

3.34 Scleromalacia perforans in rheumatoid arthritis. Long-standing inflammation of the sclera (scleritis) has resulted in thinning, which exposes the underlying choroid to secondary infection and the risk of eyeball perforation.

- Cardiac and pulmonary complications are usually limited to pericardial and pleural involvement (**3.35**); rare cardiac complications may include constrictive pericarditis, myocarditis and endocarditis; rheumatoid nodules may occur in the lung (**3.36**, **4.132**); diffuse fibrosing alveolitis (**3.35**, **3.36**), Caplan's syndrome (**4.147**) and obliterative bronchiolitis are uncommon pulmonary complications.
- Neurological manifestations include mononeuritis, which is a true extra-articular complication, and carpal tunnel syndrome and cervical myelopathy, which are compression neuropathies secondary to the arthritis process; involvement of the cervical spine can result in cord transection and sudden death if the neck is manipulated inadvertently, for example under an anaesthetic.
- In the kidneys there may be amyloid deposition, but clinical manifestations are usually limited to mild proteinuria with only very few patients developing nephrotic syndrome or renal failure.

Immunological investigations show a positive rheumatoid factor (a circulating immunoglobulin of the IgM type) in about 80% of patients. The most common haematological manifestation is a normochromic, normocytic anaemia (*see*

periarticular osteoporosis followed by joint-space narrowing and periarticular erosions. In long-standing cases subluxation, secondary OA and bony ankylosis are seen (**3.37**).

The principles in the management of all forms of arthritis are similar. The main object is to reduce pain and enable the

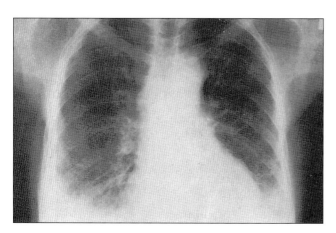

3.35 Pleural effusion is a common complication of rheumatoid arthritis, and it may precede joint symptoms. In this patient it occurred later in the disease, and was accompanied by some reticular nodular shadowing, representing early fibrosing alveolitis, in both lower zones. Pleural effusions should usually be drained to prevent fibrosis.

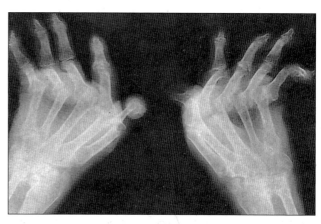

3.37 Radiographic appearance of severe rheumatoid arthritis in the hands. The bones are severely osteoporotic and there are extensive destructive changes with subluxation of many of the finger joints. This radiograph corresponds with the degree of clinical change seen in **3.24** (*see* **3.15** for the appearances at earlier stages).

patient to maintain as near normal a life as possible. Physiotherapists can recommend appropriate exercises to maintain full joint movement and strengthen weak muscles. Wax baths, ice packs, ultrasound and weak electrical current stimulation (interferential therapy) may also alleviate some of the joint symptoms. Aspiration of effusions, for example from the knees (**3.12**), followed by intra-articular steroid injection (**3.38**) may be of short-term value. Occupational therapists can

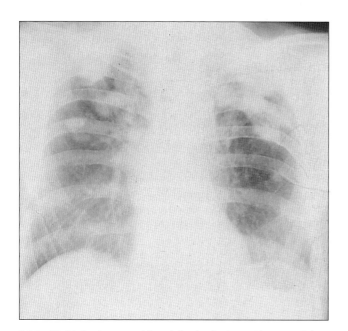

3.36 Multiple rheumatoid nodules in the lung. These nodules are more common in men. They may cavitate; they may require further investigation to exclude the possibility of malignancy. This film also demonstrates some fibrotic changes in both lungs.

p. 412), but hypochromic anaemia may occur, especially if NSAID therapy has caused gastrointestinal blood loss (**3.9**, **8.51**, *see* **p. 410**). The platelet and white cell count may be high and the ESR and plasma viscosity may be raised. Some patients may develop Felty's syndrome, which is an association of splenomegaly and neutropenia with RA.

There may not be any radiological changes in the early stages (**3.15**), but later there is soft-tissue swelling and

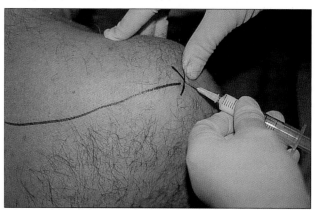

3.38 Intra-articular joint injection with steroid is often of symptomatic benefit in patients with non-infective arthritis. In this patient with RA, the shoulder joint is being injected. The line to the left of the injection site marks the upper border of the scapula.

advise on joint protection and can provide splints and other aids and appliances which allow sufferers to be independent.

The two main types of drug treatment used in RA are the non-steriodal anti-inflammatory drugs (NSAIDs) and the so-called 'slow-acting anti-rheumatic drugs' (SAARDs):

- NSAIDs are the mainstay of treatment but may produce upper gastrointestinal side-effects.
- SAARDs include gold in oral and injectable forms, penicillamine, sulphasalazine and hydroxychloroquine. They induce remission of the arthritis, but gold and penicillamine are particularly associated with high side-effect profiles such as bone marrow suppression, nephrotoxicity and hepatotoxicity. SAARDs should therefore be used only when first line treatment fails or when patients develop extra-articular complications.

In advanced cases, immunosuppressive drugs such as low-dose methotrexate and azathioprine may be used. Corticosteroids have potent anti-inflammatory effects and may be useful in the treatment of an acute flare, although long-term use should be actively discouraged. Intra-articular injections of steroids are also useful in these cases (**3.38**), as is bed rest.

Surgery may have an important role, especially in the more advanced stages of RA. Useful operations range from the removal of local areas of diseased synovial tissue (**3.39**), to the removal of subluxed metatarsal heads, and the total replacement of hip, knee, shoulder and elbow joints or the small joints of the hands (**3.40**).

Felty's syndrome

Felty's syndrome is a complication of long standing, seropostive, nodular deforming RA (**3.24**) in which splenomegaly of various degrees develops and is accompanied by severe leucopenia and a normochromic normocytic anaemia. In addition there may be weight loss, ulceration in the lower limbs (**3.30**) lymphadenopathy, hyperpigmentation, high titres of IgM rheumatoid factor and antinuclear antibodies.

As a conseqence of severe leucopenia, infection is a common presenting feature. It is also a common cause of death, especially in those who have skin ulcers, are on steroids, or have low levels of complement factors and high levels of immune complexes.

There is often suppression of all marrow elements (**3.41**) with diminished red and white cell and platelet production. The ESR, plasma viscosity and CRP are elevated and there are low levels of components of the complement system. The level of rheumatoid factor, cryoglobulins and circulating immune complexes is high. A low serum albumin is a reflection of chronic disease.

Management of Felty's syndrome requires optimal management of rheumatoid disease with SAARDs. Steroids are contraindicated in the presence of neutropenia or overt infection. Splenectomy may be of value, especially in those with recurrent infection and perhaps also in those with leg ulceration.

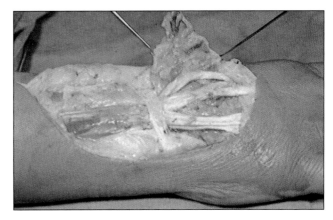

3.39 Surgical removal of diseased synovial tissue in a patient with rheumatoid arthritis.

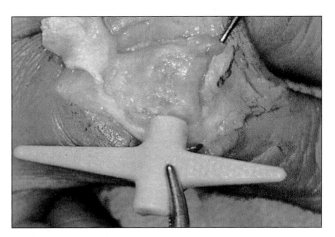

3.40 Proximal interphalangeal joint replacement. A prosthesis is assessed for size.

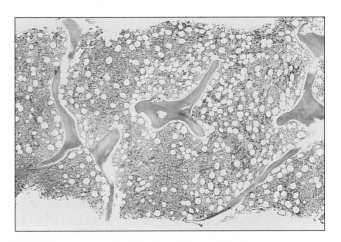

3.41 Bone marrow in Felty's syndrome. This low-power trephine biopsy shows general hypoplasia with a lymphocytic focus. The patient was anaemic, had intractable vasculitic ulceration of the legs and suffered from recurrent infections.

JUVENILE CHRONIC ARTHRITIS (JCA OR STILL'S DISEASE)

Arthritis is uncommon before the age of 16 years (incidence 0.7–1 per 1000) although arthralgia is a common problem. The essential criterion for juvenile chronic arthritis (JCA) is persistent synovitis in one or more joints for at least 3 months.

There are five main types of JCA:

- systemic Still's disease, which has an equal sex incidence and is most common in 2–3-year-olds; it is characterized mainly by systemic features, including a high spiking fever, morbilliform rash, lymphadenopathy, hepatosplenomegaly and pleuro-pericarditis; arthritis is usually a minor feature
- polyarticular Still's disease, which is seronegative for rheumatoid factor (**3.42**); the features include micrognathia (secondary to temporomandibular joint involvement with abnormal mandibular growth, **3.43**), loss of neck extension (cervical spine involvement, **3.44**), unequal limb lengths (premature closure or overgrowth of the epiphyses) and fixed flexion deformities of the lower limbs

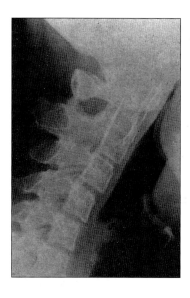

3.44　Cervical spine involvement in Still's disease. Ankylosis of the upper cervical spine is shown on this radiograph.

- pauciarticular (four joints or fewer) Still's disease, which usually affects the large joints of 2–5-year-old girls; antinuclear antibodies are usually positive and chronic iritis (**3.45**) may lead to blindness; regular slit-lamp examination is necessary, because iritis in Still's disease may be asymptomatic
- seropositive polyarthritis, which resembles adult RA
- juvenile ankylosing spondylitis, which is more common in HLA-B27-positive boys of 10–15 years of age; the clinical features resemble those of the adult form, although back pain is not prominent.

Treatment is with NSAIDs. SAARDs may be effective in the polyarticular type JCA but are associated with a high incidence of side-effects. Corticosteroids should be avoided because of their retarding effect on growth. Physiotherapy and joint protection are important. Long periods of rest may sometimes be necessary.

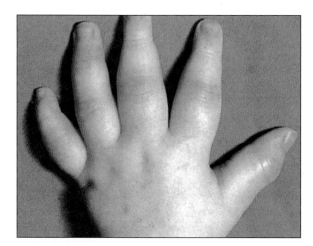

3.42　The hands in juvenile chronic arthritis. There is marked swelling of the proximal interphalangeal joints.

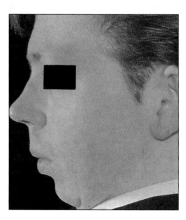

3.43　Micrognathia in a young adult who had juvenile chronic arthritis. The condition was associated with polyarticular Still's disease and with cervical spine involvement (**3.44**).

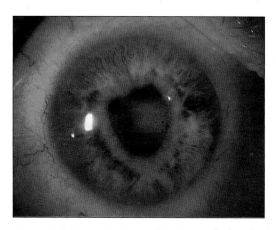

3.45　Iridocyclitis in pauciarticular Still's disease. Distortion of the pupil is caused by adhesion of the iris to the lens (posterior synechiae).

SERONEGATIVE SPONDARTHRITIS

Seronegative spondarthritis describes a group of conditions with a number of common characteristics. These include the absence of rheumatoid factor and other autoantibodies in the blood, involvement of the spine, a peripheral inflammatory arthritis, similar extra-articular features (predominantly mucocutaneous) and a high incidence of the tissue antigen HLA-B27.

Ankylosing spondylitis

Ankylosing (fusion) spondylitis (spinal vertebral joint inflammation) presents primarily in young men (9 males : 1 female), but is becoming more common in women, who tend to have milder disease. The aetiology is unknown but there appears to be a strong genetic component. A family history is common and over 90% of patients possess the HLA-B27 tissue antigen. However, 7% of the population are HLA-B27-positive and the prevalence of ankylosing spondylitis is 1%. Thus environmental factor(s) are also likely to be important.

Low back pain with morning stiffness occurs as a result of sacroiliac joint involvement. The pain is worse at rest and is often felt in the buttocks, especially when seated. It may radiate to the back of the thighs mimicking sciatica, although the latter is usually unilateral and relieved by rest. As the disease progresses upwards, pain is experienced at higher spinal levels. Patients with thoracic spine involvement may present with pleuritic chest pain but, unlike true pleurisy, it is usually bilateral. On examination, there is loss of lumbar lordosis and a fixed kyphosis usually compensated for by extension of the cervical spine, eventually producing the stooped 'question mark' posture (**3.46**). The sacroiliac joints are tender on percussion

and springing of the pelvis. Movements of the spine at various levels are restricted (**3.47**) and so is chest expansion. Changes in the peripheral joints, usually the larger ones, are similar to those seen in RA and show signs of inflammation. Extra-articular manifestions include iritis (30%) which may sometimes precede spinal involvement (**3.48**). About 4% of patients develop aortitis with signs of a collapsing pulse and the early diastolic murmur of aortic regurgitation (*see* **p. 224**). Cardiac conduction defects occur in 10% of patients. Pulmonary restriction resulting from chest wall involvement and lung fibrosis (**3.49**) may also occur.

Blood tests are often not very helpful. ESR and plasma viscosity may be raised but rheumatoid factor is not present in the blood. HLA-B27 tissue type is found in 95% of cases. Radiological changes of sacroiliitis include widening of joint space and juxtarticular erosion and sclerosis (**3.50**). In the spine there is squaring of the vertebrae caused by erosion of their

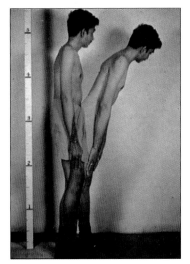

3.47 Ankylosing spondylitis. At an earlier stage the deformity is much less marked, but these superimposed pictures show gross loss of forward flexion on attempted toe-touching as a result of severe spinal involvement.

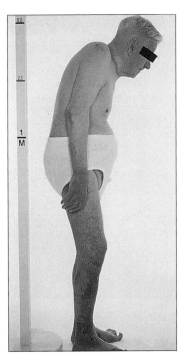

3.46 Advanced ankylosing spondylitis. Eventually, the trunk may become fixed in a fully bent position, so that the patient cannot see directly ahead – the classic 'question mark' posture.

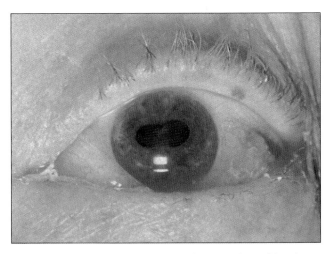

3.48 Acute iritis or iridocyclitis may be an early problem in ankylosing spondylitis. Note the irregular pupil and the haziness in the anterior chamber of the eye.

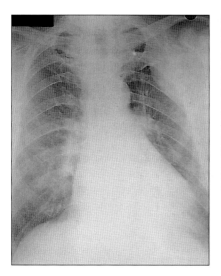

3.49 Pulmonary fibrosis in a patient with ankylosing spondylitis. The combination of pulmonary fibrosis and restricted movement of the chest wall may lead to respiratory failure in a small proportion of patients with ankylosing spondylitis.

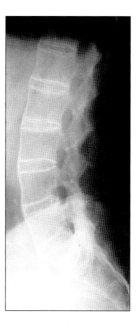

3.51 'Bamboo spine'. This lateral X-ray of the lumbar spine in advanced ankylosing spondylitis shows rigid ankylosis resulting from calcification of the spinal ligaments.

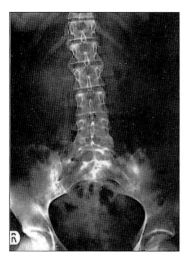

3.50 Sacroiliac joint involvement in ankylosing spondylitis is often the earliest objective evidence of the disease. Initially there is blurring and later obliteration of the sacroiliac joints. This radiograph also shows a relatively early stage of syndesmophyte formation with ankylosis between lumbar vertebrae.

irradiation, which was popular in the 1950s, is not used now because of risks of the later development of malignancy.

Psoriatic arthropathy

Psoriatic arthropathy occurs in 7–8% of patients with psoriasis. There is a strong genetic influence and a family history is common. Skin psoriasis usually precedes the onset of the arthritis, but the reverse may happen occasionally. Skin lesions may be found on the scalp, behind the ears, in the umbilicus and the natal cleft, as well as in the common places such as the extensor aspect of the elbows and knees and the trunk (**3.52** and *see* **p. 69**).

corners. Syndesmophytes (bony deposition) form at the margins of the vertebrae. These may join together and produce the classic appearance of a 'bamboo spine' (**3.51**). There may also be radiological evidence of enthesopathy (calcification and new bone formation in the soft tissues) with erosions, sclerosis and soft-tissue calcification around the ischial tuberosities, iliac crests, greater trochanters, patellae and calcanea. CT and MRI can show early inflammatory changes, and are required in teenagers whose growth is incomplete, as plain radiographs are uninterpretable in this group.

Physiotherapy is most important, and appropriate back exercises should be done daily in order to avoid spinal deformities. Hydrotherapy is also valuable. Pain control can usually be achieved by NSAIDs. Other drugs, including sulphasalazine and methotrexate, may sometimes be used in advanced cases, although their role is not fully confirmed. Iritis may be recurrent, leading to severe ocular damage, and should be treated vigorously with topical steroids. Patients should not smoke, to minimize the impactf any lung involvement. Spinal

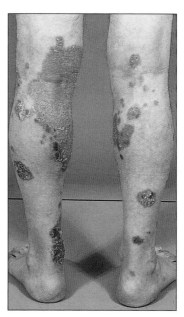

3.52 Typical psoriatic skin lesions on the legs. Not all patients with psoriatic arthropathy have such obvious skin lesions.

There are five forms of psoriatic arthropathy:

- the distal phalangeal type (**3.53**) is more common in men and is usually accompanied by nail lesions such as pitting (**3.5**), ridging, onycholysis (lifting of the nail, **2.19**) and hyperkeratosis
- the polyarthritic form may be indistinguishable from RA but it is persistently seronegative
- oligoarthritis usually affects the knees or the other large joints with an asymmetrical distribution
- a spondylitic form resembles ankylosing spondylitis and 60–70% of these patients are HLA-B27-positive
- arthritis mutilans (5%) is rare but severe (**3.54**) and is usually associated with extensive skin psoriasis.

The pathology is similar to RA but there is more fibrosis of the joint tissues resulting in ankylosis, and bony changes with periosteal inflammation produce the classic sausage-shaped

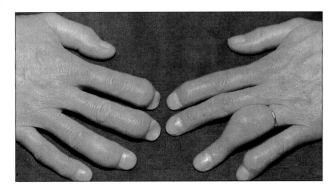

3.53   Psoriatic arthritis involving mainly the distal interphalangeal joints. There is also deformity and swelling of the left fourth proximal interphalangeal joint (dactylitis).

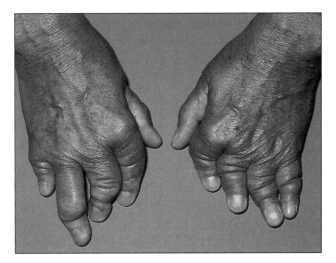

3.54   Severe psoriatic arthritis (arthritis mutilans). There is a gross destructive arthropathy, involving all joints of the hands and wrists. The phalanges have 'telescoped' (*see* **3.55**), resulting in shortening of the fingers and gross impairment of function.

digits (dactylitis, **3.53**). Extra-articular features are rare. Features in the blood are similar to those seen in ankylosing spondylitis. There are no specific radiological features, but the distribution of the arthritis can provide an important guide to the diagnosis. Periosteal new bone formation reflects periostitis. The 'pencil-in-cup' appearance of the hand radiograph is caused by periarticular bone dissolution with cupping of the proximal ends of the phalanges and whittling of the distal bone ends (**3.55**).

Most patients have mild arthritis and respond to standard NSAID treatment. In more advanced cases, corticosteroids and immunosuppressive agents such as methotrexate or azathioprine may be required. Unlike RA, patients do not respond to penicillamine.

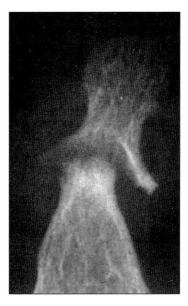

3.55   Pencil-in-cup deformity of the distal phalanx in psoriatic arthropathy. There is loss of the head and splaying of the base of the distal phalanx.

Reactive arthritis

Reactive arthritis (Reiter's syndrome) has a high male to female ratio (20:1) and up to 90% of patients possess the HLA-B27 antigen. It is likely to be a generalized reaction to an infection, either urogenital or intestinal. *Chlamydia trachomatis* has been shown to be the infective organism of the genital type, whereas the dysenteric form may follow infection with many bacteria, including *Shigella flexneri*, *Yersinia enterocolitica*, *Campylobacter jejuni* and occasionally *Salmonella* species.

The classic symptom triad comprises urethritis, conjunctivitis (**3.6**) and arthritis, although all three may not be evident. Conjuntivitis is bilateral and usually mild with few symptoms. There may be a purulent but sterile discharge. Uveitis may be found in up to 30% of long-standing diseases. The arthritis usually affects the large joints in the lower limbs. The spine is also frequently involved, especially the sacroiliac joints (20–30% of patients). Such patients develop features that are similar to those of ankylosing spondylitis. Small joints in the hands and feet may also be involved as may be tendons (especially Achilles) and the plantar fascia. Extra-articular complications are common and involve the skin (keratoderma blenorrhagicum, **3.56**), nails and mucocutaneous surface – painless mouth ulcers (**3.57**), circinate balanitis (**3.58**) and cervicitis.

The acute episode may take a month or longer to settle and patients often respond to conservative treatment such as NSAIDs. Iritis, if severe, should be treated with topical steroids. Later there may be exacerbations with remissions and up to 80% of patients may develop chronic joint disease, visual problems or urethral strictures. The urethritis can be treated by erythromycin or tetracycline, but neither alters the course of the arthritis.

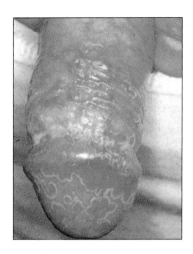

3.58   Circinate balanitis in Reiter's syndrome. Small, discrete, round or oval red macules or erosions often become confluent.

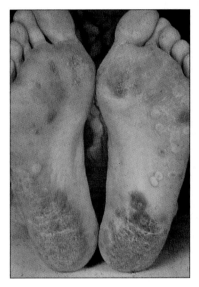

3.56   Keratoderma blenorrhagicum is a hyperkeratotic skin condition found in Reiter's syndrome. The lesions start as brown raised hyperkeratotic patches which grow and coalesce into raised yellow-brown patches. These are typically found on the soles of the feet but may be found in all skin areas, including the scalp. Pustular psoriasis may produce the same clinical and histological features (*see* **p. 70**).

Other seronegative spondarthritides

Other seronegative spondarthritides include arthritides associated with inflammatory bowel disease (Crohn's disease and ulcerative colitis) and Whipple's disease, a rare malabsorption condition. Treatment of the bowel conditions may lead to remission of the arthropathy, especially in ulcerative colitis.

INFECTIVE ARTHRITIS

Infective arthritis may be caused by bacteria, viruses or fungi that are usually borne in the blood to the joint. Arthritis may occur in viral infections with parvovirus B19, hepatitis B and HIV, and transient arthralgia may occur in many other viral infections.

In bacterial arthritis, a primary focus may be identified elsewhere, for example a boil on the skin or otitis media. The common infecting bacteria are shown in **3.59**. Arthritis may be

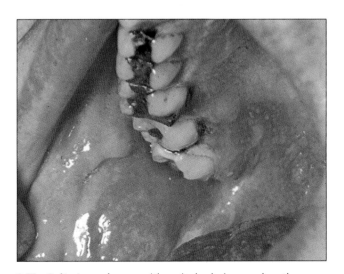

3.57   Reiter's syndrome, with vesicular lesions and erythema of the hard palate and lesions on the cheek.

THE MOST COMMON BACTERIAL CAUSES OF INFECTIVE ARTHRITIS
Staphylococcus sp.
Streptococcus pyogenes
Neisseria meningitidis
Neisseria gonorrhoeae
Salmonella spp.
Streptococcus pneumoniae
Pseudomonas aeruginosa
Borrelia burgdorferi
Mycobacterium tuberculosis
Brucella sp.

3.59   The most common bacterial causes of infective arthritis.

acute or chronic. Acute septic arthritis often involves joints that have been previously damaged by RA or OA, or occurs in patients who are immunocompromised. The patient usually presents with fever and rigors; the affected joint is swollen, tender to touch and has an effusion (**3.1**, **3.8**).

There may be other clinical clues, for example purpura (*see* **p. 437**) and the joint may be held protected in flexion. In patients with pre-existing joint disease, there is often difficulty in deciding whether the changes are caused by a flare-up of the basic disease or infection, in which case the diagnosis is made by joint aspiration of a purulent aspirate (**3.12**); there is usually systemic leucocytosis and blood culture may be positive. Acute arthritis may also be revealed by other techniques including radiography, CT and scintigraphy (**3.18**).

Establishing the diagnosis and initiating treatment is a matter of urgency. Treatment with appropriate antibiotics is mandatory to stop cartilage erosion and repeated aspiration of the effusion or surgical drainage of the joint may be required.

Chronic infective arthritis may be caused by organisms such as *Mycobacterium tuberculosis*, *Borrelia burgdorferi* (*see* **p. 41**) and a range of fungi. Arthritis may also occur in patients with bacterial endocarditis (*see* **p. 231**).

Tuberculous arthritis remains a problem in the elderly, in alcoholics, diabetics and those who are immunocompromised (including those with AIDS). In developing countries, tuberculosis remains a major public health problem associated with poverty, overcrowding and malnutrition.

Tuberculous arthritis is usually caused by dissemination of the disease from lung or kidney. It usually involves a single joint – most commonly the hip, knee (**3.60**), sacroiliac joints or intervertebral joints of the spine. The onset is insidious with systemic upset, malaise, anorexia, weight loss and night sweats followed by discomfort and swelling of the affected joint. There may be features of tuberculosis elsewhere in the patient, especially in the lung and kidney.

Diagnosis may be made by joint aspiration or synovial biopsy and culture. Radiology is unhelpful initially, showing only soft-tissue changes, but with time there is progressive cartilage and bone erosion. Treatment is to immobilize the joint in the acute phase and give the appropriate antibiotic.

OSTEOARTHRITIS (OA)

Osteoarthritis (OA), a common degenerative disease of the joints, affects approximately 10% of all adults (men and women) and the prevalence increases with age. The disease is characterized by focal areas of destruction of articular cartilage, sclerosis of the underlying bone and hypertrophy of soft tissues.

The aetiology is multifactorial, although a polygenic inheritance pattern is recognized in the generalized 'nodal' form that causes distal and proximal interphalangeal arthritis of the hands, particularly in women. Mechanical factors include obesity, previous limb trauma, abnormal joint congruity, joint hypermobility, congenital dislocation of the hip and certain occupations – 'wicket keeper's thumb', 'Zulu dancer's hip', etc. OA may also be secondary to metabolic disorders such as ochronosis, acromegaly and gout or to other inflammatory arthropathies, for example RA.

OA most commonly affects the weight-bearing joints, in particular the knees, hips and spine, and the interphalangeal joints of the hands (**3.61**). The wrists and ankles are less often involved. Not all patients with joint symptoms have radiographic changes; and not all radiographic changes are associated with symptoms. Pain can be severe and incapacitating and is worse on use of the joint and at the end of the day. Morning stiffness is not common, though stiffness after prolonged inactivity may occur. Clinical signs in advanced cases include crepitus, limitation of movement and joint deformities. The function of the hands is often affected (**3.62**). Heberden's nodes are found at the distal interphalangeal joints

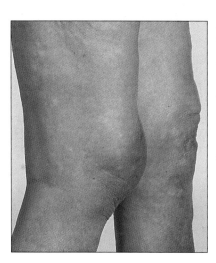

3.60 Tuberculous effusion of the right knee. In this patient, arthritis followed untreated pulmonary tuberculosis. The knee joint was destroyed and arthrodesis was required. Note the signs of weight loss in the legs.

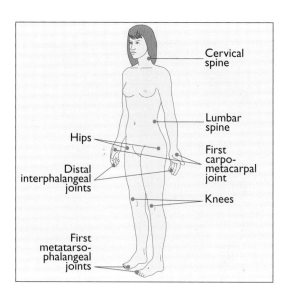

3.61 Joints commonly affected by osteoarthritis.

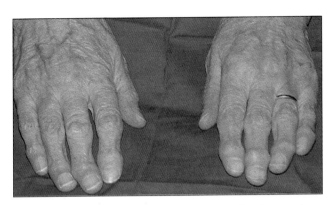

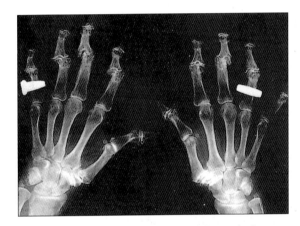

(**3.63**) and Bouchard's nodes at the proximal interphalangeal joints (**3.64**) of the hands. There may be valgus (knock knees) and varus (bow knees) (**3.65**), deformities of the knees and fixed flexion of the hip.

Blood tests are usually unhelpful, but they may sometimes reveal underlying metabolic disorders. X-rays (**3.66, 3.67**) may show loss of joint space resulting from cartilage damage. Osteophytosis (formation of new bone), altered bone contour, subchondral sclerosis (increased bone density) and cystic formation result from bony remodelling. There may also be soft-tissue swelling and periarticular calcification.

3.62 Osteoarthritis of the hands showing Herberden's nodes at the distal interphalangeal joints and Bouchard's nodes at the proximal interphalangeal joints.

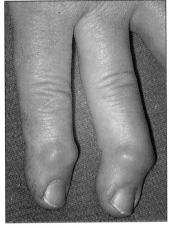

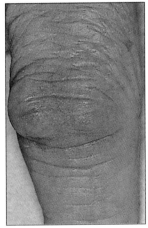

3.63 Herberden's nodes in osteoarthritis are cystic protuberances at the distal interphalangeal joints. They are usually painless, but may occasionally ache.

3.64 Bouchard's nodes in osteoarthritis are similar protuberances occurring at the proximal interphalangeal joints.

3.66 Osteoarthritis of the hands. This radiograph shows an advanced case, with severe changes in the distal and proximal interphalangeal joints and in the first carpometacarpal joints: loss of joint space, subchondral sclerosis, osteophytosis and subarticular cysts.

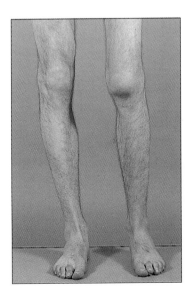

3.65 Bilateral osteoarthritis of the knees, associated with joint deformity, an effusion (confirmed clinically) in the patient's left knee and severe wasting of the quadriceps muscles in both thighs.

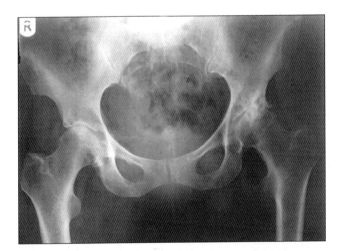

3.67 Osteoarthritis of the left hip. There is irregular narrowing of the joint space associated with thinning of the cartilage. There are osteophytes (projections of new bone) around the left femoral head and generalized thinning of the bone in the left femoral head with early bone cyst formation. The right hip shows some loss of joint space but is otherwise normal.

Treatment primarily involves pain relief, initially with simple analgesics. NSAIDs may be added if these are required, though the use of these drugs in the elderly population should be minimized. Intra-articular steroid injections are useful when there are signs of inflammation. Obese patients should lose weight. Appropriate exercises should be taught to strengthen the various muscle groups acting on the affected joint. Surgery may be considered when pain becomes intractable and severe limitation of mobility is present. Secondary causes should be sought and treated.

CRYSTAL ARTHROPATHY

Gout

Gout is most common in men and postmenopausal women, affecting up to 1 in 100 of the population. The classic history is of an abrupt onset of pain and swelling (usually at night) in the big toe with red, shiny skin overlying it (**3.1**, **3.68**), but any joint or joints may be affected (**3.69**). The serum uric acid level is often high (though it may be low during an acute attack) and joint aspiration reveals needle-shaped crystals (monosodium urate monohydrate) which appear negatively birefringent under a polarized light microscope (**3.13**). The acute episode subsides with desquamation of skin.

Uric acid is the breakdown product of the purine residues of nucleic acid. Two-thirds of it is excreted via the kidney and the rest via the gut. Most patients have primary gout, but possible secondary causes include:

- overproduction, as in the myelo- and lymphoproliferative disorders, carcinomatosis and the rare specific enzyme defects in purine biosynthesis and degradation, for example Lesch–Nyhan syndrome, a condition characterized by mental retardation and self-mutilation
- decreased renal excretion in renal failure and with inhibition of the renal tubular excretion pathway, for example the use of thiazide diuretics, lead poisoning and in conditions causing acidaemia (diabetic ketoacidosis, starvation and excessive alcohol ingestion)
- Increased dietary intake of purines, for example from offal.

Not all patients with hyperuricaemia have gout. However, the likelihood of crystal formation increases as the uric acid level increases, more so at low temperatures, and this explains the peripheral distribution of gout. As well as the first metatarsophalangeal joint (70%), the small joints in the hands, wrists, ankles and knees are also often involved.

Chronic tophaceous gout is characterized by the deposition of urate (chalky, toothpaste-like appearance) in the periarticular and subcutaneous tissues. The distribution of tophi is similar to that of rheumatoid nodules – the most common sites being the extensor surfaces of the elbow, the fingers (**3.69**, **3.71**), the anterior aspect of the knee, the Achilles tendon and the ear (**3.7**). Such tophi are now becoming rare as a result of the widespread use of allopurinol.

During acute gout, there may be a leucocytosis and the ESR or plasma viscosity is usually raised. Radiography of the joints may show soft-tissue swelling but may otherwise be normal in acute gout. In chronic cases, there are additional features such as joint-space narrowing, subarticular (compared with RA, which is periarticular) 'punched-out' cystic lesions and secondary osteoarthritic changes (**3.70**).

NSAIDs are useful during acute attacks. Intra-articular steroids or short course systemic steroids are also useful. Colchicine may be effective in acute gout, but side-effects are common at the necessary doses. A lower dose of colchicine may subsequently be used for prophylaxis. The xanthine oxidase inhibitor allopurinol is effective in the prophylactic reduction of serum urate, but it must not be used in acute gout or in renal failure, and it may precipitate an attack of gout even when started at other times.

Pseudogout

Pseudogout is characterized by the deposition of calcium pyrophosphate dihydrate crystals in the cartilage and synovium

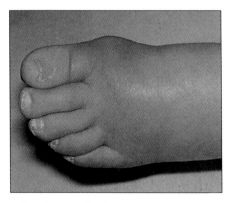

3.68 **Gout.** A classic attack of acute gout affects the big toe (see also **3.1**).

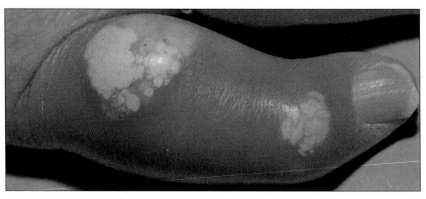

3.69 **'Acute on chronic' gout in the little finger.** The tophi helped to confirm the diagnosis. On aspiration, they were found to contain monosodium urate monohydrate crystals (see **3.13**).

(**3.72**). There is no evidence of an underlying disease in most patients, but a metabolic disorder, for example hyper-parathyroidism or haemochromatosis, may be found in some patients. Calcium pyrophosphate dihydrate crystals are rhomboid and weakly positively birefringent (**3.14**). The clinical features are similar to those seen in gout, although the onset is slower and the course milder. Conservative treatments such as NSAIDs and intra-articular steroid injections are usually effective.

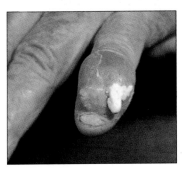

3.70   Gout. This radiograph of the hand shows destructive changes in the proximal and distal interphalangeal joints with multiple punched-out areas caused by urate deposition.

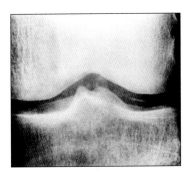

3.71   Chronic gout with a discharging tophus in the finger.

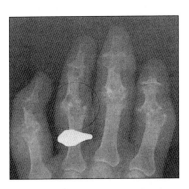

3.72   Chondrocalcinosis of the knee. The radiograph shows calcification in cartilage and synovium.

CONNECTIVE TISSUE DISEASES

The term 'connective tissue diseases' is synonymous with 'collagen vascular diseases'. Both describe a group of conditions characterized by the occurrence of vasculitis, multisystem involvement, arthritis or arthralgia and abnormal immuno-logical features, for example autoantibodies and immune complex deposition.

SYSTEMIC LUPUS ERYTHEMATOSUS (SLE)

Systemic lupus erythematosus (SLE), an autoimmune disorder, is uncommon in Caucasians (prevalence 0.1%), although it is being diagnosed more often with the development of increasingly sensitive diagnostic tests. It is more common in other races, with a prevalence of up to 1 in 250 among black women (**3.73**). The peak age of onset is 20–40 years and women are more often affected than men. The aetiology is unknown, but there is a slight increase in incidence in the families of patients with SLE and in individuals with the histocompatibility markers DR2 and DR3. The aetiological role of environmental factors, such as exposure to sunlight and certain viral infections, is being investigated but is not yet clear. Some drugs may produce a lupus-like syndrome, including hydralazine, procainamide, phenothiazines, isoniazid and oral contraceptives. Almost all patients possess an antibody against nuclear antigens (ANA; **3.10**). This is, however, a non-specific marker and may be found in other connective tissue disorders. The antibodies to double stranded DNA (anti-dsDNA) and Smith antigens (anti-Sm) are found less frequently (40–70%) but are very specific for SLE. Antiphospholipid antibodies (e.g. anticardiolipin) may also be found, and there may be associated thrombophilia (*see* **p. 442**). The primary pathology is that of a multisystem inflammatory process, probably secondary to antigen–antibody reactions.

Patients may present with constitutional symptoms, such as anorexia, tiredness, fever and weight loss, and many organ systems may be involved:

• Skin involvement is most common; rashes may be local or generalized; the classic 'butterfly rash' on the face may occur in isolation (**3.73, 3.74**), but a more generalized rash may also occur – usually in sun-exposed areas (**3.75**). The inflammatory process may manifest itself as a vasculitis, with

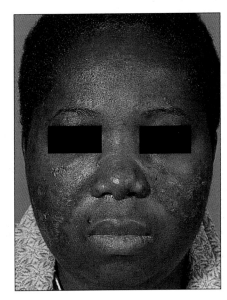

3.73   Systemic lupus erythematosus is most common in black women of child-bearing age, such as this 33-year old West Indian woman who presented with a rash over her cheeks.

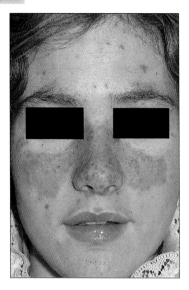

3.74 Systemic lupus erythematosus. The classic bat or butterfly wing rash in a 17-year-old. The rash was accompanied by fever, weight loss and polyarthropathy.

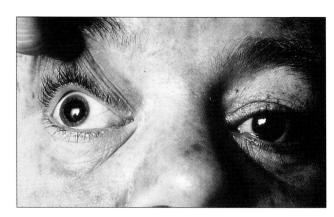

3.76 Cranial neuropathy is a frequent neural manifestation of systemic lupus erythematosus. This patient has a third nerve palsy. The right eye faces 'down and out', the pupil is fixed and dilated and the patient has a unilateral ptosis (the upper lid is lifted here to reveal the other signs).

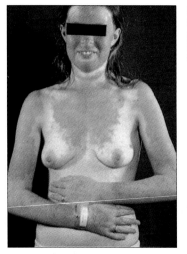

3.75 Systemic lupus erythematosus. A persistent erythematous rash may occur in sun-exposed areas.

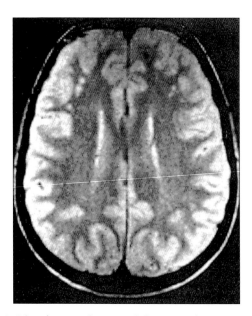

3.77 CNS involvement in systemic lupus erythematosus, as demonstrated by MRI. The numerous small white areas represent vasculitic lesions in the brain. Psychiatric symptoms (disorientation and paranoia) were an early manifestation of systemic lupus erythematosus in this patient.

periungual infarcts (**3.31**, **3.88**), erythematous nodules, palpable purpura, livedo reticularis (**2.132**, **3.95**) and Raynaud's phenomenon being common findings. Alopecia, localized or generalized, may occur (*see* **p. 89**).

- Lung involvement results in pleurisy and pulmonary infarcts.
- Cardiac involvement results in pericarditis, myocarditis and endocarditis.
- Renal involvement is often associated with a poor prognosis (*see* **p. 277**); the most common histological lesion is a diffuse proliferative glomerulonephritis.
- Neurological complications include epilepsy, focal neurological signs such as hemiparesis, aseptic meningitis, cranial and peripheral neuropathies (**3.76**) and psychiatric disturbances (**3.77**).
- Blood involvement may give rise to leucopenia, thrombocytopenia, lymphadenopathy and a thrombotic tendency (thrombophilia) which is more marked in those patients with positive anticardiolipin or antiphospholipid antibodies (*see* **p. 442**)
- Joint involvement may resemble RA, but there is usually no evidence of erosive changes on radiographs. Avascular necrosis of bone may occur.

Investigations may show a raised ESR, plasma viscosity or CRP in addition to the above. ANA is present in over 90% of patients. Anti-dsDNA may also be present, as may other subclasses of ANA such as the anti-Ro and anti-Sm antibodies. The immunoglobulin levels may also be increased. The lupus band test on a skin biopsy may be of value (**3.11**). Radiography is usually unhelpful. Advances in diagnostic techniques and monitoring systems have improved both the morbidity and mortality (there is now a 95% 5-year survival rate in SLE from diagnosis). Patients should be advised to avoid excessive sunlight exposure. Sun-blocking creams can be very useful. Mild disease usually requires only symptomatic drug treatment, for example chloroquine is useful when there are troublesome skin lesions and for suppressing moderate joint disease. When the condition becomes active, systemic steroids and immunosuppressive agents, for example azathioprine and cyclophosphamide, are the mainstay of treatment. Pregnancy is not contraindicated, but there is an increased rate of fetal loss and complications during pregnancy. SLE may flare during the post partum period.

SYSTEMIC SCLEROSIS (SSc)

Systemic sclerosis (SSc) is an uncommon idiopathic multisystem disease, also known as scleroderma, that predominantly affects the skin and blood vessels. There is a female preponderance (female:male = 3:1). Progressive fibrosis and atrophy are the main pathological features.

There are two types of SSc:

- The diffuse type is characterized by skin and vascular changes and visceral involvement is common. The skin is thickened and tight and this sometimes results in contractures (**3.78**). Telangiectasia are a common feature (**3.79**), and Raynaud's phenomenon occurs in over 95% of patients (*see* p. 243). It is only occasionally accompanied by calcinosis. Involvement of the locomotor system may manifest itself as myositis and polyarthritis. Involvement of

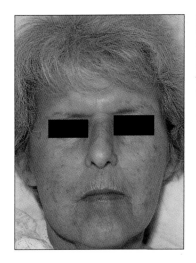

3.79 Systemic sclerosis. Puckering of the perioral skin is seen; the skin is generally waxy and shiny, and multiple telangiectasia are visible on the face and neck.

the gastrointestinal tract may appear as dysphagia (**3.84**), bowel distension, diarrhoea and weight loss resulting from malabsorption. Basal pulmonary fibrosis (*see* p. 183) develops in 45% of patients. Cardiac involvement may result in a restrictive cardiomyopathy or conduction defects. Renal involvement is associated with a high mortality; patients usually present with proteinuria and hypertension, which may be severe and lead to end-stage renal failure within months. (*see* p. 282).

- The limited type, which has a better prognosis, is also known as the CRST or CREST syndrome and is characterized by calcinosis, which may lead to ulceration (**3.80**, **3.81**) and autoamputation of the digits (**3.82**), and may also be found elsewhere (**3.83**), Raynaud's phenomenon, oesophageal involvement (**3.84**), sclerodactyly and telangiectasia (**3.79**). All of the visceral manifestations of diffuse scleroderma may also occur in the 'limited' disease, with the exception of renal disease, which is very rare.

There are no specific diagnostic tests. The ESR may be slightly raised and the full blood count may show an anaemia of chronic disorder. Both RA latex and ANA may be positive. The anti-scl 70 and anti-centromere antibodies are more specific autoantibodies and have been shown to be present in some but not all patients with the diffuse and limited types of SSc, respectively.

Treatment is symptomatic. Raynaud's phenomenon may be controlled by simple measures such as stopping smoking and using warm gloves. In more severe cases, vasodilator drugs such as nifedipine can be used. Antacids or H$_2$-antagonists, or both, are useful for patients with dyspeptic symptoms. Oesophageal dilatation may be useful in patients who have developed a stricture. Hypertension should be treated aggressively, usually with angiotensin-converting enzyme inhibitors. Specific treatment for SSc has been disappointing. Penicillamine has been tried, but it probably has only a limited use in patients with rapid skin progression.

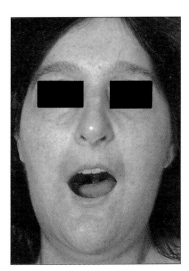

3.78 Systemic sclerosis. The skin around the mouth is tight, and the patient has opened her mouth as far as possible. Her skin is generally waxy and shiny.

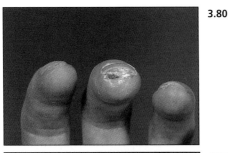

3.80

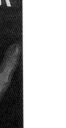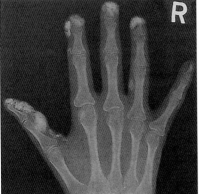

3.81

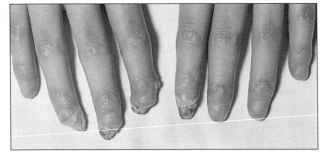

3.82

3.80, 3.81 and 3.82   In the calcinosis of systemic sclerosis the calcium deposits are characteristically seen in the fingers. The size of these hard, nontender nodules varies from a few millimetres to several centimetres. If very small they may not be visible under the skin (but can be palpated) or they may ulcerate through the skin (**3.80**). X-ray examination may show extensive calcinosis even in the absence of marked ulceration (**3.81**). In more advanced disease, chalk-like material is discharged through the ulcerated skin, and progressive autoamputation of the fingertips may occur (**3.82**).

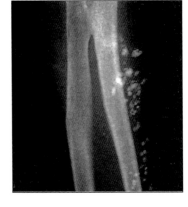

3.83   Calcinosis in the forearm of a patient with advanced systemic sclerosis.

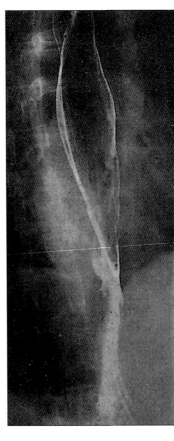

3.84   Systemic sclerosis affecting the oesophagus. The oesophagus is rigidly dilated, and there is loss of peristaltic movement.

POLYMYOSITIS AND DERMATOMYOSITIS

Polymyositis and dermatomyositis are closely related to each other and are uncommon. The incidence is not known, but is probably similar to that of SSc. There are five types:

- primary dermatomyositis
- primary polymyositis
- secondary dermatomyositis or polymyositis (90% of cases have an underlying malignant condition)
- childhood dermatomyositis or polymyositis
- dermatomyositis or polymyositis associated with a collagen vascular disease.

The cause is unclear, but a viral aetiology has been suggested, such as rubella, influenza and coxsackie infections.

The proximal (shoulder and pelvic girdle) muscle groups are commonly affected and patients may have difficulty lifting their arms and getting up and down stairs. Involvement of the skin gives rise to a heliotrope rash on the eyelids with periorbital oedema (**3.85**, **3.86**). This rash may spread to the shoulders, chest, arms and hands. In the hands, Goddron's patches (**3.87**) may be found: these are scaly, erythematous lesions on the dorsum of the hands, knuckles and extensor surfaces of the other small joints. Nail-fold infarcts are common (**3.88**). Other features include dysphagia, arthralgia, calcification of the

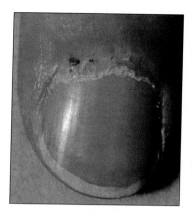

3.88 Erythema, telangiectasia and a small periungual infarct, together with ragged cuticles. These appearance are commonly seen in dermatomyositis and in SLE. Violaceous plaques and papules may occur also on the knuckles, knees, and elbows in dermatomyositis.

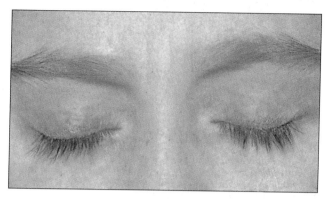

3.85 Dermatomyositis. Slight oedema of the eyelids with a red-mauve discoloration and some telangiectasia.

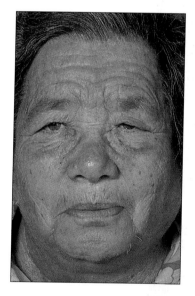

3.86 Dermatomyositis. This elderly lady has characteristic erythema and oedema of the face. She also complained of proximal muscle weakness. Investigation revealed that she had an underlying carcinoma of the bronchus.

subcutaneous tissues and muscles (**3.83**), Raynaud's phenomenon, and myocarditis. Pulmonary involvement, in the form of fibrosing alveolitis or aspiration pneumonia, is accompanied by a high mortality. In childhood, a systemic vasculitis is common.

Laboratory investigations reveal raised muscle enzyme levels, abnormalities in the electromyograph and inflammatory cell infiltration in muscle biopsy. Treatment is with high-dose steroids, or immunosuppressive drugs such as azathioprine, cyclophosphamide and methotrexate, or both. Bed rest is imperative in the acute phases. A search for an underlying malignancy is mandatory in all adult cases.

SJÖGREN'S SYNDROME

Sjögren's syndrome is characterized by dryness of the eyes (sicca syndrome) and mouth (xerostomia) caused by chronic dysfunction of the exocrine glands. Women (age 40–60 years) are more often affected (female:male = 9:1). It may occur alone or in association with RA or other connective tissue disorders.

Patients complain of a burning and itchy sensation in the eyes and there is impaired tear production. Involvement of the salivary glands results in xerostomia (**3.89**) with difficulty in speaking and swallowing, a high incidence of dental caries (**3.90**) and a predisposition to oral candidiasis. The parotid glands may be enlarged. Any mucous membrane covered areas may also be affected, for example nose, throat, larynx, bronchi and vagina. Other features include pancreatitis, pleuritis, vasculitis, renal tubular acidosis and chronic interstitial nephritis. There is an increased incidence of malignant lymphomas.

Rheumatoid factor (70%) and other autoantibodies (anti-Ro and anti-La antibodies) may be present. Schirmer's tear test, a simple bedside test, can be performed to detect the diminished tear production (**3.91**). Slit-lamp examination of the eyes is essential, and staining with rose bengal solution may also be diagnostic, as the superficial ulcers take up the stain (**3.92**).

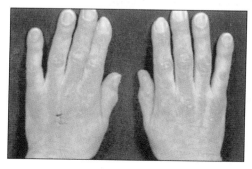

3.87 Goddron's patches in a patient with dermatomyositis. Note the scaly, erythematous nature of the lesions on the dorsa of the hands.

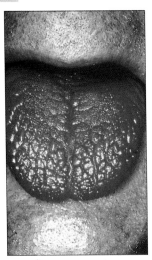

3.89 A dry tongue – xerostomia – in Sjögren's syndrome. Xerostomia results from the involvement of the salivary glands.

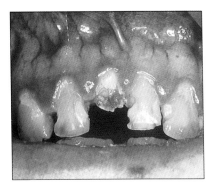

3.90 Severe dental caries in a patient with Sjögren's syndrome.

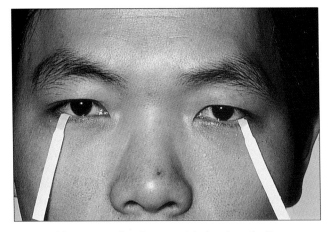

3.91 Schirmer's test for dry eyes. A strip of sterile filter paper of standard pore size is placed over the lower lid. The patient is asked to close the eyes gently, and after 5 minutes the length of the wet area is measured. Diminished tear production is present if it is less than 15 mm.

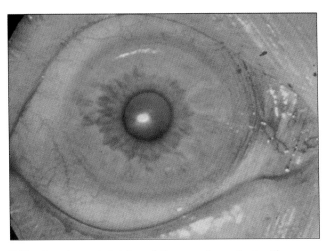

3.92 Rose bengal staining of the eye of a patient with Sjögren's syndrome. Tiny superficial ulcers have taken up the pink stain and are seen on the nasal side.

No specific treatment is available, but artificial tears can be used to lubricate the eyes with good effect though artificial saliva (hypromellose or polyvinyl alcohol) is less effective. Attention should be paid to oral hygiene, to minimize the risk of oral candidiasis and dental caries.

RELAPSING POLYCHONDRITIS

Relapsing polychondritis is a rare condition in which there is softening and collapse of cartilaginous structures. Patients often present with painful swollen ears (**3.93**) and the disease may also involve cartilage in the nose, respiratory tract and joints, and the fibrous tissue in the globe of the eye. Steroid therapy may control symptoms.

3.93 Relapsing polychondritis causing painful ears in a 58-year-old man.

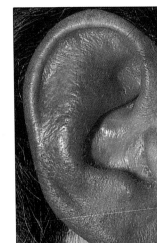

OVERLAP SYNDROMES AND MIXED CONNECTIVE TISSUE DISEASE (MCTD)

Occasionally, patients may present with a constellation of clinical and laboratory abnormalities which fit into more than one disease profile. These patients are said to have an overlap syndrome and most common among these are disorders with features of RA combined with those of SLE, or of SSc associated with those of SLE and of polymyositis. In the latter group, antibodies to the n-ribose nucleoprotein (nRNP) may be found. These cases are often referred to as mixed connective tissue disease (MCTD). This condition has a more favourable prognosis than that of SLE or SSc alone and often responds to small doses of prednisolone.

THE VASCULITIDES

The vasculitides comprise a mixed group of conditions characterized by inflammatory infiltration of the blood vessels. They may be localized or systemic and the pathology may range from simple inflammation to necrotizing arteritis or granuloma formation. Blood vessels of all sizes may be affected, so there is a wide spectrum of presentation. Most cases are idiopathic, but some complicate other conditions as in the case of rheumatoid vasculitis, SLE and dermatomyositis or polymyositis.

POLYARTERITIS NODOSA

Polyarteritis nodosa (PAN) is a rare condition that primarily affects young men (age 20–50 years). Any small or medium-sized arteries may be affected. There is fibrinoid necrosis and polymorphonuclear-cell (in some cases eosinophil) infiltration with narrowing of the lumen and thrombosis. Local ischaemia and healing by fibrosis leads to the formation of small aneurysms (nodosa). The aetiology is unknown, but 20–40% of patients possess the hepatitis B antigen (*see* **p. 386**).

Clinical features include general malaise, weight loss and arthralgia. A purpuric vasculitic skin rash is common (**3.94**). Vasculitic digital infarcts are common (**3.31**, **3.32**, **3.88**). Patients may also present with livedo reticularis (**3.95**), and this may progress to severe ulceration of the limbs (**3.96**). Cardiac involvement may appear as pericarditis, myocardial infarction or a persistent tachycardia. Pulmonary infiltration may occur (**4.131**). In the gastrointestinal tract there may be small bowel infarcts, haemorrhage and intussusception. Infarction of the gall bladder and pancreatitis may also occur. Neurological complications include mononeuritis multiplex, polyneuritis and occasionally subarachnoid haemorrhage. One-half of these patients are hypertensive; this is often related to renal involvement, which is associated with a poor prognosis (*see* **p. 275**).

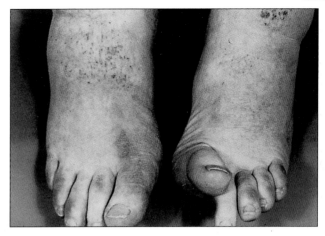

3.94 Polyarteritis nodosa. A vasculitic purpuric rash has developed over the dorsum of both feet and the patient has developed a mononeuritis – he is unable to dorsiflex his right toe.

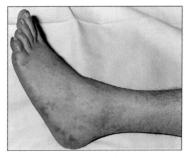

3.95 Livedo reticularis usually results from vasculitis at a deeper level in the dermis than that which leads to a purpuric rash (**3.94**).

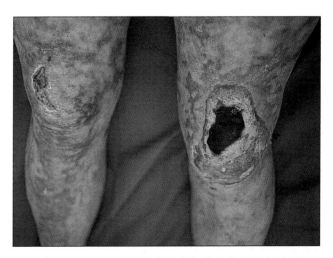

3.96 Severe, necrotic ulceration of the legs in a patient with polyarteritis nodosa. Note the underlying marble-like pattern of livedo reticularis. Patients with skin involvement of this type rarely have severe systemic involvement and have a generally good prognosis when compared with those with a purpuric rash, which is more likely to be associated with renal involvement.

Investigations reveal an elevated ESR and a high white cell count, anaemia, hyperimmunoglobulinaemia and sometimes hepatitis B antigen. Biopsy of muscle or kidney shows fibrinoid necrosis of the wall of medium-sized arteries and arterioles with cellular infiltrates. Visceral angiography may reveal characteristic aneurysms (**6.70**).

Treatment is with high-dose corticosteroids, usually in combination with an immunosuppressive agent, for example azathioprine. The prognosis is variable. Although spontaneous remission is possible, death usually occurs in months to years as a result of renal complications.

WEGENER'S GRANULOMATOSIS

Wegner's granulomatosis is another uncommon condition of unknown aetiology. Small to medium arteries are affected and the pathology is that of necrotizing granuloma formation. Wegener's granulomatosis consists of the clinical triad of upper respiratory tract granuloma, fleeting lung shadows and necrotizing glomerulonephritis. Initial presentation may be with rhinorrhoea and nasal mucosal ulceration followed by collapse of the nasal septum (**3.97**). There is later involvement of the lungs (*see* **p. 182**) and kidneys (*see* **p. 277**). Anti-neutrophil cytoplasmic antibodies (ANCA), though not specific, may be present.

Corticosteroid therapy and cyclophosphamide may be of benefit, and a number of other therapies have recently been investigated.

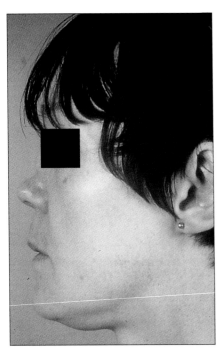

3.97 Wegener's granulomatosis. The classic appearance after collapse of the nasal septum resulting from granulomatous infiltration.

CHURG–STRAUSS SYNDROME

Churg–Strauss syndrome (allergic granulomatosis) is less generalized than polyarteritis nodosa. The small arteries and veins are predominantly involved and there may be extravascular granuloma formation. Patients present with asthma and hypereosinophilia, and chest radiographs show pneumonic-like shadows (*see* **p. 183**). There may also be peripheral nerve involvement but renal complications are less common. The condition often responds well to steroids.

POLYMYALGIA RHEUMATICA (PMR) AND TEMPORAL ARTERITIS (TA)

Polymyalglia rheumatica (PMR) is a disorder that affects middle-aged or elderly patients. It is twice as common in women as in men. It is often of abrupt onset and presents with fever, malaise, weight loss and pain and stiffness in the proximal (shoulder–pelvic girdle) muscles. Patients have difficulty getting out of bed and walking up and down the stairs. Full blood count reveals a normochromic, normocytic anaemia and the ESR, plasma viscosity and CRP are almost always elevated. The course of treated PMR is usually limited to 1–2 years, with subsequent full remission or full control on a continued low dose of steroid.

PMR and temporal arteritis (TA) are described together because they often coexist. About one in six patients with PMR has TA, and one in four patients with TA has PMR. TA is a synonym for giant-cell arteritis, which affects mainly the large arteries, most frequently the temporal artery, with inflammatory cell infiltration and giant-cell formation in all layers of the vessels. Involvement of the ophthalmic artery in TA may lead to blindness; stroke is a much rarer complication. Additional symptoms that may be present include headache, which is usually unilateral and throbbing, visual disturbance, scalp tenderness and jaw claudication. The temporal artery may appear thickened, tender and non-pulsatile (**3.98**). The ESR is characteristically over 100 mm in the first hour and the plasma viscosity and CRP are grossly elevated. Temporal artery biopsy may show giant-cell lesions (**3.99**), but these are patchy and a negative biopsy does not rule out the diagnosis.

If TA is suspected, treatment with high-dose corticosteroids (e.g. prednisolone 60 mg/day) should be started immediately, before any biopsy results are available, in order to prevent irreversible blindness. The dose should be continued for several weeks before tapering down. Lower doses of steroid (e.g. prednisolone 10–15 mg/day) may be used with good response if there is polymyalgia without cranial symptoms. The steroid dose should be very slowly reduced over the course of 1–2 years, using ESR, plasma viscosity or CRP, and clinical symptoms as guides to disease activity. Steroid-induced osteoporosis is a significant risk, particularly as patients with PMR and TA are commonly relatively immobile, elderly and female. The risk may be reduced by the addition of calcium and vitamin D supplements, or by the use of bisphosphonate therapy if long-term steroid therapy is required.

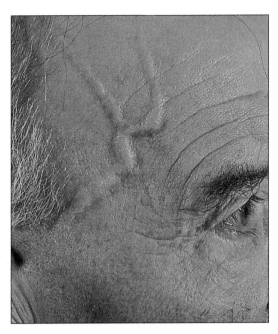

3.98 Temporal arteritis. The right temporal artery is dilated in this 74-year-old man who had severe headache, burning and tenderness over the artery and visual disturbance. Biopsy was diagnostic of temporal arteritis.

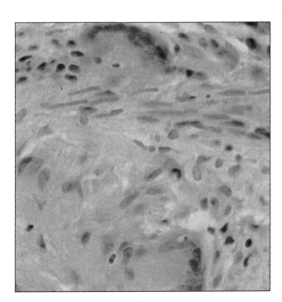

3.99 Temporal arteritis. The histological appearance of a temporal artery biopsy is diagnostic. All layers of the vessel are involved with inflammatory cell infiltration and this high-power view shows two characteristic giant cells. Biopsy gives a positive result in 60–80% of patients with temporal arteritis.

BEHÇET'S SYNDROME

Behçet's syndrome is a rare syndrome of unknown aetiology in which small blood vessels, especially small venules, become acutely inflamed (vasculitis). This results in areas of recurrent ulceration in many organs of the body, especially in the mouth and genitalia, inflammation in the eyes, acute inflammatory joint disease and CNS and gastrointestinal involvement. The disease has a worldwide distribution with a high incidence in Japan and the Middle East and this is associated strongly with HLA-B51.

Men tend to be more severely affected than women but the distribution is equal. The usual age of onset is between 20 and 35 years of age.

The common clinical manifestations are painful oral aphthous ulcers (**3.100**) which are recurrent and often heal without scarring. These are accompanied by genital ulceration (**3.101**, **3.102**) and ocular symptoms caused by uveitis (**3.103**). An excessive subacute inflammatory reaction of the skin and other tissues to non-specific injury (pathergy) is a usual feature of Behçet's syndrome in countries such as Turkey and Japan, though it is rarely seen in Northern Europe and the USA.

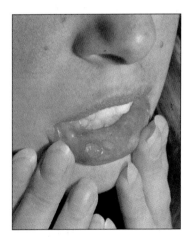

3.100 Behçet's syndrome. Acute ulceration of the lip, accompanied by scarring from previous episodes.

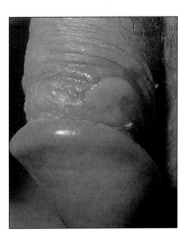

3.101 Behçet's syndrome. A typical penile ulcer, with an eythematous margin.

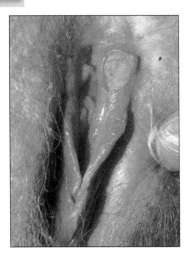

3.102 Behçet's syndrome. Ulceration of the labium minus in the same patient as in **3.100**.

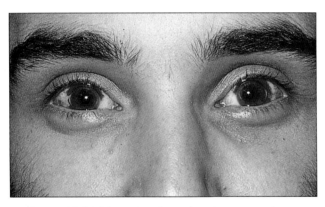

3.103 Uveitis in Behçet's syndrome is most common in patients who have HLA-B51. In this patient, there are severe changes with scleral haemorrhage.

Joint involvement is usually asymmetrical, acutely affecting the large joints of the lower limb, which are not permanently damaged.

Superficial thrombophlebitis may occur in 25% of cases and deep vein thrombosis in 5%, usually in the lower limbs. Large and small, arteries may also be acutely occluded (3–5%).

The presence of uveitis and other CNS involvement carries a poor prognosis with a high incidence of blindness and death.

Otherwise, the natural history is one of fluctuating disease activity with general abatement of activity over many years. There is no specific therapy for the disease. Anti-inflammatory therapy with steroids and immunosuppressant therapy are of some value, especially in the prevention and management of acute uveitis.

SOFT-TISSUE DISORDERS

Soft-tissue disorders are a major cause of morbidity in the general population. Most result from trauma or strain and fall

outside the remit of this book, but some are covered briefly here.

FIBROMYALGIA

This is a vague syndrome of chronic musculoskeletal aches and pains in which there is no evidence of synovitis or myositis. Using clinical diagnostic criteria, it is now felt to be present in up to 10% of the population, and it therefore represents a very significant part of the medical workload. The usual clinical features are localized tenderness at specific places (tender points).

Common precipitating factors probably include:

- viral type illnesses
- physical trauma
- depression
- steroid withdrawal
- chronic fatigue syndrome
- possibly Lyme disease (Lyme borreliosis) (*see* **p. 41**).

Rheumatologists have defined 18 sites (i.e. nine sites bilaterally) of which 11 should be tender for confirmation of the diagnosis. These are occipital, low cervical, trapezius, supraspinatus, second rib at costochondral junction, lateral epicondyle, gluteal, greater trochanter and knee. There is a great range of declaration of pain intensity.

Fatigue associated with sleep disturbances is also commonly reported. Headache, migraine, irritable bowel syndrome, Raynaud's phenomenon and depression are present in up to 50% of patients. Chronic fatigue syndrome coexists in 70% of cases.

Clinical examination is generally unhelpful except for the finding of 'tender spots'. In addition, muscle spasm may sometimes be found with skin hypersensitivity and dermatographism. Laboratory tests should be aimed at excluding other relevant pathology. Treatment is aimed at physical, psychiatric and social support. Patient and family education on the lack of sinister significance of the symptoms may be helpful.

REPETITIVE STRAIN INJURY (RSI)

Repetitive strain injury (RSI) is a poorly understood condition that can only be diagnosed clinically. Chronic pain develops during repetitive movements or as a result of the requirements of a job to hold a static posture. RSI is often associated with compensation claims against employers for working practice deficits leading to disability, but as yet there is no accepted definition and no relevant laboratory or imaging tests. There may be a psychological component to the disease, as very few self-employed workers complain of symptoms.

There is usually no history of direct muscle, bone or joint trauma, but ergonomic factors such as abnormal posture, heavy lifting or excessive continuous movements are implicated. Such people often have a history of a low pain threshold and abnormal stress responses. The dominant clinical presentation is with pains and aches, often in the shoulder girdle and upper limb. The pain is usually constant but may be exacerbated by weather, physical activity and stress. There may be local features in the limb such as 'pins and needles', heaviness and numbness. In addition there may be central features such as excess tiredness, altered sleep pattern and related behavioural problems.

Clinical examination may be unhelpful, but there may be skin tenderness, skin vasomotor disturbance (increased swelling, palmar erythema), some general joint tenderness, dermatographism and some localized increase in muscle tone, especially in the neck muscles.

Investigations should be directed at the exclusion of other better defined pathology. Management is directed towards relief of symptoms, especially pain. If the symptoms involve the upper limb, a soft cervical collar worn during sleep may be helpful. General physical fitness and mobility should be encouraged. There is no evidence that anti-inflammatory drugs are of value.

BACK PAIN

Back pain is epidemic in most industrialized countries, especially where industrial compensation is available. It is estimated that up to 65% of the population will have back pain at some time and low back pain is the single commonest cause of time lost from work in many countries.

It is likely that the most common cause is mechanical, causing soft-tissue injury, facet joint damage or disc protrusion. Ageing is also relevant, as the various tissues become less elastic and less pliable with age. Most cases show little on initial investigation, especially in the young, and the majority (90%) resolve with adequate analgesia and rapid, progressive return to normal activity, which has now been shown to be better than bed rest, physiotherapy or exercise therapy. Some patients progress to overt clinical evidence of root compression, and this is usually associated with a herniated intervertebral disc.

HERNIATED INTERVERTEBRAL DISCS

Herniation of an intervertebral disc is common and its accurate diagnosis and treatment has financial and social, as well as medical, implications.

The material from the central portion of the disc (nucleus pulposus) may herniate through the annulus in two directions: lateral to the posterior longitudinal ligament, to compress the spinal roots; or posteriorly, to compress the cord or the cauda equina. The acute protrusion may follow trauma, abnormal movement or weight-bearing, but other factors such as

degeneration of the disc, spondylosis or congenital abnormalities of the vertebrae may also be relevant. The common sites affected are the cervical and lumbar spine and the signs and symptoms depend on the site(s) and extent of the disc protrusion. If the protrusion is large, several adjacent nerve roots may be affected.

In the cervical spine, the most common sites are between C5/C6 and C6/C7. In the lumbar spine, the common sites are L4/L5 and L5/S1. Thoracic disc herniations are not common.

Local pain is common and may be exacerbated by movement, coughing or sneezing. There is usually associated local spasm and the patient resists all movements. Compression of the associated nerve results in pain referred along its distribution. Stretching of the nerve root exacerbates the pain and this forms the basis of the straight-leg raising test (**3.104**).

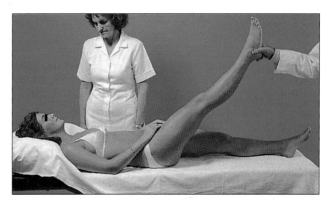

3.104   Straight-leg raising is a test that stretches the sciatic nerve roots. The patient is asked to relax, and the heel is lifted by the examiner with the knee kept straight until pain is felt. If pain is felt in the back or buttock, a central disc prolapse may be the cause. If pain is felt at the back of the thigh, the only abnormality may be tight hamstrings. If pain is felt below the knee, its location may correspond to the lumbosacral dermatomes and is an important localizing sign. If pain is felt in the opposite leg as well, this may be an indication of abnormalities within the spinal canal. In the absence of spinal or hip abnormality, straight-leg raising may usually be carried to the vertical position without pain.

Local pain may also be induced by pressing over the back. Sensory and motor symptoms and signs may identify the root involved. Herniation of the disc into the cord may produce remarkably few local signs, and the patient may present with symptoms and signs of cord compression – muscle weakness, sensory loss and upper motor neuron signs.

Diagnosis is usually made on clinical examination and straight X-ray of the spine. CT and MRI may help to identify more accurately the size and site of the herniation (**3.105**, **3.106**) and these have replaced myelography as the investigations of choice.

Adequate analgesia and early mobilization are now seen as the most important forms of treatment. Local injection of

3.105   3.106

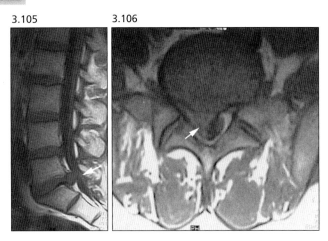

3.105 and 3.106   Prolapsed intervertebral disc. Axial and sagittal MRI show a large disc protrusion at the L5/S1 level (arrows), with resultant compression of the right S1 nerve root.

3.107   3.108

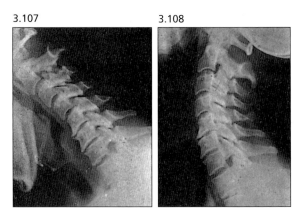

3.107, 3.108   Cervical spondylosis at the most common level (C5/C6) demonstrated by X-rays taken in full flexion and extension. Note the narrowing of the intervertebral spaces and the prominent osteophyte formation that leads to obvious abnormalities in the shape of the vertebral bodies. This appearance is very common in patients over the age of 50 years, and it is often asymptomatic.

steroids, manipulation and traction may all have a place. Surgery is indicated for intractable pain, or when the cord is involved, and consists of removal of the central portion of the disc. An alternative to surgery is the injection of proteolytic enzymes into the disc space.

SPONDYLOSIS

Spondylosis is the term applied to chronic degenerative changes that occur with ageing in the intervertebral discs and the associated changes in the adjacent ligaments and vertebral bodies, including the outgrowth of osteophytes. In most instances changes are found incidentally on a routine examination and do not produce symptoms. However, in the cervical and lumbar spine there may be sufficient new growth to cause pressure on nerves or on the cord itself. Symptoms and signs are usually slowly progressive, in contradistinction to those of a disc protrusion, which are acute. Radicular compression produces pain, which may be referred, and there may be associated muscle spasm. Lower motor neuron weakness and wasting may also occur in the same distribution. Spinal movement may be reduced and movement may exacerbate pain. The patient may be aware of 'creaking' or 'clicking' on movement. If the cord is involved, there may be myelopathy with progressive upper motor neuron weakness of the upper and lower limbs, with sensory signs, including loss of vibration sense and proprioception, and with sphincter disturbance.

Osteophytic outgrowth may also involve the vertebral canal, so that movements of the neck constrict the vertebral arteries and produce cerebellar ischaemia. These patients present with dizziness or drop attacks ('vertebrobasilar syndrome').

Straight X-ray of the cervical spine shows the typical degenerative changes with osteophyte formation (**3.107**,

3.108). Of greater importance is an assessment of the diameter of the spinal canal in cases in which myelopathy is present. This is best done by myelography or CT scan (**3.109**). In the cervical canal, a reduction to 10 mm is diagnostic of cord compression caused by spondylosis – a diameter greater than 15 mm suggests that spondylosis is not the cause of the myelopathic symptoms.

Spontaneous resolution of symptoms of radiculopathy and myelopathy occurs frequently in cervical spondylosis and

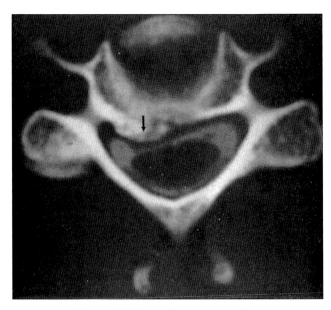

3.109   Cervical spondylosis. CT demonstrates that spur formation (arrow) is distorting the thecal sac; but, although the spinal cord is slightly displaced, it is not compressed.

treatment with a collar and analgesia is often helpful. Some patients benefit from bed rest with neck traction. Progression of the symptoms and signs of myelopathy requires urgent surgery for decompression.

HYPERMOBILITY SYNDROMES

Hypermobility syndromes are a range of inherited disorders in which there is musculoskeletal hypermobility as a result of ligamentous laxity, and in which there is no systemic rheumatological disease. Over the course of a lifetime a range of clinical features may become apparent, including:

- hyperextensible skin
- joint hypermobility
- increased incidence of synovitis
- increased incidence of OA and stress fractures.

Hypermobility is a recognized part of the spectrum of features of the Marfan and Ehlers–Danlos syndromes. Clinically the features fall into articular and non-articular groups. Articular features include joint instability, recurrent dislocation, subluxation, inflammatory synovitis, osteoarthritis, rotator cuff lesions and disc prolapse. Extra-articular features may include skin laxity, mitral valve prolapse, aortic root dilatation, muscle weakness – especially of the pelvic floor, with rectal and uterine prolapse – and fragile bones with stress fractures.

The diagnosis of hypermobility depends on the clinical picture, as hypermobility is not always associated with Ehlers–Danlos or Marfan syndromes, which can also be identified by genetic methods. Investigations in 'pure' hypermobility are usually negative except for X-rays, which may show the complications of joint damage.

There is no specific treatment but awareness of the disease and its implications is important. Mitral valve prolapse (*see* **p. 222**) requires the use of prophylactic antibiotics to cover dental extraction and other procedures (*see* **p. 231**).

EHLERS–DANLOS SYNDROME

The Ehlers–Danlos syndrome is a group of rare inherited disorders of connective tissue in which patients have hyperextensible skin, hypermobile joints, fragile tissues and a bleeding diathesis associated with poor wound healing. There are many subtypes associated with a range of collagen defects; the common ones are transmitted as autosomal dominant traits. Type 1 has been widely described clinically and has the most severe manifestations. The extremely hyperextensible skin (**3.110**) and the hypermobile joints (**3.111**) were often features found in side shows (India-rubber man). With time, the skin becomes redundant and sags, particularly over joints. It is liable to bleed and wound healing is defective; this results in large pigmented scars especially over the knees and elbows. As all

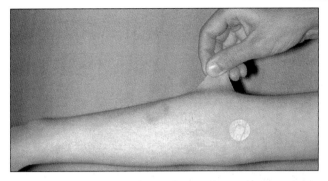

3.110 Ehlers–Danlos syndrome showing hyperelasticity of the skin.

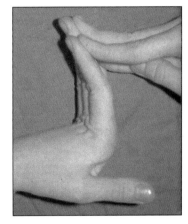

3.111 Ehlers–Danlos syndrome showing extreme extensibility of the fingers.

tissues are involved, a wide range of signs may be found, including retinal detachment, blue sclerae, dislocated lens, mitral valve prolapse, conduction defects, and aneurysm formation caused by defects in large arteries. No specific treatment is available to correct the defects, but advice should be given for skin and joint protection.

MARFAN SYNDROME

Marfan syndrome is the most common inherited connective tissue disorder (1:10 000) and is due to a defect in the production of fibrillin, an extracellular matrix glycoprotein that is critical to the physical strength and elasticity of skin, ligaments, tendons, periosteum, aortic wall and ciliary body of the eye. The fibrillin genes have been identified on chromosomes 15 and 5. Transmission is by an autosomal dominant route with almost full penetrance (**3.112**).

The physical features of a typical patient with Marfan syndrome include:

- skeletal
  - tall stature (**3.113**)
  - scoliosis

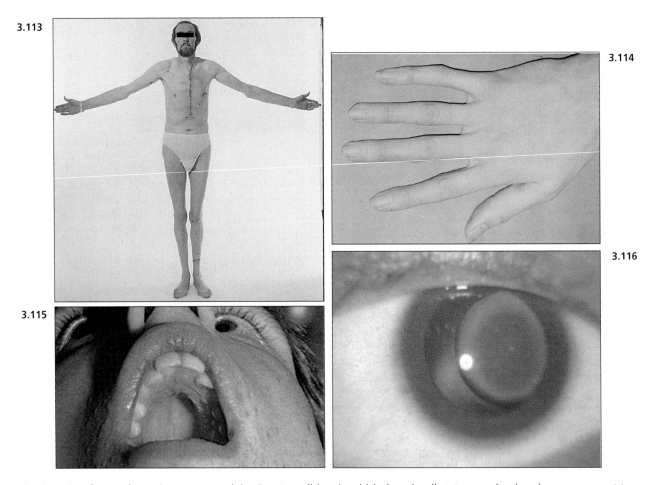

3.112 **Marfan syndrome.** A typical family pedigree showing autosomal dominant inheritance.

- long arms
- arachnodactyly (**3.114**)
- chest wall deformity
- laxity of joints (especially knees)
- high arched palate (**3.115**)
- cardiovascular
    - mitral valve prolapse (*see* **p. 222**)
    - aortic dissection (*see* **p. 247**)
    - aortic regurgitation (*see* **p. 224**)
- ocular
    - subluxation of the lens (**3.116**)
    - myopia.

A firm diagnosis should be made if there are features in three different systems, or a positive family history and features from two systems.

There is no specific treatment. One of the most common causes of death is aortic root dissection and annual ultrasound examinations are of value to measure the aortic diameter.

3.113–3.116 **Marfan syndrome** is an autosomal dominant condition, in which there is tall stature, and reduced upper segment to lower segment ratio (**3.113**), long fingers (**3.114**) and toes (arachnodactyly), and often a high arched palate (**3.115**). It is commonly associated with laxity of the joints, dislocation of the lens in the eye (**3.116**), dissecting aneurysm of the aorta, aortic regurgitation and a floppy mitral valve. The patient in **3.113** has undergone surgery for aortic dissection.

β-blockers may be of value in preventing this complication by reducing blood pressure, and they should be started by the age of 8 years. Prophylactic aortic surgery is required if the root diameter reaches 6 cm. Mitral valve disease, most commonly mitral valve prolapse and mitral regurgitation, is common. Antibiotic prophylaxis is indicated for dental procedures.

Pregnancy represents a particular hazard. Such patients should have regular routine ultrasound of the aortic root and delivery should be carefully supervised to ensure that blood pressure is not elevated during labour; caesarian section has been advocated.

Genetic counselling should be offered to all parents.

DISEASES OF BONE

Bone is a collagen-based matrix with mineral laid upon it, and its strength depends on both components. The mineral phase is composed mainly of calcium, magnesium and phosphorus. Vitamin D, parathyroid hormone (PTH) and calcitonin are important factors in bone mineralization. New bone is deposited by osteoblasts and old bone resorbed by osteoclasts. Bone is a living and dynamic tissue, constantly remodelling itself throughout life.

OSTEOGENESIS IMPERFECTA

Osteogenesis imperfecta (brittle bone disease) is a genetically determined disease in which an abnormal bone matrix and secondary osteoporosis are associated with the likelihood of recurrent bone fractures (**3.117**), small stature, joint laxity and soft discoloured teeth. Blue sclerae are a reflection of the generalized collagen defect (**3.118**).

There is no specific treatment. Attention must be paid to the prevention of fracture by the use of safety appliances, while keeping the patient mobile. Fracture-associated deformities must also be prevented when possible.

Genetic advice is required, and patients and families should be seen in a specialized unit because of the range of possible

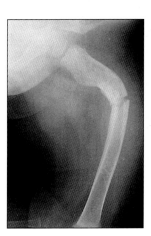

3.117 Osteogenesis imperfecta led to multiple fractures in this typical infant, including the femoral fracture shown here.

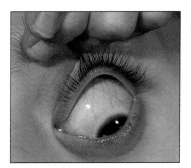

3.118 Blue sclerae are commonly seen in osteogenesis imperfecta. They are a reflection of the underlying collagen defect in the disease. Similar blue sclerae may be seen in patients with rheumatoid arthritis complicated by scleritis.

genetic defects. Accuracy of diagnosis is of great importance to prevent the risk of either missing or falsely diagnosing non-accidental injury (child abuse), which is the other major cause of multiple fractures in infants and young children.

OSTEOPOROSIS

Osteoporosis is the most common metabolic bone disease. Its frequency increases with age, and women are more commonly affected than men. The weakened bone fractures easily, and this accounts for much morbidity and indirect mortality in the elderly. There is an absolute decrease in bone mass (both mineral and non-mineral) resulting from an increased bone resorption rate (**3.119**, **3.120**). The aetiology of most cases

3.119
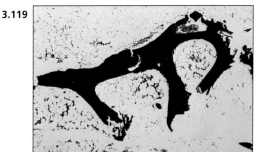

3.120
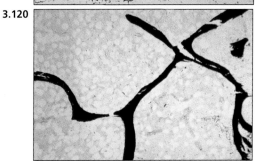

3.119 and 3.120 Trephine bone biopsies of normal bone (3.119) and bone in osteoporosis (3.120). These sections are biopsies from the iliac crest and have been stained by a silver method for calcified bone. Loss of cortical and trabecular bone in osteoporosis (**3.120**) leads to loss of bone strength and increases the liability to fracture.

remains unclear, but the effects of ageing, failure of oestrogen secretion at the time of menopause and lack of physical activity are probably of particular importance. Known risk factors for osteoporosis are listed in **3.121**, and diseases associated with osteoporosis are shown in **3.122**.

RISK FACTORS FOR OSTEOPOROSIS

Genetic	Excess alcohol intake
Female sex	History of amenorrhoea
Deficient diet	Underweight
Increased age	Systemic corticosteroid use
Sedentary occupation	Long-term heparin therapy
Caucasian race	Pregnancy
Premature menopause	Lack of hormone replacement therapy
Cigarette smoking	

3.121   Risk factors for osteoporosis.

DISEASES ASSOCIATED WITH OSTEOPOROSIS

Multiple myeloma	Chronic renal failure
Thyrotoxicosis	Hypogonadism
Cushing's syndrome	Hypopituitarism
Osteogenesis imperfecta	Post gastrectomy

3.122   Diseases associated with osteoporosis.

Asymptomatic osteoporosis is common. In patients who are symptomatic, backache is a frequent complaint. There may be episodes of severe pain caused by fractures of the weakened bones. Collapse of vertebrae may result in loss of height (**3.123**). The lumbar and thoracic vertebrae, the upper end of the humerus (**3.124**), the lower end of the radius and the neck of the femur are the most common sites of fracture (**3.125**). The bone radiographs show loss of bone density, reduction in the number and size of trabeculae and thinning of the cortex. The lumbar and thoracic vertebral bodies become biconcave in shape, with anterior wedging caused by compression or collapse (**3.126, 3.127**). Blood levels of calcium, phosphate and alkaline phosphatase are normal.

Reversal of osteoporosis is unlikely once the condition is established and prophylaxis is preferable. Bone density can now be measured and repeatedly monitored by dual energy X-ray absorptiometry (DEXA scanning) (**3.128**), and this

3.123   Osteoporosis results in loss of height, and vertebral collapse is associated with chronic backache, bouts of severe back pain and kyphosis (dowager's hump). Creases often appear in the skin, and the ribs may rub on the iliac crest.

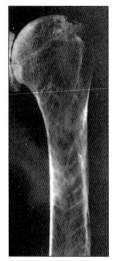

3.124   Osteoporosis has caused a loss of cortical thickness and an opening up of the trabecular pattern in this radiograph of the humerus.

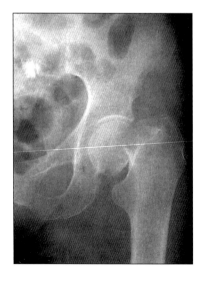

3.125   Osteoporosis is the usual underlying disorder in fracture of the neck of the femur in the elderly. This patient has a subcapital fracture, which may lead to osteonecrosis of the femoral head.

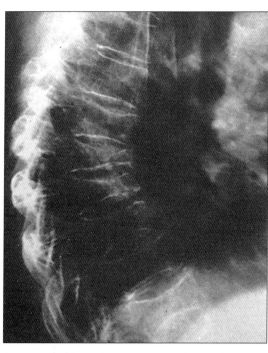

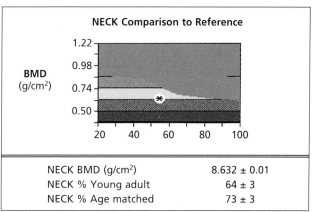

NECK Comparison to Reference		
NECK BMD (g/cm²)		8.632 ± 0.01
NECK % Young adult		64 ± 3
NECK % Age matched		73 ± 3

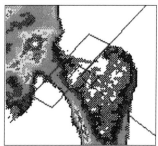

3.128 Dual energy X-ray absorptiometry (DEXA scanning) is a technique for measurement of bone mass at both axial and appendicular sites using a very low dose of radiation. Bone density values are expressed in relation to reference data as standard deviation scores. DEXA has a precision error of 1% for spine and 2–3% for the femoral neck and greater trochanter, and is useful in screening patients at risk of osteoporosis.

3.126 Osteoporosis leads to vertebral collapse. This radiograph shows wedge-shaped flattening of the vertebral bodies in the midthoracic region.

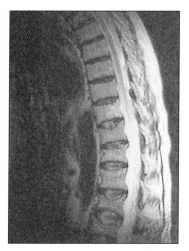

3.127 Vertebral thinning and collapse in osteoporosis demonstrated by MRI. The wedging and collapse is similar to that seen in **3.126**. The patient experienced repeated episodes of severe back pain, radiating anteriorly on occasions as a result of nerve root compression.

OSTEOMALACIA AND RICKETS

Deficiency of vitamin D, causing osteomalacia in adults and rickets in children, is now fairly uncommon in the Western world although it may occur in Asian immigrants and the elderly, as a result of a combination of dietary insufficiency and lack of exposure to sunlight. Other causes of osteomalacia and rickets are summarized in **3.129**.

The main function of vitamin D is to ensure an adequate concentration of calcium for the formation of calcium salts in bone. Deficiency results in poor bone mineralization and a reduction in tensile strength.

Childhood rickets usually manifests itself as bony deformity or failure of adequate growth. Signs include bossing of the frontal and parietal skull bones (**3.130**), delayed closure of the anterior fontanelle, rickety rosary (enlargement of the epiphyses at the costochondral junctions of the ribs), pigeon deformity of the chest and bowing or other deformities of the legs (**3.131**).

In the adult, osteomalacia may produce skeletal pain and tenderness and spontaneous bony fractures. Muscle weakness is often present and there may be a marked proximal myopathy.

In both conditions, tetany may be manifest by carpopedal spasm and facial twitching. Investigations show low or low-

technique has a role in screening and follow-up for osteoporosis. Any primary factor, such as endocrine disease or the use of long-term corticosteroids, should be corrected if possible. Hormone replacement therapy in the postmenopausal woman is helpful if started early. Other prophylactic measures include regular exercise and adequate intake of vitamin D and calcium.

CAUSES OF OSTEOMALACIA AND RICKETS

Vitamin D deficiency
Deficiency of sunlight
Defective diet
Malabsorption

Metabolic defects
Chronic renal failure
Drugs, especially anticonvulsants
Aluminium exposure
Fluoride excess
Bisphosphonates

Low phosphate
Renal tubular acidosis
Fanconi syndrome
Hypophosphataemic syndromes
Mesenchymal tumours

3.129 Causes of osteomalacia and rickets.

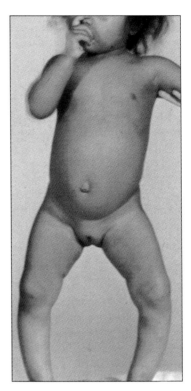

3.131 **Rickets.** Weight-bearing bones in the arms and legs show lateral and forward bowing.

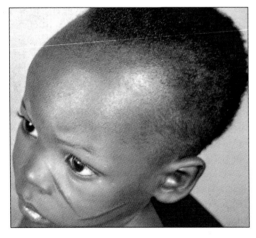

3.130 **The skull in rickets.** In infancy, the frontal bones are prominent and bossed. There is delayed closure of the fontanelles. The entire skull is soft to the touch and it can be distorted in a way that resembles a table tennis ball to which pressure has been applied.

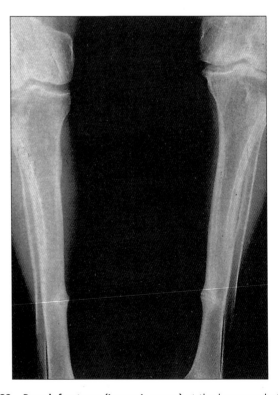

3.132 **Pseudofractures (Looser's zones)** at the lower end of both tibias in osteomalacia.

normal plasma calcium, low serum phosphate and increased alkaline phosphatase. Radiographs show rarefaction of bone (defective mineralization) and translucent bands (pseudo-fractures, Looser's zones), especially in the pelvis, ribs and long bones (**3.132**). In children, there may be additional changes in the epiphyseal zone which becomes broadened (**3.133**). Bone biopsy may sometimes be required for diagnosis in adult cases (**3.134**).

Prevention is better than cure. Education and living standards should be improved in the susceptible populations. Free access to and adequate dietary intake of vitamin D should be ensured. Supplements should be given to epileptic patients on long-term anticonvulsants. High replacement doses are required in patients with renal disease and those with vitamin D resistance.

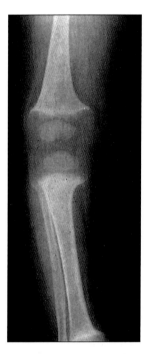

3.133 Rickets. In this radiograph of the right leg of a child, there is widening and cupping (a champagne glass appearance) of the ends of the long bones, increased space between diaphysis and epiphysis and poor mineralization of the bones.

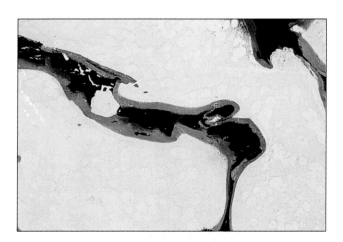

3.134 Trephine bone biopsy from the iliac crest in osteomalacia. As in the biopsy of normal bone (**3.119**), mineralized bone is stained black by a silver technique and unmineralized osteoid is stained red. The bone in osteomalacia shows normal amounts of osteoid with failure of mineralization. The end result is production of bone deficient in tensile strength, which may bend or fracture easily.

HYPERPARATHYROIDISM

Parathormone (PTH), from the parathyroid glands, controls the concentration of calcium and inorganic phosphorus in the blood. It raises the plasma calcium by enhancing the removal of mineral from the skeleton, increasing absorption from the bowel and reducing tubular reabsorption in the kidneys. It also increases the synthesis of vitamin D and lowers the serum phosphate by enhancing its excretion. Under normal physiological conditions, parathyroid hormone levels rise as the plasma calcium falls. Abnormally raised PTH levels may result from a parathyroid adenoma (primary hyperparathyroidism) and conditions that cause a tendency to hypocalcaemia, for example chronic renal failure (secondary hyperparathyroidism). If secondary hyperparathyroidism becomes long-standing, the glands may become autonomous and continue to secrete excess PTH (tertiary hyperparathyroidism).

Patients with mild hyperparathyroidism may be asymptomatic. Clinical features in the more severe cases are related to hypercalcaemia and patients complain of malaise, anorexia, nausea and vomiting, drowsiness or confusion. Peptic ulceration and acute pancreatitis may be the presenting features. Kidney involvement may manifest itself as renal colic from stones, haematuria, polyuria or nocturia from tubular damage. Bone pain suggests involvement of the bones and backache is common. Pseudogout may occur (*see* **p. 121**).

The plasma calcium may be high and the phosphate level low. Alkaline phosphatase is raised, reflecting increased osteoblastic activity in response to bone resorption. Radiological changes in the early stages include demineralization or subperiosteal erosions in the phalanges (**3.135**). Cystic changes (**3.136**) are rare. A lateral skull radiograph may reveal a typical 'ground glass' appearance (**3.137**). Other radiological features include nephrocalcinosis (*see* **p. 288**) and soft-tissue calcification elsewhere. Calcification may sometimes be seen in the eye (**3.138**).

It is important to exclude other causes of hypercalcaemia such as malignancy (particularly multiple myeloma, **p. 444**), sarcoid and drugs, including excess vitamin D. Detection of PTH by radioimmunoassay in the presence of hypercalcaemia is diagnostic of hyperparathyroidism and the second stage is the localization of the tumour or tumours. The best approach is surgical exploration of the neck, which in experienced hands has a 90% success rate in locating and removing the adenoma. Other methods involve CT scanning, radionuclide scanning (**3.139**) and selective venous sampling for PTH. Definitive treatment is surgical resection.

Hyperparathyroidism may sometimes be a component of the multiple endocrine neoplasia (MEN type 1) syndrome, in which there are multiple tumours of the anterior pituitary, parathyroids, pancreatic islet cells, adrenal medulla and thyroid in association with peptic ulceration (*see also* **p. 304**). The fundamental defect in this syndrome is in the differentiation of neural crest tissue. The parathyroid glands are most commonly affected, followed by pancreatic islet cells and the anterior

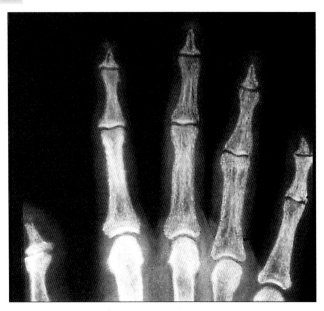

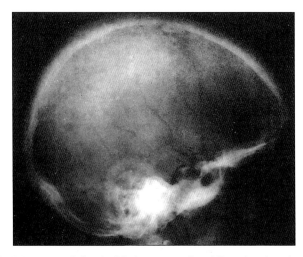

3.137 X-ray of the skull in hyperparathyroidism showing the typical granular or mottled (ground glass) appearance. Some cystic areas are also present – the so-called pepper-pot skull.

3.135 Hyperparathyroidism. There are subperiosteal erosions along the cortical surfaces of the middle and distal phalanges, especially obvious in the index finger, and gross resorption of the distal phalanges.

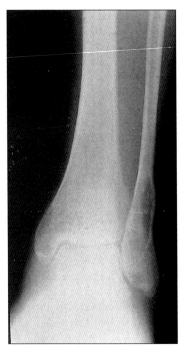

3.136 Hyperparathyroidism. A solitary bone cyst ('brown tumour') in the fibula of a patient with a large parathyroid adenoma. It is important to remember hyperparathyroidism in the differential diagnosis of bone cysts and tumours.

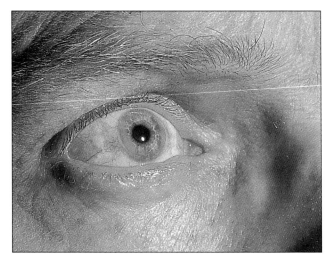

3.138 Ectopic calcification at the lateral and nasal margins of the right cornea (band keratopathy) in a patient with primary hyperparathyroidism.

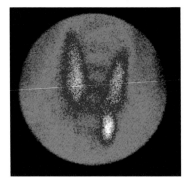

3.139 A large parathyroid adenoma below the left lobe of the thyroid, demonstrated by radionuclide scanning. This is a subtraction scan, obtained by subtracting a 99m-Tc Sestamibi scan, which shows the thyroid only, from a 99m-Tc pertechnetate scan, which shows both the thyroid and the parathyroids. The adenoma was subsequently confirmed and removed at surgery.

pituitary. All four parathyroid glands are abnormally hyperplastic or adenomatous. There are usually few clinical features at first. The patient may have had renal stones and developed renal failure as the first presentation, and hypercalcaemia may be found when calcium levels are measured.

RENAL OSTEODYSTROPHY

Patients with chronic renal failure may develop various forms of bone disease. These include osteomalacia, hyperparathyroidism (secondary and tertiary) and osteosclerosis. Osteomalacia is caused by failure of the damaged kidneys to produce the metabolically active 1,25-dihydroxycholecalciferol. Poor absorption of dietary calcium and retention of phosphate lowers the serum calcium. This leads to the development of secondary hyperparathyroidism and, if this becomes long-standing,

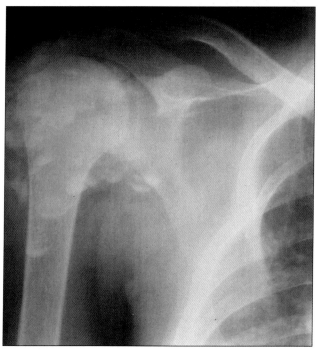

3.140 **Extensive ectopic calcification** around the soft tissues of the shoulder in a patient with chronic renal failure and renal osteodystrophy.

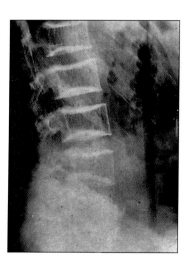

3.141 **'Rugger-jersey spine' in secondary hyperparathyroidism** caused by the demineralization of the vertebral bodies, with simultaneous new bone formation at the subchondral plates.

tertiary hyperparathyroidism. Clinical features and radiological appearances are as those described in the previous related sections and there may be extensive ectopic calcification in soft tissues (**3.140**) and arterial walls. The cause of osteosclerosis, the third type of bone lesion, is less clearly understood, although it may be a direct result of excess parathyroid hormone. It produces the characteristic 'rugger-jersey spine', a radiographic appearance caused by the formation of alternate bands of sclerotic and porotic bone in the vertebrae (**3.141**).

Renal osteodystrophy can be partially prevented and treated. Aluminium hydroxide gel given by mouth binds phosphate and lowers its concentration, and vitamin D resistance can be overcome by giving the newer biologically active derivatives. Resection of the parathyroid glands is now rarely indicated.

OSTEONECROSIS (AVASCULAR NECROSIS)

Osteonecrosis is the final common pathway of a series of physical and chemical disturbances that lead to the cell death of both bone and marrow. The femoral and humeral heads are the most common sites.

The disease progression is often slow in onset and insidious. Pain over the affected joint is often low grade and may be present for many weeks in which the standard X-ray appearances are normal. There is then limitation of joint movement with shortening of the limb as the bone structure collapses.

MRI shows early changes before CT or radionuclide imaging, and ultimately changes are also visible on plain X-ray (**3.142**). Some aetiological factors are shown in **3.143**.

Treatment involves preventing the affected joint from bearing weight and stopping its use, removing or treating any obvious causative factor and resting the part until healing takes place in 6–8 weeks. Occasionally surgery and bone grafting are necessary.

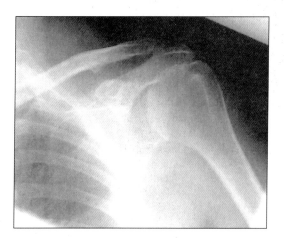

3.142 **Osteonecrosis (avascular necrosis) of the head of the humerus** in a patient who had been treated with long-term systemic steroid therapy for Takayasu's arteritis.

AETIOLOGICAL FACTORS IN OSTEONECROSIS	
Causative	Trauma – fracture or dislocation
	Radiotherapy
	Caisson disease
	Sickle-cell disease
	Gaucher's disease
Associations	Cushing's disease or high-dose steroid use
	Occlusive arterial disease
	Diabetes mellitus
	Osteomalacia
	Hyperuricaemia
	Pregnancy
	Connective tissue diseases
	Vasculitis
	Pancreatitis

3.143 Aetiological factors in osteonecrosis.

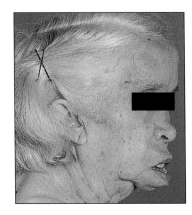

3.144 Paget's disease. Frontal bossing of the skull leads to a distorted facial appearance. This patient has gross changes and she presented with deafness secondary to ossicular involvement.

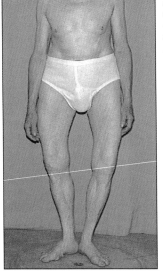

3.145 Paget's disease. Bone deformity has led to bowing of the legs and compression of the trunk, giving the appearance of relatively long arms.

PAGET'S DISEASE OF THE BONE (OSTEITIS DEFORMANS)

Paget's disease of the bone (also known as osteitis deformans), is common in the elderly (up to 10%). The aetiology is unknown, but there is a weak familial tendency. Geographical clustering of this condition emphasizes the importance of environmental factors. There is an increase in osteoclastic activity, compensated for by an increase in osteoblastic activity which results in disorganization of the normal bone architecture and an increase in bone vascularity. Any bone can be affected, including especially the pelvis, lumbar spine, femur, thoracic spine, skull and tibia.

Patients are often asymptomatic and Paget's disease of the bone is commonly an incidental finding. Those who are symptomatic complain of constant and localized bone pain, unrelieved by posture or rest. There may be bone deformities such as frontal bossing (**3.144**) and platybasia, distorted facial features and bowing of the tibia (**3.145**). The affected bone may feel warm on palpation and a bruit may be heard. Complications include blindness caused by nerve compression, deafness secondary to ossicular involvement or to nerve compression by the enlarging bone, secondary OA, and pathological fractures (**3.146**). High-output cardiac failure and osteosarcoma are rare but serious complications.

Investigations show raised alkaline phosphatase, reflecting the compensatory increase in osteoblastic activity, but normal calcium and phosphate levels. There is also an increase in urine excretion of hydroxyproline. Radiographs show lucency zones, caused by bone resorption and osteolysis, and areas of increased

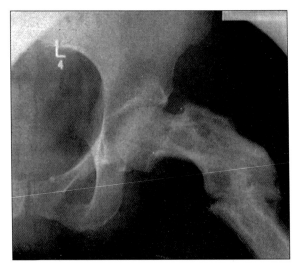

3.146 Paget's disease, with a pathological fracture of the upper femoral shaft. Lucency zones and areas of increased bone density are seen.

bone density (**3.146**, **3.147**). Bone scans with 99m-technetium-labelled bisphosphonates are useful and may show the extent of disease more effectively than other techniques (**3.148**).

Drug treatment is indicated only when patients become symptomatic or develop complications. In such cases, calcitonin and bisphosphonates may be used. Conservative measures, such as the use of simple analgesics, physiotherapy and correction of inequality of leg length, are also required.

OSTEOMYELITIS

Infection in bone may result from bloodborne or direct spread of a number of microorganisms (**3.149**) and various conditions predispose to bone infection (**3.150**). Direct spread of infection

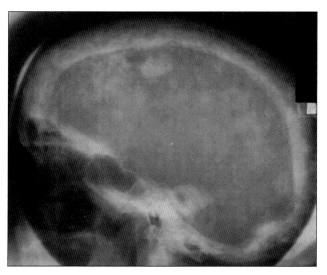

3.147   Skull X-ray in Paget's disease. Areas of lucency and increased bone density are seen. There is frontal bossing, new bone accretion on the cortex and platybasia (flattening of the base of the skull).

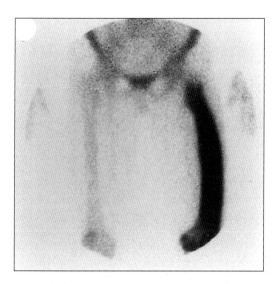

3.148   Paget's disease. In this isotope bone scan, utilizing 99m-technetium-labelled methylene diphosphonate (^{99m}Tc-NMDP), the dark areas indicate bone that is affected by Paget's disease. In this view, the pelvis and the left femur can be seen to be involved, with gross bowing of the femur.

ORGANISMS THAT MAY CAUSE ACUTE OSTEOMYELITIS
Staphylococcus aureus
Pseudomonas aeruginosa
Salmonella sp.
Gram-negative bacilli
Neisseria gonorrhoeae
Pasteurella multocida
Mixed aerobic and anaerobic organisms
Streptococci
Brucella sp.
Candida sp.

3.149   Organisms that may cause acute osteomyelitis.

OSTEOMYELITIS: PREDISPOSING CONDITIONS
Acute osteomyelitis
Bloodborne
Skin sepsis and ulcers (especially in diabetes)
Intravenous drug abuse
Sickle-cell disease
Chronic urinary tract infection
Chronic diverticulitis
Gonorrhoea
Malnutrition
Immunodeficiency
Direct spread
Open fractures
Penetrating trauma, e.g. animal bite
Prosthetic joints
Penetrating ulcer, e.g. in diabetic neuropathy
Finger pricks for blood sampling in diabetes
Chronic osteomyelitis
Inadequately treated acute disease
Tuberculosis

3.150   Predisposing conditions for osteomyelitis.

to the bones occurs most commonly in diabetics with neuropathic foot ulcers (**3.151**, **3.152**) and in patients with penetrating bed sores.

Acute osteomyelitis is usually caused by *Staphylococcus aureus*. Patients often present with fever, pain and tenderness over the affected bone, but the presentation may be more non-specific, without initial localizing features. Blood culture or needle biopsy are usually required for definitive diagnosis, but treatment can sometimes be started on clinical grounds alone.

Chronic osteomyelitis results from undiagnosed or inadequately treated acute osteomyelitis. Within 2 weeks of onset of acute osteomyelitis, radiographic changes can often be seen, and these progress to include periosteal elevation, bone erosion, areas of sclerosis and areas of cystic degeneration (**3.152**). Avascular necrosis of the bone leads to the development of a bony sequestrum (**3.153**). Intermittent episodes of acute flare-up of the disease may occur over many years, with fever, local pain and sinus formation.

Treatment of chronic osteomyelitis often involves a combination of surgery and antibiotic therapy. Patients with sickle-cell disease should receive long-term penicillin prophylaxis to prevent *Salmonella* osteomyelitis (**3.153**).

Chronic tuberculous osteomyelitis results from blood or lymphatic spread. The long bones and vertebral bodies are most commonly involved. Tracking of pus produces a 'cold' abscess

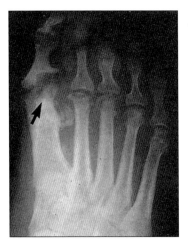

3.151 A purulent discharging ulcer at the base of the big toe in a diabetic patient. The ulcer is associated with osteomyelitis of the first metatarsal head (*see* **3.152**).

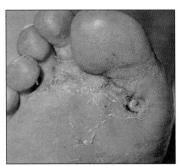

3.152 Osteomyelitis at the base of the ulcer seen in **3.151**, associated with X-ray changes, including bone erosion and sequestrum formation.

(**3.154**) and destruction and subsequent collapse of the vertebrae leads to gross kyphosis (Pott's disease of the spine). Surgery and antituberculous therapy are commonly required.

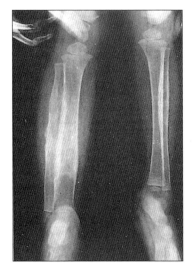

3.153 *Salmonella* osteomyelitis is a common complication of sickle-cell disease. In this child, extensive unilateral osteomyelitis has caused long bone sequestrum formation and a 'bone within a bone' appearance.

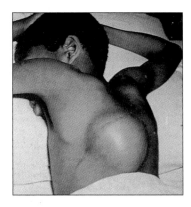

3.154 A 'cold' abscess may be the presenting feature of tuberculosis of the spine, as in this child who presented with a painless loin swelling. Such abscesses may be associated with tuberculosis of the intervertebral joints or with osteomyelitis of the spine.

TUMOURS OF BONE

Primary tumours of bone are rare and occur mainly in the young (**3.155**).

Secondary metastases in bone are common, especially from malignant tumours of the lung, breast, prostate, thyroid and kidney. Most metastases are osteolytic (**3.156**), but secondaries from carcinoma of the prostate are often sclerotic in character (**3.157**). Multiple metastases are common (**3.156**, **3.158**), and lytic bone lesions are also a feature of multiple myeloma (*see* **p. 444**).

Bone secondaries are often painful and may cause hypercalcaemia. Symptomatic treatment is usually necessary, and specific hormone treatment or chemotherapy may be helpful in some cases.

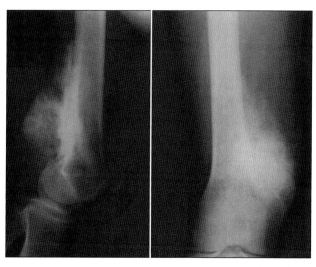

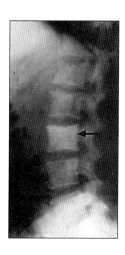

3.157   A sclerotic secondary deposit (arrowed) occupying the body of the third lumbar vertebra. The primary tumour is carcinoma of the prostate.

3.155   Parosteal osteogenic sarcoma in the distal femur of a young adult. The radiographs show periosteal new bone formation and a characteristic 'sunray' spiculation in the tumour tissues.

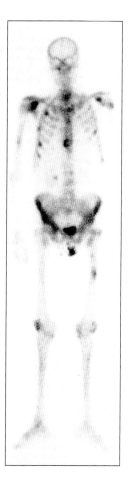

3.158   Multiple bone metastases are seen in this 99m Tc-MDP bone scintigram of a 46-year-old woman with lung cancer. A similar appearance may occur with other metastases, for example from tumours of the breast or kidney.

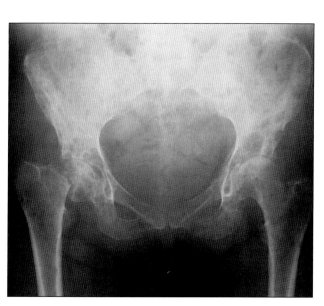

3.156 Multiple osteolytic metastases and a pathological fracture of the right femoral neck in a middle-aged woman with carcinoma of the breast. The lytic secondaries are widespread throughout the pelvis and the proximal femora.

4 Respiratory

HISTORY

A full medical history is important in any patient with respiratory symptoms or signs. Specific questions should always be asked about:

- cough
- sputum – production, volume and colour
- breathlessness – onset, duration and positional variations
- wheezing
- exercise tolerance
- fever
- chest pain
- nasal or upper respiratory tract symptoms
- weight loss
- smoking history
- occupation.

EXAMINATION

On general examination, there may be clues to the underlying disease:

- cachexia (**4.1**) may occur in malignant disease, and in severe chronic lung diseases, including fibrosis, infection and emphysema

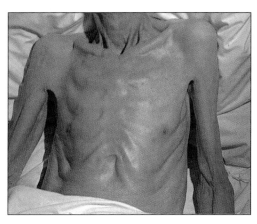

4.1 Cachexia may occur in a number of severe disorders, including chronic lung diseases such as pulmonary fibrosis, tuberculosis and emphysema, malignant disease, including bronchial carcinoma, and systemic infection, especially with HIV ('slim disease'). Note the obvious signs of weight loss, with widespread muscle and soft-tissue wasting.

- tar-stained fingers occur in heavy smokers (**4.2**), and typical pigmented scars may occur in coal miners (**4.3**); in association with finger clubbing (**2.59, 2.104, 2.105, 4.2, 4.95, 11.111**), either sign suggests underlying bronchial carcinoma, pulmonary fibrosis, bronchiectasis or chronic sepsis
- cyanosis – best seen in the lips (**4.92**), tongue (**4.4**) and fingers – indicates significant desaturation of circulating haemoglobin
- a plethoric appearance may result from polycythaemia (**4.5**) most commonly secondary to chronic hypoxia in lung disease.

On examination of the chest:

- distortion of the thoracic cage suggests chronic disease and may take many forms; look for
    - barrel-shaped chest in obstructive airways disease (**4.6**)
    - flattening of the chest wall overlying lung damage or collapse
    - kyphosis or kyphoscoliosis, which may be a primary abnormality (**4.7**), or secondary to other disease (**3.46, 3.123, 4.38**)
    - scars from previous thoracic surgery
- the respiratory rate and depth may be raised or lowered
    - is there hypoventilation or hyperventilation?
    - are the accessory muscles of respiration in use?
    - is the patient fatigued?
    - does the patient breathe out through pursed lips (**4.8**)?

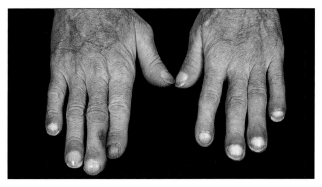

4.2 Tar-stained fingers – This patient smoked 40 cigarettes per day, but staining is more dependent on the action of smoking cigarettes right to the stub than on the total number smoked. This patient also has acute, recent onset clubbing (note the reddening and swelling of the nailfolds). He had bronchial carcinoma.

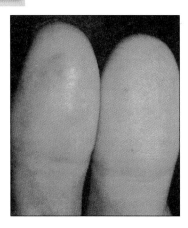

4.3   Impregnation with coal dust is commonly found in the hands of coal miners, and may give a clue to the presence of occupational lung disease (pneumoconiosis).

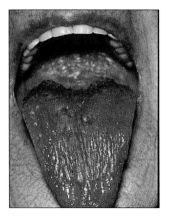 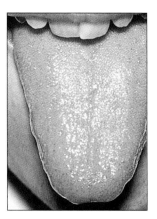

4.4   Central cyanosis is seen in the tongue, lips and earlobes. It is caused by the presence of high levels of deoxygenated haemoglobin. Here, the cyanotic patient's tongue (left) is compared with that of a normal individual (right). The blue appearance is characteristic, and may occur in severe respiratory or cardiovascular disease.

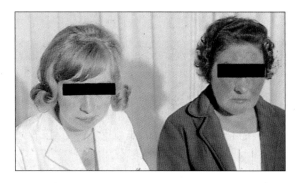

4.5   Secondary polycythaemia has developed in the patient on the right as a consequence of chronic hypoxic lung disease. Compare her appearance with that of the normal woman on the left.

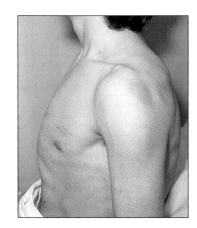

4.6   Barrel-shaped chest in a patient with chronic asthma. The hyperinflation results from air-trapping associated with inflammatory changes, hypersecretion of viscid mucus and smooth muscle contraction in the small airways. Note the associated indrawing of the intercostal muscles. Similar changes are seen in patients with chronic bronchitis and emphysema.

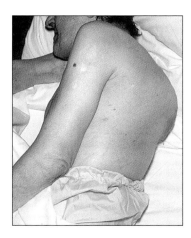

4.7   Severe kyphoscoliosis of unknown aetiology. Flexion (kyphosis) and lateral deviation (scoliosis) of the spine have the combined effect of reducing chest volume (*see* **4.38**). This compromises respiratory function, so that otherwise minor chest infections may precipitate respiratory failure.

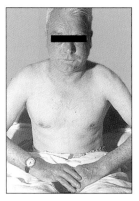

4.8   Pursed lip expiration is a common manoeuvre adopted by patients with severe chronic obstructive pulmonary disease. The patient starts to breathe out against closed or nearly closed lips to keep the intrabronchial pressure high and prevent collapse of the bronchial wall and expiratory obstruction. Later in expiration the lips are blown forwards and open, often with a grunt ('fish-mouth breathing').

- respiratory movements may be asymmetrical
- cervical lymph nodes may be visible (**4.9**) or palpable
- look and palpate for a goitre
- feel in the suprasternal notch for tracheal deviation
- examine a sputum sample if possible.

Key findings in the main groups of lung disease on palpation, percussion and auscultation are summarized in **4.10**.

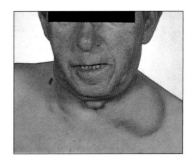

4.9 Gross enlargement of supraclavicular and cervical lymph nodes. This appearance may develop in tuberculosis and similar enlargement may occur with lymphomas, chronic lymphatic leukaemia and disseminated malignant disease. Biopsy is usually necessary for definitive diagnosis.

PHYSICAL SIGNS IN RESPIRATORY DISEASE

Lung pathology	Chest expansion	Mediastinal shift	Percussion note	Breath sounds	Voice sounds	Added sounds
Asthma	Reduced on both sides	Nil	Normal	Vesicular with prolonged expiration	Normal	Expiratory wheeze
Chronic bronchitis	Reduced on both sides	Nil	Normal	Vesicular with prolonged expiration	Normal	Expiratory wheeze and crackles
Consolidation (lobar pneumonia)	Reduced on affected side	Nil	Impaired	Bronchial	Increased	Crackles
Lung or lobar collapse	Reduced on affected side	Towards affected side	Impaired	Diminished vesicular	Reduced	Nil
Bronchiectasis	Normal or reduced on both sides	Nil	Normal	Normal	Normal	Coarse mid-inspiratory crackles
Fibrosing alveolitis	Reduced on both sides	Nil	Normal	Diminished vesicular (especially at bases)	Normal	Late inspiratory crackles
Localized fibrosis	Reduced on affected side	Towards affected side	Impaired	Bronchial	Increased	Crackles
Pneumothorax	Reduced on affected side	To opposite side	Hyper-resonant	Diminished vesicular	Reduced	Nil
Pleural effusion	Reduced on affected side	To opposite side	Stony dull	Diminished vesicular, occasionally bronchial at air fluid margin	Reduced	Rarely a pleural rub

4.10 Physical signs in respiratory disease.

INVESTIGATIONS

SPUTUM

Naked-eye examination of the sputum can give vital clinical information:

- consistently large volumes (at least 1/2 cup/day) suggest bronchiectasis
- rupture of an abscess, empyema or cyst into a bronchus may produce a sudden increase in volume
- infected sputum is usually yellow or green because of the large number of polymorphs it contains
- blood in the sputum produces a pink tinge in the typical frothy sputum of left ventricular failure, deep red flecks in bronchial carcinoma and pulmonary embolism, and a rusty colour in pneumococcal pneumonia (**4.11**)
- black sputum may be found in workers in a dusty environment or after smoke inhalation
- thick viscid sputum, sometimes taking the form of bronchial casts, is often seen in asthma and in allergic bronchopulmonary aspergillosis (**4.12**)
- rupture of a hepatic amoebic abscess into the lung gives an 'anchovy sauce' appearance to sputum

- rupture of a hepatic hydatid cyst into a right lower lobe bronchus produces bile-stained sputum.

Microscopic examination of sputum may show asbestos fibres (**4.13**), Charcot–Leyden crystals derived from eosinophils, fungal spores or clumps of pathogenic bacteria (**4.14**).

Sputum culture is of value in identifying bacteria and fungi and in testing for drug sensitivity. Culture normally takes 24–48 hours for pyogenic bacteria (up to 8 weeks for mycobacteria). Therapy should often be started without waiting for the results of culture.

For sputum cytology, as much sputum as possible should be sent fresh to the laboratory. The results are excellent with central tumours (80–90% positive, **4.15**), but much less successful with peripheral tumours.

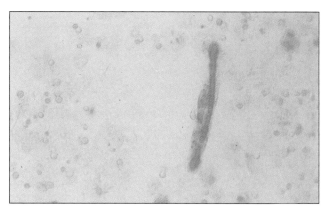

4.13 Asbestos body in sputum. The typical drumstick appearance represents an asbestos fibre surrounded by a ferroprotein complex. It is indicative of asbestos exposure with associated increased risks of bronchial malignancy and (with blue asbestos) mesothelioma.

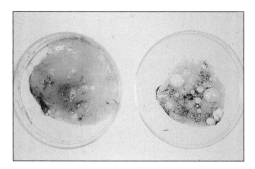

4.11 Rusty-red sputum (left) compared with fresh haemoptysis (right) in two sputum samples. The rusty red sputum comes from a patient with pneumococcal pneumonia, whereas the haemoptysis occurred in a patient with small-cell lung cancer.

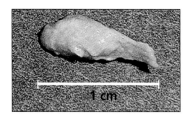

4.12 Typical sputum plug of allergic bronchopulmonary aspergillosis. These are usually brownish and firm or rubbery. On microscopy or culture they show *Aspergillus*. This plug was aspirated at fibreoptic bronchoscopy in a patient with segmental collapse on the chest radiograph. Similar plugs may be seen in patients with asthma but without aspergillosis.

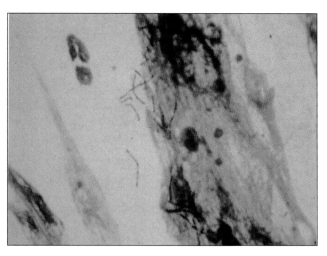

4.14 Ziehl–Neelsen staining of sputum showed many red-staining tubercle bacilli in this patient with pulmonary tuberculosis.

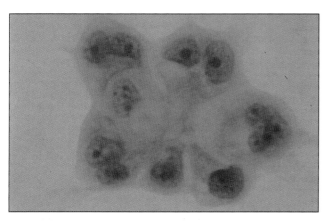

4.15 Adenocarcinoma cells in a sputum smear. The assessment of the appearances on sputum cytology is a very specialized field, and an expert opinion is essential for the definitive diagnosis of malignancy.

SKIN TESTS

Skin-prick testing may be useful in establishing the patient's immediate (type I) sensitivity to common allergens, thus confirming the patient's atopic state, and providing useful information about the possible role of allergens in disease.

Skin-prick testing may be useful in asthma, rhinitis, allergic conjunctivitis, urticaria and other allergic conditions, though false positive results are common in atopic eczema.

In skin-prick testing, a tiny quantity of allergen is introduced into the superficial layers of the stratum corneum (**4.16**).

A true-positive skin-prick test reaction (**4.17**, **4.18**) indicates that specific IgE is fixed to mast cells in the skin and has led to a vasoactive response caused by release of histamine. When the allergen concentration is high, or the patient's sensitivity is extreme, a late skin reaction may also follow 4–6 hours (or even as late as 24–48 hours) after the test, with erythema, swelling and induration.

When performed in patients with asthma, with appropriate positive (histamine) and negative (diluent) controls, skin test results correlate well with the results of bronchial challenge testing with the allergens (which is not performed routinely), and thus give useful information on the allergens involved; however, the results must always be correlated with clinical history. For inhaled allergens, up to 15% of positive results are false-positives, but fewer than 5% of negative results are false-negatives. However, skin testing is relatively unreliable for ingested allergens including food, partly because of the nature of the available allergen preparations and partly because reactions to ingested substances are not always mediated by IgE.

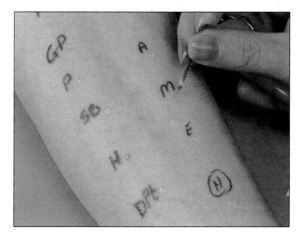

4.16 Skin-prick testing. The volar surface of the forearm is cleaned, prick sites are marked, and drops of allergen extract in appropriate concentration are placed on the skin. The test should always include a negative control of 0.5% phenol saline, the suspending solution for the allergens, and histamine 1% as a positive control. A lance or a standard needle is introduced through each drop at 45° to the skin surface to a depth of about 1 mm, the skin is lifted slightly, and the lance withdrawn. The procedure is painless, and the puncture sites should not bleed. The skin is blotted dry, and the resultant reaction is assessed at 15–20 minutes (*see* **4.17**).

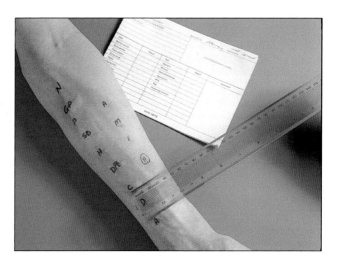

4.17 Reading the skin-prick test results. The maximum reaction is usually seen after 15–20 minutes. The saline control (N) should be negative (unless the patient has dermographism; **2.40**). The histamine control (H) should be positive; recent antihistamine administration may cause a negative result, and this invalidates other negative reactions. The presence of a positive skin response indicates the presence of specific IgE antibody in the blood, and there is a reasonable correlation between the size of the weal and the significance of different inhaled allergens in a single patient. Positive results are best recorded by measuring the diameter of the weal in millimetres, using a transparent gauge or a ruler. Here the strongest reaction is to grass pollen (GP), and significant positive reactions are also seen to cat (C) and the house-dust mite *Dermatophagoides pteronyssinus* (Dpt). The interpretation of the response depends on the clinical history.

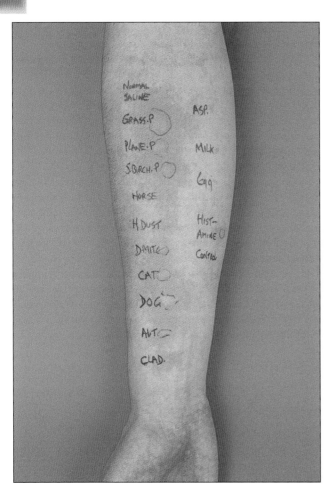

Normal
Saline
GRASS.P
PLANE:P
S.BIRCH.P
HORSE
H.DUST
D.MITE
CAT
DOG
ALT
CLAD.

ASP.
MILK
Egg
Hist-
Amine
Control

ALLERGEN EXTRACTS COMMONLY USED IN SKIN TESTING

Routine short screen for atopy:
Phenol saline (negative control)
Histamine (positive control)
House dust mite*
Grass pollen**
Aspergillus fumigatus
Cat

Additional allergens which may be used:
Tree/weed/other plant pollens
Alternaria
Cladosporium
Dog
Any other relevant animals
Any relevant foods
Any other relevant inhaled allergens

* Mixed 'house dust' extracts may be used in the routine screen; alternatively, specific allergens from Dermatophagoides pteronyssinus and/or Dermatophagoides farinae may be used.

** In some regions it is appropriate to include an alternative pollen antigen in the routine screen (e.g. birch in Scandinavia, ragweed in North America). The mix of grass pollens used may also vary between regions.

4.19   Allergen extracts commonly used in skin testing.

4.18   Multiple positive skin test results. Many asthmatics have multiple positive skin test reactions to common allergens, showing the ease with which they make IgE antibodies to common allergens in the environment. This British patient had positive reactions to grass, plane and silver birch pollens, cats, dogs and *Alternaria*. All may contribute to his asthma, which is perennial with a tendency to seasonal exacerbations during the period from April to August. The other allergens gave negative results; the flare reactions should be regarded as non-specific (a common reaction in patients with eczema), and there was no measurable weal.

Only a small number of allergens are needed for routine skin-prick testing in patients with asthma or rhinitis. A typical skin test battery can include four antigens, together with positive and negative controls (**4.19**). Additional antigens can be added when there is a clear possibility of the involvement of other antigens. The role of some allergens cannot be successfully investigated by skin-prick testing, and occupational allergens are also usually better identified by other means.

Strongly positive tuberculin tests (**1.104**) are of value in diagnosing tuberculosis in individual patients, and tuberculin testing also has a role in screening contacts and in pre-BCG (Bacillus Calmette–Guérin) assessment.

BLOOD TESTS

Venous blood samples taken for automated blood counts may provide major clues or confirmation of a suspected respiratory disease. A high haemoglobin concentration may be a reflection of polycythaemia, either primary or secondary (**4.5**) and a low haemoglobin may cause breathlessness. The total white cell count may be elevated in a range of acute bacterial infections and its subsequent fall is a reflection of successful therapy. Normal or low white cell counts are found in mycoplasma or viral infections. Eosinophilia suggests an allergic component or parasitic infection.

A range of serological tests that depend on agglutination, precipitation and complement fixation provide evidence of the presence in the patient's serum of specific antibodies against viral, bacterial, fungal, protozoal and helminth infections. Samples of blood should be tested on admission and repeated after 10–14 days to detect a rising titre.

Radioallergoabsorbent tests (RASTs) on venous blood are an alternative to skin-prick tests as a method of identifying specific IgE antibodies.

BLOOD GASES

The presence of respiratory failure may be suspected by the signs of central cyanosis. It is important to define the type and extent of failure of oxygenation and this is best done by measurement of arterial blood gas tensions (PaO_2 and $PaCO_2$), oxygen saturation (SaO_2) and pH (**4.20**). The response to drugs and the therapeutic response to oxygen can then be monitored easily. Haemoglobin saturation reflects oxygen carriage by the

blood and thus the adequacy of tissue oxygenation (if perfusion is satisfactory) and the requirement for oxygen therapy. This can be measured noninvasively by pulse oximetry (**4.21, 4.22**). The arterial partial pressure of carbon dioxide ($PaCO_2$) is a good indication of ventilation, low values indicating hyperventilation and vice versa; it is often more important than the PaO_2 in assessing the need for assisted ventilation.

PULMONARY FUNCTION TESTS

Simple pulmonary function tests may easily be done at home or at the bedside using a peak flow meter or gauge (**4.23**). This gives reasonably reliable and repeatable results and can be used to monitor therapy in asthma and chronic obstructive airways disease.

By use of a spirometer (**4.24**) and other equipment, a number of volume and flow rates can be estimated (**4.25**):

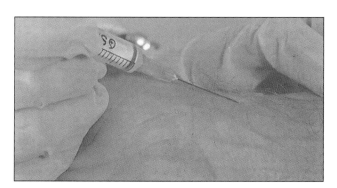

4.20   Arterial blood sampling can be carried out from the femoral, brachial or radial arteries, but the most common site is the radial artery in the patient's non-dominant arm. Firm pressure should be applied after withdrawal of the needle to prevent local haematoma formation.

4.21
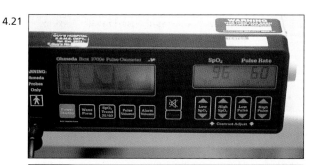

4.22
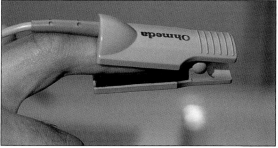

4.21 & 4.22   Pulse oximeter. The widespread introduction of pulse oximeters has been a great benefit in many areas of medicine, as oxygen saturation may be monitored non-invasively via a probe on a finger or earlobe. The estimation of oxygen saturation is not accurate at very low levels but, in the usual range for all but the most severe respiratory failure, oximeters are accurate if cardiac output and local circulation are adequate.

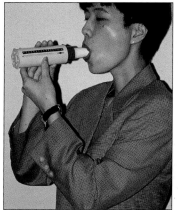

4.23   Mini peak flow meter in use. The patient takes in a deep breath, and then makes a maximal expiratory effort through the instrument. The procedure is repeated three times and the highest peak expiratory flow (PEF) is recorded. This can be compared with a nomogram that shows the patient's sex, age and weight, and plotted on a chart to show the progress or response to treatment.

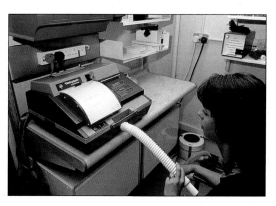

4.24   A spirometer provides a simple means of assessing air flow obstruction. The patient takes a maximal inspiration and then exhales as fast as possible for as long as possible. The volume expired against time is measured, and the forced expiratory volume in one second (FEV$_1$) and the forced vital capacity (FVC) can be simply calculated from the graph produced (**4.27**).

COMMON TESTS OF RESPIRATORY FUNCTION

Test	Abbreviation
Peak expiratory flow	PEF
Forced expiratory flow in 1 second	FEV_1
Forced vital capacity	FVC
Relaxed vital capacity	RVC
Total lung capacity	TLC
Residual volume	RV
Functional residual capacity	FRC
Maximum expiratory flow at lower lung volumes (50%, etc.)	MEF_{50}, etc.
Airways resistance	Raw
Specific conductance	sGaw
Transfer factor	TL_{co}
Transfer factor per unit lung volume (diffusion coefficient)	K_{CO}

4.25 Common tests of respiratory function.

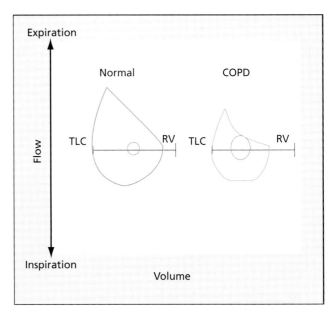

4.26 Flow-volume loop on spirometry in COPD compared with a normal flow-volume loop. The normal individual performs a full inspiration, followed by a linear expiration pattern. In COPD, by comparison, the expiratory part of the curve has a characteristic concave appearance, representing the effect of small airway obstruction during the forced expirator manoeuvre. TLC = total lung capacity (full inspiration); RV = residual volume (at full expiration).

- The peak expiratory flow (PEF) is the fastest flow rate recorded during expiration.
- The forced expiratory volume in 1 second (FEV_1) is the volume of gas expired in the first second of expiration.
- The forced vital capacity (FVC) is the total volume of gas expired.
- Flow-volume loops are particularly helpful in the assessment of airway obstruction (**4.26**).
- After a full expiration, some gas remains in the lung, the residual volume (RV); in order to measure this it is necessary to measure the volume of gas in the lungs at full inspiration (total lung capacity, TLC) and obtain the residual volume by subtracting the vital capacity; TLC is usually measured by helium dilution; a subject rebreathes a known volume and concentration of helium, which is diluted in the lung so that the TLC can be calculated by measuring how much the helium has been diluted.
- Airways resistance can be measured by body plethysmography.
- There are methodological difficulties in measuring oxygen transfer from lung to blood, so carbon monoxide transfer factor (TL_{CO}) is commonly measured; the transfer of carbon monoxide depends on how much haemoglobin can be 'seen' by the inspired gas; therefore transfer is low when the pulmonary capillary bed is damaged or obscured by inequalities of ventilation or perfusion; it is also low in anaemia and can be increased with polycythaemia or if haemorrhage into the lungs has occurred.

The results of simple spirometry provide much useful information (**4.27**) and simple lung function tests are of great

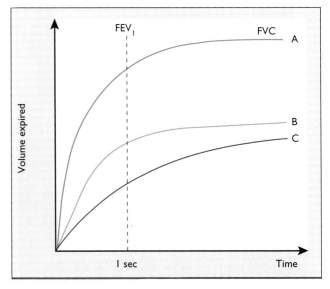

4.27 Typical results of spirometry in a normal patient (A), a patient with a restrictive defect (B) and a patient with an obstructive defect (C). In a restrictive defect (B), the FEV_1/FVC ratio is preserved at the normal level, but both absolute values are reduced. In an obstructive defect (C), both absolute values are again reduced, but the FEV_1/FVC ratio is considerably reduced, as the forced expiratory time required to reach the FVC is greatly prolonged.

value in following the course of many lung diseases and their response to treatment.

Bronchial challenge testing with histamine or methacholine is valuable in the assessment of airway hyperresponsiveness in asthma. The technique is widely used in assessing the effects of asthma therapy in clinical trials, but is not in routine clinical use in most centres.

IMAGING

A posteroanterior (PA) chest X-ray will often provide valuable diagnostic information about the nature and location of respiratory disease (**4.28–4.36**).

A lateral chest X-ray is helpful in identifying the position of abnormalities seen on the posteroanterior film (**4.37–4.40**) and may occasionally show significant abnormalities not seen on the standard film.

Tomography allows a radiograph of a specific slice of the chest; it is particularly useful for demonstrating lung cavities

(**4.41, 4.42**), the lumen of the trachea and major bronchi, and the position and nature of abnormal shadows noted on the plain radiograph.

Computerized axial tomography (computed tomography, CT) of the lung is most commonly used for the assessment of the extent of lung cancer (**4.43, 4.44**) but is being increasingly used in diffuse lung disease (**4.89, 4.117, 4.149**), has replaced bronchography as the first-line investigation of suspected bronchiectasis (**4.103**) and has largely replaced conventional tomography in other conditions..

MRI shows cardiovascular structures in the chest. Its role in pulmonary disease is still developing.

Pulmonary and aortic angiography may be used to define the anatomy of the arterial tree (**5.200**).

Radionuclide scans of lung (V/Q scan) are particularly useful in suspected pulmonary embolism (**4.45, 4.46, 5.199**). In this

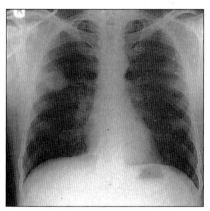

4.28 An early peripheral bronchial carcinoma in the right mid-zone, found by chance on a chest X-ray. The hilum appears normal, and this was confirmed by CT. This patient underwent a successful, and probably, curative lobectomy.

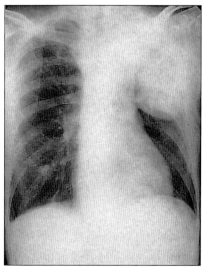

4.30 Left upper lobe opacity. The patient presented with pain in the chest and haemoptysis (**4.11**), and the underlying diagnosis proved to be small-cell carcinoma of the bronchus. Much of the shadowing is the result of infection and collapse of the lung distal to the point at which the tumour causes bronchial obstruction. Note the extensive calcification in the right hilum and lower zone – the result of healed tuberculosis.

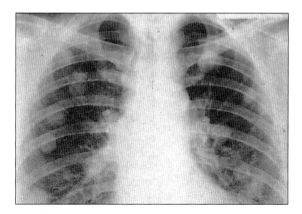

4.29 Cannonball metastases in both lung fields. Single or multiple round, discrete shadows resulting from secondary deposits occur with a number of tumours, including those of the kidney, ovary, breast, pancreas and testicle, and they are also seen in malignant melanoma.

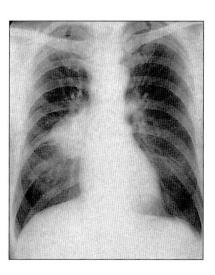

4.31 Carcinoma of the bronchus involving the right hilum and mediastinum. Bronchoscopy showed widening of the carina, which suggested lymph node involvement in the mediastinum and a friable, bleeding tumour in the right main bronchus. CT confirmed involvement of the great vessels. The tumour was thus inoperable.

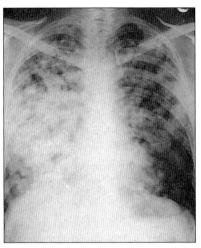

4.32 'Snowstorm' mottling in both lung fields. In this case, the underlying diagnosis was testicular seminoma, with disseminated haematogenous metastases. Such an extreme picture is usually the result of malignant disease, but the chest X-ray may look similar in a number of infectious conditions, especially miliary tuberculosis (*see* **1.101**), and in dust diseases.

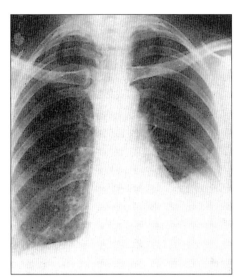

4.34 Left pleural effusion, which developed during an influenza-like illness in a young woman, and was associated with fever and pleuritic pain.

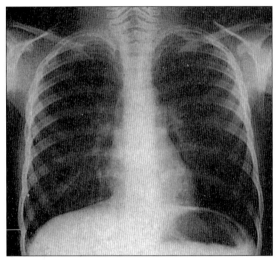

4.33 The chest X-ray is a poor guide to the severity of asthma. Although this patient had acute severe asthma requiring urgent treatment, his chest X-ray showed nothing more than mild hyperinflation with horizontally aligned ribs.

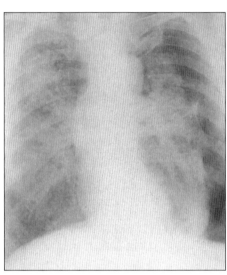

4.35 Left pneumothorax developed in this former coalminer with known pneumoconiosis. Note the obvious lung edge in the left chest and the diffuse miliary mottling of pneumoconiosis in both lungs.

4.36

4.37

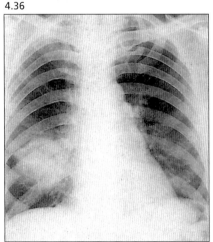

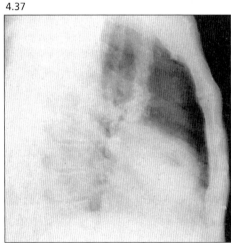

4.36 & 4.37 Staphylococcal lung abscess in the right lung of an intravenous drug misuser. The abscess is in the lower zone on the posteroanterior film, and the lateral film shows that it is above the oblique fissure, that is in the middle lobe of the lung. Note that there is also extensive calcification of the left hilum, which results from healed tuberculosis.

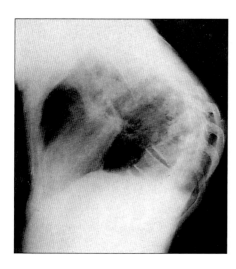

4.38 Kyphosis resulting from tuberculosis involving the thoracic vertebral bodies (T6–8). The significant reduction of lung volume is obvious (*see* **4.7**).

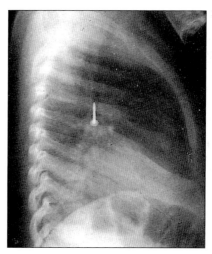

4.40 An inhaled foreign body – a nail – impacted in the right lower lobe bronchus. This young patient presented with a persistent cough and wheeze, but did not realize that he had inhaled a nail. Foreign bodies should always be borne in mind as a differential diagnosis of wheezing, especially in children.

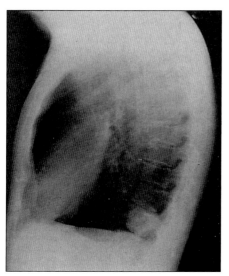

4.39 An opacity in the posterior segment of the left lower lobe shows clearly in this left lateral film, but was barely visible on the standard posteroanterior film, as it was behind the heart shadow. The lesion proved to be a benign hamartoma.

4.41

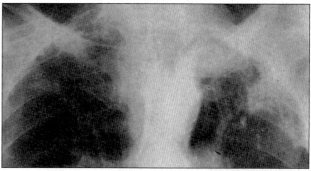

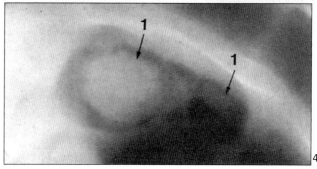

4.42

technique, xenon gas is inhaled and a gamma-camera image is produced of the alveolar distribution of the radioactivity (**4.45**). Then an intravenous injection of macroaggregates of human albumin labelled with ^{99m}Tc is injected. These microspheres embolize harmlessly in the lung vessels and the distribution of the radioactivity is a reflection of the pulmonary blood supply (**4.46**).

4.41 & 4.42 Tuberculous cavities containing aspergillomas at the left apex. This patient's left apical shadowing was further investigated by tomography, which clearly demonstrated the round mycetomas or fungus balls (1) within the chronic tuberculous cavities. CT would now be a more usual alternative to tomography.

BRONCHOSCOPY

Using a flexible fibreoptic (**4.47**) or video-bronchoscope, excellent views of all major and segmental bronchi (**4.48**) can be easily obtained and samples of mucus collected via the aspiration channel. In addition brush biopsies, suction catheters and biopsy forceps can be passed through this channel and bronchoalveolar lavage can be performed. Samples

suitable for culture, cytology and histology can be easily obtained.

Bronchoscopy is the investigation of choice for mass lesions on the central and mid-zones, especially if carcinoma is thought to be obstructing bronchi (**4.49**). In those who are very frail, however, sputum cytology may be the investigation of

4.43

4.44

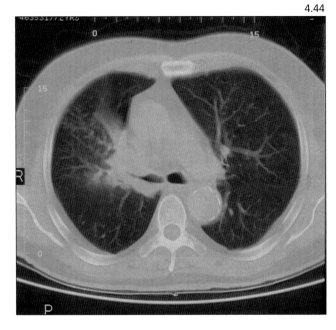

4.43 & 4.44 **Bronchial carcinoma,** revealed on chest X-ray and confirmed by CT. The reference chest X-ray (**4.43**) shows a mass adjacent to the upper right hilum. The transverse CT at level 9 (**4.44**) shows a tumour surrounding and narrowing the right upper lobe bronchus, with obstructive changes peripheral to it. Note the incidental presence of calcification in the wall of the descending aorta.

4.45

4.46

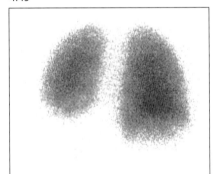

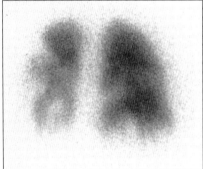

4.45 & 4.46 **Radionuclide ventilation (4.45) and perfusion (4.46) scans. 4.45** shows a normal distribution of xenon during ventilation, whereas **4.46** shows multiple perfusion defects in both lung fields when ^{99m}Tc-albumin microspheres were injected. This 'unmatched' perfusion defect is typical of multiple pulmonary emboli.

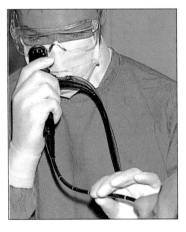

4.47 **Fibreoptic and video-bronchoscopy** are simple techniques that can be performed on the conscious patient. The bronchoscope is usually passed through the nose. This picture demonstrates the gown, mask, gloves and eye protection that are required if the patient is HIV positive. These patients often require bronchoscopy for the diagnosis of opportunistic lung infections.

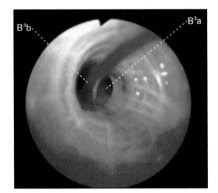

4.48 **Tracing the source of haemoptysis is often possible using the fibreoptic bronchoscope.** Here it has been traced to a subdivision of the right upper lobe bronchus labelled B³b.

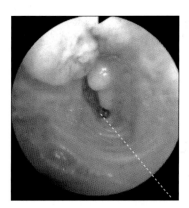

4.49 Squamous cell carcinoma seen through the fibreoptic bronchoscope at the opening of the left upper lobe bronchus (indicated by tip of dotted line). The white tumour has a relatively smooth surface. Biopsy through the bronchoscope is simple.

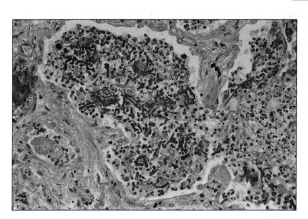

4.51 *Candida* pneumonia demonstrated on lung biopsy (PAS stain). *Candida* pneumonia is usually only found in patients who are immunosuppressed (by chemotherapy, radiotherapy or by HIV disease). The presentation is with a patchy bronchopneumonia which does not resolve with conventional antibiotics. This biopsy was taken from a patient with HIV infection and shows an alveolus filled by an inflammatory exudate in which the typical hyphae and budding forms of *Candida albicans* are seen.

choice. Lung biopsy is possible by advancing the biopsy catheter through the lung parenchyma under fluoroscopic control (**4.50, 4.51**). The use of bronchoscopy to obtain good specimens for microbiology and lung histology has reduced the requirement for open lung biopsy in patients with pulmonary infiltrates. Bronchoscopy can be useful therapeutically in the removal of secretions or foreign bodies causing airways obstruction, and some central tumours are amenable to laser resection via the bronchoscope.

Mediastinoscopy and thoracoscopy are other techniques that are of value in the investigation of selected patients with mediastinal and pleural disease.

PLEURAL ASPIRATION AND BIOPSY

Aspiration of pleural fluid is of major value for both diagnostic and therapeutic reasons. Naked-eye inspection may suggest the presence of pus, the effusion may be blood stained (**4.52**) suggesting carcinoma or pulmonary embolism, or milky white (chylous) as a result of obstruction of the thoracic duct, usually by tumour (**4.53**).

- pleural transudates are associated with generalized oedema and are pale in colour (**4.54**) with a specific gravity of less than 1015, total protein less than 2.5 g/100 ml
- pleural exudates represent inflammation and are usually darker in colour with a specific gravity above 1018 and a total protein greater than 3 g/100 ml
- total white cell count and cell type are of value; polymorphs indicate bacterial infection and lymphocytes suggest tuberculosis; culture of the fluid may show the organism responsible and cytology the diagnosis of tumour.

At the time of pleural aspiration, it is often convenient to carry out a pleural biopsy (**4.56**) with a side-cutting needle (**4.55, 4.57**). This is 'blind', but relatively atraumatic. Pleuroscopy and mediastinoscopy can be used to provide direct vision for biopsy. If the diagnosis is already made, antibiotics, cytotoxics or sclerosants may be instilled if appropriate.

Pleural aspiration and biopsy are not always harmless procedures. They may result in damage to the lung or abdominal organs, pneumothorax or haemothorax. In the longer term, biopsy of a mesothelioma may result in spread of the tumour (**4.58**).

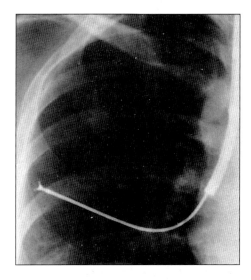

4.50 Biopsy of the peripheral lung through the flexible bronchoscope. Direct vision is not possible, but the forceps have been positioned under radiographic control and an alveolar biopsy should be obtained when their jaws are closed.

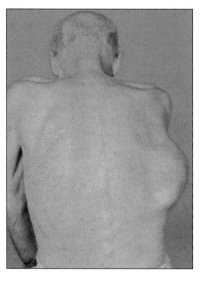

4.58 Mesothelioma has invaded down the needle track of a previous pleural biopsy into the subcutaneous tissues of this patient with an asbestos-linked pleural plaque (see **4.152**).

4.52 **4.53** **4.54**

4.52 Blood-stained pleural aspirate. This patient had pleural secondaries from carcinoma of the breast.

4.53 Chylous pleural effusion. This patient had bronchial carcinoma, which had invaded and obstructed the thoracic duct.

4.54 Pleural transudate. This pale effusion is typically found in patients with heart failure or other causes of generalized oedema.

LYMPH-NODE ASPIRATION AND BIOPSY

Aspiration of a palpable node, usually in the neck, may provide a rapid cytological diagnosis, and biopsy of a node is a further possibility in suspected malignant disease. When no nodes are felt, removal of the scalene node for culture and histology may provide diagnostic information.

INHALATION OF FOREIGN BODIES

Foreign bodies may be inhaled and lodge at any level in the respiratory system (e.g. **4.40**). Large objects may cause

4.55 **4.56**

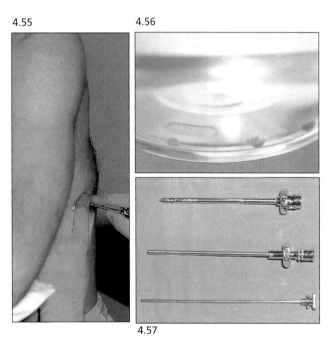

4.57

4.55, 4.56, 4.57 Pleural biopsy using an Abrams needle. As shown in **4.55** the needle is inserted into the pleural cavity and used to aspirate a pleural effusion. It then is turned round so that the notch present in the shaft engages with the parietal pleural surface. The inner cutting trocar is advanced to cut a small biopsy that may include the intercostal muscle as well as pleura and any tumour present. Examples of pleural biopsies are shown in **4.56**. This is an effective way of diagnosing pleural involvement by malignant disease. The component parts of the Abrams needle are shown in **4.57**.

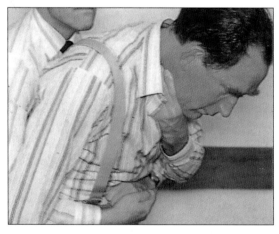

4.59 The Heimlich abdominal thrust manoeuvre can be used in an attempt to dislodge an inhaled foreign body in a conscious patient. One fist is clenched and positioned in the epigastrium and the other hand is placed on top. The patient is squeezed suddenly so that the fist moves backwards and upwards, causing a violent expulsion of air from the lungs.

potentially fatal obstruction at the level of the larynx. Such obstruction may often be dislodged by finger sweeps in the mouth, by sharp blows to the back or by use of abdominal thrust techniques (**4.59**, **4.60**).

If these techniques fail, emergency cricothyrotomy using an intravenous cannula (**4.61**) or even a sharp knife and the empty shaft of a ball-point pen may re-establish an airway.

At lower levels in the respiratory tract, inhaled foreign bodies are not usually immediately life-threatening (**4.40**); but failure to diagnose and remove foreign bodies may lead to traumatic damage to the lungs or to the collapse of segments of the lung distal to the obstruction with subsequent lobar pneumonia.

Chest X-ray is diagnostic for radio-opaque objects and bronchoscopy often allows removal of the foreign body.

UPPER RESPIRATORY TRACT DISORDERS

The common cold is discussed on **p. 10**, and rhinitis, sinusitis, tonsillitis, pharyngitis and laryngitis may also occur as part of a number of the childhood exanthemata such as measles (**p. 14**), and in infectious mononucleosis (**p. 22**) and streptococcal infection (**p. 25**).

Other medical disorders of the upper airway include other forms of rhinitis (**4.62**). Allergic rhinitis (**4.63**) may be

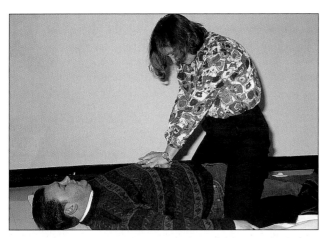

4.60 Abdominal thrust in an unconscious patient should be performed with the patient lying flat on a hard surface. Kneel over the patient and thrust upwards with both hands from below the xiphisternum. The technique should result in a violent expulsion of air from the lungs and may be repeated. Any dislodged foreign body should be removed from the mouth or pharynx by a finger sweep.

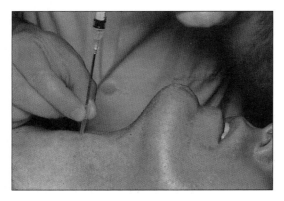

4.61 Cricothyrotomy is indicated in obstructive asphyxia when endotracheal intubation is impossible because of a foreign body, oedema or the absence of equipment. The surface marking for insertion of the needle is the space between the thyroid and cricoid cartilages. The syringe is aspirated to ensure that the needle and cannula are in the tracheal lumen, and the syringe and needle are then withdrawn, leaving the cannula in place.

SOME COMMON CAUSES OF RHINITIS
ALLERGIC
Perennial
House dust mite
Pets
Occupational causes
Seasonal
Pollens
Moulds
NON-ALLERGIC
Infections
Acute
Chronic (consider immunodeficiency/mucociliary problems)
Nasal hyperreactivity
Drugs
Aspirin
ß-blockers
Systemic diseases
Hormonal
Hypothyroidism
Pregnancy
Irritant
Irritant
Mucosal atrophy
Unknown cause

4.62 Some common causes of rhinitis.

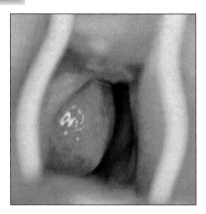

4.63 **Allergic rhinitis** produces a greyish appearance in the nasal mucous membrane, especially when chronic.

seasonal, most commonly caused by allergy to grass or other pollens (hayfever), or perennial, most commonly caused by allergy to proteins in the faecal particles of the house-dust mite. Skin-prick testing is often helpful in confirming the responsible allergens (*see* **p. 151**).

Non-allergic rhinitis produces similar symptoms, but the cause is usually obscure.

Allergic rhinitis is often associated with other atopic disorders, including conjunctivitis, urticaria and eczema, and is very commonly associated with hyperreactivity of the lower airways or asthma. Like asthma, allergic rhinitis is characterized by eosinophilic inflammation of the nasal mucosa and usually responds to topical corticosteroid therapy. Most of the symptoms of allergic rhinitis also respond to antihistamine

therapy, but this has little or no effect on the underlying inflammation.

Nasal polyps are benign, oedematous, inflammatory swellings, which originate in the mucosa of the ethmoid sinuses or middle turbinates and protrude into the nasal cavity, causing obstructive symptoms. They are particularly common in patients who also have asthma and are sensitive to aspirin and dietary salicylates, and are also associated with other respiratory tract disorders (**4.64**). They may be viewed via a nasal speculum or endoscopically (**4.65**), and their extent may be assessed by CT scan. Occasionally they may be large enough to distort the external appearance of the nose (**4.66**). They usually respond to topical steroid therapy, but systemic steroids or surgical removal may sometimes be needed to control obstructive symptoms, although recurrence is common.

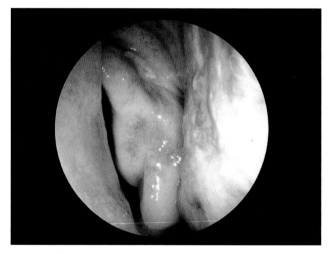

4.65 **An endoscopic view of nasal polyposis.** This is a relatively frequent accompaniment of asthma and is particularly common in adult asthmatics with sensitivity to aspirin. Polyps may be reduced in size by topical or oral steroid therapy.

THE PREVALENCE OF NASAL POLYPOSIS IN VARIOUS DISORDERS	
Disorder	**Prevalence of nasal polyps**
Aspirin intolerance	36–72%
Asthma	7%
– non-atopic	13%
– atopic	7%
Chronic rhinosinusitis	2%
– non-atopic	5%
– atopic	1.5%
Childhood asthma/ rhinosinusitis	0.1%
Cystic fibrosis	10% (children) – 50% (adults)
Young's syndrome	5%
Primary ciliary dyskinesia	5%

4.64 **The prevalence of nasal polyposis in various disorders.**

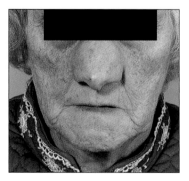

4.66 **Nasal polyps** produced near-total nasal obstruction and anosmia in this patient who had chronic aspirin-sensitive asthma. This degree of nasal enlargement is unusual. Polyps may exist in an externally normal nose.

ASTHMA

DEFINITION AND EPIDEMIOLOGY

Asthma is most simply defined as a disorder characterized by narrowing of airways that is reversible with time, either spontaneously or as a result of treatment.

A more detailed definition is that used in an International Consensus Report:

'Asthma is a chronic inflammatory disorder of the airways in which many cells play a role, in particular mast cells and eosinophils. In susceptible individuals, this inflammation causes symptoms that are usually associated with widespread but variable airflow obstruction that is often reversible either spontaneously or with treatment and causes an associated increase in airway responsiveness to a variety of stimuli.'

This more detailed definition is valuable in focusing on both the inflammatory nature and the potential reversibility of asthma, and thus in suggesting the most appropriate forms of therapy. At present, it is not possible to characterize asthma by biochemical or genetic features, but there is much continuing research in these fields.

Asthma is a common disorder. It has been estimated that its total prevalence is around 7% of the world population (about 100 million individuals), with a world population prevalence of about 6% in adults and 10% in children. At least 40 000 deaths per year worldwide can probably be attributed to asthma.

The estimated prevalence of asthma varies in different regions of the world, and in different parts of each country. In general, asthma is more common in urban than rural areas. In developing countries, asthma becomes more common in areas that adopt a 'developed' form of housing and lifestyle. The prevalence of asthma is increasing worldwide, but the reasons for this increase are unclear. It is likely that the initial sensitization process which results in asthma takes place in early infancy or even in utero, and much current research focuses on the identification and modification of the factors involved in this process.

Atmospheric pollution is probably not the major factor in the increased prevalence of asthma, but indoor air pollution resulting from house dust mite faecal particles and low rates of air exchange in modern buildings may be more significant. Occupational asthma is a well recognized problem in those exposed to sensitizing substances in industry.

MECHANISMS

Many patients develop symptoms in response to allergens such as house-dust mites (**4.67**), domestic animals or, less commonly, pollen grains; but often, especially in adult patients, there are no obvious underlying allergies. Many provoking factors are involved in the development of asthma symptoms, and these can be divided into two main groups: inducers and triggers:

- Inducers of asthma include genetic factors, allergies, infections and, probably, other factors related to occupational background or environment; they act mainly by inducing airway inflammation, which leads to airway hyperresponsiveness (AHR) and asthma symptoms.
- Triggers of asthma are factors which cause airway smooth muscle contraction and asthma symptoms on a background of pre-existing airway inflammation and airway hyperresponsiveness; these include a wide range of stimuli such as exercise, cold air, irritants, smoke, pollutants, β-blocking drugs and stress and, in susceptible individuals, drugs such as aspirin and other non-steroidal anti-inflammatory drugs, foods and other inhaled or ingested substances.

Asthma is a complex inflammatory condition involving many inflammatory cells, which release a wide variety of mediators. These mediators act on cells of the airway leading to smooth muscle contraction, mucus hypersecretion, plasma leakage, oedema, activation of cholinergic reflexes and activation of sensory nerves, which can lead to amplification of the ongoing inflammatory response. Chronic inflammation also leads to structural changes, such as subepithelial fibrosis and smooth muscle hypertrophy and hyperplasia, which are less easy to reverse than the acute processes. Inadequately treated chronic asthma is thus associated with structural changes in the lungs.

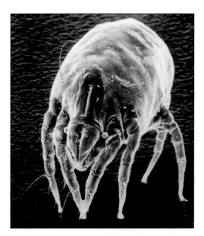

4.67   The house-dust mite, *Dermatophagoides pteronyssinus*. The faecal particles of this and related mite species are the most common cause of allergic asthma worldwide. The faecal particles are small enough to be inhaled into the peripheral airways in the lung. Dust mites are most common in moist, temperate environments. They feed on shed scales of human and animal skin, and commonly infest mattresses, pillows, carpets and soft furnishings. Their growth is encouraged by the low rate of air turnover in modern insulated houses. They are about 0.5 mm in length and invisible to the naked eye. Dust-mite allergy also plays a major role in perennial rhinitis and possibly in eczema.

TYPES OF ASTHMA

Typically, most children with asthma have identifiable trigger factors, whereas most patients with asthma that begins in adult life do not, and asthma is often classified as 'extrinsic', in which identifiable external trigger factors are present, or 'intrinsic', in which no such factors are identified. However, non-atopic patients may develop asthma in middle age from extrinsic causes such as sensitization to occupational agents, intolerance to aspirin, or the use of β-blockers for the treatment of hypertension or angina. Extrinsic causes should thus be considered in all cases of asthma and avoided whenever possible.

Current understanding of the role of genetic factors, inducers and triggers in asthma has made it obvious that this classification is an over-simplification. It is more clinically useful to consider a number of different variants of asthma (**4.68**).

Well over 200 different causes of occupational asthma have been recognized, and some are of major importance in industry. Some occupational materials produce asthma by a classic type I immunological mechanism, and specific IgE antibody can be found in the serum. In other cases, the precise mechanism has still to be determined.

Clinical assessment

The spectrum of clinical presentation of asthma ranges from very mild symptoms (**4.69**) to an acute life-threatening illness (**4.70**). A commonly used grading of asthma is shown in **4.71**.

Physical signs are of relatively little value in the diagnosis and assessment of asthma. Chest expansion may be reduced, and there may be chest deformity if asthma has been poorly controlled for many years, especially during childhood (**4.6**). In atopic individuals, signs of other allergic disorders such as rhinitis or atopic dermatitis (eczema) may be present. Skin-prick testing may be helpful in confirming atopy or suggesting relevant allergens (*see* **p. 151**). Expiratory wheezing may be heard over both lung fields, but wheezing may be absent in severe asthma, and it is important to realize that patients with asthma may show few specific signs. Even in severe asthma (**4.69**), the chest X-ray may appear normal or show no more than the signs of hyperinflation (**4.33**), though it may show complicating conditions such as pneumonia or pneumothorax (**4.175**).

Simple respiratory function tests are very helpful in the diagnosis and management of asthma, but it is usually important that they are repeated. Even repeated measurement

TYPES OF ASTHMA	
Type	**Common features**
Childhood onset	Patient usually atopic, marked variability, obvious trigger factors
Adult onset	Demonstrable atopy uncommon, usually persistent, infection a common trigger, but other identifiable triggers uncommon
Occupational	Under-diagnosed, careful assessment needed
Nocturnal	May occur with all types of asthma, indicates poor overall control and increased airway hyperresponsiveness
Prominent cough	A common presentation in childhood, may precede significant airflow obstruction, responsive to anti-inflammatory treatment
Exercise-induced	A common precipitant of other types of asthma, especially in childhood. May be the main problem in childhood

4.68 Types of asthma. More than one of these patterns may coexist in the same patient.

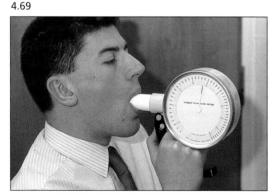

4.69

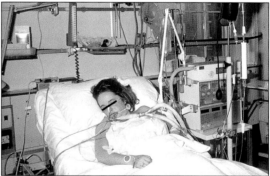

4.70

4.69 & 4.70 The range of presentation of asthma. The patient in **4.69** was found incidentally to have a degree of reversible airways obstruction during a medical examination for other reasons. He had never been aware of symptoms. The patient in **4.70**, by comparison, presented as a medical emergency with acute severe breathlessness and required immediate intensive care including intermittent positive-pressure ventilation.

SEVERITY OF ASTHMA: CLASSIFICATION AND FREQUENCY

Severity (% of total asthma population)	Features
Very severe (2%)	Disabling disease Numerous exacerbations with hospital admission Much time off work or school Life-threatening attacks
Severe (18%)	Daily wheezing Severe nocturnal symptoms Poor quality of life Off work or school for several weeks per year Hospital admission common
Moderate (20%)	Daily symptoms, but no significant diurnal variation Occasional nocturnal symptoms Patient avoids exercise
Mild (20%)	Periodic symptoms Patient reacts to triggers (e.g. pollen or cold air) Symptoms restrict activity 2–3 times per week
Very mild (40%)	Occasional cough or wheezing that does not cause major impairment Respiratory tract sensitive to infections and intense cold Allergens may cause symptoms

4.71   Severity of asthma: classification and frequency.

at the same time of day may mask regular variations in PEF (**4.72**), so several measurements per day are needed for full assessment. Reversibility of airway obstruction after inhalation of a test dose of bronchodilator (usually a β₂-agonist) is indicative of asthma. Measurement following simple provocation tests, (e.g. exercise) may also be very useful (**4.73**).

Some patients, especially children, may exist at low levels of PEF without complaint, but if this is recognized and treated there may be major quality-of-life benefits.

The assessment of patients with severe asthma is of critical importance in reducing the mortality of asthma (**4.74**).

MANAGEMENT OF ASTHMA

The treatment of severe acute asthma usually requires hospital admission for oxygen therapy, nebulized bronchodilators and systemic steroids (**4.75**). Intermittent positive-pressure ventilation may be required in very severe cases (**4.70**). It is essential that the patient's maintenance therapy is established, with evidence of adequate control, before the patient is discharged from hospital.

Currently available drug therapy for asthma is summarized in **4.76**. Numerous national and international guidelines have been developed, which share many common features. The mainstay of treatment for persistent asthma is regular inhaled steroid therapy, supplemented if necessary in moderate and severe asthma by an inhaled long-acting β₂-agonist, oral theophylline, or an oral leukotriene antagonist. The long-term use of oral steroids should be avoided because of the risk of side-effects, and a steroid-sparing agent such as methotrexate may be used in very severe asthma. Inhaled rapid-acting β₂-agonist therapy is the mainstay for immediate symptomatic relief in asthma at all grades of severity, but this should be supplemented by preventive therapy if required more than three times per week.

Inhaled drugs may be administered via a confusing number of devices, which have differing performance characteristics (**4.77**). Nebulized therapy has a role in severe asthma (**4.78**), but the three main types of inhaler are the pressurized metered-dose inhaler (pMDI; **4.79**), the pMDI with a spacer device (**4.80**) and dry powder inhalers (DPI; **4.81**). Some advantages and disadvantages of these devices are summarized in **4.82**.

Patient education in all aspects of asthma, including inhaler use, is of great importance in long-term care.

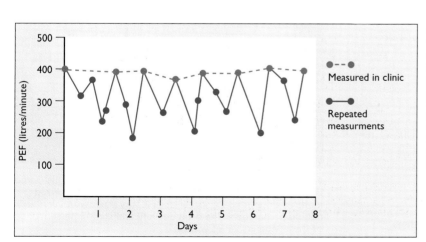

4.72   Diurnal variation in peak expiratory flow (PEF). Even daily measurements of airflow obstruction in a hospital or general practice setting may not show any evidence of airflow obstruction, because the typical morning 'dip' in PEF usually occurs between 4.00 a.m. and 7.00 a.m., with spontaneous improvement in peak flow over the next few hours. In these circumstances only home monitoring of PEF reveals the extent of the patient's asthma. In well controlled asthma, the circadian variation in PEF should be no more than 20%.

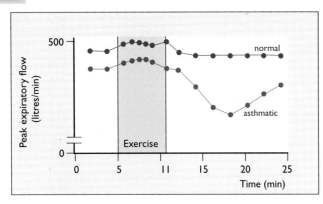

4.73 Peak expiratory flow responses to an exercise test. In normal and asthmatic patients there is a small degree of bronchodilatation during exercise, but in asthmatic patients this initial bronchodilatation is followed by bronchoconstriction, reaching its maximum 5–10 minutes after the end of exercise. A 15% drop from baseline levels of PEF is considered a positive test, and the fall in PEF can be rapidly reversed with an inhaled bronchodilator. Exercise-induced asthma is a particularly common problem in childhood.

THE ASSESSMENT OF PATIENTS WITH SEVERE ASTHMA

Patients have asthma that has deteriorated with increased wheeze, breathlessness, chest tightness or coughing, sleep disturbance, or failure to respond to usual treatment

Features of uncontrolled asthma

• peak expiratory flow (PEF) > 50% of predicted normal or best
• respiratory rate < 25 breaths/minute
• pulse rate < 110 beats/minute
• speech normal

Features of acute severe asthma

(Any one of the following indicates a severe attack)
• PEF ≤ 50% of predicted normal or best
• respiratory rate ≥ 25 breaths/minute
• cannot complete sentences in one breath

Life-threatening features

(Any one of the following indicates a very severe attack)
• PEF < 33% of predicted or best
• silent chest, cyanosis or feeble respiratory effort
• bradycardia or hypotension
• exhaustion, confusion or coma

Arterial gas markers of a very severe attack

(Measure if SaO_2 < 92% or any life-threatening features are present)
• normal or high $PaCO_2$ (> 5.0 kPa, 40 mmHg)
• low PaO_2 (< 8.0 kPa, 60 mmHg)
• low pH (<7.36)

4.74 The assessment of patients with severe asthma.

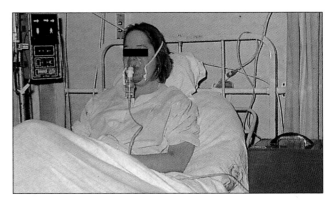

4.75 An acute asthmatic patient in hospital, receiving nebulized β_2 agonist (the nebulizer is driven by oxygen) and intravenous hydrocortisone. Careful monitoring of therapy is required.

DRUG THERAPY IN ASTHMA

Preventive therapy

Inhaled steroids	Oral theophylline*
Inhaled long-acting β_2-agonists	Oral leukotriene antagonists
	Oral steroids
Inhaled cromones	Oral steroid-sparing agents

Reliever therapy

Inhaled β_2-agonists	Oral (or injected) β_2-agonists
Inhaled anticholinergics	Oral theophylline

* Theophylline is used principally as reliever therapy, but may also exert some preventive, anti-inflammatory effect.

4.76 Drug therapy in asthma.

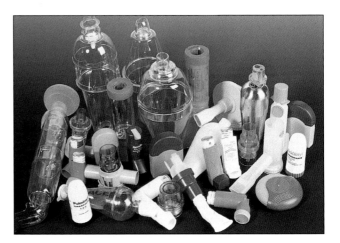

4.77 Inhaler devices in asthma. This picture includes just some of the many devices available, including various pressurized metered-dose inhalers, spacer devices, dry powder inhalers and nebulizer chambers. The drug delivery and clinical performance of these inhalers varies widely.

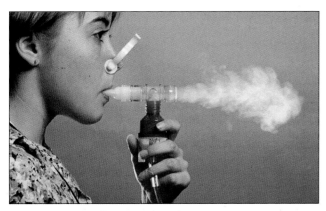

4.78   Nebulized therapy may be helpful in severe asthma.
High doses of bronchodilators may be delivered by this method
in carefully defined circumstances. Nebulized steroid therapy
may provide an alternative to oral steroid therapy, or an aid to
oral dose reduction.

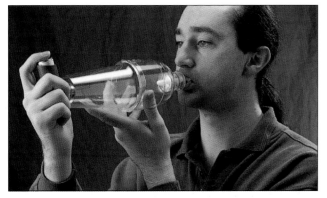

**4.80   Large volume 'spacer' or extension chamber added to a
pressurized metered-dose inhaler.** Large volume spacers allow
the aerosol cloud to slow down, and overcome problems of
patient coordination. They may increase lung deposition and
reduce oral impaction, a potentially useful feature with inhaled
steroid therapy. They may also be used in acute attacks of
asthma to deliver repeat aerosol doses of bronchodilator every
few minutes. Smaller metal spacer devices may achieve the
same effect while eliminating the unpredictability of dose
which may result from static charging of polycarbonate spacers.

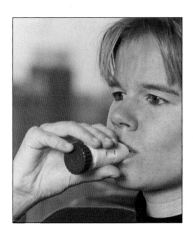

**4.81   A dry-powder,
multidose inhaler
(Turbohaler or
Turbuhaler).** Dry-powder
inhalers are inspiratory
flow-actuated and driven,
so they overcome the
coordination problems of
pMDIs. The performance
of different dry-powder
inhalers varies, but
Turbohaler achieves a
substantially higher lung
deposition of drug than
many pMDIs, and a single
inhaler holds up to 200
doses of the drug.

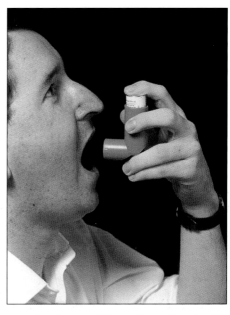

4.79   A pressurized metered-dose inhaler (pMDI). All
commonly used inhaled therapy for asthma is available in this
form. Although convenient and portable, the pMDI requires
good coordination between actuation and inhalation by the
patient. The drug delivery characteristics of many pMDIs have
changed recently, as new propellant gases (HFAs) have replaced
CFC gases for environmental reasons.

**SOME ADVANTAGES AND DISADVANTAGES OF THE THREE
FORMS OF PORTABLE INHALER**

Advantages	Disadvantages
pMDI	
Quick to use	Difficult inhalation technique
Compact and portable	Propellants required
Multidose	High oropharyngeal deposition
Often inexpensive	
pMDI + spacer device	
Practical advantages as for pMDI	More bulky than pMDI
Easier to use effectively than pMDI	Propellants required
Reduced oropharyngeal deposition	Static charge on wall may affect delivered dose
Dry-powder inhaler	
Practical advantages similar to pMDI (if multidose or multiple single-dose)	Some may be moisture sensitive
No propellants needed	Inspiratory flow driven (potential problem at low inspiratory force)
Inspiratory flow-actuated	Patient may be unsure whether dose delivered
Easier to use than pMDI	

**4.82   Some advantages and disadvantages of the three forms
of portable inhaler.**

The aim of asthma management is to achieve good, long-term control of the disease and its manifestations. The features of good control of asthma are shown in **4.83**.

FEATURES OF GOOD CONTROL IN ASTHMA

Minimal (ideally no) chronic symptoms

No nocturnal symptoms

No acute exacerbations

Minimal need for 'reliever' bronchodilators

No limitation of activity, including exercise

Circadian variability of peak flow < 20%

Peak flow > 80% of predicted or best achievable

Minimal (ideally no) adverse effects from treatment

4.83   **Features of good control in asthma.**

ANAPHYLAXIS

Anaphylaxis is an acute medical emergency characterized by bronchoconstriction, laryngeal oedema, urticaria, angioedema and hypotension. These features are often severe, and the associated respiratory obstruction and shock may be rapidly fatal. Immediate recognition and urgent treatment are required to ensure survival. Fatal anaphylaxis is, fortunately, rare, but less major reactions are much more common and probably under-reported.

Anaphylaxis results from a type I (immediate) hypersensitivity reaction, which involves a generalized IgE-mediated response to an allergen to which the patient has previously been sensitized, and results in the release of vasoactive and bronchoconstricting mediators including histamine and bradykinin. The patient may be aware of sensitivity to the provoking agent, but anaphylaxis may be its first manifestation.

Prodromal symptoms occur in some patients, and may include light-headedness, anxiety, local pruritius and paraesthesiae, and acute allergic reactions in the mouth (especially if the allergen was ingested), eyes and nose. Later (usually within a few minutes) the patient develops:

- generalized flushing, pruritus and urticaria (**2.41**)
- oedema of the mouth, pharynx and larynx (**4.84, 8.126**), wheezing and ultimately respiratory arrest
- hypotension, arrhythmias, myocardial ischaemia (especially in older patients) and ultimately cardiac arrest
- often nausea, vomiting, tenesmus and diarrhoea
- sometimes convulsions.

Anaphylaxis is most likely to lead to death in younger patients with asthma, in older patients with cardiovascular or cerebrovascular disease and in any patient receiving beta-blocker therapy (which intensifies the reaction to mediator release).

It is important to distinguish anaphylaxis from vasovagal attacks, hyperventilation, myocardial infarction, hypoglycaemia and other causes of shock. This is usually straightforward when the patient can give a history of known sensitivity, or is carrying evidence of a known allergy. Without this history, the presence of urticaria and angioedema in a patient with shock or respiratory obstruction is strongly suggestive of anaphylaxis.

Milder reactions may respond to systemic H_1-antihistamine therapy. However, the key to successful treatment of severe anaphylaxis is the immediate administration of intramuscular or subcutaneous adrenaline (epinephrine). Patients who have a predominantly airway response may benefit from inhaled adrenaline (epinephrine), but this should be followed by systemic adrenaline (epinephrine) unless there is an immediate response. Intubation may be necessary for upper airway oedema (**4.84**). Oxygen, bronchodilator treatment, blood volume expanders and intensive care are required in severe reactions, and systemic corticosteroid therapy may lessen the chance of late relapse.

The commonest causes of anaphylaxis are penicillins, bee and wasp stings and food allergy (*see* **p. 371**), but many other factors may lead to anaphylaxis in sensitized individuals (**4.85**). In developed countries, allergy to peanuts is one of the commonest causes of anaphylaxis. In the UK, for example, over 1% of children are now estimated to be allergic to peanut protein, and the ingestion of – or in some cases even oral contact with – peanuts can provoke a severe reaction in many such patients.

Education of patients (and parents, teachers, etc.) in the avoidance of provoking allergens is essential for the prevention of future attacks, and the food industry and the medical profession also have a duty to avoid exposure of individuals to

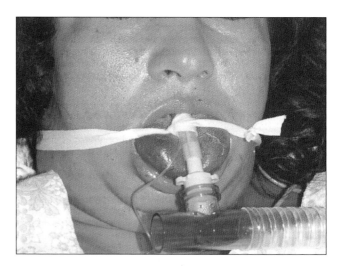

4.84 Severe angioedema in a 43-year-old woman with anaphylaxis. She required endotracheal intubation to overcome laryngeal obstruction. Note the oedema of her mouth and face.

PRECIPITATING FACTORS IN ANAPHYLACTIC REACTIONS	
Factor	**Examples**
Drugs	Aspirin, NSAIDs, anaesthetics, antibiotics, induction agents and muscle relaxants
Diagnostic agents	Radio-opaque dyes
Vitamins	Folic acid, thiamine
Hormones	ACTH, insulin, methylprednisolone, parathormone, estradiol
Enzymes	Asparaginase, chymopapain, chymotrypsin, penicillinase, trypsin
Allergen extracts	Epidermal extracts, house dust mite, pollens
Horse antiserum	Antilymphocytic globulin, venom antitoxin
Blood products	Blood, cryoprecipitate, immunoglobulin
Venoms	Bee and wasp venom
Foods	Peanut, egg, milk, nuts, shellfish, soy bean
Miscellaneous	Dextran, seminal fluid, latex

4.85   Precipitating factors in anaphylactic reactions.

allergens to which they are known to be sensitized. Patients at risk of severe attacks should always wear an identifying bracelet or carry an identifying card. They should also carry an adrenaline (epinephrine) syringe or 'pen', for the self-administration of subcutaneous adrenaline (epinephrine) and be trained in its use. Unfortunately the severity of one attack is not a guide to the likely severity of future attacks.

CHRONIC OBSTRUCTIVE PULMONARY DISEASE (COPD)

Chronic obstructive pulmonary disease (COPD, a term that embraces chronic bronchitis, chronic bronchiolitis and emphysema) is the fourth most common cause of death worldwide, and its prevalence is increasing. It is currently more common in men than women and most frequent in industrialized countries. However, it becomes more common wherever the prevalence of smoking in men and/or women increases – as currently in much of the developing world. COPD is very rare in non-smokers. Airway obstruction in a non-smoker or light smoker is usually caused by asthma, rarer causes being emphysema in α_1-antitrypsin deficiency, obliterative bronchiolitis or industrial lung disease.

Chronic bronchitis is defined clinically by the daily production of sputum, associated with cough, which persists over 3 months in each of at least 2 consecutive years. Pathologically there is large airway inflammation with goblet

cell hyperplasia. Excessive mucus secretion by bronchial goblet cells stimulates the cough reflex, so that sputum is produced. There are often episodes of superimposed viral or bacterial infection in which the sputum may be yellow or green and often contains a fleck of blood. Many patients also have an intermittent wheeze with objective evidence of airway obstruction on pulmonary function tests and some may have acute severe bronchoconstriction in response to respiratory infections or to irritants or allergens (asthmatic bronchitis).

Chronic bronchiolitis and alveolitis (small airways disease) affect many smokers and may lead to microscopic emphysema, impaired gas mixing and exchange, and ultimately to pulmonary hypertension and cor pulmonale.

Emphysema is a pathological or radiological rather than a clinical diagnosis and is commonly associated with chronic bronchitis. Destruction of the alveolar septae results in the formation of multiple bullae in the lungs, with hyperinflation of the chest (**4.86–4.89**) and impaired respiratory function.

169

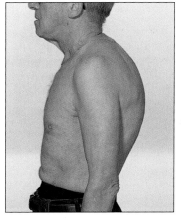

4.86   Emphysema. The hyperinflation of the chest and associated kyphosis are typical but not diagnostic. A similar appearance may be seen in any chronic respiratory disorder. Note the typical 'pursed lip' appearance (**4.8**).

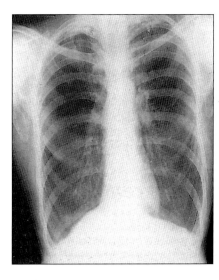

4.87   Emphysema. The PA chest X-ray shows hyperinflation of both lung fields, producing depression of both diaphragms and a characteristic long, thin mediastinum. There are also calcified lesions and some scarring at both apices and both hila as a result of old, healed tuberculosis.

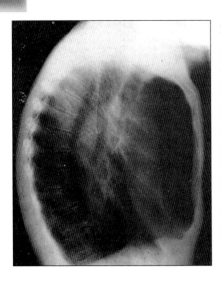

4.88 Emphysema. The right lateral chest X-ray shows hyperinflation of the chest with sparse lung markings. There is a marked increase in the posteroanterior diameter of the chest, and the diaphragmatic depression is again seen. In this patient the hilar calcification resulting from old, healed tuberculosis is also well seen in the lateral view.

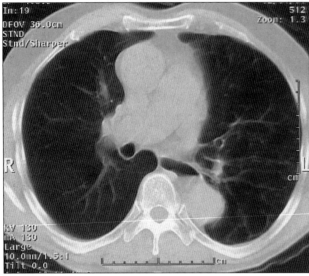

4.89 CT of emphysema, predominantly in the left lung in this view. Bullous areas and reduced density of the lung structure are well shown on thin slices of lung in a CT scan. This has emerged as the best method for quantification of the extent of emphysema. The measurements of lung density correlate well with histological findings.

The symptoms are usually worse in winter and exacerbated by atmospheric pollution, dry air, intercurrent infections and industrial exposure to irritant gases or dusts. Some patients present with the complications of later stage COPD (**4.90**), not having sought medical help at the earlier stages.

In early COPD, there are usually few abnormal findings on examination, but in more advanced disease there is commonly hyperinflation of the chest, with reduced breath sounds and wheezing.

The diagnosis of COPD should be confirmed by spirometry, which demonstrates airflow obstruction by an FEV_1:FVC ratio of less that 70%, and shows a characteristic abnormality in the computerized flow-volume loop (**4.26**). PEF is reduced in severe COPD, but this is of little value in the diagnosis and management of milder COPD, as it seriously underestimates the degree of airflow obstruction.

The FEV_1 (expressed as a percentage of the predicted value) can be used to assess the severity of COPD. Precise values vary between different sets of guidelines, but broadly:

- FEV_1 > 80% predicted – mild COPD
- FEV_1 30–80% predicted – moderate COPD
- FEV_1 < 30% predicted – severe COPD.

Pulse oximetry (**4.21**, **4.22**) should be performed on those with severe COPD and an oxygen saturation of less that 92% is an indication for full arterial blood gas measurement, to identify those with impending respiratory failure.

Other relevant investigations may include a full blood picture, to exclude polycythaemia, α_1-antitrypsin level and a chest X-ray, which may reveal hyperinflation (**4.87**, **4.88**) or large emphysematous bullae or demonstrate associated lung cancer or tuberculosis. CT of the thorax is useful in selected patients to define the extent of emphysema (**4.89**), and to investigate associated pathology including lung cancer or bronchiectasis.

At a later stage in the disease, two common clinical pictures represent opposite ends of the spectrum of COPD:

- the 'pink puffer' (**4.91**) usually has significant emphysema with a barrel-shaped chest, but is thin and maintains a normal $PaCO_2$ by increasing his or her respiratory rate

PRESENTATIONS AND COMPLICATIONS OF COPD	
Clinical presentations	**Complications**
Cough and sputum	Weight loss
Breathlessness	Cough syncope
Wheezing	Cor pulmonale
Chest tightness or discomfort	Respiratory failure
	Psychosocial problems

4.90 Presentations and complications of COPD.

Chronic bronchitis, chronic bronchiolitis and emphysema commonly coexist in COPD. Chronic bronchitis occurs in the majority of heavy smokers, but significant airways obstruction, chronic bronchiolitis and emphysema occur in only a minority.

CLINICAL ASSESSMENT OF COPD

The characteristic clinical features of COPD are cough, productive of sputum, progressive breathlessness, wheezing and sometimes a feeling of chest tightness or discomfort (**4.90**).

- the 'blue bloater' (**4.92**) tends to be fatter, polycythaemic, centrally cyanosed and to show signs of pulmonary hypertension (**4.93**, **4.94**, **5.120**, *see* **p. 230**). As the disease progresses, the $PaCO_2$ rises and leads to a compensated respiratory acidosis (**4.95**, **4.96**).

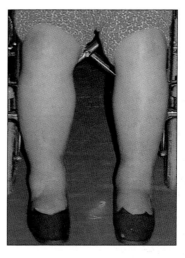

4.93 Chronic bronchitis with right heart failure causing gross peripheral oedema. The patient was a typical 'blue bloater' and he was not unduly breathless.

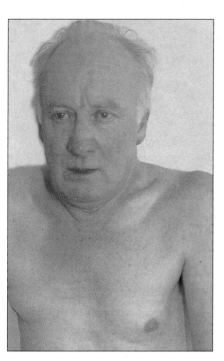

4.91 A 'pink puffer'. Some patients with severe long-standing chronic bronchitis and emphysema are breathless and have a hyperinflated chest, but a well maintained PaO_2 and a low $PaCO_2$. These patients are not cyanosed but are breathless, hence the term 'pink puffer'.

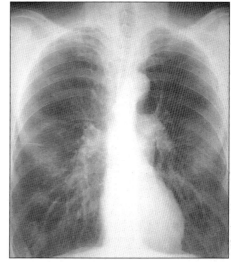

4.94 Cor pulmonale in a patient with COPD. Both pulmonary arteries are enlarged, and there is marked peripheral pruning of the pulmonary vessels. There is also a small pleural effusion on the right in the horizontal fissure.

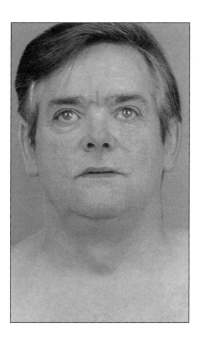

4.92 A 'blue bloater'. In these patients, the $PaCO_2$ has risen, and the PaO_2 has fallen. Breathlessness at rest is not prominent, and the patient looks more comfortable than the 'pink puffer'; 'blue bloaters' have right heart failure, which results in peripheral oedema. The combination of this oedema and the cyanosis accounts for the term 'blue bloater'. Many patients with chronic bronchitis and emphysema fall between the two extremes demonstrated here and in **4.91**.

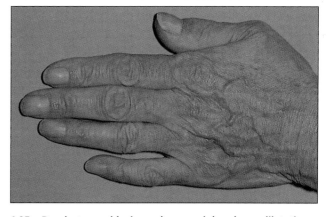

4.95 Respiratory acidosis produces peripheral vasodilatation, giving hands which are warm and dry, cyanosed and show features of a hyperkinetic circulation: a bounding pulse and tachycardia, with dilatation of the peripheral veins. A flapping tremor of the hands may also develop. This patient also has early finger clubbing, which is an indication for further investigation.

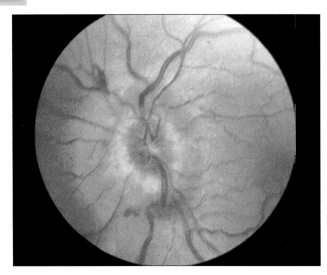

4.96 **Papilloedema occurs in respiratory failure** as a result of the increased cerebral and retinal blood flow caused by CO_2 retention, though it is often less marked than here. This papilloedema is similar to that seen in raised intracranial pressure of other causes.

MANAGEMENT OF COPD

The most important step in management is to persuade the patient to stop smoking, though this may be difficult. Treatment of established COPD is palliative rather than curative (**4.97**), and the prognosis is little changed by current therapies. Nevertheless the effect of some pharmalogical and non-pharmacological interventions on symptoms and quality of life can be very beneficial. These interventions have been evaluated in a number of national and international guidelines:

- In patients with mild COPD the main recommendation is avoidance of noxious agents, and particularly smoking cessation. A rapid-acting bronchodilator may be used as needed.

AIMS OF LONG-TERM TREATMENT IN COPD

Prevention of disease progression

Relief of symptoms

Improvement in exercise tolerance

Improvement in health status

Prevention and treatment of exacerbations

Prevention and treatment of complications

Prevention of mortality

Minimization of side-effects from treatment

4.97 **Aims of long-term treatment in COPD.**

- For patients with moderate COPD, who constitute the majority of patients encountered in routine clinical practice, regular bronchodilator treatment is recommended, together with a rapid-acting bronchodilator as needed and inhaled steroids in selected patients. In addition, pulmonary rehabilitation is recommended for patients whose general health and exercise capacity is severely impaired.
- In patients with severe COPD, attention should be paid to managing exacerbations and complications. Inhaled steroids may have a role in this group of patients, and pulmonary rehabilitation and long-term oxygen therapy are also useful.

Long-term oxygen therapy (LTOT) for more than 15 hours daily has been shown to improve mortality and morbidity in some severely affected patients. There are four main types of LTOT equipment:

- compressed oxygen (in cylinders)
- liquid oxygen
- molecular-sieve oxygen concentrators
- membrane separator oxygen enrichers.

Oxygen is usually given via nasal cannulae (**4.98**), which are more comfortable than wearing a face mask over many hours. Occasionally transtracheal oxygen therapy (TTOT) via a small polyethylene catheter introduced directly into the trachea via the second tracheal interspace is of value.

Infections are frequent in COPD, and it is important to educate patients in the early recognition of symptoms and signs, for example change of sputum colour and quality, fever or increasing wheeze. Many patients should be given a supply of antibiotics to keep at home for self-medication. There is little evidence that long-term antibiotic prophylaxis is of value, but influenza vaccination each winter is helpful, and vaccination against *Streptococcus pneumoniae* infection may also be of value. Surgical removal of large bullae is occasionally beneficial in emphysema, and lung volume reduction surgery may benefit selected patients with hyperinflation. Complications of COPD

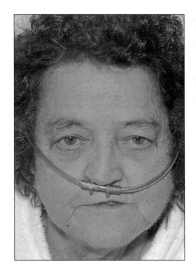

4.98 **Long-term oxygen therapy** from cylinders or an oxygen concentrator may be of value in patients with chronic stable respiratory failure. The flow rate and concentration are adjusted to relieve arterial hypoxaemia while avoiding carbon dioxide narcosis.

such as right heart failure and polycythaemia (**4.5**) may also require treatment.

MACLEOD'S SYNDROME

In Macleod's syndrome, unilateral emphysema may develop in association with hypoplasia of one lung (**4.99**). This abnormality probably results from infective lung damage in childhood.

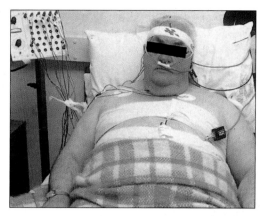

4.100 Sleep apnoea under investigation in a sleep laboratory. Note the presence of an ear oximeter, and ECG and EEG monitoring. The syndrome should always be considered in patients with chronic respiratory disease who complain of daytime somnolence, or whose partners complain about the patient's snoring or apnoeic episodes at night. Alarming falls in arterial oxygen saturation may be found during sleep apnoea, and the syndrome is a cause of sudden death at night.

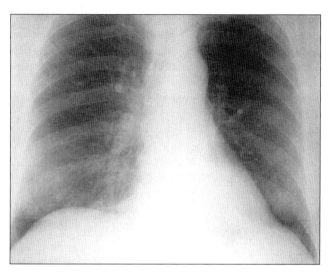

4.99 Macleod's syndrome. The left lung is smaller in volume than the right and is emphysematous. Hypoplasia of the lung is associated with a small left pulmonary artery and decreased peripheral vasculature.

these is oximetry, which may show alarming falls in oxygen saturation during apnoeic episodes. However, many patients require overnight admission with recording of EEG, respiratory and oxygenation patterns in specialized units.

Treatment consists of weight loss, avoidance of evening alcohol and withdrawal of any sedatives. The keystone of treatment is continuous positive airway pressure (CPAP) therapy administered by a tight-fitting nasal mask which blows the throat open so that recurrent arousals are abolished, as is the loud snoring. This often results in dramatic cessation of daytime symptoms and may also reduce morbidity and mortality.

SLEEP APNOEA SYNDROME

With the aid of sleep laboratories, a variety of disturbances in sleep patterns have now been recorded. The most common is the sleep apnoea syndrome, which occurs as a result of intermittent pharyngeal obstruction during REM sleep. It is most common in grossly obese chronic bronchitics who have nasal obstruction and abuse alcohol or take hypnotics. Most patients (80%) are male and many are obese (50%). However, the syndrome is now being recognized more frequently in thinner men of all ages. The clinical presentation is often from the spouse who complains of explosive episodes of snoring or snorting; general poor sleep quality and recurrent daytime tiredness are the patient's major complaints, but other symptoms may include nocturnal choking, morning headache, nocturia, reduced libido, depression and personality changes.

Suspicion of the syndrome should be followed by appropriate tests in a sleep laboratory (**4.100**). The simplest of

RESPIRATORY INFECTIONS

ACUTE BRONCHITIS

Viral infections of the upper respiratory tract often lead to secondary bacterial infection of the lower respiratory tract, especially in patients with pre-existing respiratory disorders. These infections may damage bronchial epithelium, leading to exacerbations of asthma or obstructive airways disease and to bronchitis and pneumonia, most commonly with *Streptococcus pneumoniae* or *Haemophilus influenzae*.

BRONCHIECTASIS

Damage to the elastic and muscle fibres in the bronchial wall may lead to bronchiectasis – the abnormal dilatation of a bronchus (or bronchi). The pathological process by which the damage is initiated is often not clear, but a number of conditions are associated with subsequent development. These include

- impairment of mucociliary function as seen in primary ciliary dyskinesia (**4.101**) and cystic fibrosis (**p. 101**)

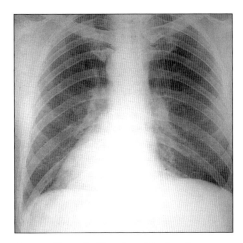

4.101   Primary ciliary dyskinesia, with situs inversus (Kartagener's syndrome). This rare autosomal recessive condition is associated with male infertility and chronic infection of the upper and lower respiratory tract, leading to nasal polyposis (**p. 161**) and bronchiectasis. In this patient there are some bronchiectatic changes in the left middle lobe and the situs inversus is obvious.

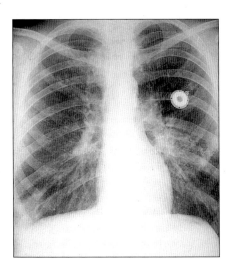

4.102   Cystic fibrosis. Widespread bronchiectatic changes are present, with an area of consolidation at the right costophrenic angle representing acute infection. An indwelling intravenous catheter for antibiotic administration is present. In such patients the common colonizing organisms are *Staphylococcus aureus*, *Haemophilus influenzae* and *Pseudomonas aeruginosa*, and these may require intensive parenteral antibiotic therapy.

- impairment of immunity as in hypogammaglobulinaemia, which predisposes to recurrent infection
- acute suppurative or necrotizing pneumonia resulting from viral or bacterial infections, including tuberculosis
- persistent infection with *Aspergillus*, as in asthmatics
- bronchial obstruction by lymph nodes or by a foreign body
- inhalation of corrosive materials, for example gastric contents or industrial hydrocarbons
- in some races there may be a hereditary element to bronchiectasis.

The end result of all these processes is a vicious circle of events in which there is alteration of normal drainage and mucus production, recurrent bacterial superinfection and acceleration of the lung damage.

The onset is usually insidious and the symptoms and signs are progressive. The first features include a chronic cough productive of increasing volumes of sputum that is intermittently infected (yellow or green) and often tinged with blood. Basal bronchiectasis may be associated with sudden coughing up of large volumes of sputum on changing posture. Episodes of superinfection may be associated with fever, signs of pneumonia, lung abscess, empyema and septicaemia. Copious foul-smelling sputum may be produced and occasionally major haemoptysis may lead to exsanguination. In the quiescent phase residual signs often persist, especially showers of coarse crepitations associated with areas of bronchial breathing. Finger clubbing (**2.104**, **2.105**) is usual and may be progressive.

The clinical course is often progressive, with gradual loss of respiratory function and cor pulmonale is found in the late stages of the disease. Chronic disease may rarely be associated with secondary amyloid, which is associated with peripheral oedema and proteinuria (*see* **p. 278**).

Diagnosis is made on history and examination, and the disease localized by plain X-ray (**4.102**), tomogram, bronchogram or CT (**4.103**). Monitoring of respiratory function tests, blood gases and renal function is important. The white cell count and erythrocyte sedimentation rate (ESR) are raised in acute exacerbations.

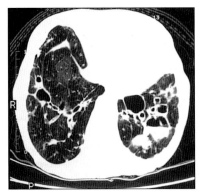

4.103   Bronchiectasis. Florid cystic bronchiectasis demonstrated on CT. Fluid levels are present in grossly dilated lower lobe bronchi. CT is now the imaging technique of choice in most patients with bronchiectasis.

Treatment consists of intensive physiotherapy and postural drainage. Antibiotics may be given for acute exacerbations or for prolonged periods as prophylaxis. Bronchodilators are of value when indicated by pulmonary function tests, and surgery should be considered for localized disease if the rest of the lung tissue is reasonably normal. Vaccination against influenza is probably of value as many acute exacerbations are precipitated by virus infections.

CYSTIC FIBROSIS

Cystic fibrosis is the most common fatal inherited disease in European populations; with a carrier frequency of 1:20, it affects 1:2000 children. The abnormal gene is located on chromosome 7 and the structure of an abnormal protein has been identified. Prenatal diagnosis can now be made precisely and population screening for heterozygotes is theoretically possible.

The disease is characterized by production of mucus of high viscosity and a severe biochemical derangement of the sweat glands, which secrete an excess of sodium and chloride (3–5 times greater than normal). A major clinical feature of the disease is bronchiectasis (**4.102** and *see* **p. 174**); and the majority of patients have pancreatic malabsorption (**4.104**). Other complications include meconium ileus presenting at birth (**4.105**), pneumothorax, haemoptysis, cor pulmonale and diabetes mellitus.

Investigations include chest X-ray, lung function tests and a sweat test. Measurement of immunoreactive trypsin allows detection at birth, before sweating is established.

In the past, most patients died in childhood from severe respiratory involvement, but the life expectancy of patients has increased with early diagnosis and prophylactic treatment. This has highlighted additional problems such as stunting of normal

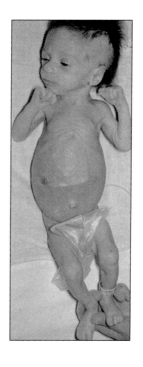

4.105 Cystic fibrosis presenting in the neonate. Note the emaciated appearance and distended abdomen, which follow surgery for meconium ileus. The meconium in cystic fibrosis is abnormally sticky, and this may result in intestinal blockage and peritonitis.

growth (resulting from malabsorption), infertility (because of lack of ciliary movement in the vas deferens), gallstones and eventually cirrhosis of the liver.

Treatment of bronchiectasis with physiotherapy and antibiotics (**4.102**), and attention to nutrition are the mainstays of therapy. Nutritional treatment involves a high calorie, high fat diet with enteric-coated pancreatic enzymes (pancreatin) plus a broad range of vitamins. Some patients receive a successful heart–lung transplant, but many still die early from respiratory failure, although current treatment allows some to survive well into adult life. In affected families, genetic counselling is important and prenatal diagnosis should be offered.

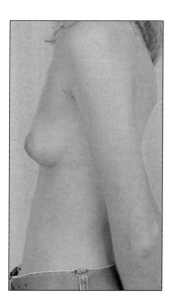

4.104 Cystic fibrosis presenting at the age of 18 years. This girl had previously been diagnosed as asthmatic, but she presented with weight loss (note the loose trousers and belt), and a sweat test confirmed the diagnosis. Her malabsorption was corrected by pancreatic enzyme supplements.

PNEUMONIA

Pneumonia is an inflammation of the lung, usually caused by bacteria, viruses or protozoa. If the infection is localized to one or two lobes of a lung it is referred to as 'lobar pneumonia' and if the infection is more generalized and involves primarily the bronchi it is known as 'bronchopneumonia'. The World Health Organization estimates that pneumonia kills 3.5 million people per year worldwide, the majority of whom are children. Pneumonia is also a common cause of death in old age, in the debilitated and in those with HIV infection.

A wide range of infecting organisms has been implicated (**4.106**). In up to 30% of patients in developed countries no organism is identified, usually because of prior antibiotic administration. In many patients there is a preceding history of an upper respiratory virus infection. Most community-acquired

PNEUMONIA: INFECTING ORGANISMS IN APPROXIMATE DESCENDING ORDER OF FREQUENCY

Community acquired
Streptococcus pneumoniae
Mycoplasma pneumoniae
Influenza virus A
Haemophilus influenzae
Legionella pneumophila
Staphylococcus aureus
Coxiella burnetii
Chlamydia psittaci

Hospital acquired
Gram-negative bacilli
Staphylococcus aureus
Streptococcus pneumoniae
Legionella pneumophila
Haemophilus influenzae
Pseudomonas spp.

Immunocompromised patients
Pneumocystis carinii
Cytomegalovirus
Mycobacterium avium-intracellulare
Mycobacterium tuberculosis
Streptococcus pneumoniae
Haemophilus influenzae
Legionella pneumophila
Actinomyces israelii
Aspergillus fumigatus
Nocardia asteroides

4.106 Pneumonia: infecting organisms in approximate descending order of frequency.

pneumonia can be managed at home, and has a low mortality; studies of patients admitted to hospital have shown a mortality of 6–24% depending on the population studied and the presence or absence of such risk factors as old age and underlying disease.

The usual clinical presentation in pneumonia caused by *Streptococcus pneumoniae* is acute, with the abrupt onset of malaise, fever, rigors, cough, pleuritic pain, tachycardia and tachypnoea, often accompanied by confusion, especially in the elderly. The signs include a high temperature, consolidation and pleural rubs, and herpetic lesions may appear on the lips. There may also be signs of pre-existing disease, especially chronic bronchitis and emphysema or heart failure in the elderly. The sputum becomes rust coloured over the following 24 hours (**4.11**). The diagnosis is made on clinical grounds and confirmed by chest X-ray (**4.107–4.109**, **4.156**). The white cell count and ESR are usually elevated. Blood should be sent for culture before antibiotic therapy is given and a baseline blood sample taken for serology. Sputum should be sent for culture.

Direct Gram-staining of a fresh sputum sample may show the organism. Pneumococcal antigen can be identified in sputum, urine or serum. Antibiotic therapy should not be delayed while awaiting sputum culture results.

The symptoms usually resolve rapidly over 7–10 days and the signs over a slightly longer period. Radiological resolution

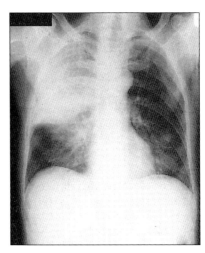

4.107 Pneumonia in the right upper lobe caused by *Streptococcus pneumoniae*. The consolidation involves the whole of the right upper lobe, and a small amount of fluid is present in the horizontal fissure. There are also some areas of consolidation in the right and left lower zones, probably as the result of transbronchial spread of infection. This patient produced typical rusty-red sputum (**4.11**).

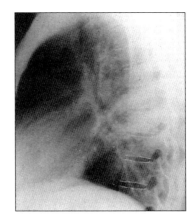

4.108 Pneumonia caused by *Mycoplasma pneumoniae*. This patient presented with fever and left lower posterior pleuritic chest pain. There is patchy consolidation in the upper part of the left lower lobe, as seen in this left lateral film.

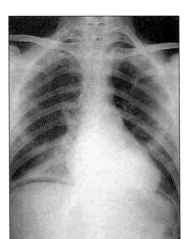

4.109 Postoperative pneumonia is common after abdominal surgery. This patient underwent urgent surgery for a perforated duodenal ulcer. Note the gas shadows below both diaphragms. He has a right basal consolidation, which results from a combination of aspiration and poor chest movement postoperatively.

should be complete by 12 weeks. Persistence of changes in the X-ray after this, or recurrence of pneumonia, suggests some other pathological process and should trigger a search for underlying carcinoma. Careful examination should be made at presentation for clinical features of HIV infection (see p. 5).

Mycoplasma pneumoniae (p. 43) is the most common cause of the 'atypical' pneumonias. Infection usually occurs in older children and young adults, who present with pharyngitis and bronchitis; pneumonia occurs in the minority and is rarely severe (4.108). Psittacosis (p. 42) is acquired from birds and Q-fever (p. 44) from animals, commonly farm livestock; they also cause atypical pneumonia, although the Q-fever organism, *Coxiella burnetii*, may also cause endocarditis. The diagnosis of the atypical pneumonias is usually made by serology.

Staphylococcal pneumonia typically occurs as a complication of influenza, especially in the elderly and, although uncommon, is important because of the attendant high mortality. It is a destructive pneumonia, which frequently leads to the formation of cavities within the lung (1.53, 1.78, 4.36, 4.37). Such cavitating pneumonia was most frequently caused by tuberculosis in the past but now staphylococci, *Klebsiella* and anaerobic organisms are the most common causes.

Legionnaires' disease is pneumonia caused by *Legionella pneumophila* (see p. 38 and 1.115). Infection is most common in debilitated or immunocompromised patients. Most cases are sporadic, but outbreaks occur from contaminated water droplet sources. Patients may present with a wide spectrum of additional symptoms, such as headache, cerebellar ataxia, renal failure or hepatic involvement. Special medium is necessary for the culture of the organism and the diagnosis is usually made by serology.

Aspiration pneumonia results from the aspiration of gastric contents into the lung and is associated with impaired consciousness (e.g. anaesthesia – 4.109, epilepsy, alcoholism) or dysphagia. Multiple organisms may be isolated.

Nosocomial pneumonia occurs when infection takes place in hospital; patients may be debilitated, immunocompromised or have just undergone a major operation. The causative organism(s) are often Gram-negative or the Gram-positive coccus, *Staphylococcus aureus*. The high mortality is usually related to the severity of the underlying disease.

Lung abscess or empyema (a collection of pus within the thoracic cavity), or both, may be caused by specific organisms or may complicate any aspiration pneumonia. Septic pulmonary emboli can lead to multiple lung abscesses, pulmonary infarcts may become infected cavities and abscesses can develop distal to lesions obstructing a bronchus.

Treatment of all pneumonias should be started immediately and the antibiotic chosen should be the 'best guess' (decided on by the origin of the pneumonia and its clinical severity). If community-acquired, then a high-dose parenteral penicillin (or erythromycin) will usually be effective. If legionnaires' disease is suspected on epidemiological grounds, rifampicin should be given with erythromycin. If staphylococcal pneumonia is suspected, because of preceding influenza, flucloxacillin should be added to the regimen. In hospital-acquired pneumonia,

combination therapy is required to cover the range of possible pathogenic organisms (especially Gram-negative bacilli). Combinations such as gentamicin with piperacillin or a cephalosporin may be used. In aspiration pneumonia, in which anaerobes may be present, metronidazole should be added to these combinations. Supportive measures should include oxygen, intravenous fluids, inotropic agents when necessary, bronchial suction and assisted ventilation. Physiotherapy and bronchodilators are of value in pneumonia complicating chronic bronchitis and emphysema.

Lung infections in the immunocompromised host

There has been a steady increase in the number of patients whose immune system has been damaged by malignancy, organ failure, drugs or the HIV virus. In such immunocompromised patients, infections of the lung are common and may be caused by organisms that are not usually pathogenic in the normal host. Invasive fungal infections tend to occur in neutropenic patients, whereas T-cell defects often lead to infection with viruses, mycobacteria and protozoa such as *Pneumocystis carinii*. The tempo of infection in the immunocompromised patient can be extremely rapid; it is important to take steps to identify the pathogen and to start therapy as soon as possible.

Pneumocystis carinii

Pneumocystis carinii is the most important cause of fatal pneumonia in immunosuppressed patients. It is believed that the infection is acquired in early childhood, and that reactivation occurs when the immune system becomes damaged. The incubation period is approximately 1–2 months before the insidious appearance of a low-grade progressive pneumonia, which manifests itself as severe dyspnoea with, at first, only minimal chest signs and X-ray changes (4.110). The

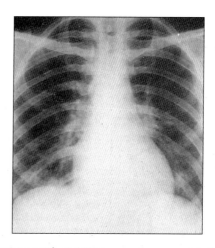

4.110 *Pneumocystis carinii* pneumonia on presentation in a patient with AIDS. The changes on X-ray (at the right base) are very minor, but the patient was markedly hypoxic and a transbronchial biopsy revealed *P. carinii*. Unless the infection is treated promptly, more severe pneumonic changes follow (see 1.25).

pneumonia progresses rapidly, and within a few days obvious pneumonic changes may be seen on the chest X-ray (**1.25**). Diagnosis depends on demonstrating the organism in sputum, bronchial lavage or lung tissue, which may require a lung biopsy (**4.50**). Treatment is with co-trimoxazole or pentamidine; both of these may be used in prophylaxis. Mortality remains high despite treatment.

PULMONARY TUBERCULOSIS

Tuberculosis may infect many parts of the body (*see* **p. 32**) but pulmonary infection is its most common manifestation.

Primary infection usually involves the lungs (**1.99, 1.100**). Within months, further pulmonary complications may occur, including lobar collapse, bronchiectasis, miliary tuberculosis (**1.101**) or the development of a pleural effusion (**4.111**).

More commonly, the 'primary complex' in the lung heals and calcifies. The patient remains well, often for many years or even for life. However, if host resistance is lowered later in life by malignant disease or its treatment, diabetes mellitus, malnutrition or HIV infection, or if reinfection with large numbers of organisms occurs, the patient may develop active adult pulmonary tuberculosis.

Pulmonary tuberculosis is characterized by fever, tiredness, malaise, anorexia and weight loss, associated with an increasingly productive cough. There may be few or no signs on examination, but X-ray changes are always present, and may include patchy or nodular pneumonic shadowing in the upper zones (**4.112**), cavitation (**4.112–4.114**), calcification (**4.115**), fibrosis (**4.116**) and lymph node enlargement (**1.102, 1.103, 4.9**). Pleural effusion (**4.111**) and calcification may also be seen. CT may also show changes (**4.117**).

The diagnosis may be strongly suggested by the X-ray appearances. However, microbiological confirmation is necessary to exclude chronic necrotizing pulmonary aspergillosis, which produces a similar picture, histoplasmosis (**p. 44**) and coccidioidomycosis (**p. 46**) – especially in those who live in or who have visited an endemic area for these diseases –

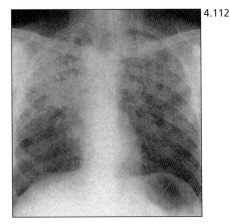

4.112

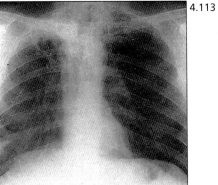

4.113

4.112 & 4.113 Active tuberculosis in a Greek immigrant to the UK (**4.112**), who presented with weight loss, low-grade fever and fresh haemoptysis. He gave a family history of tuberculosis. This film shows multiple areas of shadowing, especially in the upper lobes, and several lesions have started to cavitate. Despite the extensive nature of the disease, chemotherapy resulted in dramatic healing of the lesions as seen in a film taken 3 years later (**4.113**), which shows only minimal residual scarring at both apices.

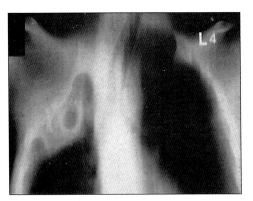

4.114 Cavitating right apical tuberculosis revealed on tomography. This 'slice' shows three separate cavities, surrounded by dense inflammation and fibrosis, with pulling of the trachea to the right. The chest wall has been surgically collapsed (thoracoplasty). This obsolete technique was used before effective chemotherapy became available in an attempt to accelerate the healing of the cavities.

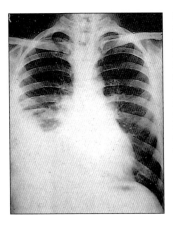

4.111 Tuberculous effusion. This patient presented with a 6-month history of malaise and weight loss, but no symptoms directly referable to the chest. The large right pleural effusion is accompanied by fluid in the horizontal fissure. Aspiration and culture confirmed the diagnosis.

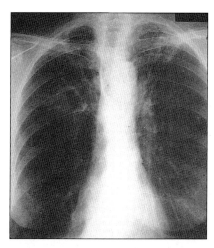

4.115 Bilateral apical fibrosis resulting from pulmonary tuberculosis. The hila are elevated, and streaky linear shadows extend from the hila to the apices. Scattered calcified upper zone nodules are also present bilaterally.

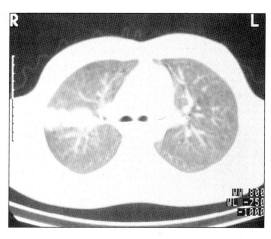

4.117 Tuberculous pneumonic consolidation and hilar node enlargement demonstrated by CT. The consolidation can be seen to extend from the hilum to the pleura.

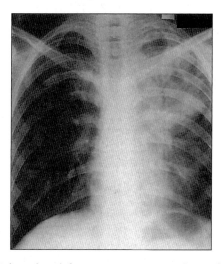

4.116 Tuberculous left upper zone pneumonia, confirmed by sputum examination. The presence of an air bronchogram in the left upper zone confirms that the underlying pathology is consolidation rather than collapse.

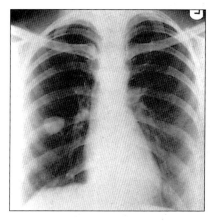

4.118 Tuberculoma. This solid, calcified lesion in the right lower lobe (as confirmed by a lateral film) represents the healed stage of tuberculosis. There is associated bilateral hilar lymph node calcification. It is important to exclude the possibility of lung cancer whenever solitary lesions are seen.

and cryptococcosis in immunocompromised patients. Similar appearances may also occur with non-tuberculous mycobacterial infections in normal and immunocompromised patients (*see* **p. 34**).

Pulmonary tuberculosis requires treatment with antituberculous chemotherapy for a period of 6–9 months (*see* **p. 33**). Investigation and immunization of contacts is essential (*see* **p. 34**), and in many countries tuberculosis is a notifiable disease. Patients with signs of previous tuberculosis (as in **4.112, 4.118**), who are about to undergo immunosuppressive drug treatment or manoeuvres such as haemodialysis for renal failure, should be given prophylactic antituberculous therapy.

PULMONARY INFILTRATIONS

SARCOIDOSIS

Sarcoidosis, a multisystem disorder, has a prevalence of 15–20 per 100 000 people, with the highest prevalence between the ages of 25 and 35 years. It is most often found in the lung parenchyma and related lymph nodes, but it can involve the skin, eyes, peripheral lymph nodes, gut, liver, bone and CNS. The pathological process is a granulomatous reaction of the type seen with insoluble antigens, but as yet no single factor has been positively identified. It is not contagious, but there is a slightly increased incidence within families and in women. In the USA it is much more common in black patients.

The most common clinical presentation of sarcoidosis is respiratory. It is often found on chest X-rays in patients with non-specific features such as tiredness, weight loss or recurrent fever. The characteristic lesions are:

- bilateral hilar lymphadenopathy (**4.119**), usually asymptomatic, which will subside without treatment in about 80–90% of patients
- pulmonary infiltration with bilateral hilar lymphadenopathy (**4.120**, **4.121**), which may cause symptoms such as dyspnoea, cough and fever, but which subsides in 40% of patients
- pulmonary fibrosis after diffuse infiltration, ultimately leading to bullae formation or fibrosis (**4.122**, **4.123**), or

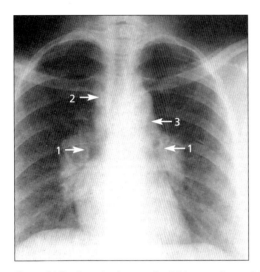

4.119   Bilateral hilar lymphadenopathy (1) in a patient with sarcoidosis. Note that there is increased right paratracheal shadowing (2) and shadowing in the aorticopulmonary window (3). These shadows indicate more widespread lymph node enlargement, but the prognosis at this stage is good, even without treatment.

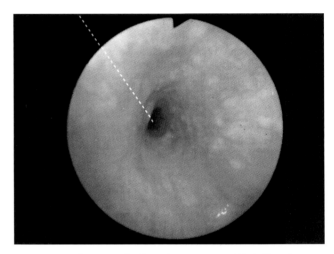

4.121   Bronchoscopic findings in a patient with infiltrative sarcoidosis. The lumen of the left main bronchus (indicated by tip of dotted line) is so narrowed that a fibreoptic bronchoscope can hardly pass through it. There are dilated mucosal vessels, and multiple sarcoid nodules in the mucosa.

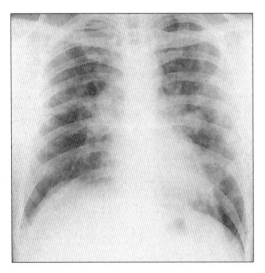

4.120   Pulmonary infiltration with bilateral hilar lymphadenopathy in a patient with sarcoidosis. Note the nodular pattern in both lung fields with relative sparing of the apices in this patient. In this young man, the important differential diagnosis included secondary deposits, especially as a cystic testicular swelling was found; but in this case the diagnosis of sarcoidosis was confirmed by lung biopsy, and the swelling was a simple hydrocele.

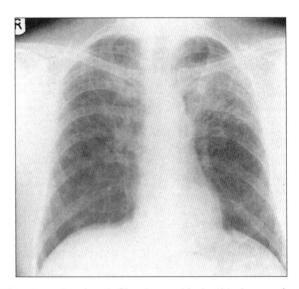

4.122   Extensive chronic fibrotic sarcoidosis. This degree of fibrosis results in severe irreversible impairment of respiratory function.

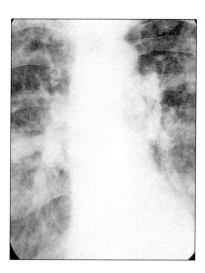

4.123 Calcification is often seen in chronic sarcoidosis, as in the left hilar nodes in this patient.

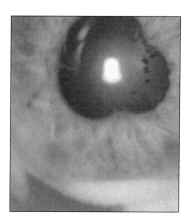

4.126 Acute anterior uveitis occurs in up to 25% of patients with sarcoidosis. Note the fluid level of pus in the anterior chamber (hypopyon) and the distortion of the pupil caused by the development of posterior synechiae. A cataract may form if this eye involvement does not receive prompt treatment.

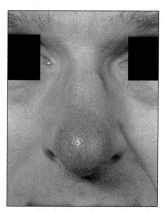

4.124 Lupus pernio is the term used to describe a dusky-purple infiltration of the skin of the nose in chronic sarcoidosis. It is important to distinguish this appearance from rhinophyma (see **2.85**) and acne rosacea.

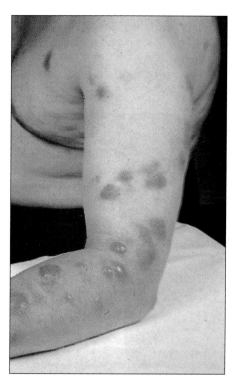

4.125 Sarcoid lesions may occur in the skin at any site, and they may take noular, papular or plaque forms. Biopsy is usually necessary for diagnosis.

both, associated with symptoms and a restrictive defect on respiratory function testing.

Evidence of the disease should be sought in the skin, eye and peripheral lymph nodes.

The most common skin lesion in sarcoidosis is erythema nodosum (**2.45**). However, this is a non-specific sign. Sarcoid nodules may be found in the skin in about 5% of cases particularly on the face, especially the nose (lupus pernio) (**4.124**), in scars and elsewhere (**4.125**).

Patients with eye involvement may present acutely with a painful eye and acute impairment of vision (**4.126**). More often there is progressive visual impairment from posterior uveitis (**4.127**). There may also be involvement of the lacrimal glands (producing dry eyes) and of both parotids (uveoparotid fever) producing a dry mouth. The seventh cranial nerve may be involved by this process and sarcoidosis may affect other parts

181

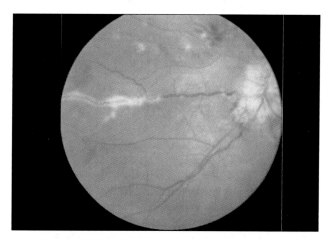

4.127 Posterior uveitis is a relatively common complication in sarcoidosis, and may cause choroiditis, retinitis and even blindness. In this patient, a focal retinal periphlebitis alternates with stretches of unaffected vein.

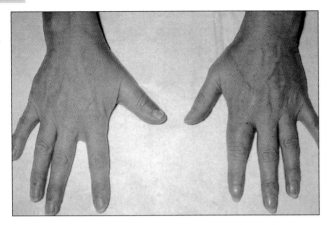

4.128 Dactylitis in sarcoidosis. The left index finger shows obvious signs of inflammation and swelling, particularly of the proximal phalanx and interphalangeal joint, and the other digits are also involved.

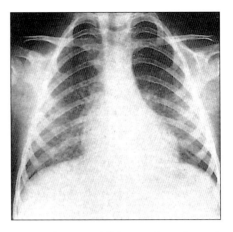

4.129 Histiocytosis X in a child. Granuloma formation has produced generalized miliary mottling.

of the CNS (**11.29**). Localized involvement of bones may give tender swellings (**4.128**) and X-rays may show localized bone cysts. Involvement of heart, gut and liver are rare.

Hypercalcaemia is often found in established disease as a result of additional α-hydroxylation occurring in the sarcoid lesions in the lung. This may result in metastatic calcification or stone formation in the urinary tract (*see* **p. 287**).

The diagnosis is made by biopsy of lymph nodes, skin or lung. Lung function tests often show a restrictive defect and the Mantoux test is often negative. The Kveim test is now of largely historical interest; the theoretical possibility of HIV transmission limits its use.

Treatment of sarcoidosis depends on the extent of the disease and the tissues involved. Parenchymal lung disease, acute eye involvement and CNS or heart signs require a prolonged course of steroids. Minor skin or lymph node involvement can be watched over a period of months for spontaneous resolution. The level of angiotensin-converting enzyme is often raised and may be used to follow the course of disease activity, but this is not a specific diagnostic test.

HISTIOCYTOSIS X

Histocytosis X is a disease of unknown aetiology, which is associated with the presence of granulomas that are rich in eosinophils. There are two forms found in young children (Letterer–Siwe and Hand–Schüller–Christian disease) and one in adults (eosinophilic granuloma). The granulomas may be found in bones and in the lung parenchyma where they produce progressive restrictive lung disease and may produce pneumothorax (**4.129**). Hypothalamic–pituitary axis involvement may lead to diabetes insipidus, panhypopituitarism or obesity.

VASCULITIS

The vasculitic diseases most commonly affecting the lung are Wegener's granulomatosis and allergic granulomatosis. Classic polyarteritis nodosa rarely affects the upper and lower respiratory tracts; renal involvement (*see* **p. 275**) is much more common.

WEGENER'S GRANULOMATOSIS

Classic Wegener's granulomatosis consists of the clinical triad of upper respiratory tract granulomas (**3.97**), fleeting lung shadows and necrotizing glomerulonephritis (*see* **p. 277**), but solitary lung lesions may also occur without renal involvement.

Chest X-rays show nodular masses and pneumonic infiltrates (**4.130**). Cavitation may also occur. In the early stages, the chest X-ray changes are 'fleeting': lesions clear from one area as new lesions appear elsewhere. Immunosuppressive

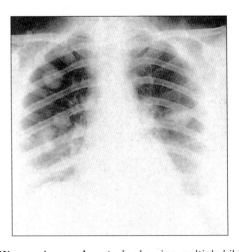

4.130 Wegener's granulomatosis, showing multiple bilateral nodular lesions and pneumonic infiltration in both lower zones.

therapy may help to reverse the lung changes, but renal involvement usually requires complex therapy (*see* **p. 128**).

Midline granuloma (known also as lethal midline granuloma) is a variant of Wegener's granulomatosis in which progressive nasal ulceration is associated with lung and renal involvement. It carries a poor prognosis.

ALLERGIC GRANULOMATOSIS

Allergic granulomatosis (Churg–Strauss syndrome) occurs on a background of asthma that has usually been difficult to control and present for a year or more. Recently some cases have been reported to follow a reduction in inhaled steroid dose and the addition of antileukotriene therapy in patients with asthma, probably representing the 'unmasking' of the condition rather than a true drug side-effect. A high blood eosinophilia is found, and tissue eosinophilia, granulomata and vasculitis develop in various organs. The lungs, nervous system, skin and heart are often involved, whereas renal involvement is not usually significant (unlike other forms of vasculitis). Treatment is with systemic steroids, with the addition of azathioprine if necessary.

POLYARTERITIS NODOSA

Polyarteritis nodosa is a multisystem disorder characterized by widespread vasculitis (*see* **p. 127**). Pulmonary involvement may rarely occur, presenting with cough, haemoptysis, fever or asthmatic symptoms. Chest X-ray may show pneumonic infiltration (**4.131**) and biopsy of lung or other tissue may be required for definitive diagnosis.

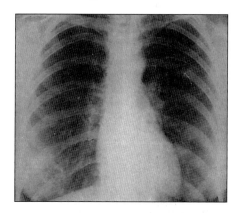

4.131 Polyarteritis nodosa with pulmonary infiltration in both lower zones. The appearance is not diagnostic, and the diagnosis must be based on the clinical picture and confirmed by angiography or biopsy, or both.

PULMONARY COMPLICATIONS OF THE CONNECTIVE TISSUE DISEASES

Fibrosing alveolitis, indistinguishable from the cryptogenic variety (**4.139**) (*see* **p. 185**), may occur in any collagen disease,

but is most commonly seen in rheumatoid arthritis (**3.36**). There is an excess mortality from respiratory infection in rheumatoid arthritis. Other pulmonary complications also occur, including bronchitis, obliterative bronchiolitis and bronchiectasis, multiple (**3.36**) or single (**4.132**) pulmonary nodules, which may cavitate, and pleural effusions (**3.35**), which occur predominantly in men. In Caplan's syndrome, pulmonary lesions occur in a patient with rheumatoid arthritis who has been exposed to dust as a coal miner or in an industrial setting; they may progress to massive pulmonary fibrosis (**4.147**). Complications seen in other connective tissue diseases include pleurisy, pleural effusions and lung atelectasis in systemic lupus erythematosus and pulmonary hypertension and basal fibrosis (**4.131**) in systemic sclerosis.

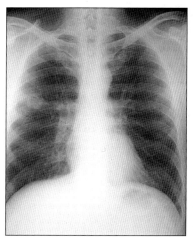

4.132 A single rheumatoid nodule in the right mid-zone in a 55-year-old man with rheumatoid arthritis. Rheumatoid nodules are more common in men than in women, and solitary nodules often require biopsy to exclude malignancy.

PULMONARY INFILTRATION WITH EOSINOPHILIA

The association of blood eosinophilia and pulmonary shadowing may occur in a number of situations, some of which are imperfectly characterized (**4.133**).

Simple pulmonary eosinophilia is a short-lived illness in which cough and a slight fever are associated with transient

CAUSES OF PULMONARY EOSINOPHILIA
Allergic bronchopulmonary aspergillosis (ABPA)
Worm infestation
Drugs
Eosinophilic myalgic syndrome
Acute or chronic eosinophilic pneumonia
Allergic granulomatosis

4.133 Causes of pulmonary eosinophilia.

pneumonic shadowing (**4.134**, **4.135**) and blood eosinophilia. It appears to be an allergic response, and the provoking allergen may be the result of worm infestation or drug therapy, though often no allergen can be identified. The condition is usually self-limiting.

Allergic aspergillosis (*see* **p. 45**) occurs in asthmatics and may produce chronic symptoms with the risk of permanent lung damage (**1.134**), as may tropical pulmonary eosinophilia, which is probably usually caused by a reaction to *Wuchereria bancrofti* infection (*see* **p. 51**), and the 'hypereosinophilic' syndrome, in which the provoking cause is unknown.

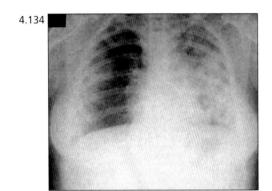
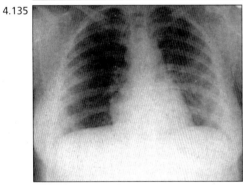

4.134 & 4.135   Pulmonary infiltration with eosinophilia (also known as Löffler's syndrome) (4.134). In this patient the infiltration was mainly in the left lung, and it persisted for 2–3 weeks. The patient had a mild fever and a cough, but no other symptoms. **4.135** shows the appearance of the chest 4 weeks after **4.134**. Spontaneous clearing of the lung shadowing within 1 month is usual, and the condition produces few, if any, symptoms.

GOODPASTURE'S SYNDROME

Goodpasture's syndrome is a disease of unknown aetiology that often occurs after an upper respiratory infection. The patient usually has small repeated haemoptyses with progressive dyspnoea and cough, followed by massive intrapulmonary bleeding, and may present acutely with dyspnoea and massive

haemoptysis (**4.136**). These appearances may precede the development of acute glomerulonephritis, which often progresses to renal failure (*see* **p. 275**). The disease is mediated by anti-glomerular basement membrane antibodies. Treatment is generally unsatisfactory in the established case.

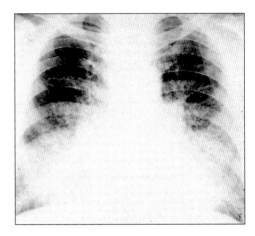

4.136   Goodpasture's syndrome. Massive intrapulmonary bleeding has led to opacities ('white-out') of both mid and lower zones on chest X-ray. The mortality rate is high as a result of pulmonary and renal involvement.

PULMONARY OEDEMA: CARDIOGENIC AND NON-CARDIOGENIC

In patients with heart disease, a rise in the hydrostatic pressure within the pulmonary capillaries produces pulmonary oedema. This is most commonly seen acutely, after a myocardial infarction, pulmonary embolus, arrhythmia or hypertension, or may happen chronically in patients with valve disease or a rise in pulmonary or systemic pressure (**5.15**, **5.28**).

Acute pulmonary oedema may also be the result of a range of non-cardiac conditions (**4.137**), the end result of which is to increase the permeability of the pulmonary capillaries. Most of these patients are admitted with an acute medical or surgical condition that is later followed, in hours or days, by progressive hypoxia, and dyspnoea associated with scattered rhonchi and crepitations over the lung fields (the adult respiratory distress syndrome; ARDS). X-rays show diffuse patchy 'infiltrates' (**4.138**), and high resolution CT may show evidence of pulmonary fibrosis or other treatable complications. These findings often progress rapidly to cardiorespiratory failure and death, and assisted ventilation and haemodynamic support may be urgently required to prevent this. Other important therapy may include effective antimicrobial treatment, nitric oxide (NO), surfactants and high dose systemic steroids. Survivors of ARDS commonly have long-term physical and psychological impairment, with a reduced quality of life.

CAUSES OF THE ADULT RESPIRATORY DISTRESS SYNDROME (ARDS)

Inhaled smoke
Overwhelming infections
Aspiration of gastric contents
Drowning
Uraemia
Pancreatitis
Massive blood transfusion
Disseminated intravascular coagulation (DIC)
Poisoning with paraquat and other toxins/drugs
Post cardiopulmonary bypass
Acute radiation pneumonia
Trauma
Other causes of shock

4.137　Causes of the adult respiratory distress syndrome.

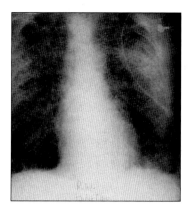

4.138　Adult respiratory distress syndrome. The chest X-ray appearances in this portable anteroposterior (AP) film are similar to those seen in cardiogenic pulmonary oedema, but the condition results from an increase in pulmonary capillary permeability rather than from heart failure. This patient had inhaled smoke in a domestic fire.

PULMONARY FIBROSIS

Many different lung diseases may result in pulmonary fibrosis, which may be localized or generalized. For example:

- localized unilateral fibrosis may result from a destructive pneumonia
- localized bilateral fibrosis may occur in tuberculosis, histoplasmosis and other chronic infections
- generalized fibrosis may occur as the end-stage of a range of parenchymal lung disorders, including industrial lung diseases, connective tissue diseases, ankylosing spondylitis (3.48) and sarcoidosis; and in cryptogenic fibrosing alveolitis and extrinsic allergic alveolitis.

CRYPTOGENIC FIBROSING ALVEOLITIS (CFA)

Cryptogenic fibrosing alveolitis (CFA, idiopathic pulmonary fibrosis) is the most common of the interstitial lung diseases, affecting between 5 and 10 per 100 000 people, men more often

than women (2:1), and most commonly seen in those over 65 years of age. Alveolitis leads to the destruction of alveoli and the laying down of scar tissue (fibrosis), which further disrupts the function of the lung. There is wide variation in the tempo of the illness. Patients may die from respiratory failure within a few months of presentation, or the disease may be identified by chance on chest X-ray and show little progression over many years. Most commonly, the disease progresses to respiratory failure over a few years. The principal symptoms are dyspnoea, cough, generally unproductive, and arthralgia. Gross clubbing of the fingers is common (2.103, 2.104) and late inspiratory crackles are heard, particularly at the lung bases. Chest X-ray shows widespread shadowing (4.139), which is often most marked in the lower zones, and comparison of X-rays over time often shows a loss of lung volume (if taken correctly, in full inspiration, the chest X-ray is an indicator of total lung capacity). CT shows a characteristic 'honeycomb' appearance (4.140). Pulmonary function tests show a restrictive defect, often with a greater reduction in transfer factor than would be expected for the loss of lung volume. The ESR, CRP or plasma viscosity is usually moderately raised. Blood tests may show positive autoantibodies and there is an association with other autoimmune diseases. Lung biopsy may be necessary for diagnosis and shows characteristic changes (4.141). Systemic corticosteroids lead to improvement in 75% of patients and must be continued for many months. The alternative option is immunosuppression with cyclophosphamide and azathioprine. The response to treatment

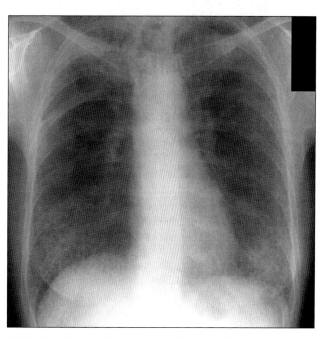

4.139　Cryptogenic fibrosing alveolitis typically causes predominantly basal pulmonary shadowing, and in this patient this has progressed to generalized shadowing. Note that the appearance is very similar to that found with pulmonary fibrosis complicating rheumatoid arthritis and other collagen diseases.

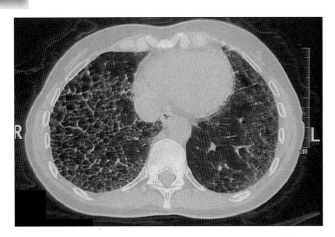

4.140 **Cryptogenic fibrosing alveolitis** as demonstrated by high-resolution CT in the patient shown in **4.139**. The 'honeycomb' appearance on high-resolution CT is characteristic of fibrosing alveolitis.

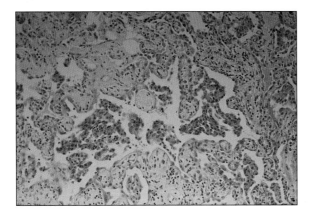

4.141 **Lung biopsy in cryptogenic fibrosing alveolitis (H&E)** showing diffuse infiltration of the alveolar walls with lymphocytes and plasma cells and the alveolar spaces filled with an inflammatory exudate of macrophages and lymphocytes. There is also extensive fibrosis of the alveolar walls. In earlier disease, electron microscopy may show collagen deposition in the basement membrane of the alveolar epithelium and pulmonary vessels, and in the alveolar wall interstitium.

is better if inflammation is more marked than fibrosis in the lung histology. The course of the disease is monitored by signs and lung function tests. The mean survival is 5 years from diagnosis. The causes of death are supervening infection, cor pulmonale or respiratory failure and bronchial carcinoma. Younger and otherwise fit patients with severe disease should be considered for heart–lung transplantation.

EXTRINSIC ALLERGIC ALVEOLITIS (EAA)

Extrinsic allergic alveolitis (EAA, allergic bronchioalveolitis, hypersensitivity pneumonitis) develops as a result of a

hypersensitivity reaction in the lungs, provoked by a wide range of organic dusts. Many of these are encountered at work, and a large number of occupational lung diseases fall within this classification, whereas other causes relate to hobbies, especially the keeping of birds. Farmer's lung is the most common cause, accounting for 50% of cases of extrinsic allergic alveolitis. About 1 in 10 homes in the UK keep a bird and extrinsic allergic alveolitis ('bird fancier's lung') is found in about 5% of bird owners and 20% of pigeon keepers.

Repeated exposure of a susceptible individual to the offending antigen leads to the production of circulating precipitating antibodies and immune complexes and ultimately to macrophage activation and epithelioid cell granuloma formation.

The factors that predispose to allergic alveolitis are poorly understood. There is some evidence of genetic susceptibility, but no link with atopy, or with elevated IgE or eosinophil levels.

Symptoms may develop within 6 hours of heavy exposure to the antigen or may appear insidiously over years. The most common presentation is with breathlessness, dry cough and influenza-like symptoms (malaise, fever and muscle pains). Chest X-ray in the acute phase shows a fine nodular shadowing (**4.142**), but repeated exposure may lead to chronic respiratory impairment caused by pulmonary fibrosis, which radiologically tends to be more marked in the upper zones, as with sarcoidosis, than in the lower zones, as with cryptogenic fibrosing alveolitis. Lung function shows restricted ventilation (reduced TLC and FVC), accompanied by reduced compliance and gas transfer.

In the acute stage the provoking factor must be identified and removed. This alone may result in rapid control of

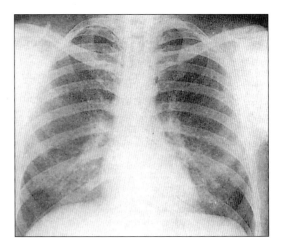

4.142 **Acute extrinsic allergic alveolitis** – in this case pigeon fancier's lung. This man presented with acute symptoms after cleaning out his pigeon loft. The X-ray shows diffuse, hazy opacification in both lung fields, which partially obscures the normal vascular markings.

symptoms. In very severe cases, systemic corticosteroids may accelerate recovery.

In the more chronic form removal of the stimulus is important but may not be practicable. In this situation, an alternative way of reducing exposure should be implemented, for example by better ventilation and extraction of air. Systemic corticosteroids may reduce symptoms.

IATROGENIC LUNG DISEASE

The most common iatrogenic lung lesion results from radiotherapy, usually given for diseases such as cancer of the breast, bronchus, thymus or lymph nodes. The determining factors in lung damage are total radiation dose, duration of time over which the dose is given and the number of treatments. Acute radiation pneumonitis occurs a few days to some weeks after exposure and presents with a cough, fever and progessive dyspnoea. Systemic corticosteroids may ameliorate these acute symptoms. Fibrosis may develop over many months (**4.143**) and there is evidence of a progressive restrictive defect in the pulmonary function tests with a decreased transfer factor.

A large number of drugs, alone or in combination, may produce a range of respiratory problems that include:

- asthma (e.g. β-blockers)
- infiltration or fibrosis (e.g. bleomycin, methotrexate)
- eosinophilia (e.g. nitrofurantoin)
- systemic lupus erythematosus-like syndromes (e.g. hydralazine)
- respiratory depression (e.g. opiates, barbiturates)
- opportunistic infection (e.g. high dose steroids, immunosuppressives).

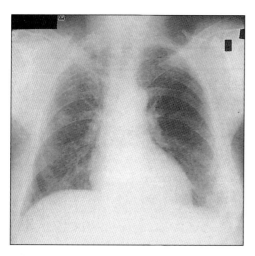

4.143 Radiation fibrosis. This patient had undergone a right mastectomy for breast cancer, followed by a course of radiotherapy. There are fibrotic changes in the lung, with upper lobe shrinkage, especially on the right, and the trachea is pulled to the right. She also had some ununited rib fractures on the right, resulting from secondary deposits.

OCCUPATIONAL LUNG DISEASE

Lung diseases associated with industrial exposure are a common problem. They can be avoided if appropriate occupational regulations are enforced, especially efficient ventilation and individual protection by ventilators or masks. A range of common disorders related to dust inhalation are listed in **4.144**. Asthma (**p. 163**) and extrinsic allergic alveolitis (**p. 186**) are other common occupational problems.

SOME LUNG DISEASES CAUSED BY DUST INHALATION	
Disease	**Dust**
Coal workers' pneumoconiosis	Coal
Silicosis	Crystalline silica
Asbestosis	Serpentine (chrysolite), amphibole (crocidolite, amosite, anthophyllite)
Pneumoconiosis	Talc, slate, kaolin
Stannosis	Tin oxide
Baritosis	Barium sulphate
Berylliosis	Beryllium

4.144 Some lung diseases caused by dust inhalation.

COAL WORKERS' PNEUMOCONIOSIS (CWP)

Pneumoconiosis is lung disease resulting from exposure to dust. Coal workers' pneumoconiosis (CWP) was commonplace until dust exposure was reduced. Initially, it was believed that the disease was caused by the inhalation of silica (silicosis), but it is now clear that the disease can be caused by silica-free coal dust, although the mineral make-up of the dust influences the incidence and progression. CWP and silicosis are defined radiologically as simple if there is fine micronodulation, usually in the upper lobes (**4.35, 4.145**), or as complicated if the nodules coalesce to masses greater than 1 cm in diameter causing lung damage and significant functional impairment (**4.146**). These diseases attract industrial compensation in many countries, and a spectrum of functional and radiological lung changes is recognized for this purpose. Tests of lung function may show a reduction in lung volume, especially when nodules are present, with some obstruction and restrictive defects. Patients who are developing complicated CWP complain of progressive dyspnoea on exertion and eventually at rest. Cough with black sputum is a common feature (melanoptysis). No treatment prevents the progression of the disease. The picture is often complicated by the effects of chronic cigarette smoking and in some cases by coincidental

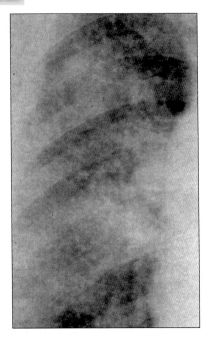

4.145 Simple pneumoconiosis. A close-up view shows the fine, reticular pattern associated with the repeated inhalation of coal dust. The appearance is very similar to that of other forms of miliary mottling. It may not be associated with symptoms.

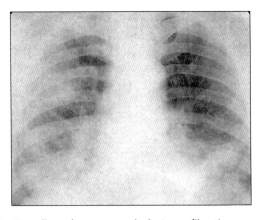

4.146 Complicated pneumoconiosis. Large fibrotic masses, which are irregular in shape, are present, mainly in both lower zones and on the right. Similar appearances may occur in complicated silicosis.

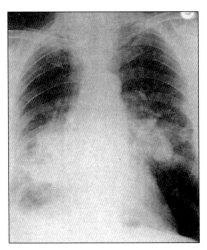

4.147 Progressive massive fibrosis (PMF) in Caplan's syndrome. There is progression in the formation of fibrotic tissue to form large masses, as seen in both mid-zones. Central necrosis has led to a fluid-filled cavity in the right lung, and the necrotic material may be coughed up.

SILICOSIS

Silicosis is a disease of miners, tunnellers and stonemasons, which results from inhalation of crystalline silicon dioxide (quartz). The result is progressive pulmonary fibrosis that ranges in appearance from micronodular fibrosis to progressive massive fibrosis, as in coal workers' pneumoconiosis. The time taken for development of the changes depends on the amount of inhaled silica. With simple silicosis there are usually no clinical features and the condition is diagnosed on routine X-ray. Complicated silicosis is associated with progressive fibrosis over many years, and presents clinically with dyspnoea, weight loss, cough and recurrent chest infections, especially tuberculosis and other mycobacterial infections. The X-ray appearance is of progressive fibrosis (**4.146**); there may be a pleural reaction and the hilar lymph nodes may be enlarged and calcified. Pulmonary function tests become abnormal as the disease progresses and the defects are a mixture of restriction and obstruction. The disease may be compounded by cigarette smoking and infection with tuberculosis, fungi or bacteria. There is no specific treatment for the fibrous reaction. Prevention of exposure to silica dust is the key to prevention, and masks and respirators may aid this process.

ASBESTOS-RELATED DISEASE

Asbestos exists in a variety of chemical forms which have been widely used for insulation in building, pipe-lagging and shipbuilding. Inhalation of the fibres by workers during construction and demolition is the most common cause of lung disease, but it can also occur in the public living close to factories producing asbestos products, in the partners of asbestos workers and in those living in houses insulated with asbestos.

The risks of disease are greatest with crocidolite (blue asbestos) and chrysolite (white asbestos). When inhaled, most fibres are cleared by microcirculatory action and some by macrophages. Fibres which remain in the lung become coated

infection with tuberculosis. Many of these patients also have COPD.

Caplan's syndrome is the association of rheumatoid arthritis (or rheumatoid factor) with CWP. The lung nodules may enlarge rapidly and may cavitate (**4.147**). These appearances are usually associated with the presence of subcutaneous nodules, active rheumatoid joint disease and high titres of rheumatoid factor.

There is no specific treatment, but prevention is possible by reducing exposure to dust and by the use of respirators. Complications such as infection and heart failure require treatment.

with ferroproteins and may be seen in sputum (**4.13**). Such fibres after a long latent period cause a range of effects, including pulmonary fibrosis (asbestosis), pleural effusion, and eventually calcified pleural plaques, mesothelioma and bronchial carcinoma.

The clinical features of asbestosis at presentation may include an irritant cough and progressive shortness of breath. Examination shows finger clubbing in 50% of patients and diffuse fine crepitations over both bases, which spread with time. A history of cigarette smoking is important, as tobacco smoke and asbestos exposure seem to have a synergistic action in promoting the subsequent onset of bronchial carcinoma.

Lung function tests reflect the diffuse fibrosis with evidence of restrictive lung disease and impairment of gas transfer.

X-ray of the chest shows a spectrum of abnormalities in the early stages of asbestosis, which include irregular opacities in the lower zones (**4.148**, **4.149**) and later pleural thickening and calcification that is usually bilateral (**4.150**, **4.151**). Later features include mesothelioma (**4.152**) and bronchial carcinoma (**4.153**).

Mesothelioma is a highly malignant tumour of the pleura, which is diagnosed by pleural biopsy, a procedure that may occasionally lead to local spread of the tumour (**4.58**). Mesotheliomas may also develop in the peritoneum.

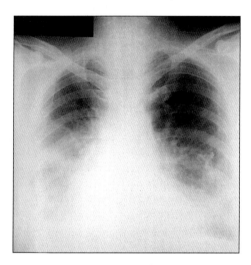

4.148   Asbestosis. The advanced fibrotic changes in the lungs are best seen around the heart and in the lower zones. The patient's occupational exposure was as a shipyard worker.

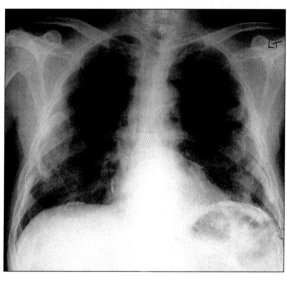

4.150   Extensive pleural and pericardial calcification after long-term industrial asbestos exposure.

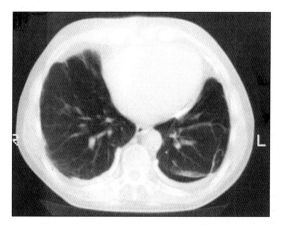

4.149   CT in asbestosis. There are widespread fibrotic changes in both lungs and some patchy pleural calcification is seen.

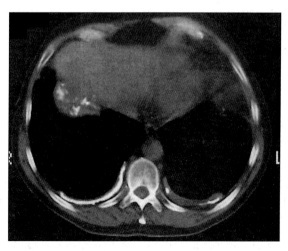

4.151   Pleural calcification shown by CT. The pleural calcification is particularly obvious in this cut posteriorly on the right; and anteriorly, the calcification in the right diaphragmatic pleura is clearly seen.

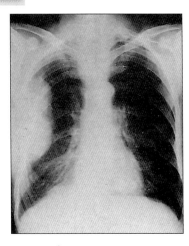

4.152 Mesothelioma of the right pleura. The patient had a long history of asbestos exposure and has now developed a large pleural mass, which can be seen by soft-tissue shadowing to have extended through the chest wall (*see* **4.58**).

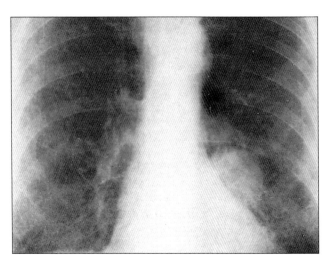

4.153 Carcinoma of the bronchus in asbestosis. Reticulonodular shadowing was present throughout both lungs, especially basally. A mass is seen behind the heart in the left lower lobe. Percutaneous needle biopsy showed a squamous cell carcinoma. The patient was a smoker and a retired shipbuilder.

Treatment of asbestos-related disease is ineffective and this underlines the importance of preventing exposure. Compensation schemes for the effects of asbestos exposure exist in many countries. About 50% of the patients with asbestosis who also smoke die of bronchial carcinoma and 10% die of mesothelioma.

TUMOURS OF THE LUNG

BENIGN TUMOURS

Benign tumours of the lung account for about 2% of all tumours of lung and present either as solitary nodules on the

chest X-ray or, if endobronchial, with cough, haemoptysis or pneumonia. The most common type is a hamartoma, which is usually found as a solitary nodule in a young asymptomatic adult (**4.39**). Other benign tumours are rare. Endobronchial carcinoid tumours may give rise to atelectasis, recurrent infections and sometimes bronchiectasis. The carcinoid syndrome may occasionally be seen, and carcinoid tumours may ultimately metastasize.

The treatment of all these tumours is surgical removal whenever possible.

BRONCHIAL CARCINOMA

Bronchial carcinoma (lung cancer) is the most common type of malignant disease worldwide. It causes about 35 000 deaths annually in England and Wales, almost 80% of which are in men. In the last few years the steady rise in male mortality from bronchial carcinoma seems to have peaked and begun its decline, but female mortality continues to increase. The development of lung cancer has been associated with exposure to a number of substances, but the overriding aetiological agent is tobacco. Cigarette smoking is associated with about 85% of bronchial carcinoma, but as only a minority of smokers develop bronchial carcinoma other factors must be important. There is some evidence that genetic and dietary factors may play a role, and exposure to asbestos and possibly to other inhaled substances may have a synergistic effect with smoking.

Presentation

Intrathoracic manifestations
The clinical presentation of bronchial carcinoma can vary enormously:

- In about 5% of patients, a symptomless abnormality is found on a routine chest X-ray (**4.28**) and confirmed by CT (**4.43**, **4.44**), bronchoscopy (**4.49**, **4.154**) or lung biopsy, whereas other patients present with extensive disease and die rapidly (**4.155**).
- Cough is the most common presenting symptom; because the majority of cases are in smokers, a change in the

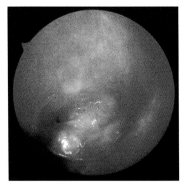

4.154 Left upper lobe bronchial carcinoma seen on bronchoscopy.

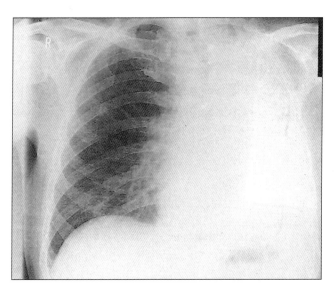

4.155   Carcinoma of the bronchus presenting with complete collapse of the left lung as a result of total occlusion of the left main bronchus. Note the marked deviation of the trachea and mediastinum to the left, and the compensatory hyperinflation of the right lung. The patient presented with rapid-onset dyspnoea.

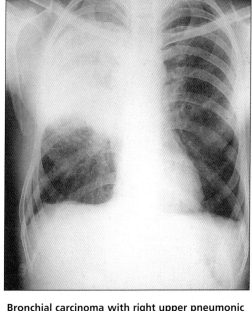

4.156   Bronchial carcinoma with right upper pneumonic consolidation. The consolidation follows obstruction of the right upper lobe bronchus.

character of the cough is more important than the cough itself.
- Haemoptysis occurs as an initial symptom in up to 50% of patients, and in a smoker over the age of 40 years is an indication for bronchoscopy (**4.48**), even in the absence of a radiological abnormality.
- Dyspnoea occurs commonly and may be caused by large airway obstruction with tumour, the development of pneumonia or collapse distal to the tumour (**4.43**, **4.44**, **4.155**, **4.156**), the development of a large pleural effusion or, more rarely, involvement of the lung lymphatics (lymphangitis carcinomatosa, **4.157**) or pericardium.
- Chest discomfort is a common symptom; it is often of an ill defined aching nature, but may be localized to the chest wall if there is direct invasion of the chest wall, metastasis to the ribs or pleurisy associated with infection.
- Pain in the shoulder, radiating down the upper inner arm, can be the first sign of a Pancoast tumour situated in the apex of the lung, causing symptoms by invasion of the ribs, vertebrae, sympathetic trunk, brachial plexus and artery (**4.158–4.161**).
- Wheeze is described by 10% of patients, and is often stridor caused by the narrowing of a major airway.
- A hoarse voice may be caused by paralysis of the left recurrent laryngeal nerve as it loops round the arch of the aorta; in contradistinction to the hoarse voice of chronic laryngitis associated with smoking, the patient with a paralysed vocal cord is unable to produce an explosive cough, producing instead a 'bovine' cough (**4.162**).

- Superior vena caval obstruction is most commonly caused by small-cell carcinoma, and presents with swelling of the head and neck, engorgement of the neck veins without visible pulsation and the development of collateral venous circulation over the chest wall (**4.163**, **4.164**).

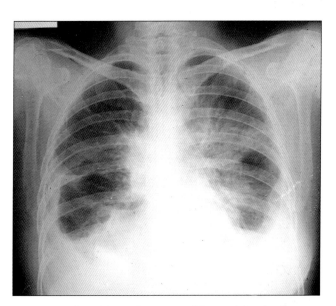

4.157   Lymphangitis carcinomatosa. Micronodular shadows are seen throughout the lungs especially on the left, and there is a streaky appearance, which results from tumour infiltration of lymphatic vessels.

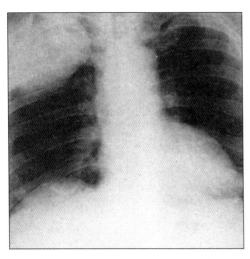

4.158 Right apical carcinoma of the bronchus (Pancoast tumour). In this location, the tumour may cause other symptoms (*see* **4.159–4.161**).

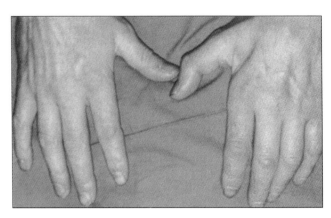

4.160 Wasting of the small muscles of the left hand (most noticeably the first dorsal interosseus) as a consequence of a left apical tumour.

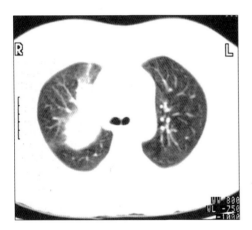

4.159 Right apical bronchial carcinoma invading the hilum and lung substance revealed by CT. This cut is at T4 level, just below the carina.

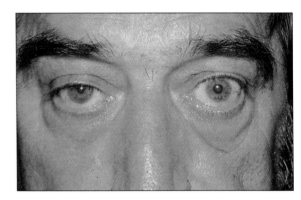

4.161 Horner's syndrome resulting from a right Pancoast tumour. The patient had a right ptosis and a constricted right pupil, caused by tumour infiltration of the inferior cervical sympathetic ganglia.

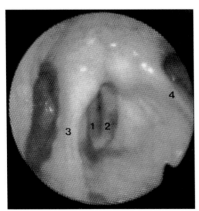

4.162 Left vocal cord paralysis during phonation in a patient with recurrent laryngeal nerve involvement by a bronchial carcinoma. This endoscopic view shows that during phonation the normal right vocal cord (1) adducts to the midline, whereas the left vocal cord (2) appears bowed and lies at a lower level than the right vocal cord. Adduction to the midline is partial, resulting in incomplete glottic closure, so the patient has a breathy voice and a bovine cough. The right aryepiglottic fold (3) is tense and appears in the normal position during phonation, whereas the left aryepiglottic fold (4) has lost its tone and cannot conform to the normal position.

- Another feature of mediastinal glandular involvement is compression of the oesophagus causing dysphagia.

Extrathoracic manifestations

About one-third of patients present with symptoms resulting from metastases; 20% of patients have bone pain at presentation (*see* **p. 145**). The lung is the most common origin of cerebral metastases (**4.165**, **11.37**); liver (*see* **p. 395**), adrenal and para-aortic lymph node involvement is also common and skin secondaries may occur (**4.166**).

A number of non-metastatic syndromes are associated with bronchial carcinoma. Inappropriate secretion of antidiuretic hormone (ADH) and ectopic adrenocorticotrophic hormone

(ACTH) secretion are seen with small-cell lung cancer (**4.167**), whereas hypercalcaemia and more rarely gynaecomastia (**4.168**) and hyperthyroidism are associated with squamous cell cancer. Neuromyopathies (**11.111**, **11.112**), dermatomyositis,

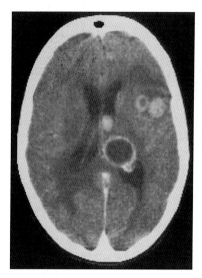

4.165 Multiple cerebral metastases in a patient with carcinoma of the bronchus, demonstrated by enhanced CT. The patient was a 47-year-old woman smoker, and the primary tumour was a small-cell carcinoma.

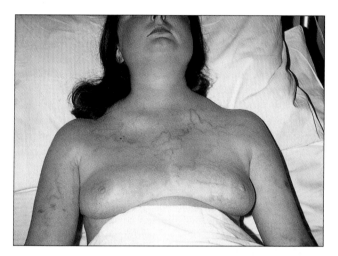

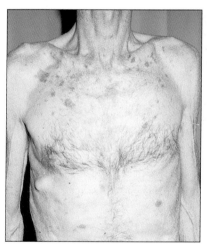

4.166 Multiple secondary deposits in the skin in a patient with carcinoma of the bronchus. Note the signs of weight loss and the subcutaneous nodule on the right.

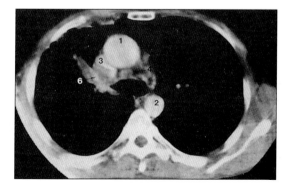

4.163 Superior vena caval obstruction in bronchial carcinoma. Note the swelling of the face and neck and the development of a collateral circulation in the veins of the chest wall.

4.164 Superior vena caval obstruction caused by bronchial carcinoma. The superior vena cava (3) is invaded and compressed by the tumour (6), which has also invaded and enlarged a pretracheal lymph node (4). The ascending aorta is marked 1 and the descending aorta is marked 2. The mediastinal involvement demonstrated by this CT scan shows that the tumour is inoperable.

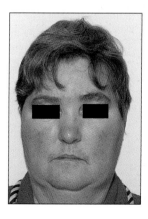

4.167 Cushing's syndrome resulting from ectopic adrenocoticotrophin hormone (ACTH) secretion by a small-cell bronchial carcinoma. The facial appearance is similar to that of Cushing's disease of other causes (*see* **p. 299**), but the disease often runs a very rapid course.

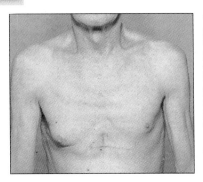

4.168 Unilateral gynaecomastia developed in this male patient with squamous cell carcinoma of the bronchus. Note the positioning line for radiotherapy. The patient shows signs of weight loss and possible early generalized hyperpigmentation.

encephalopathy and myelopathy have all been associated with bronchial carcinoma. Finger clubbing (**2.104**, **2.105**, **4.2**) is common, except in small-cell cancer, and may progress to hypertrophic pulmonary osteoarthropathy, in which there is pain in the wrists and ankles associated with periosteal new bone formation in the long bones (**4.169**, **4.170**). Anaemia and weight loss are common accompaniments of bronchial carcinoma. Thrombophlebitis, venous thrombosis and skin lesions such as acanthosis nigricans occur much less commonly.

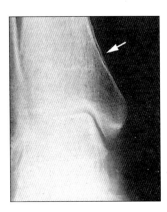

4.169 Hypertrophic pulmonary osteoarthropathy (HPOA) at the ankle in a patient with bronchial carcinoma. New bone formation is shown by the double margin seen at the medial border of the tibia (arrowed).

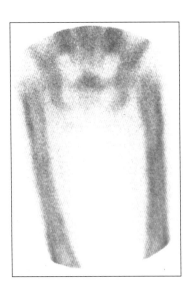

4.170 Hypertrophic pulmonary osteoarthropathy (HPOA) in bronchial carcinoma, demonstrated by radionuclide bone scan. Extensive cortical new bone formation is demonstrated by the 'tramline' appearance of both femurs.

Diagnosis and treatment

Most tumours are visible on chest X-ray, and a firm diagnosis is made by microscopic examination of sputum (**4.15**) or of specimens obtained at bronchoscopy, or by the biopsy of metastatic lesions. Occasionally, closed or open lung biopsy is required. Although there are many types of lung tumour, the simplest, clinically useful classification is to distinguish between small-cell lung cancer, non-small-cell lung cancer and benign tumours:

- Small-cell carcinoma (**4.171**) has almost always metastasized by the time of diagnosis, and it is rare for surgical resection to be performed if this diagnosis is known; the tumour is sensitive to chemotherapy and radiotherapy, both of which can lead to a significant prolongation of useful life but rarely a cure.
- In non-small-cell lung cancer (**4.172**), the patients with the best outcome are those who undergo a successful resection; two criteria must be satisfied before a patient undergoes surgery: firstly, they must be fit enough to survive the operation and have sufficiently good lung function to have good-quality survival after lung removal; secondly, the surgery must be likely to remove all of the tumour and therefore it is usual to perform scanning before operation to identify metastases; radiotherapy is valuable for the treatment of bronchial bleeding, superior vena caval obstruction, and painful bony metastases.

Many patients with cancer fear a painful death, but simple analgesics, morphine, radiotherapy and techniques such as transcutaneous nerve stimulation will control pain in almost all patients. The prognosis of bronchial carcinoma is poor. About 5% of patients will survive 5 years, and the majority of these are patients who undergo successful surgery.

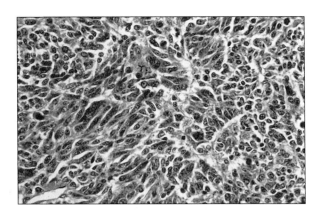

4.171 Small cell anaplastic ('oat-cell') lung cancer (H&E) arises from the bronchial epithelium and differentiates into neuroendocrine cells containing neurosecretory granules. This type of tumour grows rapidly and metastasizes rapidly to the regional lymph nodes and via the bloodstream. The typical appearance shown here is of dark, tightly-packed sheets of cells (like grains of oats). The nuclei contain nucleoli and the cytoplasm is scanty. The cells often form into rosettes. Chemotherapy and radiotherapy is the best treatment option.

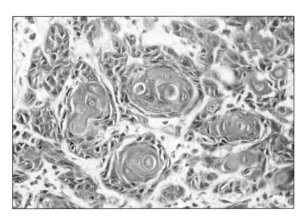

4.172 Squamous carcinoma of lung (H&E) is a form of non-small cell lung cancer that develops following metaplasia of airway epithelium to a squamous type, a change which results from chronic irritation by cigarette smoke. In this picture there are many well differentiated foci (cell nests) of tumour cells producing keratin in layers. Such tumours develop centrally, close to the carina, are slow-growing and are often amenable to surgery.

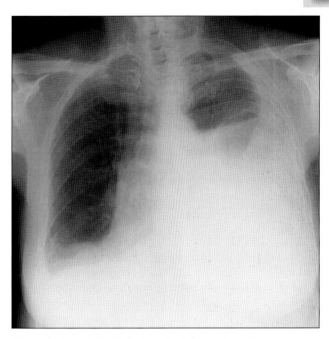

4.173 A large left-sided pleural effusion. The patient presented with breathlessness, and had previously undergone 'lumpectomy' for carcinoma of the left breast. On aspiration, the effusion was bloodstained (**4.52**).

SECONDARY TUMOURS

Metastases in the lung are common. They may occur as one or more discrete nodules (**4.29**), as a finer pattern of multiple metastases (**4.32**) or as lymphangitis carcinomatosa (**4.157**). The most common primary sites are the kidney, breast, prostate, gut, cervix and ovary. Discrete metastases are often asymptomatic, but their presence is generally a bad prognostic sign. Surgical removal of secondaries is only very rarely possible.

DISEASES OF THE PLEURA
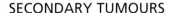

PLEURAL EFFUSIONS

Pleural effusions are a common clinical problem (**4.34**, **4.173**) and can be classified as transudates and exudates (*see* **p. 160**).

- Transudation of fluid (**4.54**) occurs with increased capillary pressure and reduced plasma oncotic pressure, and therefore is most common in cardiac failure and hypoalbuminaemic states.
- An exudative pleural effusion is caused by an inflammatory process, such as carcinoma, pneumonia (**4.34**), tuberculosis (**4.111**), rheumatoid arthritis (**3.35**), asbestosis or pulmonary infarction; pleural fluid cytology, Gram stain, culture, glucose, amylase, lactate dehydrogenase (LDH), pH and pleural biopsy can all contribute to the identification of aetiology.
- A bloody effusion (**4.52**) is most commonly seen with tumour involvement of the pleura (**4.152**), but can also occur

in pulmonary infarction, tuberculosis, trauma, coagulation disorders or ruptured aneurysm.
- Damage to the thoracic duct, usually by trauma or mediastinal malignancy leads to drainage of chyle into the pleural cavity, a chylothorax (**4.53**).

Large pleural effusions may require aspiration to improve the patient's respiratory state (*see* **p. 196**), but in general, it is most important to treat the underlying condition.

PNEUMOTHORAX

In pneumothorax air leaks into the pleural cavity, usually from the lung but occasionally from penetration of the chest wall (during surgery, penetrative trauma, etc.). The most common medical problem is a 'spontaneous' pneumothorax. This results from rupture of a congenital 'bleb' in the lung, which is usually apical and may be multiple. These are relatively common in young, tall, thin, healthy athletic men and pneumothoraces may come on at rest or after some major respiratory effort. Spontaneous pneumothorax also occurs in other medical disorders (**4.174**).

Clinical presentation is often dramatic, with the sudden onset of unilateral pain of a pleuritic type and sometimes progressive dyspnoea. It is probable that most small pneumothoraces remain undiagnosed and resolve rapidly.

CAUSES OF SPONTANEOUS PNEUMOTHORAX

Primary	Due to apical subpleural blebs
Secondary to	Asthma
	COPD
	Bacterial pneumonia or pleurisy
	Lung abscess
	Whooping cough
	Malignancy
	Marfan's syndrome

4.174 Causes of spontaneous pneumothorax.

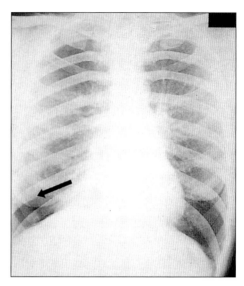

4.175 **Right-sided pneumothorax** in an adult woman with asthma. The edge of the collapsed lung is not so obvious as in **4.35**, and it is important to consider pneumothorax whenever examining the chest X-ray of a patient with an acute respiratory problem. The edge of the collapsed lung is marked with an arrow.

Larger ones can be readily diagnosed by clinical examination, and chest X-rays usually confirm the diagnosis (**4.35**, **4.175**). Usually a pneumothorax occupying less than 20% of the hemithorax may safely be left to resolve in an otherwise healthy individual as the ruptured bleb seals itself. Rarely, rupture of a bleb may leave a valve-like abnormality on the pleural surface, so that air continues to fill the pleural space, which expands and pushes over the mediastinum (tension pneumothorax). Urgent decompression is necessary and this may be done with an intrapleural catheter attached to an underwater seal drain. After conservative treatment the recurrence rate can be as high as 30%. Such patients should have thoracoscopy, which may identify a bleb or blebs that can be dealt with by oversewing using a minimally invasive technique. If the lung is apparently normal then talc may be inserted (poudrage) to achieve adhesion of the parietal and visceral pleura (pleurodesis).

4.176

4.177

4.178

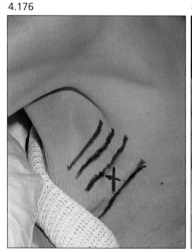
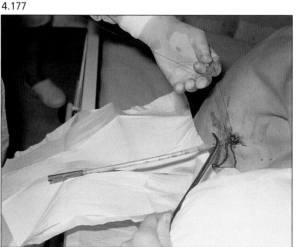
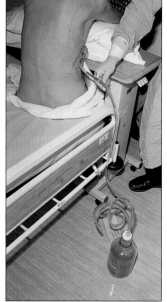

4.176, 4.177, 4.178 **Insertion of an intercostal drain.** The chosen site in the sixth intercostal space (**4.176**) is injected with local anaesthetic, a small incision is made through the skin, and a suitable drainage tube introduced with the aid of a trochar. The tube is held in place with a suture (**4.177**). The drainage tube can be attached to a one-way valve or, as here, to an underwater seal drain. If a tension pneumothorax is present, or if a large air leak from the lung persists, suction may be applied to the underwater seal. In this patient, drainage was required for symptomatic relief of a large pleural effusion.

Intercostal drainage

In the presence of an enlarging pneumothorax, or one with which significant dyspnoea is present, a tube should be inserted into the pleural space. Similar drains may also be used for very large or persistent pleural effusions. If there is a haemothorax, early removal of blood prevents later fibrosis.

The optimum site for drain insertion is in the axilla in the so-called triangle of safety – the three sides of which are the anterior axillary line, the lateral margin of pectoralis major and a horizontal line at the nipple level (**4.176**).

Silastic catheters of reasonable size are optimal as they cause less tissue reaction and are readily inserted (**4.176-4.178**).

Possible complications of chest drain insertion include:

* haemorrhage from damaged intercostal vessels
* injury to abdominal and thoracic organs
* wrong placement – usually too low
* blockage of tube with fibrin, blood clot, or pus
* kinking or migration of tube
* subcutaneous (surgical) emphysema (**4.179**).

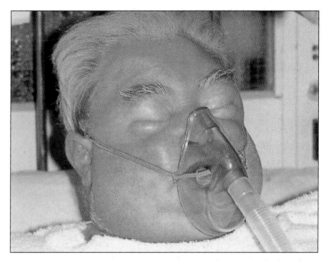

4.179 Severe subcutaneous (surgical) emphysema, which developed after the insertion of a chest drain for the treatment of pneumothorax in a patient with COPD. The condition resolved spontaneously after repositioning of the catheter. Though usually of minor clinical importance, subcutaneous emphysema may occasionally compress vital structures with life-threatening consequences.

197

5 Cardiovascular

HISTORY

Many patients with heart disease are symptom free until a relatively late stage in the illness when a catastrophic event may occur. This is particularly the case when the progression of atheroma is concerned. Early lesions may be present from the early teens, but patients usually present with myocardial infarction, sudden death, stroke or peripheral arterial disease in middle or old age. Valve diseases, congenital lesions, hyperlipidaemia and hypertension may also be asymptomatic for many years.

Most of the symptoms of heart disease result from myocardial ischaemia, abnormalities of rhythm or impaired pumping action. Many patients have non-specific symptoms such as tiredness, easy fatiguability and anorexia, but the two main symptoms are chest pain and breathlessness.

There are two main causes of cardiac pain: myocardial ischaemia and pericarditis. Ischaemic pain is usually of sudden onset, located centrally and constricting; it may radiate to the left arm, occasionally to the right, into the neck and to the back. It may be brought on by exercise, emotion, fright or sexual intercourse. Angina pectoris usually lasts less than 30 minutes and may be relieved by rest or administration of glyceryl trinitrate (GTN). The pain of myocardial infarction usually lasts for more than 30 minutes, often as long as several hours.

Failure of the heart to pump efficiently may lead to the accumulation of blood in the lungs and dyspnoea (breathlessness). Heart failure should be defined in the four categories of the New York Heart Association (5.1).

Orthopnoea is the feeling of being out of breath when lying flat, which improves on sitting up.

Paroxysmal nocturnal dyspnoea occurs when the patient lies flat in bed at night; as a result of redistribution of oedema from the periphery to the lungs there is sudden dyspnoea which makes the patient sit up or lean out of the window to get 'fresh air'.

Palpitations are an awareness of the heart beating. They can be normal in excitement, anxiety or after exercise, and may be provoked by excessive intake of caffeine, nicotine or chocolate, by heavy meals and indigestion or by sympathomimetic or vasodilator drugs; however, they may also result from cardiac rhythm disturbances.

Syncope results from failure to maintain an adequate circulation to the brain. The attacks may come on suddenly without any warning and result in sudden collapse. Syncope may have a number of causes (5.2).

Always note any family history of congenital heart disease or other genetic disorders with cardiac implications. Premature death (age < 55 years in males; < 65 years in females) in near relatives from myocardial infarction or stroke, or hyperlipidaemia or hypertension in family members are important findings.

The most acute presentation of heart disease is cardiac arrest. The patient collapses and becomes unconcious, respiration ceases and no pulse can be felt (5.3). Death results unless resuscitation is carried out successfully (see p. 215).

EXAMINATION

Examination should start with the general appearance. There may be obvious breathlessness, even at rest, as a result of heart

FUNCTIONAL GRADING OF HEART DISEASE (NEW YORK HEART ASSOCIATION)	
Grade I	No limitation of activities, i.e. free of symptoms
Grade II	No limitation under resting conditions, but symptoms appear on severe activity
Grade III	Limitation of activities on mild exertion
Grade IV	Breathlessness at rest, restricting the person to bed or a chair

5.1 Functional grading of heart disease (New York Heart Association).

CAUSES OF SYNCOPE
Vasodilatation – vasovagal attack, drugs, micturition syncope
Cardiac causes – heart block, paroxysmal tachycardia
Outflow obstruction – aortic stenosis, hypertrophic obstructive cardiomyopathy (HOCM)
Reduced ventricular filling – pulmonary embolism, atrial myxoma
Reduced blood volume – bleeding

5.2 Causes of syncope.

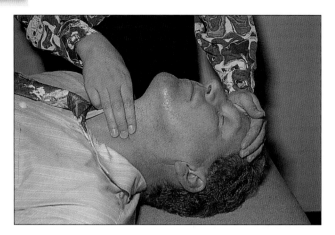

5.3   Cardiac arrest. The diagnosis is established clinically by feeling for the carotid pulse. The head should be slightly extended if possible, and the neck should be palpated for evidence of a carotid pulse on one side of the thyroid cartilage for 10 seconds. An absent carotid pulse indicates probable cardiac arrest, but peripheral pulselessness or the absence of heart sounds are unreliable signs.

failure; this may make the patient sit up in bed, propped up on pillows. The skin of the face may have the bluish discoloration of cyanosis. Severe central cyanosis, best seen in the tongue and lips, is often a feature of congenital heart disease (**4.4**). A facial flush may be present. Arcus cornealis in a young patient (**6.43**, **7.107**), xanthelasmas (**7.108**) or skin and tendon xanthomata (**7.109–7.112**) point to hyperlipidaemia. Jaundice may reflect hepatic disturbance from heart failure.

Finger clubbing (**2.104**, **2.105**) may be caused by infective endocarditis or cyanotic congenital heart disease. Infective endocarditis may cause splinter haemorrhages in the nails (**3.32**) and tender nodules in the tips of fingers and toes (**5.124**).

Distended internal and external jugular veins (**5.4**) and abnormalities of the jugular venous waveform occur in right heart failure, with abnormalities of the tricuspid valve, and in arrhythmias in which the right atrium contracts against a closed tricuspid valve.

Patients with the disproportionately long arms and fingers of Marfan's syndrome (**3.113–3.116**), are susceptible to the development of aortic aneurysm and aortic regurgitation.

The abdomen may be distended in chronic heart failure, because of the presence of ascites, and there may be pitting oedema of the legs (**5.5**, **5.6**) and the skin over the sacrum. Unilateral leg swelling is suggestive of deep venous thrombosis (**5.191**). Arterial embolism into the legs causes gangrene, which may also result from diffuse atherothrombotic arterial disease.

Examination of the radial artery pulse gives information about heart rate and rhythm, and the character of the pulse may suggest abnormalities of the aortic valve or pericardium, or cardiomyopathies.

The position of the apex beat can indicate cardiac enlargement, and auscultation of the heart allows the detection of abnormal heart sounds and murmurs caused by valve disease and congenital malformations (**5.7**).

Crepitations in the lung fields that persist after coughing may indicate cardiac failure. In hypertensive patients, the fundi may show evidence of retinal arterial damage (*see* **p. 238**).

Blood pressure should always be measured, using correctly calibrated equipment and paying strict attention to correct technique. The value of single casual readings is low, and high readings should be repeated or followed up by 24-hour ambulatory blood pressure monitoring. National and international guidelines on the interpretation and management of blood pressure measurements are helpful.

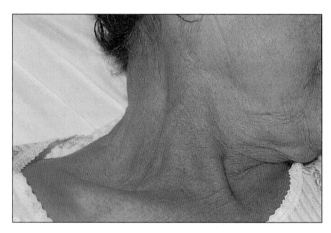

5.4   Elevated external jugular venous pressure (JVP). The pressure in the internal and external jugular veins is elevated in right heart failure. Abnormalities in waveform may provide evidence of tricuspid valve disease or cardiac arrhythmia, although these abnormalities are more reliably noted in the internal than the external jugular vein, which may be affected by position.

5.5   5.6

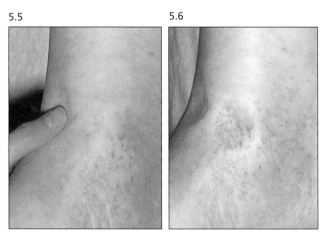

5.5 & 5.6   Pitting oedema in a patient with cardiac failure. A depression ('pit') remains in the oedema for some minutes after firm fingertip pressure is applied.

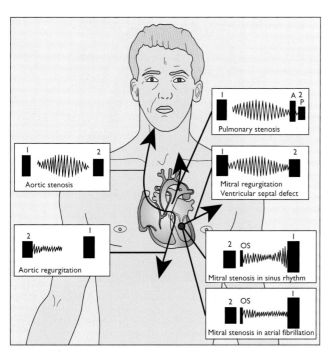

5.7 **Common systolic and diastolic murmurs and their radiation patterns.** 1: First heart sound; 2: second heart sound; A: aortic component; P: pulmonary component; OS: opening snap.

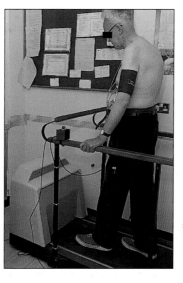

5.8 **The exercise treadmill test** may reveal signs of ischaemia on the ECG when the resting trace is normal (**5.10**).

BRUCE PROTOCOL FOR EXERCISE TOLERANCE TEST

Phase 1 – slow walk (1.7 mph) at 10° incline increasing in six more stages at 3 minute intervals to

Phase 7 – running (6 mph) at 22° incline

Negative test

Absence of chest pain, ischaemia or arrhythmia when the patient reaches 80, 90 or 100% of target heart rate (220 minus age)

Positive test

Presence of chest pain, ischaemia or arrhythmia. Ischaemia is at least 1–2 mm depression of down-sloping ST segment

5.9 **Bruce protocol for exercise tolerance test.**

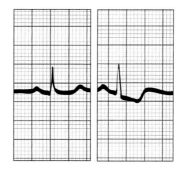

5.10 **A positive exercise test as shown in lead II.** The trace taken before exercise is normal, but the second trace, recorded 2 minutes after the end of exercise, shows ST segment depression with T-wave inversion. Analysis of the full trace may show further evidence of ischaemia (**5.63**).

INVESTIGATIONS

The main investigatory techniques in cardiovascular disorders are electrocardiography, chest radiography, echocardiography, colour-flow Doppler, nuclear cardiology, cardiac catheterization, angiography and MRI.

The heart generates electrical activity that can be recorded on an **electrocardiogram** (ECG or EKG):

- The resting ECG is useful in the diagnosis of myocardial infarction, cardiac hypertrophy or abnormalities in rhythm; characteristic ECG abnormalities usually develop soon after coronary artery occlusion occurs, and some abnormalities usually persist after the patient's recovery (*see* **p. 214**); the resting ECG can also detect ventricular hypertrophy and abnormalities of conduction, such as bundle branch block.
- The resting ECG is often normal in patients with angina pectoris, but a recording during exercise, on a bicycle or treadmill, usually reveals characteristic changes indicating myocardial ischaemia (**5.8–5.10**).
- Ambulatory electrocardiography is useful when heart rhythm disturbances occur only intermittently. The recording is made on a portable tape recorder (**5.11**), usually over 24 hours, and it can be analysed in a computer. Correlation is made between symptomatic episodes, for example palpitations, and the ECG record.

Ambulatory blood pressure monitoring (**5.12**, **5.13**) records blood pressure over a 24–48 hour period, to take account of changes due to sympathetic overactivity, posture, muscle activity and state of hydration It is valuable in identifying patients with labile blood pressures and those with 'white coat' hypertension.

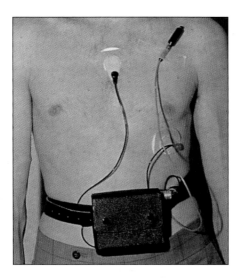

5.11   Ambulatory electrocardiography ('Holter monitoring'). The patient undertakes a range of normal activities over a 24-hour period while wearing this lightweight ECG monitoring equipment. He can mark symptomatic episodes on the recording tape by pushing a button on the recorder, and the entire 24-hour recording can then be analysed for ischaemia or arrhythmias in a computer.

The **chest X-ray** is important in diagnosing and assessing the severity of many cardiac abnormalities (**5.14**). It is superior to the stethoscope in revealing heart failure and shows characteristic features of pulmonary congestion and oedema (**5.15**). It indicates whether the heart and great vessels are enlarged and whether there is calcification (**5.141**) or fluid in the pericardium.

Echocardiography, Doppler flow studies and colour-flow Doppler involve the analysis of reflected high-frequency sound directed at the heart from a transducer on the chest wall. They permit real-time visualization of the heart valves, to determine whether they are stenosed or incompetent, and examination of the walls of the left ventricle, providing an index of the function of the left ventricle during systole or diastole:

- The original technique, M-mode echocardiography, is one-dimensional, but it allows the assessment of intracardiac dimensions and the simultaneous monitoring and visualization of the ECG (**5.16**).
- Doppler flow studies can be combined with M-mode or two-dimensional echocardiography to provide further dynamic information (**5.17**) and to study the function of the left ventricle during diastole.
- Two-dimensional imaging produces clearer anatomical images (**5.18**), and allows simple diagnosis of a range of cardiac abnormalities, including valvular heart disease, congenital abnormalities, cardiac tumours and pericardial effusions.
- Colour-flow Doppler echocardiography allows further evaluation of blood flow within the heart; it has particularly

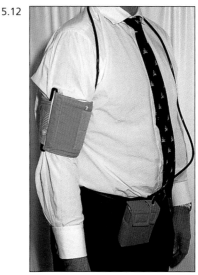

5.12

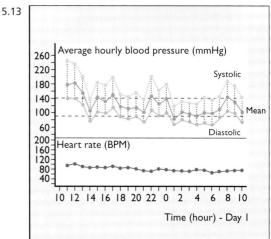

5.13

5.12, 5.13   Ambulatory blood pressure monitoring. These lightweight monitoring devices consist of a cuff applied to the upper arm, connected to a monitor attached to the belt (**5.12**). The air pressure cuff is inflated automatically and the Korotkoff sounds are recorded electronically with the heart rate and time. A typical tracing is shown in **5.13**. In the initial part of the trace the blood pressure has fallen dramatically after the patient left the clinic (suggesting 'white coat' hypertension), but the blood pressure was also elevated several times over the next 24 hours. It is important to obtain a proper baseline value for BP before starting therapy with hypotensive agents.

aided the diagnosis of valvular stenosis and incompetence (**5.19**).

- Transoesophageal echocardiography (TOE) utilizes an ultrasonic window to the heart that avoids the problems of chest wall, ribs and lung; it is of value for patients whose transthoracic echocardiograms are unsatisfactory and who have lesions of the left atrium (**5.126**), the ascending aorta,

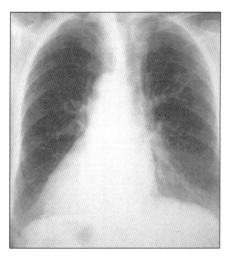

5.14 Situs inversus revealed by chest X-ray. The apex of the heart lies in the right side of the the thorax (dextrocardia). The left dome of the diaphragm is higher than the right, because the liver is on the left and the spleen and the stomach are on the right. Situs inversus is usually a harmless abnormality with a normal life-expectancy, but it may be associated with ciliary abnormalities in Kartagener's syndrome (**4.101**), a hereditary disorder in which the patient also has sinusitis, bronchiectasis and, if male, infertility resulting from immotile spermatozoa. Isolated dextrocardia is usually associated with other major congenital heart disease.

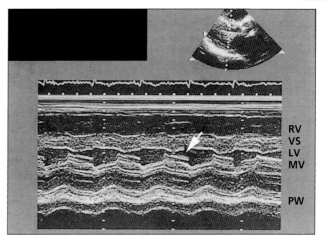

5.16 M-mode echocardiogram in mitral stenosis. Ultrasound waves are transmitted into the body in a one-dimensional ('ice-pick') form. They are reflected back each time they reach an interface between tissues of different acoustic impedance. This allows an assessment of the relative movement of different parts of the heart. This tracing shows impaired movement of the mitral valve leaflets, which is revealed as flattening of the normal mitral valve trace (arrow). The orientation of the view across the mitral valve is shown in the small two-dimensional view above, and the structures are labelled in the M-mode view (RV = right ventricle; VS = ventricular septum; LV = left ventricle; MV = mitral valve; PW = posterior wall of left ventricle).

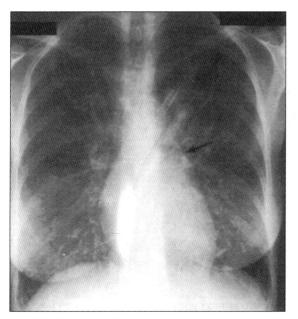

5.15 Heart failure in a patient with mitral stenosis. The left atrial appendage is enlarged (arrowed), the upper zone blood vessels are distended and there are linear densities in the periphery of the lower zones (interstitial or Kerley B lines). The lung-field changes are typical of moderate pulmonary oedema (*see* **5.97** for a further example).

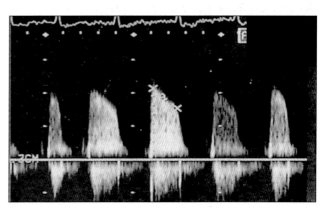

5.17 Doppler flow in mitral stenosis. Using Doppler, it is possible to measure the velocity of blood flow and calculate the instantaneous pressure difference across valves. The mitral valve orifice area can then be estimated by measuring the pressure half time, the time taken for the pressure difference to fall to half its value. In this example (the same patient as in **5.16**) the estimated valve area is 0.75 cm^2, which suggests significant mitral stenosis (the normal area is 3.5 cm^2).

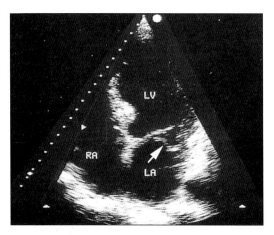

5.18   Two-dimensional cardiac ultrasound allows imaging that can be monitored in real time. This long axis view is from a patient with mitral valve prolapse. The posterior cusp of the mitral valve (arrow) is seen to prolapse into the left atrium in this systolic frame (LV = left ventricle; LA = left atrium; RA = right atrium).

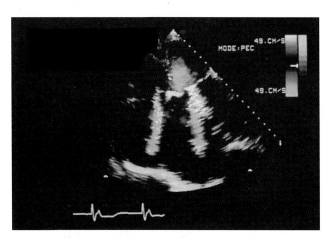

5.19   Colour-flow mapping results from the parallel processing of both two-dimensional and Doppler flow data, which are combined in real time to provide a dynamic image of anatomical, functional and haemodynamic status. This systolic apical four-chamber view shows both mitral and tricuspid regurgitation. The left ventricle is the blue area at the top of the image, and the regurgitant flow through the mitral valve is seen on the right. Tricuspid regurgitation is seen as a narrower band of flow on the left.

handled like potassium by the body) or technetium-tetrofosmin, which behaves similarly, may be injected intravenously. Radioactivity can be assessed from within the cavities of the heart (technetium erythrocyte or albumin technique), permitting evaluation of cardiac function (**5.20**), or from the walls of the heart (thallium or tetrofosmin technique), allowing assessment of ischaemia and infarction (**5.21**).

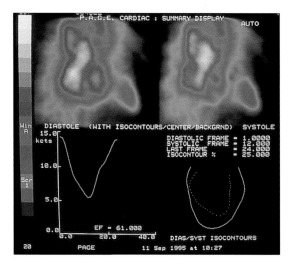

5.20   Technetium blood pool study in a patient with chest pain but normal ventricular function. Typical diastolic and systolic frames are shown top left and top right, and the contours of the left ventricle are displayed graphically at bottom right. The area of the blood pool at each of 16 frames of the cardiac cycle is plotted bottom left and allows the calculation of the left ventricular ejection fraction, which is normal at 61%.

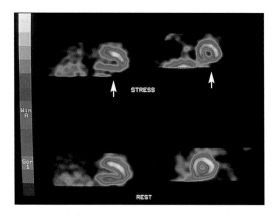

5.21   Nuclear tomograms after the injection of Tc-tetrofosmin, demonstrating myocardial perfusion. During exercise (stress), the inferior wall of the left ventricle is poorly perfused, as shown in the ventricular long axis (top left) and short axis (top right) views (arrows). After rest, a greater though still abnormally low level of perfusion is seen.

the aortic valve (especially vegetations), and in atrial and ventricular septal defects; it may also be used intraoperatively and in intensive care, especially in dissection of the root of the aorta (**5.178**).

Nuclear cardiology is a useful method of assessing the function of cardiac muscle. Technetium-99m may be bound to albumin or red cells from the patient's blood and thallium-201 (which is

Cardiac catheterization and angiography are invasive techniques (**5.22**). Catheters are advanced to the right and left heart under X-ray screening. Pressures are measured at the tips of the catheters, permitting evaluation of valvular stenosis (**5.23**), and oxygen saturations can be assessed to diagnose septal defects. During angiography, radio-opaque contrast medium is injected through the catheters into the heart or vessels. Left ventriculography outlines the inside of the left ventricle and assesses systolic function and mitral regurgitation. Many of these catheter techniques have been largely superseded by (non-invasive) echocardiography, but coronary angiography is still the only accurate method of assessing the severity and extent of coronary disease – an essential preliminary to coronary

artery surgery. A catheter is inserted into the coronary artery ostia and the vessels are injected with radio-opaque contrast material (**5.24**). Coronary angioplasty may be carried out in the same session (**5.25**). Digital subtraction angiography permits the use of smaller amounts of contrast medium, which can be given intravenously. This is useful in imaging peripheral arteries.

MRI is a further non-invasive tool that can be synchronized with the ECG to allow diastolic and systolic images to be produced (**5.26**).

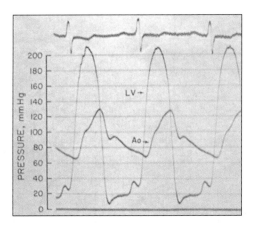

5.22   The cardiac catheter laboratory. Catheters may be advanced to the left and right heart in aseptic conditions and under X-ray control. Angiography and an increasing number of interventional techniques, including ablation of abnormal conduction pathways, may be performed, in addition to pressure and oxygen saturation studies.

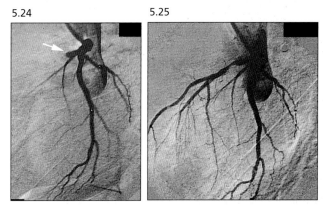

5.24   5.25

5.24 & 5.25   Coronary angiography and angioplasty. The coronary angiogram in left lateral projection shows complete occlusion of the left anterior descending coronary artery. Only a stump is seen (**5.24**, arrow). After coronary angioplasty (*see* **p. 213**), there is good perfusion of the left anterior descending artery, although a residual stenosis is seen (**5.25**). This can, if necessary, be dealt with electively at a later stage by further angioplasty, stenting or surgery.

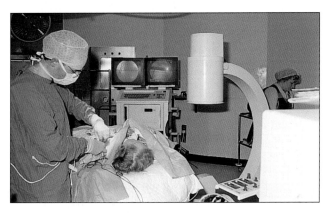

5.23   Pressure gradient across the aortic valve in aortic stenosis, as measured at cardiac catheterization. Note the low aortic (Ao) pressure compared with the left ventricular pressure (LV) and the delayed peak in aortic pressure – both characteristic of severe aortic stenosis. Such pressure studies are less commonly performed than in the past, because echocardiography and Doppler flow studies can provide much of the relevant information non-invasively.

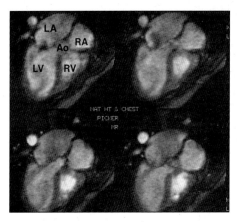

5.26   Magnetic resonance cine gradient echo scan (horizontal long axis plane) in dilated cardiomyopathy showing a grossly hypertrophied left ventricle (LV) that contracts poorly. These four frames show extremely poor systolic left ventricular thickening and motion, and a small jet of mitral regurgitation can be seen in the top right image by virtue of loss of signal (black) from the turbulent jet (LV = left ventricle; LA = left atrium; RV = right ventricle; RA = right atrium; Ao = aortic root).

CIRCULATORY FAILURE

Circulatory failure is an extremely common problem, with an incidence of 2% at age 50 years, rising to 10% at age 80 years. There is still a high mortality: 10–30% per year.

Circulatory failure occurs when an adequate blood flow to the tissues cannot be maintained. This may be caused by inadequate cardiac output (heart failure) or by a markedly reduced intravascular volume, for example after major haemorrhage, acute dehydration or in septicaemic shock.

Heart failure may develop because the heart muscle itself is diseased or because excessive demands are placed on it. The main myocardial disease is ischaemia resulting from atheromatous narrowing of the coronary arteries. Features of heart failure develop when about 40% of the myocardium has been damaged. Other causes include cardiomyopathies, hypertension and the conditions listed in **5.27**. Excessive demands on the heart may occur with regurgitant or stenotic valves, atrial fibrillation, outflow tract obstructions and with obstruction caused by cardiac tamponade or constrictive pericarditis. High-output states such as anaemia, thyrotoxicosis, beri-beri and Paget's disease have a similar effect.

When cardiac output is inadequate, compensatory mechanisms develop in an attempt by the body to maintain blood flow. These mechanisms are responsible for many of the signs of heart failure and may have other deleterious effects. Increased sympathetic tone causes tachycardia, and increased aldosterone levels stimulate salt and water retention. The signs of heart failure depend to a great extent on its chronicity. Conventionally heart failure is described as mainly right-sided or left-sided, but usually features of both are present.

In left ventricular failure, the dominant symptom is dyspnoea, which may be present at rest or after exercise, or may be associated with paroxysmal nocturnal dyspnoea. There may be episodes of acute pulmonary oedema during which the patient coughs up copious volumes of frothy white sputum that may be tinged with blood, and Cheyne–Stokes respiration may

also be observed. The clinical signs in the heart vary with the cause of the failure, but most patients have a marked tachycardia and occasionally pulsus alternans and a third heart sound during diastole (gallop rhythm). The basal areas of both lungs may reveal fine moist crepitations.

In right heart failure there is engorgement of the venous tree. This leads to distension of the jugular veins (**5.4**); distension of the liver, which is enlarged and tender and retention of fluid, producing dependent oedema of the legs (**4.93**, **5.5**), ascites, hydrothorax and sometimes pericardial effusion. The patient may be deeply cyanosed (**4.4**).

The degree of failure can be confirmed by chest X-ray (**5.15**, **5.28**). ECG may demonstrate arrhythmia or ischaemia, and echocardiography demonstrates reduced motion of the walls of the failing heart during systole. Doppler echocardiography can demonstrate impaired filling of the ventricles in diastole. Other important investigations include a full blood count to exclude anaemia, urea and electrolytes, thyroid function tests, liver function tests and cardiac enzymes if recent myocardial infarction is suspected.

The drug treatment of heart failure is largely concerned with improving or abolishing the unwanted effects of pulmonary congestion and fluid retention. In heart failure, an attempt is also made to increase cardiac output.

Diuretics, nitrates and angiotensin-converting enzyme (ACE) inhibitors reduce cardiac work, and other drugs, including β-blockers and digoxin, have a role in selected patients. Cardiac transplantation should be considered in unresponsive cases, and implantable 'artificial hearts' or left ventricular assist devices have a developing role (**5.29**, **5.30**).

COMMON CAUSES OF HEART FAILURE
Ischaemic heart disease
Hypertension
Dilated cardiomyopathy
Valvular heart disease
Toxic (especially alcohol)
Untreated arrhythmias
Thyrotoxicosis

5.27 Common causes of heart failure.

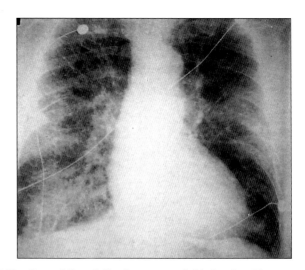

5.28 Heart failure following myocardial infarction. The changes are more severe than in **5.15**: there is distension of the upper zone vessels, interstitial (Kerley B) lines are present at both bases; and there are some areas of apparent consolidation, indicating alveolar pulmonary oedema.

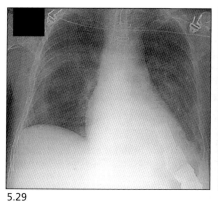
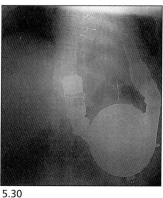

5.29 & 5.30 A left ventricular assist device implanted in a patient with previously intractable heart failure. The pneumatically driven pump is implanted in the abdomen. Blood flows from the apex of the left ventricle, through a porcine valve into the pump, and from there through an outlet porcine valve to a Dacron conduit attached to the ascending aorta. Electrically driven pumps are also available.

5.29   5.30

ARRHYTHMIAS

Abnormal heart rhythms may be classified according to the mechanism of origin of the rhythm disturbance, by the site of origin or by their effect on heart rate. Because the mechanisms are often not clear and the precise site is often unknown, this section will classify those rhythms into tachycardias (heart rate greater than 100 bpm) and bradycardias (heart rate less than 60 bpm). The rhythm is usually investigated by a standard 12-lead ECG with a rhythm strip (usually a prolonged section of lead II).

Typical examples of ECG traces in the tachycardias are seen in **5.31–5.36** and **5.38–5.45** and typical bradycardia traces are seen in **5.46–5.48**. The causes of atrial fibrillation, one of the commonest arrhythmias, are listed in **5.37**.

Heart block, a failure of conduction, may occur at the atrio-ventricular node (**5.49–5.53**). When complete, it may need to be treated by cardiac pacing (**5.54–5.58, 11.2**). Intraventricular block may be the result of conduction failure in the right or left branches of the His bundle, or in the hemi-branches of the left branch. Left bundle branch block (**5.59**) and right bundle branch block give typical ECG appearances, but these may often be modified by myocardial infarction or other underlying causes. Bifascicular block (in which any two of the three main intraventricular conduction pathways are wholly or partially blocked) may also occur. The treatment of bundle branch block is usually that of the underlying disease and its haemodynamic complications.

Recurrent tachyarrhythmias which are associated with abnormal conducting pathways in the heart may be identified by cardiac mapping and such pathways may sometimes be destroyed by radiofrequency catheter ablation techniques. When this is not possible, ventricular fibrillation may be detected and reversed in selected patients by an automatic implantable cardioverter-defibrillator (**5.60, 5.61**).

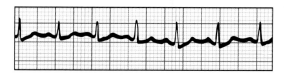

5.31   Sinus tachycardia – a regular tachycardia in which the beats originate in the sino-atrial node. This may represent a physiological response to exercise, emotion, fear or anxiety; or it may accompany fever, blood loss, thyrotoxicosis, a falling blood pressure or heart failure. Each beat is preceded by a normal P wave, the upper limit of rate is about 180 bpm and, in contrast to paroxysmal tachycardia, the rate tends to fluctuate. Carotid sinus compression usually slows the rate transiently.

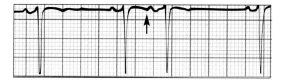

5.32   Atrial ectopic beat. The ectopic is arrowed. Its QRS complex is identical to those of normal beats, but the P wave differs slightly in shape and deforms the T wave of the preceding beat. The next sinus beat follows after an interval that is close to the inter-beat interval of the basic sinus rhythm. Like other ectopics, atrial ectopics are caused by an electrical discharge from an irritable focus, but atrial ectopics are usually of little clinical significance.

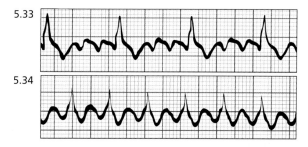

5.33

5.34

5.33 & 5.34   Atrial flutter is always associated with organic heart disease and is characterized by a rapid regular atrial rate between 220 and 360 bpm. There is a fixed or variable degree of atrioventricular block, which results in one, two or three atrial impulses being blocked for each one transmitted. On the ECG the flutter (F) waves produce a 'saw tooth' pattern, though some may be buried in the QRS complex. **5.33** shows atrial flutter with 4:1 atrioventricular block. **5.34** shows atrial flutter with 2:1 atrioventricular block. The usual associations are with ischaemic heart disease, rheumatic valvular disease and cor pulmonale.

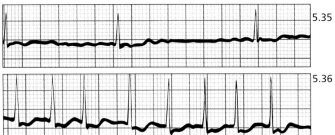

5.35

5.36

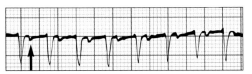

5.35 & 5.36 Atrial fibrillation. There is chaotic atrial activity at a frequency of 400–600 bpm. There is little or no mechanical activity of the atria and few of the beats are conducted by the atrioventricular node, so the ventricular response is totally irregular and may be slow (**5.35**) or as rapid as 200 bpm (**5.36**). The pulse is 'irregularly irregular' on palpation and the ECG has absent P waves, which are replaced by rapid irregular waves (f waves). Note the irregularity of the QRS response. This is one of the most common arrhythmias and has many potential causes (**5.37**). It is also found in about 15% of elderly people who are otherwise symptom-free. Atrial fibrillation of acute onset can often be reversed by DC shock or drug therapy, but in chronic atrial fibrillation, drug therapy may be used to modify the ventricular response. Because of the high incidence of cerebral embolism, a decision must be taken about long-term anticoagulation with warfarin.

5.38 Junctional tachycardias are brought about by re-entry of the cardiac impulse often via an accessory pathway between atria and ventricles. These rhythms are usually paroxysmal, and they may be precipitated by coffee or alcohol. The patient may be aware of palpitations, and the tachycardia may lead to dyspnoea and polyuria. There is usually no major structural heart disease. In atrioventricular re-entry tachycardia (**5.38**) there is a large circuit comprising the atrioventricular node, the His bundle, the ventricle, an abnormal connection and the atrium. The rhythm is absolutely regular, but the rate may vary from 140 to 280 bpm. In **5.38**, inverted P waves can be seen buried in the QRST complex (arrowed), so there has been retrograde atrial activation. **5.39** is an example of atrioventricular nodal re-entry tachycardia where no P waves are visible. These tachycardias may be terminated by vagotonic manoeuvres such as carotid sinus massage, by drug therapy (**5.40**) or, occasionally, by DC shock. Prophylactic therapy is indicated if the arrythmias occur frequently or are symptomatically very troublesome. Verapamil, flecainide, propafenone, disopyramide, digoxin and beta-blockers can all be used. Amiodarone may also be effective but should be used only for the most refractory arrhythmias because of its long-term toxic effects. If the arrhythmia does not respond to treatment or there are side-effects from the drug therapy radio-frequency ablation of the abberant pathway may be effective.

THE MOST COMMON CAUSES OF ATRIAL FIBRILLATION
Rheumatic heart disease – especially mitral valve
Ischaemic heart disease
Sick sinus syndome
Thyrotoxicosis
Alcohol abuse
Cardiomyopathies/myocarditis
Thoracotomy
Atrial septal defects
Pulmonary embolism
Acute infections
Trauma
Cor pulmonale
Idiopathic

5.37 The most common causes of atrial fibrillation.

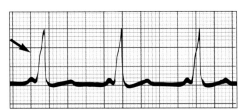

5.39 Wolff–Parkinson–White (WPW) syndrome. In this congenital condition, there is an abnormal myocardial connection between atrium and ventricle (the bundle of Kent). The activating impulse from the atria can pass down this pathway, as well as across the atrioventricular node, so the ventricles are activated without the usual delay introduced by the atrioventricular node, and the PR interval is short. There is a characteristic wide QRS complex that begins as a slurred part, the 'delta wave' (arrowed). WPW may be associated with re-entrant tachycardia or atrial fibrillation. With severe or frequent paroxysmal attacks, patients require treatment, which may involve surgery or electrical ablation of the aberrant pathway.

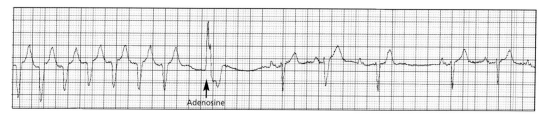

5.40   Termination of an episode of supraventricular atrioventricular nodal re-entry tachycardia by an intravenous bolus of adenosine. This patient had WPW syndrome, and was awaiting elective ablation of the aberrant pathway.

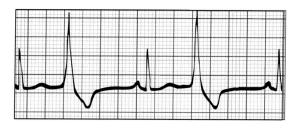

5.41   Ventricular ectopic beats are beats resulting from an abnormal irritable focus in the ventricle. Occasional ectopics are usually of little clinical significance, but in acute abnormalities such as myocardial infarction they may be the prelude to the 'coupled' ectopic beats seen here (where each sinus beat is followed by an ectopic) and to ventricular tachycardia or fibrillation. Coupled beats like this can cause serious disturbance of cardiac performance, as the ectopic beat may contribute little or nothing to cardiac output.

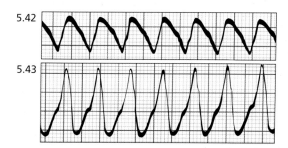

5.42 & 5.43   Ventricular tachycardia. This serious arrhythmia may have a range of appearances and two examples are shown here. The QRS complexes are broad and they merge into one another, and the heart rate is commonly in the range 150–200 bpm. Ventricular tachycardia may be caused by the repetitive discharge of an irritable focus in the ventricles; it may be sustained or end rapidly in ventricular fibrillation. Ventricular tachycardia occurs in ischaemia, rheumatic heart disease, cardiomyopathy, digoxin toxicity and in the presence of healed myocardial infarction and requires urgent treatment.

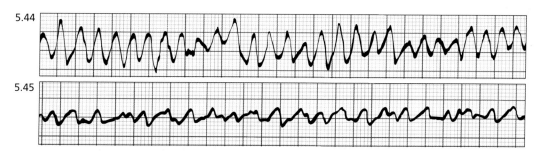

5.44 & 5.45   Ventricular fibrillation. This is a terminal rhythm in which coordinated activity of the ventricles ceases. Despite continuing electrical activity, the heart does not pump. The patient rapidly becomes unconscious and pulseless, and emergency treatment for cardiac arrest is essential. The ECG shows irregular, ill-defined waves that vary in size. In **5.44** the fibrillation waves are of good amplitude and there are periods suggestive of ventricular flutter. Defibrillation by DC shock is more likely to be successful with this appearance than with that seen in **5.45**, where there are very variable low-voltage waves.

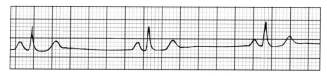

5.46   Sinus bradycardia. The complexes are normal, but the heart rate is below 60 bpm (here about 44 bpm). This may be a normal finding in healthy athletes, but after myocardial infarction it may be more sinister, producing a reduction in coronary blood flow, hypotension and decreased cardiac output. In these circumstances it can be treated with atropine.

5.47
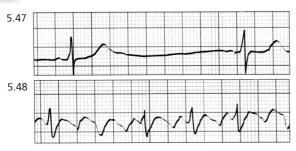

5.48

5.47 & 5.48   Sinus node disease (the 'sick sinus syndrome'). This syndrome is caused by ischaemia, infarction or degenerative disease of the sinus node, and is characterized by long intervals between consecutive P waves. These intervals may allow tachycardias to emerge, often resulting in alternating periods of bradycardia and tachycardia (the tachy-brady syndrome). In this patient, extreme sinus bradycardia (**5.47**) was followed by atrial flutter with 2:1 block (**5.48**).

5.49
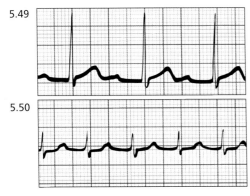

5.50

5.49 & 5.50   First degree atrioventricular block. The PR interval exceeds 0.22 seconds, so there is a delay in atrioventricular conduction, but all impulses pass on and result in a QRS complex and ventricular contraction. In **5.49** the PR interval is easily measured, but in **5.50** the P wave is hidden in the T wave of the preceding beat and could easily be missed.

5.51
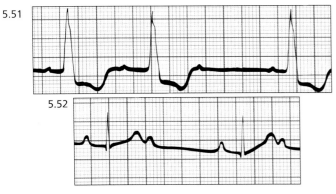

5.52

5.51 & 5.52   Second degree atrioventricular block occurs in two forms. In the first, there is progressive lengthening of the PR interval until finally one P wave is not conducted (the Wenckebach phenomenon, 5.50). In the second form, there is intermittent blockage of P-wave conduction to the ventricles without any preceding lengthening of the PR interval, as in 5.51 which shows regular 2:1 conduction. This type is particularly likely to be followed by complete heart block.

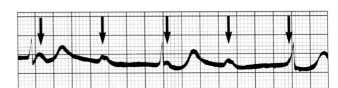

5.53   Third degree atrioventricular block, in which the atria and ventricles beat completely independently of one another and there is no transmission of atrial activity to the ventricles. The ventricular rhythm is usually regular at 40–50 bpm, and the P waves are not always easy to see (they are arrowed here). The most common causes of complete heart block are idiopathic conducting system disease and acute myocardial infarction, but it may occur in a range of other congenital and acquired conditions. Definitive treatment usually requires temporary or permanent cardiac pacing.

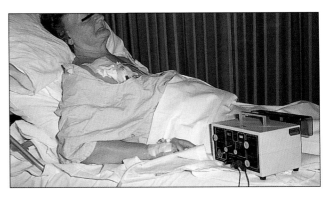

5.54   A temporary pacemaker, newly implanted in a patient with heart block following myocardial infarction. Here, the pacemaker wire is introduced via the subclavian vein, and pacing is controlled from an external source.

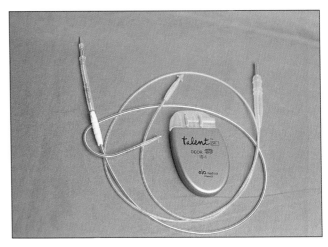

5.55   A modern permanent cardiac pacemaker unit, together with the pacing wire that leads from the pacemaker to the right ventricle. These pacemakers are small and easily and inconspicuously implantable beneath the skin. They may, however, set off security alarms and are a hazard in the presence of microwaves or MRI equipment. They should be removed before cremation.

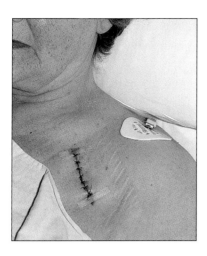

5.56 The site of implantation of a permanent pacemaker. The pacemaker is usually implanted in the left pectoral region, but may be placed elsewhere if necessary.

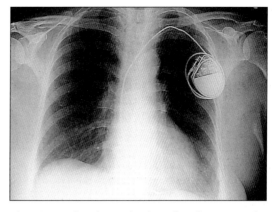

5.57 Chest X-ray showing an implanted pacing system (same patient as **5.56**). The pacemaker is in the left pectoral region, and the endocardial pacing wire is positioned at the tip of the right ventricle, in contact with the endocardium.

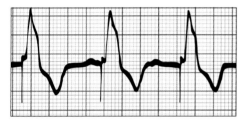

5.58 Endocardial pacing produces a pacing artefact on the ECG as here, where the patient is being paced with a unipolar electrode at the apex of the right ventricle.

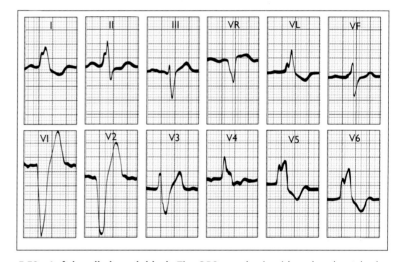

5.59 Left bundle branch block. The QRS complex is widened and notched over the left ventricle as a result of abnormal activation via the right bundle. Repolarization is also abnormal, so the T waves are sharply inverted in these leads. The small Q wave normally seen in V6 is missing, because the septum is no longer activated from the left side.

5.60

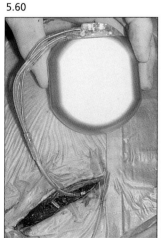

5.61

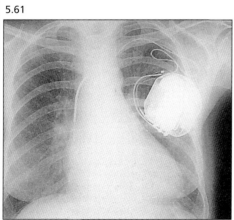

5.60, 5.61 An automatic implantable cardioverter-defibrillator (AICD). Modern AICDs can be implanted in a pectoral pocket in the same way as implantable pacemakers (**5.60**). The AICD is connected to a single transvenous lead which bears two defibrillation coils. On implantation, one coil is in the superior vena cava (right atrium); the other is near the apex of the right ventricle (**5.61**). The AICD contains a computer which senses the onset of ventricular fibrillation and initiates defibrillation. Function of the device (number of episodes, provoking rhythms, dates of defibrillation, etc) can be interrogated by a non-invasive, external radio device.

ISCHAEMIC HEART DISEASE (IHD)

Ischaemic heart disease (IHD; also known as coronary heart disease, CHD) is usually caused by structural disorder of the coronary arteries (coronary artery disease, CAD), although disorders of small coronary vessels may occasionally lead to similar symptomatology. IHD is the main cause of death in Western society and is usually a result of a combination of genetic and lifestyle factors (**5.62**). Cigarette smoking has a major causative effect.

Ischaemic heart disease is characterized by the deposition of plaques of atheroma, a fatty deposit, in the subendothelium of the coronary arteries. Atheroma has a patchy distribution, usually in the proximal parts of the vessels, and the atheromatous plaques narrow the lumen of the arteries, limiting blood flow through them. Further narrowing can result from spasm of the vessel wall near the site of the plaques and from the formation of a platelet–fibrin thrombus on the surface. Symptoms are usually experienced when the cross-sectional area of the artery is reduced by about 75%. Atheromatous plaques may fissure and heal spontaneously or a thrombus may form on the surface of the fissure. Thrombosis usually underlies the development of unstable angina or myocardial infarction.

Ischaemic heart disease produces two main syndromes:

- angina pectoris – stable or unstable
- myocardial infarction.

Cardiac failure may accompany any of these syndromes, and sudden death may result from arrhythmia without the onset of other symptoms.

ANGINA PECTORIS

Angina is a painful constricting sensation of pressure or weight felt in the centre of the chest, which may radiate to the arms, the throat, back and epigastrium. It is usually provoked by activity that increases heart rate and blood pressure, thereby increasing myocardial oxygen demand, for example exercise, emotion, stress, fear or sexual intercourse. The pain or tightness of 'stable' angina typically starts while walking and is relieved in a few minutes by rest or sublingual glyceryl trinitrate.

Patients with stable angina frequently have a normal ECG at rest, but changes may occur during angina attacks (**5.63**) and an exercise ECG usually shows characteristic changes (**5.8– 5.10**). It is important to consider other possible causes of chest pain (**5.64**).

Drug therapy for angina may include nitrates, beta-blockers, calcium antagonists and ACE inhibitors. If optimum drug therapy does not permit a patient to lead a near-normal life, then coronary angiography should be performed to identify the site of atheromatous narrowing or occlusion of the coronary arteries (**5.24**), as a prelude to possible coronary angioplasty or bypass surgery.

Coronary angioplasty involves dilating a stenosed coronary artery with a balloon-tipped cardiac catheter (usually inserted via the femoral artery); (**5.24**, **5.25**, **5.65–5.68**). The technique often relieves angina, but 30% of patients experience recurrent

---

RISK FACTORS FOR ISCHAEMIC HEART DISEASE (IHD)

Fixed risks
Male sex
Family history of IHD
Increasing age
Social class V
Race

Modifiable risks
Cigarette smoking
High blood cholesterol level (total and LDL); low HDL
High blood triglycerides
Hypertension
Obesity
Western diet
Diabetes mellitus
Physical inactivity
Use of oral contraceptive pill
High plasma fibrinogen level
High plasma homocystine level
Unemployment
Stress
Personality

Other factors still await identification

5.62 Risk factors for ischaemic heart disease (IHD).

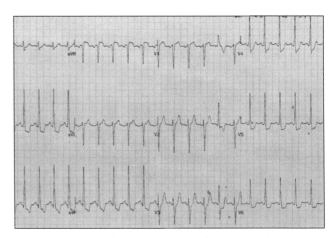

5.63 Angina pectoris associated with ECG changes. During anginal pain, there are usually ST-segment changes on the ECG. This ECG was taken during an episode of exercise-induced angina, and it shows ST-segment depression (4 mm) in leads V4–6, standard leads II and III and lead aVF.

MAJOR CAUSES OF NON-IHD CHEST PAIN

Cause	Feature	Further investigation
Oesophageal/gall bladder/ peptic ulcer	Associated with dyspepsia, waterbrash, related to food, not related to exertion, relieved by antacids	Endoscopy Ultrasound of gall bladder
Lung disease/pulmonary embolism	Pain is pleuritic; worse on breathing, coughing and sneezing. May have cough or infected sputum or blood in sputum. There may be a friction rub	Chest X-ray Ventilation/perfusion scan
Other cardiac causes	Dissecting aneurysm – very severe pain, especially in back. Patient hypotensive and may collapse	Chest X-ray CT
	Pericarditis – sharp pain worse on breathing and lying flat – better if upright. Pericardial rub may be heard	Echocardiogram
	Mitral valve prolapse – pain is often vague central chest – comes on after exercise – often present in young women	Echocardiogram
Musculoskeletal	Sharp pain related to position and movement. May be localized to chest wall – perhaps a history of injury – (includes costochondritis – Tietze's syndrome)	Chest X-ray Spine and rib X-rays
Functional	Present in anxious young women and men – no apparent cause is found. May be associated with hyperventilation (Da Costa's syndrome)	Rebreathing from bag if hyperventilation. Otherwise diagnose by exclusion

5.64 Major causes of non IHD chest pain.

5.65   5.66   5.67   5.68

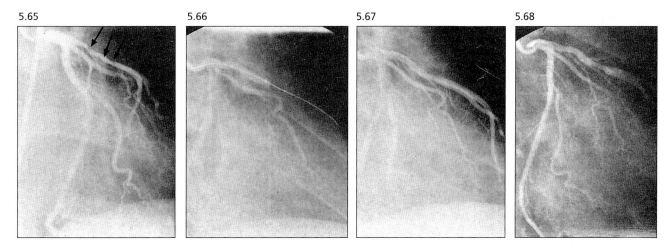

5.65–5.68 Percutaneous transluminal coronary angioplasty of a left anterior descending coronary stricture: **5.65** is the pre-angioplasty coronary arteriogram – a long stricture is arrowed; **5.66** shows the balloon of the angioplasty catheter inflated *in situ* across the stricture; **5.67** shows the coronary arteriogram taken immediately after the angioplasty catheter had been removed. The stricture has been successfully dilated; **5.68** shows the appearance 1 month after angioplasty. There is a slight residual narrowing, which is a normal finding at this stage and does not indicate re-stenosis. The patient's angina was dramatically improved by the manoeuvre.

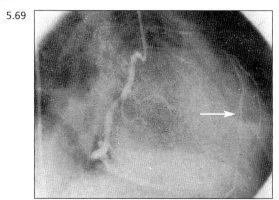

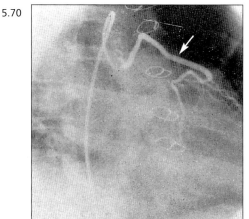

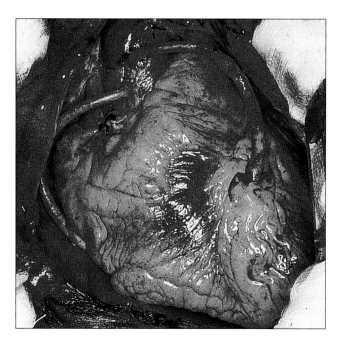

5.71   Coronary artery surgery. Bypass grafts to the right and left anterior descending coronary arteries are in position, and the anastomoses are checked for leaks immediately before closing the chest.

5.69 & 5.70   Coronary angiogram before and after saphenous vein grafting in a patient with angina. **5.69** shows the appearance before surgery. There is a significant stenosis in the right coronary artery, but this fills by the normal route. By contrast, the left anterior descending artery (arrowed) fills only by collaterals. The origin of the artery is completely obstructed. **5.70** shows the appearance after surgery. The saphenous vein graft is arrowed, and it fills the left anterior descending artery. The patient's angina was relieved.

pain within 6 months and need repeated angioplasty or coronary artery surgery. An arterial stent implant may keep the vessel patent for a much longer period.

In coronary artery surgery, the patient's own saphenous vein or internal mammary artery is used to bypass the blocked segment (**5.69–5.71**). The operation carries a mortality rate of 1–2%. After surgery, almost all patients are free of angina for several years and their life expectancy may also be improved.

UNSTABLE ANGINA

Unstable angina is identified when the typical anginal pain becomes more severe and more frequent, comes on with less exertion or occurs at rest, and is not relieved by glyceryl trinitrate. ST-segment changes are present on the ECG. Such patients should be admitted to hospital for adequate analgesia,

intravenous infusions of nitrate, intravenous heparin and aspirin. Many patients settle with this but some require immediate bypass surgery.

MYOCARDIAL INFARCTION (MI)

Myocardial infarction (MI) usually results from the occlusion of one or more coronary arteries by atheroma and subsequent thrombus. It presents with severe central chest pain, having the same site and character as the pain of angina pectoris but usually lasting for more than 30 minutes. Pallor, anxiety, sweating and vomiting are usually present. Occasionally, myocardial infarction occurs without any pain.

Acute ischaemia often provokes changes of rhythm. Ventricular fibrillation (**5.44**, **5.45**) is the most important, as it rapidly leads to death from circulatory arrest. Immediate cardiopulmonary resuscitation is required (**5.72–5.78**). More rarely, cardiac arrest is due to asystole or there is electromechanical dissociation, in which there is circulatory arrest despite continued coordinated electrical activity in the heart. The details of recommended drug and DC shock therapy differ in these groups. Acute myocardial infarction produces distinctive ECG patterns. The appearances depend upon the site and the time from the onset of the infarct. Within a few minutes, the T waves become tall, pointed and upright and ST-segment elevation follows rapidly. Within a few hours the T waves invert. With full thickness infarcts, the R-wave voltage

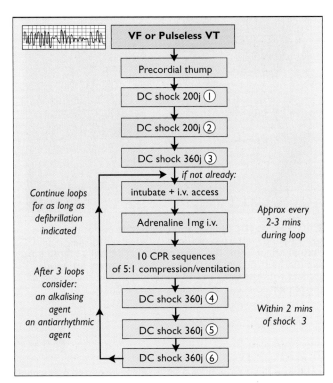

```
┌─────────────────────────────┐
│      VF or Pulseless VT      │
└─────────────────────────────┘
              ↓
┌─────────────────────────────┐
│      Precordial thump        │
└─────────────────────────────┘
              ↓
┌─────────────────────────────┐
│      DC shock 200j  ①        │
└─────────────────────────────┘
              ↓
┌─────────────────────────────┐
│      DC shock 200j  ②        │
└─────────────────────────────┘
              ↓
┌─────────────────────────────┐
│      DC shock 360j  ③        │
└─────────────────────────────┘
              ↓
        if not already:
┌─────────────────────────────┐
│    intubate + i.v. access    │
└─────────────────────────────┘
              ↓
┌─────────────────────────────┐
│     Adrenaline 1mg i.v.      │
└─────────────────────────────┘
              ↓
┌─────────────────────────────┐
│     10 CPR sequences         │
│  of 5:1 compression/ventilation │
└─────────────────────────────┘
              ↓
┌─────────────────────────────┐
│      DC shock 360j  ④        │
└─────────────────────────────┘
              ↓
┌─────────────────────────────┐
│      DC shock 360j  ⑤        │
└─────────────────────────────┘
              ↓
┌─────────────────────────────┐
│      DC shock 360j  ⑥        │
└─────────────────────────────┘
```

Continue loops for as long as defibrillation indicated

After 3 loops consider:
an alkalising agent
an antiarrhythmic agent

Approx every 2-3 mins during loop

Within 2 mins of shock 3

5.72   European Resuscitation Council recommendations for the management of ventricular fibrillation. Often preceded by rapid ventricular tachycardia, ventricular fibrillation is the most common cause of reversible cardiac arrest. The key to its successful management is defibrillation as soon as possible. In ventricular fibrillation, basic life support should cause no delay to the administration of the first three shocks, though a precordial thump is rapid and may sometimes be helpful. For refractory ventricular fibrillation adrenaline (epinephrine) is the drug of first choice. Antiarrhythmic and alkalizing agents may be valuable, but should be used much later in treatment than was recommended in earlier protocols.

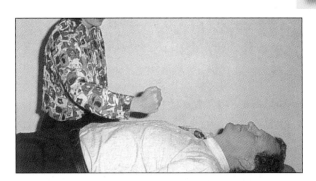

5.74   A firm blow to the sternum may sometimes restart the heart, especially when an arrest has been witnessed.

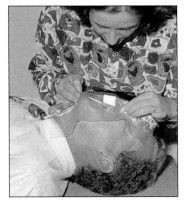

5.75   Artificial respiration should be started using the mouth-to-mouth technique. The nose is occluded with the thumb and index finger, and the movement of the chest provides an index of the efficacy of ventilation. In this case protection for the operator is provided by a simple plastic sheet with a small mesh-covered vent at the mouth (Laerdal).

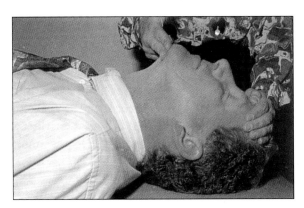

5.73   The cardiac arrest patient should be placed flat on a hard surface. His head and neck should be extended by lifting the chin with one hand and pressing the forehead with another. The airway may be cleared digitally or with suction if available at this time.

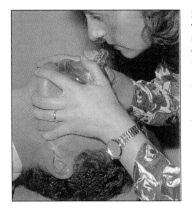

5.76   A more efficient way to avoid mouth-to-mouth contact and to ensure adequate respiration is with a Laerdal mask. These should be available in all hospital wards and carried by all members of the resuscitation team. Supplemental oxygen may be added to the inlet port.

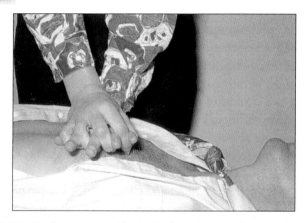

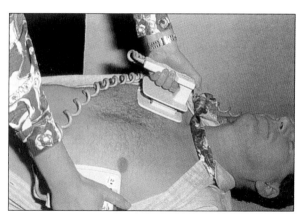

5.77 Cardiac massage. The heel of one hand is placed on the lower third of the sternum and the other hand is rested on top of the first with the arms straight. Using a sharp jerky movement, 60–90 strokes per minute are administered, aiming to move the sternum 3–4 cm at each stroke. After each stroke it is important to lift the hands quickly to allow the chest to expand and the heart to fill. An assistant should set up an intravenous line for drug administration, and the patient's ECG should be monitored as soon as possible.

5.78 External DC defibrillation should be performed if the heart has not restarted or the ECG shows ventricular fibrillation, or both. The electrodes must be well separated to avoid a short circuit, electrolyte jelly is necessary for good contact with the skin, and all personnel should stand clear of the patient to avoid receiving an electric shock.

diminishes and pathological Q waves develop (**5.79**). The ST segment usually returns to normal within a few days. The T wave usually becomes upright within a few weeks, but the pathological Q waves persist as a marker of previous infarction.

The diagnosis of recent infarction can be confirmed by detecting regulatory proteins and enzymes released from the damaged heart muscle into the blood, especially troponin T, I and C and creatine kinase (CK) and its isoenzyme (CK-MB) (**5.80**).

Myocardial infarction should usually be managed in hospital, but treatment can begin before admission. Oxygen should be administered and pain relief by morphine or diamorphine is usually necessary. Aspirin should be given immediately, and when the diagnosis has been confirmed by an ECG, a thrombolytic agent should be considered if there are no contraindications (**5.81**). This may be done *en route* to hospital by trained staff if a defibrillator is available. Thrombolysis dissolves the thrombus responsible for the occlusion in the

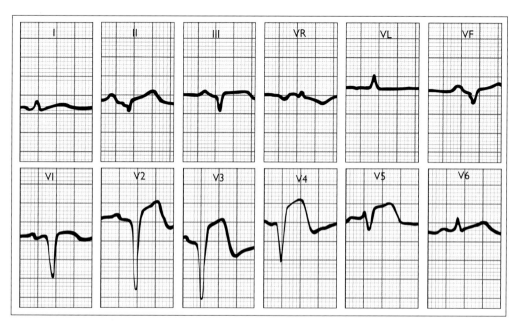

5.79 Acute anterior myocardial infarction extending inferiorly – 3 hours after onset. The changes are those of acute full-thickness infarction, with widespread ST-segment and T-wave changes and Q waves in V1–V4.

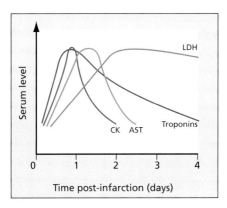

5.80 The pattern of serum markers after acute myocardial infarction. The troponins are detectable within 2–4 hours of myocardial infarction and are very specific for cardiac injury. Creatine kinase (CK), which is muscle specific, also rises rapidly and earlier than detectable changes in aspartate aminotransferase (AST) or lactate dehydrogenase (LDH). CK also rises in response to exertion or skeletal muscle injury, for example after an injection or a fall. A more specific marker is the isoenzyme CK-MB, which is expressed as a percentage of the total CK – normally this is less than 5% of the total. Peak levels are usually recorded at 10±2 hours after onset of pain. Other serum markers include myoglobin. The only justification for using AST or LDH is if the patient presents late and the peak of CK (or CK-MB) has been missed and if troponin measurements are not available.

coronary artery, improves blood flow to the myocardium, limits left ventricular dysfunction and improves the prognosis (**5.82, 5.83**). Aspirin and heparin may prevent the diseased vessel reoccluding after successful thrombolysis. Further treatment may be needed for arrhythmias.

Other complications of acute myocardial infarction

Cardiac failure and shock
Mild left ventricular failure is a common sequel to acute infarction and the only apparent features are bilateral basal

CONTRAINDICATIONS TO THROMBOLYSIS

Recent bleeding from any site
Recent surgery or childbirth
Active duodenal or gastric ulcer or recent gastrointestinal biopsy
Recent stroke (6 months)
Recent head injury
Severe uncontrolled hypertension
Renal or hepatic failure

5.81 Contraindications to thrombolysis.

crepitations that respond rapidly to diuretic therapy. More severe heart failure carries a poor prognosis and cardiogenic shock has a mortality of over 90% despite therapy (*see also* **p. 206**).

Cardiac rupture
Cardiac rupture is an uncommon feature after infarction and usually occurs about 7–10 days later as the muscle necroses. It may vary from papillary-muscle rupture, producing acute mitral regurgitation, to septal rupture with an acute left-to-right shunt (**5.84**) or, most severely, to rupture of the left ventricular wall producing acute cardiac tamponade (and rapid death).

Left ventricular thrombosis
Anterior myocardial infarction is associated with an incidence of about 30% of mural thrombus formation. This may be detected by ultrasound (**5.85**) or ventriculography. Surprisingly, only about 5% of these thrombi throw off clinically significant emboli to the brain, kidneys, mesentery or limbs. Heparin and warfarin should be given to prevent this complication.

5.82

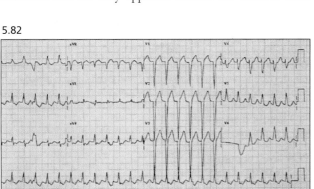

5.83

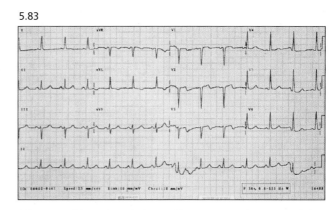

5.82 & 5.83 ECGs before and 12 hours after thrombolytic therapy with streptokinase in a patient with acute anterior myocardial infarction. **5.82** shows widespread anterior lead ST-segment and T-wave changes, with deep Q waves in V1–2. The heart rate is rapid and extrasystoles are seen. These changes are largely reversed 12 hours after streptokinase (**5.83**). Only the residual ST-segment and T-wave changes point to the diagnosis.

RESULTS OF SWAN–GANZ CATHETERIZATION	
Sample from	Oxygen saturation (%)
Superior vena cava	40
Right atrium	42
Right ventricle	84
Pulmonary artery	80
Radial artery	96

5.84   Results of Swan–Ganz catheterization, demonstrating a left-to-right shunt in a patient with ventricular septal rupture after myocardial infarction.

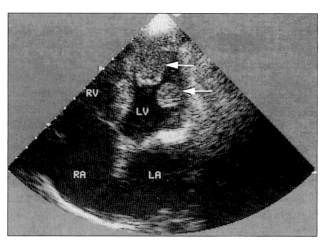

5.85   Left ventricular thrombus after myocardial infarction. The diastolic apical four-chamber view shows at least two large thrombi on the apical and anterior walls of the left ventricle (arrowed). Left ventricular thrombosis is common after myocardial infarction, and its incidence, and the risk of embolism, can be dramatically reduced by heparin therapy.

Deep vein thrombosis

Immobility associated with tissue breakdown and cardiac failure produces an incidence of venous thrombosis of 1–2% (*see* **p. 250**), and a small number of these thrombi embolize to the lung (*see* **p. 252**). These complications may be prevented by low-dose heparin therapy, which should be routinely used after myocardial infarction.

Shoulder–hand syndrome

The cause of shoulder–hand syndrome is unknown, but stiffness of the shoulder and upper arm joints may follow an infarct. Physiotherapy and non-steroidal anti-inflammatory drugs are useful in treatment.

Post-myocardial infarction syndrome (Dressler's syndrome)

Post-myocardial infarction syndrome (Dressler's syndrome) is an autoimmune response to acute myocardial infarction in which autoantibodies are formed and produce a febrile illness with pericarditis and effusion about 10–14 days after the acute episode. Treatment is with non-steroidal anti-inflammatory agents, or sometimes with a course of systemic steroid therapy.

Left ventricular aneurysm

Death of myocardial fibres and replacement by fibrous tissue may result in a severely weakened left ventricular wall that becomes aneurysmal. This produces persistent ST–T changes on the ECG (**5.86**) and a typical appearance on chest X-ray (**5.87**).

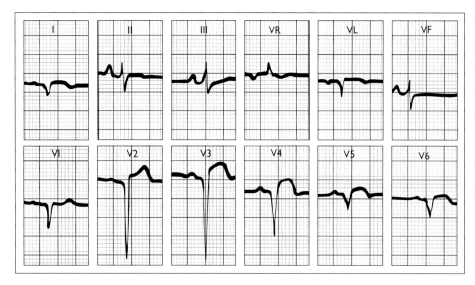

5.86   Left ventricular aneurysm produces a persistence of the pattern of acute myocardial infarction in the ECG. In uncomplicated myocardial infarction, the ST segment has normally returned to the isoelectric line within 3–6 weeks; persistence of ST elevation beyond this time is a pointer to possible aneurysm. This ECG was taken 10 weeks after infarction in a patient who had signs of heart failure. The QRS complexes in all precordial leads show that the patient had an extensive full-thickness infarct.

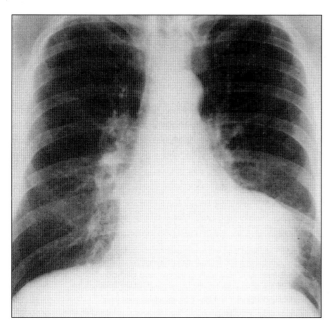

5.87 **Ventricular aneurysm,** revealed on chest X-ray 3 months after myocardial infarction. Note the bulge in the left cardiac border. On screening, this would be found to move paradoxically outwards during systole.

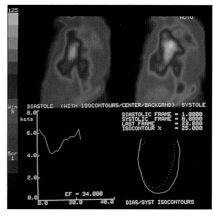

5.88 **Technetium blood pool study** in a patient with poor left ventricular function after myocardial infarction. Typical diastolic and systolic frames are shown top left and top right, and the contours of the left ventricle are displayed graphically at bottom right. The area of the blood pool at each of 16 frames of the cardiac cycle is plotted bottom left and allows the calculation of the left ventricular ejection fraction, which is very low at 34%. The left ventricular wall movement is best seen kinetically. It was poor at the interventricular septum and there was early aneurysmal dilatation at the apex.

Isotope scans (**5.88**), ultrasound or ventriculography show part of the left ventricle to be non-contractile. Some of these aneurysms can be surgically resected.

Population screening and primary prevention of ischaemic heart disease

Risk factors for IHD can be identified by mass screening projects or by the initiative of individual family or workplace doctors. The cost and logistic implications are massive and most schemes now focus on people who have a high risk, that is those with a family history of premature arterial disease in near relatives, cigarette smokers, hypertensives, diabetics and those with peripheral or cerebral artery disease.

Lifestyle changes must be emphasized, especially stopping smoking, alteration of diet to reduce the amount of saturated fat, an increase in the amount of dietary monounsaturates, fibre and fresh fruit and vegetables. Increased exercise and weight reduction are also beneficial. Drugs to control hypertension and reduce high lipid levels have a proven place in primary prevention of IHD.

Rehabilitation and secondary prevention of ischaemic heart disease

After a few days to stabilize in hospital, most patients with myocardial infarction are fit to return home, but they should be offered a rehabilitation programme of graduated exercise and lifestyle advice. Regular low-dose aspirin and other antiplatelet drugs, beta-blocker and ACE inhibitor therapy may lessen the chances of subsequent infarction. It is usually possible to identify individuals with a poor prognosis after myocardial infarction by exercise ECG, nuclear exercise tests, echo-cardiography and coronary angiography. When appropriate, coronary artery surgery may improve their prognosis.

All patients with proven coronary disease must be given appropriate lifestyle advice, as for the primary prevention of IHD, and hypertension and hyperlipidaemia should be identified and treated. There is evidence that these measures may lead to reduction in size (regression) of occluding atheromatous plaques and to an improved prognosis, especially when effective lipid-lowering agents ('statin' drugs) are included in therapy.

RHEUMATIC FEVER

Rheumatic fever is an acute inflammatory disease of connective tissue that is a sequel to infection with Group A streptococci (*see* **p. 25**) and may involve the heart, skin, CNS and joints. It is now a rare disease in the developed world but is still endemic elsewhere; even in the West there is still a large residue of patients with rheumatic valve disease that resulted from childhood infection.

The cardinal skin signs are erythema marginatum (**5.89**) and subcutaneous nodules, which are firm, painless and discrete,

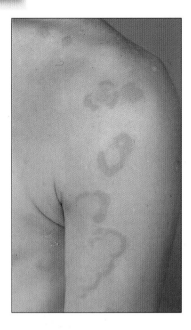

5.89 Erythema marginatum is a characteristic skin rash which may follow any streptococcal infection, especially tonsillitis. It is one of the common signs of acute rheumatic fever, and its presence should raise the possibility of cardiac involvement. The rash is similar to that seen in Lyme disease (**1.122**).

As an aid to the clinical diagnosis and more accurate classification of rheumatic fever, a range of diagnostic criteria (the Jones criteria) may be used (**5.90**).

The differential diagnosis of rheumatic fever includes juvenile rheumatoid arthritis, mixed connective tissue disease, systemic lupus erythematosus and Lyme disease.

Treatment should be directed towards the elimination of any residual streptococcal infection with penicillin. Aspirin is an effective anti-inflammatory and antipyretic agent for the other features. Prevention of recurrence may be necessary with long-term oral penicillin.

The damage resulting from rheumatic fever may require long-term treatment.

about 0.5–1 cm in diameter, and are found mainly over bony prominences and tendons. They resolve after a few weeks.

The arthritis varies from arthralgia to a flitting polyarthritis, mainly affecting the larger joints such as the knees, ankles, wrists and elbows. These joints may become acutely swollen, hot and tender, and the synovial fluid is full of polymorphs.

Carditis is the most important aspect of this disease as it has major long-term implications. Endocarditis, myocarditis and pericarditis are all often present. The diagnosis of carditis requires the finding of:

- new cardiac murmurs
- cardiomegaly
- pericarditis
- congestive cardiac failure.

The murmurs may include an apical systolic murmur (caused by mitral regurgitation), a transient apical mid-diastolic (Carey Coombs) murmur (caused by turbulent flow across the inflamed mitral valve), and a basal diastolic murmur (caused by aortic regurgitation). Other cardiac signs may include tachycardia, pericardial friction rub, muffled heart sounds resulting from pericardial effusion and evidence of heart failure.

Neurological involvement (Sydenham's chorea) is uncommon and develops after a latent period of several weeks. The patient develops rapid purposeless involuntary movements mostly in the limbs and face (*see* **p. 482**).

Investigations should include throat-swab culture and the measurement of antibody response to *Streptococcus* (anti-streptolysin 'O' titre). There is usually a leucocytosis and elevation of the ESR and C-reactive protein levels. X-ray of the chest may show a pericardial effusion and rarely pneumonia or lobar collapse. ECG often shows first degree heartblock (**5.49**, **5.50**).

CRITERIA FOR THE DIAGNOSIS OF RHEUMATIC FEVER (JONES CRITERIA)	
Major findings	**Minor findings**
Carditis	Arthralgia
Polyarthritis	Past history of rheumatic fever or rheumatic heart disease
Sydenham's chorea	
Erythema marginatum	
Fever	
plus *recent evidence of streptococcal infection i.e. ASO titre, antibodies, culture from throat or recent scarlet fever*	

5.90 Criteria for the diagnosis of rheumatic fever (Jones criteria). The definitive diagnosis requires two major findings or one major and two minor findings plus evidence of recent infection.

ACQUIRED VALVE DISEASES

The most common forms of heart valve disease affect the mitral and aortic valves, causing left heart failure and pulmonary congestion. The valves may fail to open fully (stenosis) or to close (regurgitation or incompetence). Both stenosis and regurgitation can coexist. The effects of both types of lesion are haemodynamic with major implications for cardiac function.

The presence of heart valve disease is suspected from a heart murmur. An ECG and chest X-ray may provide additional clues, but the main diagnostic technique for valve disease is echocardiography. Doppler echocardiography is particularly useful in establishing the severity of valvular stenosis or regurgitation. The diagnosis in adults is usually confirmed by cardiac catheterization and angiography, which also permits evaluation of the coronary arteries.

MITRAL STENOSIS

The most common cause of mitral stenosis is rheumatic fever, and mitral stenosis occurs in about one-half of all patients with chronic rheumatic heart disease. The mitral valve usually narrows slowly and the pulmonary vasculature adapts to the rising pressure of blood within the pulmonary capillaries, pulmonary veins and the left atrium. Symptoms develop when the valve area is reduced to 1 cm² or less.

The walls of the pulmonary vessels thicken, reducing blood flow and cardiac output but protecting the patient from pulmonary oedema. Patients notice only a gradual decline in exercise tolerance, although they may be aware of a brisk deterioration if their heart rhythm changes from sinus rhythm to atrial fibrillation. Episodes of acute pulmonary oedema occur as the cross-sectional area of the valve diminishes and the patient may have episodes of acute dyspnoea, orthopnoea and paroxysmal nocturnal dyspnoea. As the pulmonary blood pressure rises there are episodes of haemoptysis. Systemic embolism is common from thrombi in the large left atrium, especially in the presence of atrial fibrillation. The common sites for embolism are cerebral (*see* **p. 473**), mesenteric, renal and limb arteries (**5.91**).

Two-thirds of the patients are female. They may have a malar flush or central cyanosis; there may be signs of weight loss or peripheral oedema. Jugular venous pulsation becomes obvious only when right heart failure appears. The key cardiac findings are a tapping apex beat, and a rumbling mid-diastolic murmur at the apex (**5.7**). There may be pre-systolic accentuation and the murmur may be preceded by an opening snap. Exercise and positioning the patient in the left lateral position will accentuate the murmur. As pulmonary hypertension develops, the pulmonary second sound becomes accentuated and a right ventricular heave becomes apparent. Bilateral basal pulmonary crepitations may herald the onset of left heart failure.

Radiography of the chest shows a generally small heart with an accentuation of its left upper border from the enlarged left atrium and often signs of pulmonary oedema (**5.15**). The ECG shows a bifid P wave (P mitrale) (**5.92**) and there may be features of right ventricular hypertrophy and atrial fibrillation (**5.35**, **5.36**). The diagnosis should be confirmed by echocardiography, which will show the immobility of the mitral valve cusps (**5.16**, **5.17**, **5.93**), and may show atrial thrombus (**5.94**). Cardiac catheterization is usual if surgery is contemplated.

221

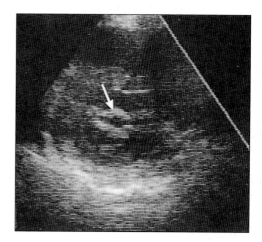

5.93   Echocardiogram (short-axis view) showing tight mitral stenosis. The tight orifice of the mitral valve is arrowed.

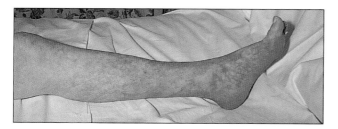

5.91   Arterial embolism causing acute ischaemia of the leg in a patient with mitral stenosis. The patient was in atrial fibrillation, and the source of the embolus was the left atrium (*see* **5.94**). Initial pallor of the leg and foot is followed by cyanosis, and by reactive hyperaemia if a collateral circulation opens up.

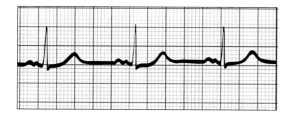

5.92   P mitrale. The P wave is bifid and has a duration of 0.12 seconds or more. The appearance results from delayed activation of the enlarged left atrium; the first peak represents right atrial, and the second left atrial activation.

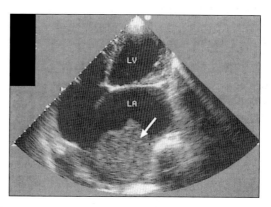

5.94   Echocardiogram (parasternal short-axis view) in a patient with rheumatic mitral stenosis, showing a very large thrombus attached to the walls of the left atrium (arrow). The patient presented with a stroke (*see* **p. 473**) and was found to have atrial fibrillation and a diastolic murmur. Anticoagulation is required to prevent further emboli.

Treatment includes diuretics for heart failure and digoxin for atrial fibrillation. Warfarin reduces the chances of thrombosis in the left atrium and of embolism. In severe cases, the fused cusps may be separated by balloon inflation or surgical valvotomy, or the valve can be replaced (**1.5**).

MITRAL REGURGITATION

There are many causes of mitral regurgitation (*see* **5.95**). The result of mitral regurgitation is dilatation of the left atrium and ventricle. Eventually this leads to pulmonary hypertension and oedema. The same picture may develop acutely with rupture of the chordae tendineae. Infective endocarditis may also occur.

Symptoms may appear only after some time has elapsed; they are usually dyspnoea on exertion (later at rest) and palpitations. With the onset of pulmonary hypertension, there may be symptoms from right heart failure.

Signs are dominated by left ventricular dilatation, with the heaving apex beat displaced to the left, a systolic thrill at the apex and a high-pitched pansystolic murmur at the apex, transmitted to the left axilla (**5.7**). Later in the disease, there may be a right ventricular heave associated with accentuation of the pulmonary second sound. The diagnosis is confirmed as follows:

- chest X-ray shows enlargement of left ventricle and atrium and sometimes calcification of the mitral valve
- ECG shows left ventricular hypertrophy (**5.147**), and often atrial fibrillation (**5.35**, **5.36**)
- echocardiography shows the position of the valve leaflets at closure (**5.96**), and colour-flow Doppler shows the regurgitant jet (**5.19**, **5.99**)
- cardiac catheterization can define the pressure differences between chambers, and ventriculography will confirm the presence of regurgitation
- coronary angiography should be performed in older patients to assess the extent of underlying IHD.

Medical treatment includes prevention of endocarditis, control of heart failure, and anticoagulation to prevent thromboembolism.

Poor prognostic factors include:

- poor left ventricular function
- age over 70 years
- New York Heart Association functional grade IV
- myocardial ischaemia
- necessity for emergency surgery.

A severely damaged valve will need surgical replacement with a mechanical valve or bioprosthesis. Rarely, the existing valve can be repaired.

MITRAL VALVE PROLAPSE

Mitral valve prolapse (floppy mitral valve, Barlow's syndrome) is the second most common valvular disorder after aortic stenosis. It is usually asymptomatic and benign and is often detected clinically at routine medicals or on routine echocardiography. The reported prevalence in women is in the range of 4–17% and in men 2–12%. The range is wide because of differing levels of awareness and the variable availability of routine echocardiography, by which the diagnosis is confirmed. During systole, especially late systole, the valve leaflets prolapse back into the left atrium (**5.18**, **5.96**).

When symptoms are present they tend to be non-specific and include vague chest pain, palpitations, syncope and effort intolerance due to breathlessness and general tiredness. The presence of these vague symptoms with valve prolapse is now

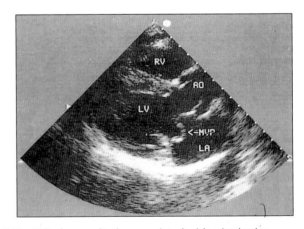

5.96 Mitral regurgitation associated with mitral valve prolapse, seen on two-dimensional echocardiography (parasternal long-axis view) in systole. Note the open cusps of the aortic valve. The posterior leaflet of the mitral valve is prolapsing backwards into the left atrium in systole (MVP). This abnormality is fairly common in young women for no obvious cause. It may also be a feature of Marfan's syndrome (**p. 150**) and other connective tissue disorders (LA = left atrium; LV = left ventricle; Ao = aorta; RV = right ventricle).

CAUSES OF MITRAL REGURGITATION

Rheumatic fever in acute phase

Post-rheumatic fever (with mitral stenosis)

Mitral valve prolapse

Ischaemic heart disease (papillary muscle dysfunction)

Infective endocarditis

Connective tissue disorders (especially systemic lupus erythematosus)

Ruptured chordae tendinae

Myxomatous degeneration

5.95 Causes of mitral regurgitation.

known as the mitral valve prolapse syndrome. The character of the pain varies greatly, ranging from an angina-like pain (in quality, duration and site) to a mild left mammary discomfort. In such patients other causes for chest pain often coexist, for example spasm of the oesophagus, peptic ulcer, chest wall pain or coronary artery disease.

Palpitations are reported by about one-half of the patients. This may sometimes be a reflection of heightened awareness in patients in whom the diagnosis has been made. Ambulatory monitoring of the ECG shows a poor correlation between reported symptoms and recorded arrythmias. Syncope commonly occurs with no change of rhythm.

It has been suggested that mitral valve prolapse may be part of a neuroendocrinopathy in which there is dysautonomia with exaggerated heart rate and blood pressure responses, postural hypotension, hyperresponsiveness to catecholamines, decreased intravascular and intraventricular volume on standing and activation of atrial natriuretic peptide. It may also be associated with hypermobility syndromes (*see* **p. 150**).

Most often a minor degree of mitral prolapse does not interfere in any way with a normal lifestyle. The usual course is benign, but complications may include mitral regurgitation and heart failure, stroke caused by emboli from atrial thrombus, infective endocarditis and ventricular tachyarrythmias.

Sudden death is rare in mitral valve prolapse and is usually due to sustained ventricular tachycardia or ventricular fibrillation. Patients who survive an arrest are candidates for an implantable defibrillator (**5.60, 5.61**).

AORTIC STENOSIS

Acquired aortic valve stenosis often results from progressive degeneration and calcification of a congenitally bicuspid valve. Rheumatic fever and arteriosclerotic degeneration are rarer causes. Aortic stenosis leads to left ventricular hypertrophy and relative left ventricular ischaemia. When the valve area is reduced to 1 cm² or less, the patient may present with angina, infarction, left ventricular failure or arrhythmias. Ventricular fibrillation is a common cause of sudden death. Calcification around the valve may extend into the conducting tissue, causing heart block and syncope.

The dominant clinical features of aortic stenosis are a low-volume, slow-rising pulse; a forceful apex beat; a systolic thrill at the base of the heart; and a mid-systolic murmur at the aortic area, which radiates to the neck (**5.7**).

The diagnosis is supported by features of left ventricular hypertrophy on ECG (**5.147**) and left ventricular dilatation on chest X-ray (**5.97**). Echocardiography confirms the diagnosis by showing thickened and calcified valve cusps (**5.98**). Doppler echocardiography (**5.99**) or cardiac catheterization (**5.23**), or both, establishes the severity of the stenosis, and Doppler echocardiography is extremely valuable in following the course of the disease in individual patients. Ultrasound has removed the need for repeated cardiac catheterization. The peak aortic

pressure gradient can be calculated, and it correlates well with the degree of severity of stenosis. Patients with a valve gradient of 50 mmHg or more should be considered for valve surgery.

The valve is usually replaced with a mechanical or biological prosthetic valve. There is an 85% 5-year survival rate following operation.

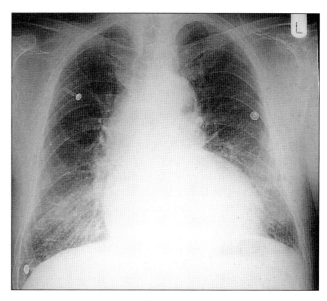

5.97 Chest X-ray (AP view) in a patient admitted with cardiac failure associated with aortic stenosis. There is gross cardiomegaly, with left ventricular dilatation and a bilateral symmetrical increase in bronchovascular markings, especially in the lower zones. Bilateral Kerley B lines are seen, which are consistent with pulmonary oedema.

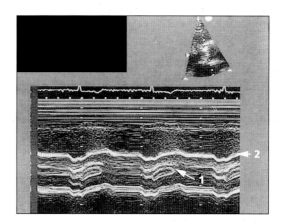

5.98 Aortic stenosis with calcification. This M-mode parasternal long-axis view shows the characteristic box shape of valve opening during systole (1). Calcification of the valve and annulus is suggested by the density of whiteness of the tracing (2).

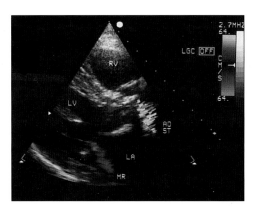

5.99 Colour flow Doppler mapping in aortic stenosis. The typical jet flow through the stenotic aortic valve is seen (AO ST), and there is also a minor degree of mitral regurgitation (MR) (RV = right ventricle; LV = left ventricle; LA = left atrium).

AORTIC REGURGITATION

Aortic regurgitation occurs if the aortic valve ring dilates, as a result of dissecting aneurysm, ankylosing spondylitis or syphilis for example, or if the valve cusps degenerate, such as after rheumatic fever or endocarditis. Aortic regurgitation leads to dilatation and hypertrophy of the left ventricle and ultimately left ventricular failure. Clinical symptoms often occur late and the patient may present with significant heart failure or angina. There may have been a preceding history of palpitations, syncope or headaches because of the high systolic blood pressure, especially during exercise.

Many of the physical signs are a reflection of the size of the leak, for example collapsing pulse, capillary pulsation, visible carotid pulsation, head bobbing and the Duroziez's murmur heard over the femoral artery. On examination, there is left ventricular hypertrophy, with the apex beat displaced to the left and an early diastolic murmur down the left side of the sternum, which is best heard by sitting the patient upright and leaning forward in full expiration. A diastolic thrill is rarely felt down the left sternal edge.

Chest X-ray (**5.100**), ECG (**5.147**) and echocardiogram show left ventricular enlargement. Aortography or colour-flow Doppler (**5.101**) shows the regurgitant jet.

Medical treatment is directed at managing the angina, correcting the failure and preventing endocarditis. Definitive treatment consists of replacing the valve with a prosthetic one.

TRICUSPID AND PULMONARY VALVE DISEASE

The tricuspid and pulmonary valves are rarely stenosed by rheumatic fever and they may be slightly incompetent in healthy individuals. Severe pulmonary regurgitation is usually secondary to left heart failure or lung disease, through the effects of a raised pulmonary arterial pressure, which causes dilatation of the pulmonary artery and stretching of the pulmonary valve annulus. The resultant murmur of pulmonary regurgitation has the same early diastolic characteristics as the murmur of aortic regurgitation, but the characteristic findings in the arterial pulse are absent.

Tricuspid regurgitation usually follows dilatation of the right ventricle. Once it develops, signs of right heart failure become

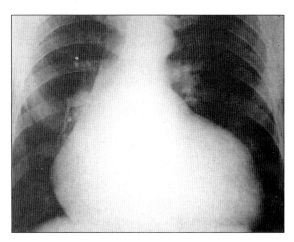

5.100 Left ventricular hypertrophy and dilatation in a patient with severe aortic regurgitation. Left ventricular hypertrophy alters the shape of the heart, making the left heart border more convex than normal, but hypertrophy alone does not increase the size of the heart. The cardiac enlargement seen here is indicative of ventricular dilatation.

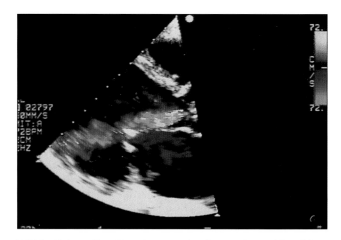

5.101 Colour–flow Doppler mapping in a patient with mild aortic regurgitation (parasternal long-axis view). The aortic regurgitant jet (in blue) is directed posteriorly at an acute angle from the aortic valve (to the right in the picture), back into the left ventricle (to the left in the picture), impinging directly on the anterior mitral valve leaflet (in the centre of the picture) immediately below the blue jet.

prominent, for example distended jugular veins, enlarged liver, ascites and oedema. A pansystolic murmur may be audible at the lower left sternal border (**5.7**). Chest X-ray may show right atrial enlargement (**5.102**). Echocardiography is the most effective method of diagnosing pulmonary and tricuspid valve disease (**5.19**).

calcifies. With advances in surgical and medical care, many patients with congenital heart disease now live into adult life.

Congenital lesions may result from a variety of maternal and fetal factors, including maternal alcohol or drug abuse, maternal rubella (diminishing in importance in the developed world), and occasionally single gene mutations. A range of syndromes, that include cardiac abnormalities, are described elsewhere, for example Down's syndrome (**p. 336**), Turner's syndrome (**p. 306***), Ehlers–Danlos syndrome (**p. 133**), Friedreich's ataxia (**p. 485**) and Noonan's syndrome (**p. 306**). Congenital cardiac lesions may also be associated with other, less well defined anomalies (**5.103**).

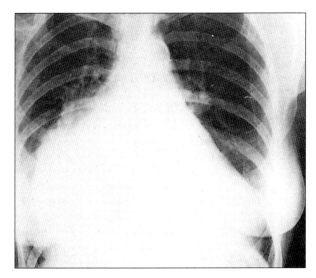

5.102 Chest X-ray in a patient with tricuspid regurgitation. The enlargement of the right heart shadow is caused by a grossly enlarged right atrium. Note also the calcified aortic arch (and the incidental bilateral hilar calcification, resulting from old tuberculosis). This woman's tricuspid regurgitation resulted from ischaemic heart disease.

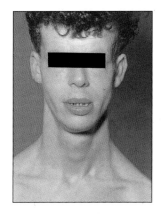

5.103 Congenital heart disease may be associated with many other congenital anomalies. This young man with congenital aortic stenosis also had a webbed neck, a small face, with a hypoplastic mandible, low-set ears and a range of other musculoskeletal abnormalities (not part of any named syndrome). Note also the presence of dental caries – a risk factor for infective endocarditis and brain abscess. Antibiotic prophylaxis should be given before dental treatment commences.

Obstruction to right ventricular outflow may occur above, below or at the level of the pulmonary valve. The clinical problems that result from pulmonary stenosis depend on the severity of the obstruction rather than on the actual site. Patients are usually asymptomatic and symptoms appear only if there is progression of the stenosis. These include fatigue, symptoms of right ventricular failure and syncope. The clinical signs are those of right ventricular hypertrophy (a right ventricular heave) and a loud systolic murmur in the second left intercostal space, with a preceding click if valvular stenosis is responsible. Chest X-ray may show right ventricular enlargement or post-stenotic dilatation. Pulmonary stenosis can be diagnosed by echocardiography and its severity assessed by Doppler. Pulmonary valvuloplasty (usually by balloon catheter) corrects valvular stenosis.

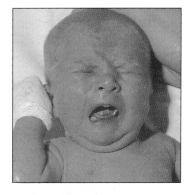

5.104 Congenital heart disease commonly presents with cyanosis at or soon after birth (a 'blue baby'). Urgent assessment and consideration for cardiac surgery is necessary, and feeding is often particularly difficult in these neonates. This baby had transposition of the great arteries (**p. 230**).

CONGENITAL HEART DISEASE

Congenital heart disease is found in 8 per 1000 live births. Congenital bicuspid aortic valve is much more common (2% of live births) but usually only becomes a problem when it

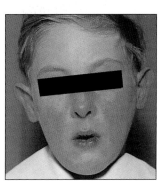

5.105 Severe central cyanosis in a boy with Fallot's tetralogy, photographed just before surgical correction. Fallot's tetralogy is the most common cause of cyanotic congenital heart disease in patients over the age of 1 year.

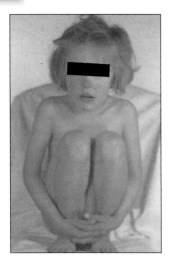

5.106 Squatting is a common feature in children with cyanotic congenital heart disease, especially Fallot's tetralogy. The child usually squats after exercise, apparently to relieve breathlessness. The mechanism by which squatting achieves symptomatic relief is not clear, but it may involve an increase in systemic vascular resistance that decreases the right-to-left shunt, a pooling of desaturated blood in the legs or an increase in systemic venous return and pulmonary blood flow.

Patients with congenital heart disease may present at birth (**5.104**), with cyanosis or associated symptoms in childhood (**5.105**, **5.106**, **7.149**), or sometimes in adult life. They commonly have finger clubbing.

The most common congenital cardiac anomalies are listed in **5.107**. Congenital cardiac anomalies may be divided into two main types:

- communications between cardiac chambers or blood vessels
- lesions that obstruct blood flow.

Combinations of both types of anomaly may occur, as in Fallot's tetralogy and other complex congenital conditions.

Communications between the left and right sides of the heart cause blood to flow from the high-pressure left side to the low-pressure right side. This happens when an atrial septal defect or ventricular septal defect is present, or if there is a patent ductus arteriosus causing blood to flow from the aorta to the pulmonary artery. Pulmonary blood flow increases and, in extreme cases, the pulmonary capillaries and arterioles may respond by thickening their walls and narrowing their lumens. This increases the work of the right ventricle, which must raise its systolic pressure to maintain normal cardiac output (pulmonary hypertension). The elevated pressure may then reverse the shunt, causing blood to flow from right to left through the abnormal communication, so that unoxygenated blood bypasses the lungs (Eisenmenger syndrome).

ATRIAL SEPTAL DEFECT (ASD)

Atrial septal defects (ASDs) most commonly occur in the middle of the interatrial septum (a secundum defect), although they may occur in the upper part (sinus venosus defect) or lower part (primum defect) where associated abnormalities of the mitral and tricuspid valves make the condition more serious. The history and findings depend on the age at presentation and the severity of the defect or defects. Children with secundum defects seldom experience symptoms, but in adult life, heart failure and cardiac arrhythmias, usually atrial fibrillation, develop, so the defects should often be closed. If presentation is late, the main features are those of right heart failure. There is usually a marked right ventricular impulse and wide fixed splitting of P2, with a systolic pulmonary ejection murmur resulting from increased flow across the normal pulmonary valve. These findings change as pulmonary vascular resistance increases and a right-to-left shunt appears. The X-ray of the chest may show evidence of right ventricular hypertrophy and dilatation, with a prominent pulmonary artery with pulmonary plethora (**5.108**). The ECG shows a characteristic right bundle branch block pattern. Echocardiography confirms right ventricular hypertrophy and dilatation of the pulmonary artery and may define the anatomical site and dimensions of the defect (**5.109**). These findings may be confirmed by cardiac catheterization or by MRI (**5.110**). Treatment is usually surgical, but devices for closure via a catheter are now used in some patients, especially children.

THE MOST COMMON FORMS OF CONGENITAL HEART DISEASE
Bicuspid aortic valve
Ventricular septal defects
Patent ductus arteriosus
Pulmonary stenosis
Coarctation of aorta
Atrial septal defects
Aortic stenosis
Tetralogy of Fallot
Transposition of great arteries

5.107 The most common forms of congenital heart disease (in descending order of frequency).

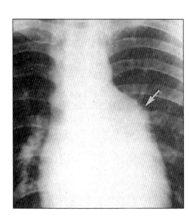

5.108 Atrial septal defect with a large left-to-right shunt. The pulmonary arteries are prominent, especially on the left (arrow).

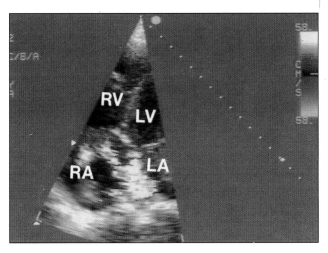

5.109 Atrial septal defect. This colour-flow Doppler apical four-chamber view shows blood flow from the left to the right atrium through a moderate-sized atrial septal defect (LA = left atrium; RA = right atrium; LV = left ventricle; RV = right ventricle).

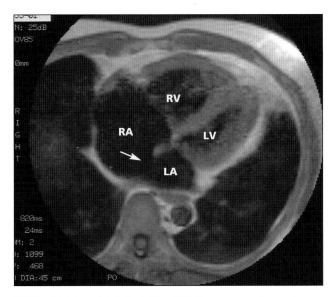

5.110 Atrial septal defect. This MRI (transverse spin echo) shows an ostium secundum atrial septal defect (arrow). The right ventricle and right atrium are dilated; there is a small part of the atrial septum present at the atrioventricular valve plane but the rest of the septum is absent (RA = right atrium; RV = right ventricle; LA = left atrium; LV = left ventricle).

and signs are dependent on the size of the defect, the state of the pulmonary vasculature and the presence of other abnormalities. Most congenital defects are small, cause no symptoms and close spontaneously during childhood. Initially, the greater pressure in the left ventricle is associated with a left-to-right shunt that is present throughout systole and is heard as a loud systolic murmur to the left side of the sternum (maladie de Roger). With moderate-sized shunts, fatigue and dyspnoea on exertion may occur, and with larger shunts there may be recurrent pulmonary infections, growth retardation and cardiac failure at an early age. Large defects cause right and left heart failure and, if they are not closed surgically, the Eisenmenger syndrome ensues, with cyanosis, finger clubbing and polycythaemia. Once this has developed survival is poor and heart and lung transplantation is the only possibility.

Clinical signs in these large defects include the signs of right ventricular hypertrophy and pulmonary hypertension. There is cardiomegaly with a forceful apex beat and a prominent systolic thrill at the left sternal edge. The pulmonary second sound is accentuated and there is a characteristic pansystolic murmur best heard at the third and fourth interspaces to the left of the sternum with radiation across the anterior chest wall (**5.7**). With a small VSD, the chest X-ray and ECG are both normal. With larger defects, the chest X-ray may show an enlarged left atrium, left and right ventricular hypertrophy, a large pulmonary artery and increased pulmonary vascular markings (**5.111**). The ECG shows evidence of biventricular hypertrophy. The diagnosis can be confirmed by echocardiography (**5.112**), colour-flow Doppler (**5.113**) or MRI and cardiac catheterization may be required if the defect is complicated by other pathology. There is a risk of bacterial endocarditis in all VSD patients, especially in those with smaller defects. Surgery is required in all patients with a moderate or large left-to-right shunt.

VENTRICULAR SEPTAL DEFECT (VSD)

Ventricular septal defects (VSDs) are common and the most frequent type is a single opening in the membranous portion of the septum. Non-congenital VSDs may also occur as a complication of septal myocardial infarction. The symptoms

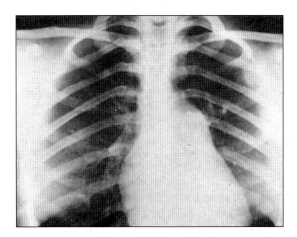

5.111 Large ventricular septal defect. The chest X-ray shows cardiomegaly with prominent pulmonary arteries and some pulmonary plethora. With a smaller ventricular septal defect, the chest X-ray may be completely normal or may simply show a slight increase in pulmonary vascular markings.

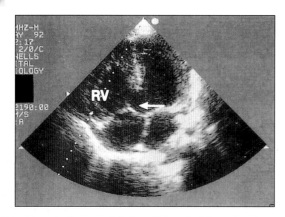

5.112   **Ventricular septal defect.** This apical four-chamber echocardiogram view clearly shows the anatomical defect in the interventricular septum (arrowed). There is also enlargement of the right ventricle (RV) due to the left-to-right shunt. This patient had Down's syndrome.

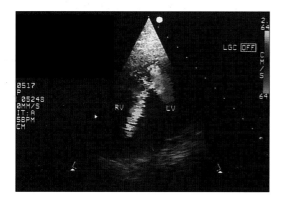

5.113   **Ventricular septal defect.** This colour-flow Doppler echocardiogram shows a high-velocity jet of blood flowing through a small septal defect from the left ventricle (LV) to the right ventricle (RV).

PATENT DUCTUS ARTERIOSUS (PDA)

Normal closure of the ductus arteriosus (joining the aorta to the bifurcation of the pulmonary artery) occurs immediately after birth, probably as a result of changes in production of vascular prostaglandins. Patency of the ductus (PDA) may be an isolated lesion or it may be combined with other lesions so that the ductus remains the only route for maintenance of the pulmonary or systemic blood flow. The amount of flow in the ductus is a reflection of its size and of the pulmonary and systemic pressures. The clinical signs depend on the extent of the pathology and its duration. With a large PDA there may be rapid onset of heart failure. Examination often shows a typical thrill at the left sternal edge and, on auscultation, there is a characteristic 'machinery' murmur at the upper left sternal border over the first intercostal space (**5.114**). In a large ductus, there is an enhanced differential in pulse pressure, felt as a

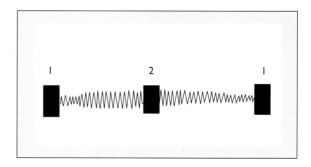

5.114   **The characteristic continuous 'machinery' murmur of patent ductus arteriosus,** which is typically loudest at the upper left sternal border over the first intercostal space (1= first heart sound; 2= second heart sound.

bounding pulse. The X-ray of the chest may show left ventricular and left atrial enlargement, a prominent aorta and pulmonary artery and pulmonary plethora (appearances similar to **5.111**). The ECG and echocardiogram show evidence of left ventricular and atrial hypertrophy and the duct may be seen on echo (**5.115**). Catheterization of the aorta may be necessary to demonstrate the defect. Heart failure indicates an urgent need for surgical correction.

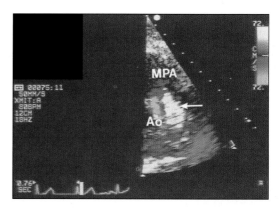

5.115   **Patent ductus arteriosus.** This colour-flow Doppler (short-axis view) shows a characteristic ductal jet (arrowed), which represents flow from the aorta (Ao) into the main pulmonary artery (MPA). The patient was a 43–year-old woman from a developing country, who presented in Dundee with shortness of breath and signs of heart failure.

COARCTATION OF THE AORTA

Coarctation of the aorta is a relatively uncommon lesion, found in 5–10% of patients with congenital heart disease. It is a congenital narrowing of the aorta that can occur at any point in its length but is usually found just after the origin of the left subclavian artery. It is often found in Turner's syndrome (**p. 306**) and may be associated with other cardiac and vascular abnormalities. Most children are asymptomatic and the patient is often found to have hypertension in the upper half of the body on routine physical examination. Severe cases may present with intermittent claudication, cold lower limbs or headache and epistaxis from hypertension. The dominant clinical feature is absence, diminution or delay of the pulse at the femoral

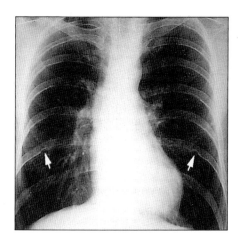

5.116   Coarctation of the aorta. The heart is not enlarged, but there is bilateral rib notching as a result of dilated intercostal arteries, which is particularly obvious in both 8th ribs (arrows). This 30-year-old man presented with hypertension, which was diagnosed at an insurance medical examination.

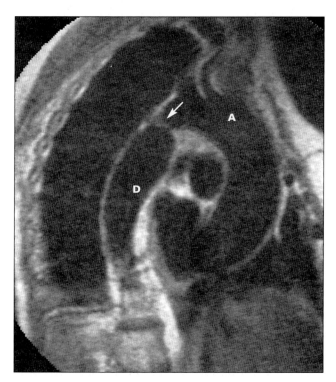

5.117   Coarctation of the aorta. This oblique MRI view through the arch of the aorta shows the coarctation as a thin shelf across the whole of the aorta (arrow). There was a small lumen, allowing blood to flow past the obstruction, which was out of plane in this view (A = ascending aorta; D = descending aorta).

artery compared with the radial artery. There is also a marked difference between the blood pressure in the upper and lower limbs. In the adult, pulsating collateral vessels may be found in the interscapular area, the axillae and the intercostal spaces. Auscultation of the heart reveals a mid-systolic murmur over the anterior chest and back.

X-ray of the chest may show left ventricular hypertrophy with a dilated ascending aorta. The stenotic area may occasionally be visible. Rib notching caused by dilated collateral vessels is common (**5.116**). The ECG shows left ventricular hypertrophy (**5.147**). Aortography is necessary to define accurately the position and length of the coarctation, though MRI can produce elegant results (**5.117**). Echocardiography and cardiac catheterization may be needed to exclude other lesions, especially bicuspid aortic valve, congenital aortic stenosis and PDA.

AORTIC AND PULMONARY STENOSIS

Aortic stenosis accounts for 2–4% of congenital heart disease. Congenital narrowing of the aortic valve is present from birth, and calcification of the valve may occur later in life (**5.98**). The signs, investigatory findings and treatment are similar to those in acquired disease (*see* **p. 223**). Pulmonary stenosis may also be an isolated congenital lesion (*see* **p. 225**) or part of a complex congenital lesion.

FALLOT'S TETRALOGY

Fallot's tetralogy forms about 10% of all cases of congenital heart disease and is the most common cardiac cause of cyanosis in infants over 1 year of age. The four characteristics of this syndrome are:

- ventricular septal defect
- overriding of the aorta over the defect
- pulmonary outflow tract obstruction
- right ventricular hypertrophy resulting from the stenosis.

Affected children are cyanosed from birth (**5.104**, **7.149**) and have dyspnoea on exertion (**5.106**) (and later at rest), retarded growth, finger clubbing (**2.104**, **2.105**) and secondary polycythaemia. The cardiac signs are those of right ventricular hypertrophy and dilatation, and a systolic thrill may be felt along the left sternal edge. There is a loud ejection systolic murmur often maximal in the second left interspace as a result of disturbed flow across the stenotic pulmonary outflow tract.

The chest X-ray shows a normal-sized heart that becomes boot-shaped (coeur-en-sabot) if the condition is not treated by early surgery because of prominence of the right ventricle and the small pulmonary arteries (**5.118**). The ECG shows right ventricular and later right atrial hypertrophy. Echocardiography may show the defect and angiocardiography is necessary to define the extent of the abnormalities.

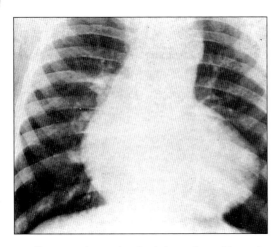

5.118 Fallot's tetralogy. The classic boot-shaped heart (coeur-en-sabot) in a child who did not receive early surgical treatment. The appearance is brought about by gross right ventricular hypertrophy, associated with small pulmonary arteries. The absence of the normal pulmonary arterial markings produces a 'bay' or indentation in the left cardiac border. The lung fields retain some vascular markings, because of their supply by systemic rather than pulmonary arteries.

Before surgery, patients are cyanosed (**5.105**, **5.106**) and require repeated venesections for polycythaemia. They are susceptible to endocarditis and cerebral abscesses. Total correction of the lesions is required and is usually carried out in infancy.

Before the advent of complete surgical repair affected children invariably died of both the septal defect and stenosis.

COMPLETE TRANSPOSITION OF THE GREAT ARTERIES

Complete transposition of the great arteries is a relatively common congenital anomaly (**5.104**) but few patients survive untreated to adult life. The aorta arises from the right ventricle, and the pulmonary artery arises from the left ventricle so that the systemic and pulmonary circulations are quite distinct. Death is inevitable without a communication between the two circulations to oxygenate systemic blood. Fortunately, many patients have an associated ventricular septal defect, and in others an atrial septal defect can be created immediately after birth, by pulling a balloon-tipped cardiac catheter across the interatrial septum. Further surgery is necessary later if life is to be maintained.

PULMONARY HYPERTENSION

Pulmonary hypertension is a common consequence of a variety of lung and heart conditions (**5.119**). The long-term result is right ventricular and atrial hypertrophy and dilatation. Such patients may present with ischaemic-type chest pain, features of right heart failure, syncope and occasionally hoarseness caused

by pressure on the left recurrent laryngeal nerve from the enlarging pulmonary artery. Sudden cardiac death is relatively common and may occur during diagnostic instrumentation. On examination, the clinical picture is that of right heart failure with a prominent right ventricular heave, jugular venous congestion with a prominent A wave, peripheral oedema and hepatic congestion. The pulmonary second sound is accentuated and may be felt. Incompetence of the pulmonary valve may be a late feature.

The chest X-ray usually shows cardiac enlargement with right ventricular and right atrial enlargement and dilatation of the pulmonary arteries. The lung fields may be oligaemic. The ECG shows features of right-axis deviation, right ventricular hypertrophy and strain (**5.120**) and occasionally right bundle

DISEASES ASSOCIATED WITH PULMONARY HYPERTENSION
Chronic obstructive lung diseases
Chronic parenchymal lung disease
Recurrent pulmonary embolism
Chronic left ventricular failure
Mitral valve disease
Congenital heart diseases (VSD, ASD, PDA and pulmonary artery stenosis)
Idiopathic (primary) pulmonary hypertension
Connective tissue diseases (SLE, systemic sclerosis, etc.)
Peripheral arterio-venous shunts
Left atrial myxoma
High altitude living
Pulmonary veno-occlusive disease

5.119 Diseases associated with pulmonary hypertension.

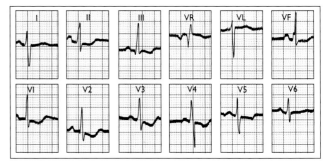

5.120 Right ventricular hypertrophy in a patient with pulmonary hypertension. Note the tall R wave (7 mm +) in V1, which is taller than the S wave, a combined voltage of R in V1 and S in V6 of 10 mm or more, and the ST depression and T-wave inversion from V1 to V5. Right ventricular hypertrophy may also be manifested as dominant S waves across all the chest leads. P pulmonale (tall, peaked P waves at least 2.4 mm in height) is another common finding, though absent on this trace.

branch block. Echocardiography and colour-flow Doppler may show the cause of pulmonary hypertension, for example atrial or ventricular septal defects or mitral stenosis. Cardiac catheterization is of value to determine the site of the lesion and measure pressures and degree of oxygenation. Treatment is directed at the underlying cause. Diuretics, oxygen, vasodilators and anticoagulants have a place in management, as does heart–lung transplantation as a last resort.

INFECTIVE ENDOCARDITIS

In infective endocarditis, a bacteraemia is complicated by the development of 'vegetations' on the endocardium of the heart (endocarditis). Vegetations usually form on aortic and mitral valves that are already damaged from rheumatic fever, but they may be associated with congenital abnormalities such as ventricular and atrial septal defects and coarctation of the aorta (in which they may cause aortitis). The organisms involved are usually commensals of the mouth and pharynx (*Streptococcus viridans*) or the bowel (*Streptococcus faecalis*). Rarely, virulent organisms such as *Streptococcus pyogenes* or *Staphylococcus aureus* may infect a previously normal heart valve, especially in intravenous drug misusers and in patients with indwelling cannulae and pacing lines. Prosthetic heart valves are more susceptible to endocarditis than normal valves and they may become infected with unusual organisms, such as *Staphylococcus epidermidis*, Gram-negative organisms and fungi such as *Candida albicans*, *Histoplasma* and *Aspergillus*. Implanted pacemakers and defibrillators may also harbour infection. Although episodes of bacteraemia may apparently occur spontaneously, especially in patients with dental caries and gingivitis (**5.103**, **5.121**), dental procedures, endotracheal intubation and bronchoscopy, genitourinary and colonic endoscopy and surgery are especially likely to provoke bacteraemia. Patients with diseased valves or congenital cardiac abnormalities should therefore be given prophylactic antibiotics before these procedures.

Infective vegetations produce clinical features in four ways:

- they induce febrile symptoms, such as sweating and weight loss
- they may erode heart valves and rupture chordae tendineae, causing valvular incompetence and heart failure; the infection may extend beyond the valve into the conducting tissue of the heart, causing heart block
- they can embolize causing stroke, limb ischaemia, renal and splenic infarcts and occasionally myocardial and pulmonary infarction
- their presence can stimulate the formation of immune complexes in the blood; these complexes can produce focal glomerulonephritis and vasculitis in the eye and skin.

Untreated endocarditis is usually fatal. Numerous signs are traditionally associated with the disorder, but many are seldom seen in modern medicine. The key features in most patients with infective endocarditis are:

- fever (often low-grade)
- a changing cardiac murmur
- embolic phenomena.

Most patients feel generally unwell, and there may be weight loss, anaemia, haematuria, an enlarged spleen, petechiae and vasculitic lesions under the nails (splinter haemorrhages, **3.32**), in the sclerae (**5.122**), conjunctivae, retinae (Roth spots) (**5.123**) and in the finger and toe pulps (Osler's nodes, **5.124**).

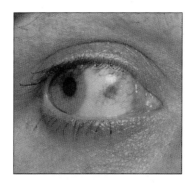

5.122 Scleral and conjunctival haemorrhages are a recognized but rare feature in established infective endocarditis. They are probably the result of infected microemboli from cardiac vegetations, but may also be associated with thrombocytopenia.

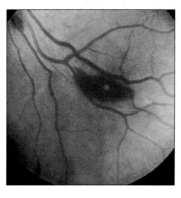

5.123 A Roth spot in the retina in infective endocarditis. These oval haemorrhagic lesions with white centres are thought to result from septic emboli, but similar appearances may sometimes occur in patients with anaemia or leukaemia.

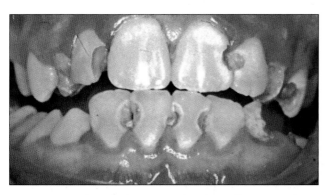

5.121 Severe dental caries and gingivitis predisposes patients to episodes of bacteraemia, and thus to infective endocarditis in the presence of a congenital or acquired cardiac abnormality. Full treatment of caries or appropriate dental extraction should be carried out with antibiotic prophylaxis in all such patients.

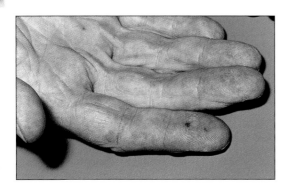

5.124 Small dermal infarcts in infective endocarditis. When palpable, these are known as Osler's nodes. These infarcts are usually tender. They may be caused by septic emboli from the cardiac vegetations, but similar appearances may result from vasculitis associated with circulating immune complexes.

Finger clubbing is now extremely rare, as patients are usually treated before it develops.

When the diagnosis is suspected, an echocardiogram should be performed. Small vegetations are often not identifiable, but large vegetations can be visualized (**5.125**) and the extent of the valvular incompetence clarified. Vegetations are particularly difficult to identify on prosthetic heart valves, and colour-flow or transoesophageal echocardiography may be valuable in these patients and for patients with lesions in the left atrium (**5.126**). Blood tests often show a normochromic, normocytic anaemia, there may be a polymorph leucocytosis and the ESR and C-reactive proteins are elevated. Circulating immune complexes are found and there is a rise in immunoglobulin levels and a fall in total complement.

Multiple blood cultures are required and sampling should coincide with peaks of fever. This permits identification of the infecting organism, so that appropriate combinations of

antibiotics can be given in high dosage intravenously for several weeks (**5.127**). Less aggressive therapy is usually ineffective. If cultures are negative, other causes of endocarditis should be sought by appropriate serological tests, for example for fungi, Q fever or psittacosis.

Antibiotics may not eradicate the infection and emergency surgery may be required. The infected valve is removed and replaced with a prosthetic one. Other indications for emergency valve replacement are the development of severe valvular incompetence causing heart failure or a dangerous embolic episode, for example cerebral embolism. The mortality rate

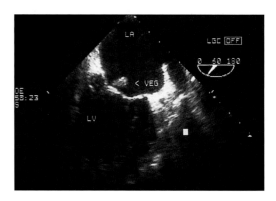

5.126 Transoesophageal echocardiography is a valuable technique for demonstrating cardiac vegetations in infective endocarditis. Here a vegetation attached to the atrial surface of the mitral valve is clearly seen. This abnormality was not visible on transthoracic echocardiography.

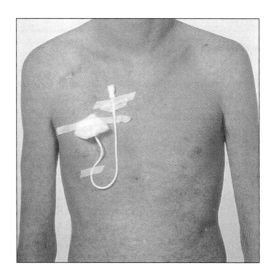

5.127 Prolonged, high-dose antibiotic therapy in infective endocarditis is best given via a central venous line. This patient has a Hickman line, which tunnels under the skin to its entry point into the venous system in the cephalic or axillary vein. The tip of the catheter is in the superior vena cava. This patient's morbilliform rash probably resulted from previous therapy with ampicillin, which also complicated the interpretation of blood cultures.

5.125 Echocardiogram in infective endocarditis. This parasternal long-axis view shows a large vegetation on the anterior leaflet of the mitral valve (arrowed). The patient had recently been unwell with diverticulitis and a local intra-abdominal abscess. *Streptococcus faecalis* was grown on blood culture (LA = left atrium; LV = left ventricle).

associated with emergency valve replacement during endocarditis is higher than for elective surgery involving a sterile valve.

MYOCARDITIS

Myocarditis is a general term for any inflammatory process involving the heart. It is usually infective but can be caused by chemicals, physical agents or drugs (**5.128**).

The history depends on the cause. The most common type of myocarditis in the developed world follows a viral infection, typically an upper respiratory tract infection. The onset is usually insidious with features of right and left heart failure, fever and general malaise. There is tachycardia with a low-volume pulse, hypotension, faint heart sounds, a third heart sound and features of pericarditis. The chest X-ray shows cardiomegaly (**5.129**), sometimes with a pericardial effusion; the ECG may show arrhythmias, diffuse ST-segment and T-wave changes and heart block. Cardiac enzymes are elevated if the acute inflammatory process is ongoing. Serology may show a rising titre of viral antibodies. Treatment involves bed rest and control of failure and arrhythmias. Steroids can be of value.

Myocarditis usually remits but it may progress and behave like a chronic cardiomyopathy.

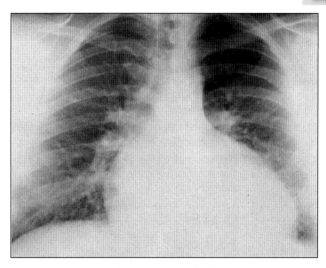

5.129   Acute myocarditis causing marked enlargement of all cardiac chambers and pulmonary venous congestion. The ECG showed generalized T-wave inversion. Serology showed the cause to be a coxsackievirus infection, and the patient made a complete recovery within a few weeks. An identical chest X-ray appearance may be seen in dilated cardiomyopathy.

CAUSES OF MYOCARDITIS		
Infections	Viruses	Coxsackie Influenza Adenoviruses Echovirus Rubella
	Bacteria	*Corynebacterium diphtheriae* *Chlamydia* *Rickettsia* *Coxiella burnetii*
	Protozoa	*Trypanosoma cruzi* *Toxoplasma gondii*
Physical	Radiation	From therapy for breast or lung cancer, lymphoma or thymoma
Toxins	Alcohol	
Drugs	Emetine	In treatment of amoebiasis
	Chloroquine	In malaria prophylaxis

5.128   Causes of myocarditis.

CARDIOMYOPATHIES

The most common causes of diseased heart muscle are coronary disease, hypertension and heart valve disease. However, the myocardium may also be damaged in other conditions, for example prolonged alcohol abuse, hypothyroidism, acromegaly, phaeochromocytoma, inherited neuromuscular disorders, connective tissue and storage diseases and by some drug therapy (e.g. doxorubicin).

Idiopathic cardiomyopathies are primary heart muscle disorders of indeterminate cause. They can be divided into three pathophysiological types that produce distinctive clinical syndromes:

- dilated cardiomyopathy
- hypertrophic cardiomyopathy
- restrictive cardiomyopathy.

DILATED CARDIOMYOPATHY

In dilated cardiomyopathy the heart muscle weakens and the chambers progressively dilate. The aetiology of idiopathic dilated cardiomyopathy is unknown, but some cases are familial and previous coxsackievirus infection may also be causally related. Patients become breathless and develop signs of right and left heart failure, with pulmonary congestion, cardiomegaly and, sometimes, arrhythmias and emboli. Ventricular dilatation may lead to functional mitral or tricuspid regurgitation.

Chest X-ray (**5.129**), echocardiography and MRI (**5.26**) confirm dilated cardiac chambers and inefficient left ventricular wall motion in systole. The ECG may show ST-segment changes and arrhythmias, but has no diagnostic value.

Patients with idiopathic dilated cardiomyopathy may fail to respond to diuretics and vasodilator drugs and the heart failure may progress to death within a few years. Cardiac transplantation is feasible in some younger patients.

HYPERTROPHIC CARDIOMYOPATHY

In hypertrophic cardiomyopathy, a localized segment of the heart muscle becomes thickened; the interventricular septum is usually involved and the abnormal muscle restricts filling of the left ventricle during diastole. If it also obstructs the flow of blood from the ventricle to the aorta during systole, the condition is termed hypertrophic obstructive cardiomyopathy (HOCM). The abnormal muscle is a focus for dangerous arrhythmias, especially ventricular tachycardia, which may convert to ventricular fibrillation. Hypertrophic cardio-myopathy is potentially fatal, and patients should avoid strenuous exercise which may provoke arrhythmias. Patients with hypertrophic cardiomyopathy may be asymptomatic. However, some have angina, as their hypertrophied muscle requires more oxygen, even in the absence of coronary disease. Some also have a low cardiac output causing dizziness and syncope. These patients may also develop an ejection systolic murmur, best heard over the left sternal border, caused by the obstruction. As the obstruction develops, it also distorts the mitral valve and a regurgitant murmur may be heard.

The diagnosis is best made by echocardiography (**5.130**, **5.131**). The ECG classically shows a combination of left ventricular hypertrophy and pathological Q waves resulting from hypertrophy of the interventricular septum. Treatment is directed at preventing serious arrhythmias and relieving angina. If there is severe obstruction to left ventricular outflow, surgical removal of the hypertrophied muscle below the aortic valve may be beneficial.

The condition is inherited as an autosomal dominant in about one-half of the reported cases, and family members should be studied by echocardiography to determine whether they have an asymptomatic form of the condition. Long-term follow-up of these family members is required for early diagnosis and treatment of complications.

RESTRICTIVE CARDIOMYOPATHY

Restrictive cardiomyopathy is very rare in developed countries. It is associated with a range of conditions, including amyloidosis, sarcoidosis and leukaemic infiltration. Endo-myocardial fibrosis is the most common cause in the tropics.

The myocardium is infiltrated by abnormal tissue, which renders the chambers stiff and non-compliant. This is particularly evident in diastole and can be confirmed by Doppler echocardiography. Patients develop congestive cardiac failure, with ascites and ankle swelling. The physical signs are similar to those of constrictive pericarditis (**p. 237**) with raised jugular venous pressure and cardiac enlargement. The X-ray (**5.129**) and ECG show cardiac enlargement. The echocardiogram shows the thickening of the myocardium with impaired ventricular filling.

5.130

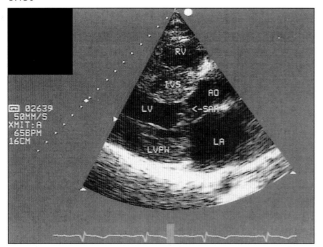

5.131

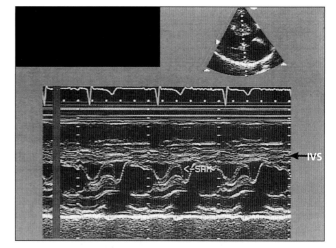

5.130 & 5.131 Hypertrophic obstructive cardiomyopathy. The two-dimensional long-axis parasternal view (**5.130**) shows the chambers of the heart (LA = left atrium; RV = right ventricle; LV = left ventricle). The left ventricle posterior wall (LVPW) is thickened, and the most striking abnormality is the hypertrophy of the interventricular septum (IVS). Another characteristic feature is a Venturi effect: as blood leaves the left ventricle it sucks the anterior leaflet of the mitral valve forward – systolic anterior motion (SAM). This phenomenon is more clearly shown (SAM) in the parasternal long-axis M-mode echocardiogram (**5.131**). The massive thickening of the septum is also obvious in the M-mode (IVS).

CARDIAC TUMOURS

Primary cardiac tumours are rare, but secondary deposits are often found incidentally at autopsy, infiltrating the pericardium and, less commonly, the myocardium. Pericardial deposits may produce a pericardial effusion that can constrict the heart and cause death from tamponade.

The most common primary tumour of the heart is an atrial myxoma. It usually grows in the cavity of the left atrium and is attached by a stalk to the left atrial wall just behind the mitral valve. If it obstructs blood flow from the left atrium to the left ventricle, syncope can occur. Portions of the tumour may also become detached and embolize. This association of peripheral emboli with a heart murmur may lead to the mistaken diagnosis of infective endocarditis, but a myxoma is easily demonstrable by echocardiography (**5.132**) or MRI (**5.133**). Myxomas can be removed surgically with good long-term results.

Tumours in the myocardium are usually secondaries and the bronchus and breast are the most common primary sites. These malignant deposits may have haemodynamic effects, and they often interfere with the conducting system, causing heart block, or may be a focus for ventricular or supraventricular tachyarrhythmias. Curative treatment is usually impossible.

PERICARDIAL DISEASE

Patients with pericardial disease may present in one of three ways: pericarditis, pericardial effusion or constrictive pericarditis.

PERICARDITIS

Causes of pericarditis include:

- acute and chronic infections
- myocardial infarction
- metabolic
- connective tissue disorders
- acute rheumatic fever
- malignancy
- radiation
- idiopathic.

The usual clinical presentation is with acute, sharp, central chest pain that may radiate to the neck and shoulders and may be brought on by movement. There is usually associated fever and occasionally myalgia. The most common causes are Coxsackie B virus infection (*see* **p. 11**) and acute myocardial infarction (**p. 214**). A friction rub may be heard. Investigations show leucocytosis and elevation of the ESR, and in the absence of myocardial infarction the ECG shows a typical pattern of ST elevation without QRS changes (**5.134**). The T wave becomes inverted in most leads after several days. There may also be an increase in levels of cardiac enzymes and echocardiography may

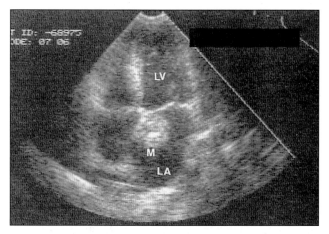

5.132   Left atrial myxoma. This apical four-chamber echocardiogram shows a circular mass (M) arising in a typical position from the interatrial septum just above the mitral valve (LA = left atrium; LV = left ventricle).

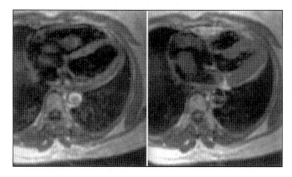

5.133   Right atrial myxoma, demonstrated by MRI. Diastolic (left) and systolic (right) transverse images show that the mass has three lobes. It prolapses through the tricuspid valve in diastole and is fully within the right atrium in systole.

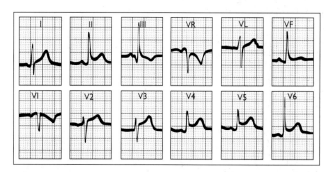

5.134   Acute pericarditis. In the first few days, the ECG shows ST elevation, concave upwards, with upright T waves in most leads. Classically it is more obvious in lead II than in I or III. There are no pathological Q waves, and the widespread distribution of ST–T changes without reciprocal depression, distinguishes acute pericarditis from early myocardial infarction. In the later stages of pericarditis, the T waves become inverted in most leads. The ECG changes in pericarditis are caused by the superficial myocarditis that accompanies it.

show an increase in pericardial fluid. The chest X-ray usually shows a normal cardiac outline, which may enlarge if the amount of pericardial fluid increases. There may also be associated inflammatory lung changes. Analgesia and anti-inflammatory drug treatment are often helpful.

PERICARDIAL EFFUSION

A pericardial effusion is an accumulation of excess fluid within the pericardium, often as a result of acute or chronic pericarditis. There are many possible causes (**5.135**). The implications for cardiac function depend on the rate at which the fluid accumulates. The first effect is to reduce the venous return to the heart; this is reflected in elevation of the jugular venous pressure (JVP), hepatic congestion and peripheral oedema. As the amount of pericardial fluid increases, cardiac filling is progressively diminished and cardiac output reduced; thus a vicious circle is established (cardiac tamponade) that leads to declining cardiac function and death. The diagnosis can be made clinically because of the features of heart failure (JVP elevation, peripheral oedema, hepatomegaly) and diminished output (thready 'paradoxical' pulse, central cyanosis, low blood pressure). There may be an increased area of cardiac dullness and the heart sounds may be muffled. Pericardial rub is usually absent.

X-ray of the chest shows an enlarged cardiac shadow (**5.136**) and may give clues to the underlying cause (**5.137**). The ECG shows low-voltage complexes, often with T-wave inversion (**5.138**). Echocardiography shows the size of the effusion (**5.139**). If there is impairment of cardiac function, urgent aspiration is required (**5.140**). Examination of the aspirate may give a clue to aetiology and the need for further treatment.

CAUSES OF PERICARDIAL EFFUSION
Neoplasia
Infection – viruses, bacteria, fungi
Idiopathic
Myocardial infarction
Heart failure
Trauma
Connective tissue disorders
Drugs
Renal failure or nephrotic syndrome

5.135 **Causes of pericardial effusion (in descending order of frequency).**

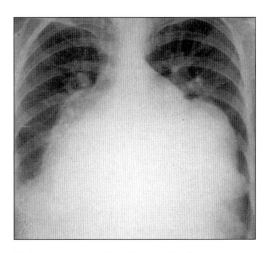

5.137 **Malignant pericardial effusion.** The heart shadow is generally enlarged, but the odd, irregular outline of the enlargement suggests the presence of secondary tumour deposits in the pericardium. This patient had a primary ovarian carcinoma.

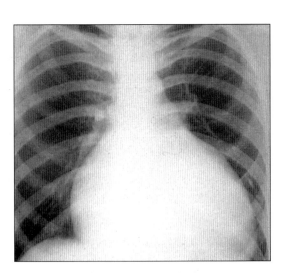

5.136 **Pericardial effusion.** The heart shadow appears generally enlarged, but the appearance is not diagnostic. A similar appearance can be seen in cardiac failure, in myocarditis or in dilated cardiomyopathy.

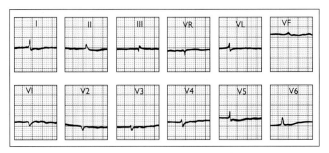

5.138 **Pericardial effusion.** Large quantities of pericardial fluid produce an ECG of generally low voltage, with generalized T-wave flattening or inversion; this is partly the result of the insulating effect of the fluid, and partly because of superficial myocarditis. Note that this patient has also developed atrial fibrillation.

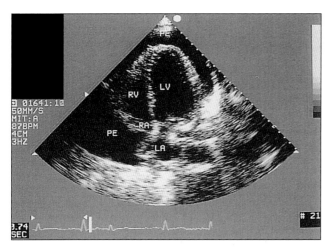

5.139 Pericardial effusion. This echocardiogram shows a pericardial effusion and also a pleural effusion – both are labelled PE; the apical PE indicates the pericardial effusion, whereas that to the left indicates pleural effusion. In addition there is a solid tissue mass invading the wall of the left atrium and ventricle, which probably represents secondary tumour. The patient also had multiple secondaries elsewhere from a primary carcinoma of the breast (LV = left ventricle; RV = right ventricle; LA = left atrium; RA = right atrium).

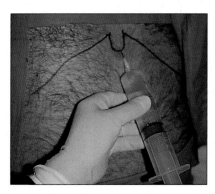

5.140 Aspiration of pericardial fluid is indicated in cardiac tamponade or to obtain fluid for diagnostic purposes. A wide-bore needle is inserted in the epigastrium below the xiphoid process and advanced in the direction of the medial third of the right clavicle. If the needle is connected to the V lead of an ECG monitor, ST elevation will usually be seen if the needle touches the epicardium. This can be useful in distinguishing a bloody pericardial effusion from accidental puncture of the heart. Other complications of the procedure may include arrhythmias, vasovagal attack and pneumothorax.

CONSTRICTIVE PERICARDITIS

Fibrosis and calcification of the pericardium may follow an episode of acute pericarditis or may develop insidiously over a period of time. The end result is impaired cardiac filling and ventricular function. The dominant features are distension of the neck veins, peripheral oedema, ascites and hepatic congestion. There may be a striking increase in jugular venous distension on inspiration (Kussmaul's sign). Pulsus paradoxus is

present. Chest X-ray shows a small heart shadow and there may be pericardial calcification (**5.141**). The ECG shows non-specific changes, often with low-voltage complexes, and atrial fibrillation is frequently found in the late stages of the disease. Echocardiography shows a thickened pericardium with small ventricular and atrial chambers. Treatment is by pericardiectomy.

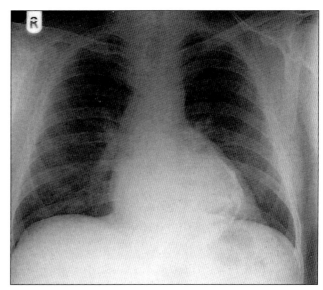

5.141 Pericardial calcification is clearly seen around the left and inferior borders of the heart. This patient has a normal-sized heart, but the calcification may progress further, leading to constrictive pericarditis.

HYPERTENSION

Hypertension is high blood pressure in the systemic arterial circulation, (> 90 mmHg diastolic and/or >140mmHg systolic). Ultimately hypertension can damage the walls of arteries, arterioles and the left ventricle of the heart with serious consequences, chiefly affecting the brain, heart, kidneys and eyes. It is one of the most common disorders in the Western world, with a prevalence of about 15%.

Large and medium-sized arteries respond to high blood pressure by thickening of the media and disruption of the elastic tissue within their walls. The vessels may become tortuous and dilated and may rupture because of the high pressure in the lumen. If this occurs in the brain, cerebral haemorrhage usually leaves the patient dead or paralysed from a 'stroke'. Hypertension also promotes the formation of atheroma in medium-sized and large arteries, so a stroke may also be caused by occlusion of a cerebral artery by thrombus formed on an atheromatous plaque, or by embolization of atheromatous material from plaques in the extracranial segments of the carotid arteries or aorta (*see* **p. 473**). Atheroma formation in the coronary arteries renders hypertensive patients susceptible to angina pectoris, myocardial infarction and sudden death.

In smaller arteries and arterioles, hypertension causes prominent thickening of the intima, in addition to medial hypertrophy. In cases of 'accelerated' or 'malignant' hypertension, in which the blood pressure is very high or has risen quickly, these intimal changes can occlude the vessels, producing distal tissue ischaemia. This particularly affects the kidneys, causing renal failure (*see* **p. 282**). The walls of the small arteries in the brain may be damaged so that their permeability is increased and cerebral oedema results, causing hypertensive encephalopathy, characterized by headache, confusion, fits and coma. There may also be visual disturbances due to retinal arterial damage, which may be seen on examination of the fundi.

The left ventricle responds to high blood pressure by hypertrophy. Initially, this increases its force of contraction and maintains a normal cardiac output, but eventually the hypertrophied muscle outgrows its oxygen supply and angina and cardiac failure result.

An identifiable cause of high blood pressure is only apparent in 1–2% of hypertensive individuals. They are said to have secondary hypertension. In the remainder, no single cause of high blood pressure has been found. These individuals are said to have primary or essential hypertension. Genetic factors are important, as shown by the relevance of a family history of hypertension and by racial variations in prevalence. Lifestyle patterns also influence blood pressure, and obesity, alcohol intake, insufficient physical activity and possibly excessive salt consumption all contribute to hypertension. Smoking does not cause hypertension, but it accelerates atherogenesis.

Many patients with hypertension are asymptomatic, and the elevated blood pressure is picked up by chance on routine screening or after a stroke, infarct or other vascular catastrophe. Those with more severe disease may not present until they have features of renal failure, heart failure or angina. Only when there is a rise in intracranial pressure is headache a feature. Blurred vision may result from retinopathy.

Examination of the patient with uncomplicated hypertension usually reveals few abnormal findings, but it is important to look for signs of end-organ damage (renal failure, cerebrovascular disease, cardiac failure) and to stage any changes in the fundi (**5.142–5.145**).

It is also important to look for signs of possible causes of secondary hypertension (**5.146**).

Investigations should usually include an ECG for signs of left ventricular hypertrophy (**5.147**) and ischaemia, and a chest X-ray for cardiac size (**5.148**) and (rarely) signs of coarctation of the aorta (**5.116**). Echocardiography can also provide an accurate assessement of the severity of ventricular hypertrophy. The extent and severity of hypertension can often be usefully clarified by ambulatory blood pressure monitoring (**5.112**, **5.113**).

Proteinuria is an indicator of possible renal disease. Plasma electrolytes, urea and creatinine will show changes if there is renal failure and these and other specific investigations may be required in patients with renal disease (**p. 282**) and to exclude other causes of secondary hypertension.

Treatment should follow appropriate national or international guidelines and must be decided on an individual basis. Decisions on treatment depend on several baseline blood pressure recordings, age, sex and whether complications of hypertension are already present. Patients with diastolic pressure consistently in excess of 90 mmHg and/or a systolic pressure consistently in excess of 140 mmHg should be treated. Many antihypertensive drugs are available and they act in different ways, so drugs may be used in combination. Reduction of blood pressure reduces the risks of stroke, myocardial infarction, heart failure and renal failure.

In those relatively rare patients in whom hypertension is secondary to an identifiable cause, there is the possibility of treatment of the cause, or of curative surgery.

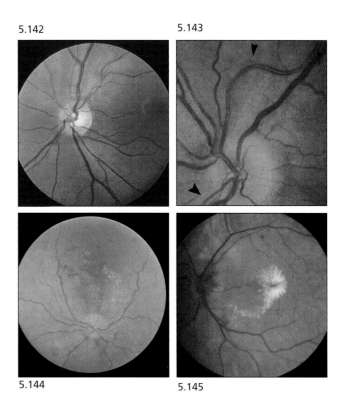

5.142–5.145 Hypertensive retinopathy is traditionally divided into four grades. Grade 1 (**5.142**) shows very early and minor changes in a young patient: increased tortuosity of a retinal vessel and increased reflectiveness (silver wiring) of a retinal artery, are seen at 1 o'clock in this view. Otherwise, the fundus is completely normal. Grade 2 (**5.143**) again shows increased tortuosity and silver wiring (coarse arrows). In addition there is 'nipping' of the venules at arteriovenous crossings (fine arrow). Grade 3 (**5.144**) shows the same changes as grade 2 plus flame-shaped retinal haemorrhages and soft 'cotton-wool' exudates. In Grade 4 (**5.145**) there is swelling of the optic disc (papilloedema), retinal oedema is present, and hard exudates may collect around the fovea, producing a typical 'macular star'.

CAUSES OF SECONDARY HYPERTENSION

Renal disease

Bilateral	Chronic glomerulonephritis
	Chronic pyelonephritis (reflux nephropathy)
	Polycystic kidneys
	Analgesic nephropathy
Unilateral	Chronic pyelonephritis (reflux nephropathy)
	Renal artery stenosis

Endocrine disorders

Conn's syndrome

Cushing's syndrome

Phaeochromocytoma

Acromegaly

Hyperparathyroidism

Cardiovascular disorders

Coarctation of the aorta

Pregnancy

Pre-eclampsia and eclampsia

Drugs

Oral contraceptives

Corticosteroids

Monoamineoxidase inhibitors (interaction with tyramine)

5.146   Causes of secondary hypertension.

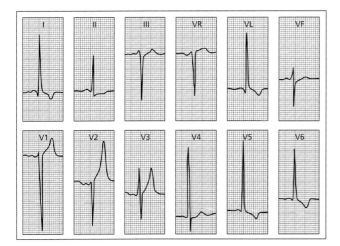

5.147   Left ventricular hypertrophy in hypertension. This ECG shows severe hypertrophy. Left ventricular hypertrophy (LVH) is present when the R wave in V4 or V6 or the S wave in V1 or V2 exceeds 24 mm in an adult of normal build. This ECG also shows T-wave inversion over the left ventricle (V5–6) and, as the heart is relatively horizontally placed, in I and VL.

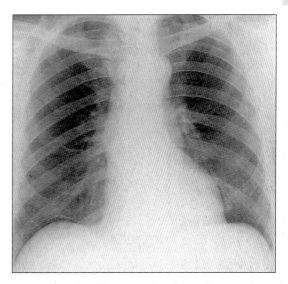

5.148   Hypertension. The chest X-ray is usually normal in mild to moderate hypertension, but cardiac enlargement associated with left ventricular hypertrophy (as here) may occur in the later stages. There is no evidence of cardiac failure in this patient.

239

PERIPHERAL ARTERIAL OCCLUSIVE DISEASE (PAOD)

Peripheral arterial obstruction in the legs is a common problem in the ageing population of the Western world, with a male:female ratio of 10:1. Long-term cigarette smoking is by far the most important underlying cause of peripheral arterial occlusive disease (PAOD), and atheroma is the major pathological process. Patients often have other arterial manifestations, including IHD, stroke, transient ischaemic attacks and intestinal ischaemia. Ischaemic heart disease is the most common cause of death in these patients. Atheroma usually has a patchy distribution in the aorta and the femoral and popliteal vessels. It is found particularly at the aortic bifurcation and around the origins of smaller vessels. The lesions tend to enlarge slowly and gradually reduce blood flow.

Symptoms usually occur when the arterial obstruction is 50–75%. The most common symptom is a cramp-like pain in the calf and thigh muscles on exercise, which disappears on resting for a few minutes (intermittent claudication). There is often a history of progressive shortening of the distance walked without pain as the disease progresses. The level of the arterial block dictates the muscle group in which pain is felt: for example, an obstructive lesion in the profunda femoris artery will present with buttock, hip and thigh claudication (and impotence).

Patients may also complain of weakness of muscle groups and numbness or paraesthesiae. Ulceration and gangrene may appear with constant pain at rest. Diabetics usually have extensive atheroma and their presentation is more complex as they often also have peripheral neuropathy and small vessel disease, and have lost deep pain sensation and sympathetic tone.

Clinical examination in PAOD shows:

- atrophy of the skin, loss of hair, trophic nail changes (**5.149**)
- a cold limb, which may be pallid or cyanosed (**5.150, 5.151**)
- slow capillary return when finger pressure is released
- loss or diminution of pulses in the affected leg (**5.149**)
- a bruit over the affected segment of vessel
- ulceration or gangrene, particularly of the toes (**5.152**)
- loss of sensation.

Special investigations include measurement of arm and leg systolic blood pressure (ankle:brachial pressure index – ABPI; **5.153**), blood pressure measurement at the ankle after exercise (it falls to very low levels) and arteriography (**5.154**) to localize the site and extent of the block and the presence of collaterals. The site of block may also be found non-invasively with colour-flow Doppler. Thermography may have a place in

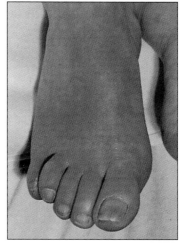

5.151 'Critical' ischaemia of the foot. The patient had sudden onset of discomfort, with coldness and loss of sensation in the toes and the dorsum of the foot. He had previously suffered from intermittent claudication and has evidence of chronic ischaemia, including absence of hair and thinness of the skin. Arteriography is necessary to define the nature of the lesion.

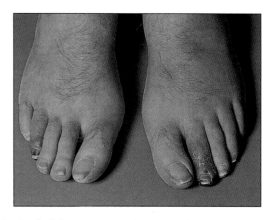

5.152 Typical dry gangrene of two toes in a patient with diffuse atheroma. The patient had a history of intermittent claudication. Note the chronic nail changes that are also seen (resembling onycholysis). The residual hair on the dorsum of the feet is unusual in chronic ischaemia; usually the hair is lost (*see* **5.151**).

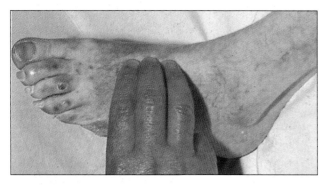

5.149 Peripheral vascular disease. Typical changes in the skin include atrophy, pallor, loss of hair and, in some patients, trophic nail changes. This patient also has early ulceration on the dorsum of three toes. It is important to examine the peripheral pulses. In this patient the dorsalis pedis pulse was impalpable.

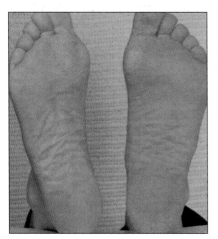

5.150 Ischaemic pallor of the patient's right foot. Note the colour difference between the two feet, which has been accentuated by elevation of the legs.

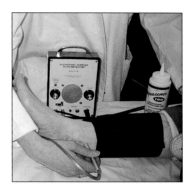

5.153 Ankle: brachial pressure index (ABPI). This is a simple screening test to determine the presence of obstruction of flow of the lower limb arteries. Blood pressure is measured accurately with the aid of a Doppler probe at the ankle and that value is compared as a ratio with the brachial artery pressure. A ratio of 0.9 or below suggests impairment.

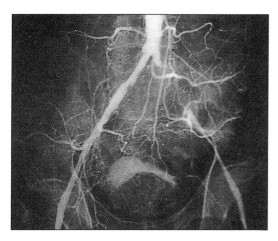

5.154 Multiple atheromatous deposits and complete occlusion of the left external iliac artery with collateral formation, in a patient with severe left-sided intermittent claudication and ischaemic skin changes.

determining skin blood flow in patients in whom amputation is being considered (**5.155**). Other investigations that may be helpful in selected patients include duplex ultrasound measurement of pressure in small arteries, oximetry on the dorsum of the foot, isotope clearance studies, plethysmography and MRI.

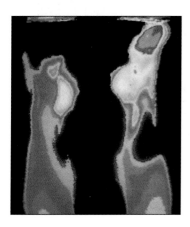

5.155 Thermography may be useful in assessing the skin circulation in ischaemic limbs. This patient has severe ischaemia of the right foot.

Treatment includes lifestyle advice about stopping smoking, weight reduction, lipid and blood pressure control, and graded exercises. Sympathectomy may have a place in selected patients. Skilled foot care is important, especially in the diabetic. Drug therapy is generally unsatisfactory. The circulation may be improved by angioplasty (**5.156**, **5.157**), stenting (**5.157**) or vessel grafting, but gangrene requires amputation (**5.158**).

5.156

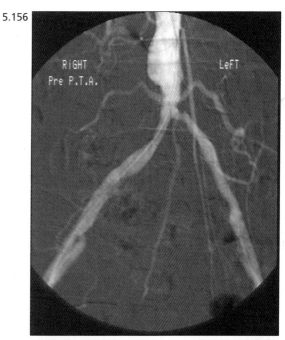

5.157

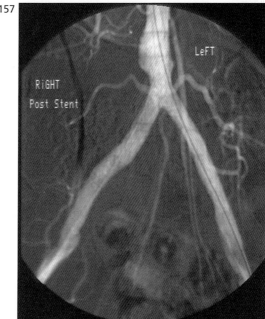

5.156 & 5.157 Percutaneous transluminal angioplasty (PTA) and stenting are routinely used in peripheral vascular disease. **5.156** shows significant narrowing of the aortic bifurcation and both common iliac arteries. The narrowing in both common iliacs was successfully treated by angioplasty and bilateral stents were inserted to maintain patency. The patient had presented with bilateral calf claudication, which was relieved by this procedure.

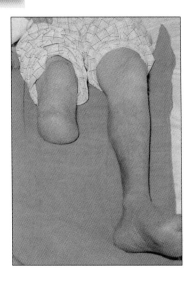

5.158 Amputation is still often necessary in patients with severe peripheral vascular disease. This patient developed massive gangrene of the leg and foot.

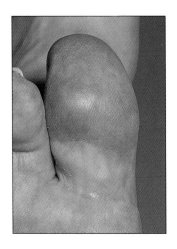

5.160 Digital ischaemia in Buerger's disease often affects the toes. Here the ischaemia is more severe than that seen in **5.159**. Again, this progressed to gangrene, and amputation of the toe was necessary to eliminate infection.

THROMBO-ANGIITIS OBLITERANS (BUERGER'S DISEASE)

Thrombo-angiitis obliterans (Buerger's disease) is a disease of young male smokers who develop ulceration and gangrene of their digits, caused by spasm of the digital arteries associated with an intense inflammatory response, which may also involve veins and nerves. There is no evidence of excessive atheroma. The major symptoms are referable to ischaemia of the fingers (**5.159**) and toes (**5.160**), but many patients also have intermittent claudication, usually affecting the calf and often the 'instep' of the foot, and also occasionally claudication of the hand. Ultimately, there may be severe rest pain and gangrene. Examination may show cold digits, digital ulcers, a migratory phlebitis of hands and feet and absent foot and hand pulses. Patients should stop all use of tobacco and may be helped by

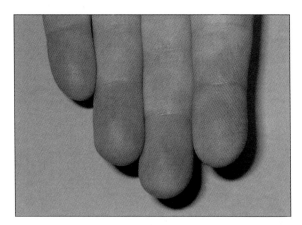

5.159 Digital ischaemia in Buerger's disease. The fingertips are cyanotic, though no irreversible changes have yet occurred. This man continued to smoke, against all advice, and subsequently developed gangrene.

vasodilator drugs. Sympathectomy may be of value, but amputation of digits may become necessary.

CRITICAL LIMB ISCHAEMIA

In critical limb ischaemia a limb's survival is compromised by its vascular insufficiency or obstruction. Thrombosis on an atheromatous plaque or embolism may produce acute ischaemia very rapidly. The sources of emboli include the left atrium when the mitral or aortic valves are damaged by rheumatic endocarditis (**5.94**), especially when the rhythm changes from sinus rhythm to atrial fibrillation; mural thrombus in the left ventricle after myocardial infarction (**5.85**); prosthetic valves (**1.15**); vegetations in infective endocarditis (**5.125, 5.126**); and atheromatous plaques or aneurysms in the aorta (**5.176**). The features are acute onset of pain, pallor of the limb and lack of pulses and capillary return, followed by reactive hyperaemia (**5.91**) or cyanosis and gangrene (**5.150–5.152**). The level of the block may be defined by colour-flow Doppler or angiography (**5.156**).

The essential principle of treatment is to revascularize the limb if possible. Distal emboli or thrombosis may be treated with a thrombolytic agent. More proximal lesions may be amenable to angioplasty or thrombectomy. Prevention of recurrence usually requires treatment with aspirin and anticoagulants.

Acute arterial occlusion may also occur when drug abusers inject intra-arterially (**5.161**).

COMPARTMENT SYNDROME

Reperfusion of an arterial bed which has been ischaemic produces local oedema due to increased capillary permeability. Where muscles have tight fascial constraints, this increase in the local pressure may lead to muscle necrosis (compartment syndrome). The symptoms are swelling, pain and tenderness on

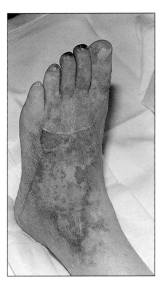

5.161 Acute arterial occlusion following deliberate intra-arterial drug injection. This 34-year-old intravenous drug abuser had run out of accessible veins following recurrent thrombosis. He injected a suspension of crushed dipipanone hydrochloride (Diconal) tablets into the dorsalis pedis artery and immediately experienced severe pain in the toes and dorsum of the foot. The early changes are shown here. The ischaemic skin was grafted but this was not successful and he eventually required amputation of the forefoot.

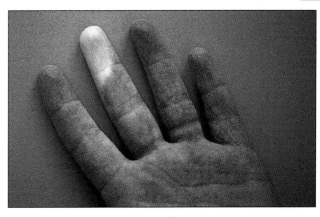

5.162 Raynaud's syndrome in the acute phase, with severe blanching of the tip of one finger. The phase of pallor is followed by a phase of reactive hyperaemia.

gentle squeezing of the muscle group. Fasciotomy is the treatment of choice (fig. **1.89**).

RAYNAUD'S SYNDROME

Raynaud's syndrome affects 5–10% of the adult population worldwide, especially young women, and is characterized by recurrent vasospastic episodes in which one or more fingers becomes white and numb, followed after a few minutes by a blue or purple cyanosis and then by redness caused by reactive arterial dilatation (**5.162**). The toes are rarely affected. The attacks are usually bilateral and symmetrical and may have a familial incidence and follow a benign course. They often start in the early teens and abate at the menopause. These attacks (primary Raynaud's syndrome) are often precipitated by exposure to cold or by emotion. Most patients have no evidence of any other disease process and are only inconvenienced by the attack. Rarely the signs progress to finger tip ulceration and gangrene (**5.163**).

Secondary Raynaud's syndrome implies that the features are a result of an underlying disease (**5.164**). This is most likely if the condition starts later in life, is seen in a man, is unilateral, or has an abrupt onset with rapid development of digital ulceration and gangrene. About 20% of patients with Raynaud's syndrome ultimately develop features of rheumatic disease or a connective tissue disorder. Examination of nailfold capillaries and a serum autoantibody profile will predict most of those who will subsequently develop systemic sclerosis.

It is important to enquire about cigarette smoking and the use of beta-blocking drugs, oral contraceptives or ergot derivatives, and about the handling of vibrating tools such as drills, chain saws or electric hammers (vibration white finger) (**5.165**). The position of the arm before the onset of symptoms may suggest a thoracic outlet syndrome (*see* **p. 249**).

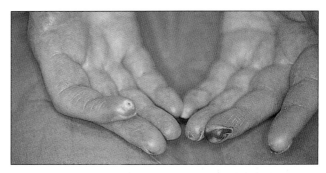

5.163 Primary Raynaud's syndrome occasionally progresses to fingertip ulceration or even gangrene. This 40-year-old woman had small, painful recurrent necrotic ulcers of the fingertips, wasting of the pulps and irregular nail growth. A larger area of gangrene has now developed.

DISEASES ASSOCIATED WITH SECONDARY RAYNAUD'S SYNDROME
Connective tissue disorders, especially SLE and systemic sclerosis
Drug or chemical associated – especially nicotine, oral contraceptives, beta-blockers, ergot derivatives, bleomycin, cisplatin
Vibration tool associated ('vibration white finger')
Thoracic outlet syndrome/carpal tunnel syndrome
Atherosclerosis
Thrombo-angiitis obliterans
Malignancy
Hyperviscosity syndromes/monoclonal gammopathy
Polycythaemia/cold agglutinin disorders

5.164 Diseases associated with secondary Raynaud's syndrome.

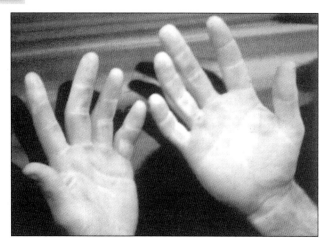

5.165 Vibration white finger. This patient developed painful vasospasm in most fingers on both hands as a result of continual use of a chainsaw. His symptoms appeared within a year of starting this work.

The extent and severity of Raynaud's disease may be assessed by thermography (**5.166**).

In the primary form, the prognosis is very good and treatment is directed at prevention of attacks by keeping the hands (and feet) warm. Electrically heated gloves are usually effective. The patient should stop smoking and stop taking any relevant drugs that predispose to the condition. Change of employment is sometimes necessary.

In secondary Raynaud's, an attempt must be made to identify and treat the underlying condition. Cervical

sympathectomy is rarely of value. Treatment with a calcium-channel blocker and transdermal prostacyclin is often effective.

COLD INJURY

Cooling of tissues produces vasoconstriction, increase in plasma and whole blood viscosity, and impairment of oxygen transport. Below freezing point, these changes are compounded by the formation of ice crystals, which produce irreversible cell death.

'Immersion' or 'trench' foot is a result of wet, cold exposure of the feet over a prolonged period. There are recognizable phases: initially, there is an ischaemic phase when the feet are cold, white and pulseless, followed by a hyperaemic response, when they become painful, red and oedematous. They may eventually recover, but superficial areas of skin gangrene may require grafting. In frostbite, the blood supply is permanently damaged and tissue necrosis occurs in the exposed extremities. The area is usually numb and bloodless. Rewarming is associated with local pain (**5.167**) and the development of a demarcation zone between viable and non-viable tissues. Gangrene may result (**5.168**). Chemical or surgical sympathectomy may be of value.

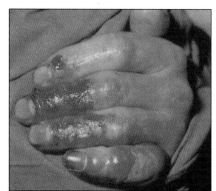

5.167 Frostbite of the hand in a mountaineer. On rewarming, the hand became painful, red and oedematous, with signs of probable gangrene in the fifth finger.

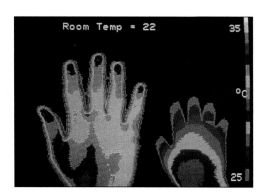

5.166 Thermography may be used to assess the extent and severity of Raynaud's disease. This is a method of displaying infrared radiation from the skin. The left picture was obtained at a room temperature of 22°C, and hand blood flow was adequate at that time, as evidenced by the full image of the hand and its colour (note the colour/temperature scale to the right of the picture). The provocative test was to immerse the hand for 2 minutes in ice-water, and the result is shown in the right picture, in which the dominant colours are blue and purple; the circulation to the distal part of the digits has totally disappeared. This is a very abnormal reaction which confirms vasospastic disease.

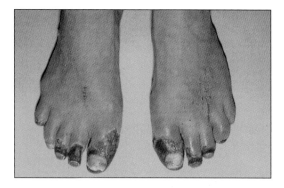

5.168 Gangrene after frostbite. The patient had been sleeping rough in the winter in London. He developed symmetrical changes in both feet, requiring the amputation of some toes.

HYPOTHERMIA

A fall in the core temperature of the body may result from a variety of illnesses such as myxoedema, Addison's disease, hyperglycaemia, stroke, myocardial infarction and the ingestion of drugs or alcohol. It is especially likely to occur in the elderly. Hypothermia may also occur accidentally in those injured or immersed in snow or icy water or exposed to cold, wet and windy conditions. Often multiple factors play a role, for example the alcoholic lying comatose outside in the winter, or the isolated elderly stroke patient falling in an unheated house. The rate of loss of heat depends on factors such as nutritional status, clothing, recent alcohol or drug ingestion and the ambient temperature.

The clinical features depend on the core temperature. Mild hypothermia (core temperature 35–37°C) usually only causes discomfort: the patient feels cold and shivers, but remains mentally alert and is often able to take appropriate action to reverse the decline in temperature. Below this level there is progressive impairment of higher cerebral function with loss of coordination, judgement and eventually loss of consciousness. Below a temperature of 32°C there is an exponential rise in mortality.

Patients usually appear cold and pale, with bradycardia, hypotension, slow respiration and an appearance of rigor mortis. Laboratory investigations show acidosis, haemo-concentration and renal impairment. There is peripheral hypoxia as the low temperature drives the oxygen dissociation curve to the left – there is decreased unloading of oxygen in the periphery. Central nervous reflexes (e.g. pupillary responses) become progressively impaired. Ventricular arrhythmias (tachycardia or fibrillation) are the common cause of death, but a variety of changes may be found on the ECG, for example bradycardia, slow atrial fibrillation and a characteristic J wave (**5.169**).

Treatment of minor degrees of hypothermia can be achieved by gradual rewarming in a heated room or bed, use of a 'space blanket' (**5.170**) and general supportive measures. Most patients with temperatures over 32°C respond to these simple measures. In severe hypothermia the patient should also be well oxygenated and attention should be paid to correction of the fluid and metabolic disturbance. External warming with an electric blanket is contraindicated, but intravenous fluids and peritoneal dialysis fluid (if needed for renal failure) should be warmed. Antibiotics should be given, as these patients are likely to develop pneumonia.

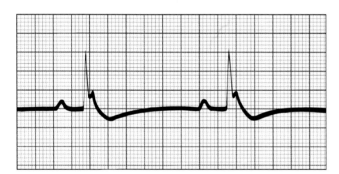

5.169 Hypothermia. The characteristic finding is the J wave (Osborne wave), a positive wave occurring on the down slope of the QRS complex. It is seen in most leads and broadens and increases its size as the body temperature drops.

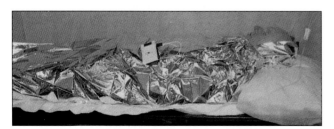

5.170 Treatment of hypothermia. A 'space blanket' is useful for slow rewarming. A constant-reading digital electronic rectal thermometer is in place. An intravenous infusion and a central venous pressure line are established, so that any hypotension caused by vasodilatation as warming occurs can be safely corrected.

AORTIC DISEASES

ANEURYSMS

An aneurysm is an abnormal widening of an artery that involves all four coats. In the aorta they may occur in the thoracic and abdominal segments.

Abdominal aneurysms

Abdominal aneurysms are most common in men aged over 50 years whose vessels are arteriosclerotic. They may be found by chance on routine abdominal palpation or on X-ray. Occasionally, patients complain of pain in the epigastrium that radiates into the flanks. Rarely, they present with a dramatic onset of abdominal pain and severe hypotension (leading to death) caused by rupture. As an aneurysm enlarges, concentric layers of thrombus are laid down; in a large aneurysm this may be the source of disseminated intravascular coagulation (DIC) with consumption of clotting factors and platelets. Multiple emboli may also originate from this thrombus and occlude the vessels of the toes and feet. Occasionally, the enlarging aneurysm may erode into the vena cava or bowel to form a fistula.

The diagnosis may be made (often coincidentally) on plain X-ray (**5.171**), but ultrasound (**5.172**) is the diagnostic method of choice, and may be used for screening purposes. CT scan (**5.173**) and (occasionally) angiography (**5.174**) may be used for presurgical assessment.

The risk of rupture increases exponentially in aneurysms above 5.5–6.0 cm in diameter and it is now usual to intervene if the aneurysm exceeds 5.5 cm. The aneurysm may be repaired by

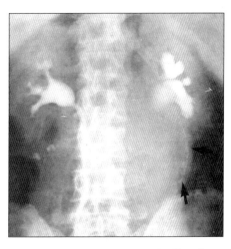

5.171 Abdominal aortic aneurysm. Aortic dilatation and calcification (arrowed) was an incidental finding during an intravenous urogram (the IVU also shows dilatation of the left renal pelvis).

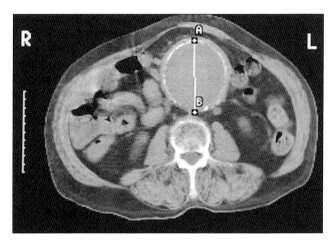

5.173 Abdominal aortic aneurysm on CT. This is a sensitive imaging method that allows precise measurement of size (point A to point B) and demonstrates the thickened wall of the aneurysm.

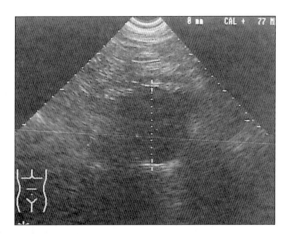

5.172 Abdominal aortic aneurysm revealed by ultrasound. The aorta is grossly and irregularly dilated. Note the presence of echogenic material in the lumen, representing layers of thrombus. The diameter of lumen was 6.2 cm (a diameter over 5.5 cm is an indication for operative intervention). Examination at a higher level showed that the aneurysm started below the renal arteries, so immediate aortic bifurcation grafting was performed.

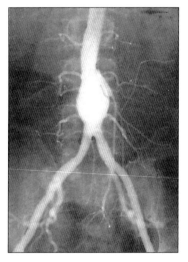

5.174 Small abdominal aortic aneurysm revealed on aortography. The diagnosis was suspected by the presence of an abdominal bruit. Ultrasound and CT now prevent the need for routine aortography.

use of an endoprosthesis delivered via the femoral artery. This is particularly valuable for patients with coexistent disease. Studies are in progress to compare this approach with conventional surgical repair. Elective surgery carries a mortality of 5–10% and emergency surgery has a mortality of over 50%.

A positive family history increases the risk of abdominal aortic aneurysm, so first-degree relatives should ideally be screened by ultrasound.

Thoracic aneurysms

Thoracic aneurysms are historically associated with the long-term complications of syphilitic aortitis (**1.192**) and may involve the ascending or descending thoracic aorta or the arch. Aneurysms of the ascending aorta may involve the ostia of the coronary arteries and the aortic valve, so that diastolic filling of the coronary arteries is defective and the patient has angina pectoris. Massive enlargement may lead to a pulsatile painful mass in the anterior chest wall as the ribs and sternum are eroded. Aneurysmal dilatation of the arch may compress the left main bronchus to produce respiratory difficulty from atelectasis, a 'brassy' cough, a tracheal tug and paralysis of the left recurrent laryngeal nerve, and occasionally a left-sided Horner's syndrome. Compression of the oesophagus may cause dysphagia, and rupture may occur into the oesophagus, bronchus or externally. The diagnosis of syphilis should be confirmed serologically and treated with an appropriate antibiotic regime. These aneurysms are now extremely rare in the developed world, but non-syphilitic aneurysms of the descending thoracic aorta may be found at routine X-ray examination (**5.175**) and are often symptomless. They may be further investigated by CT (**5.176**) or MRI.

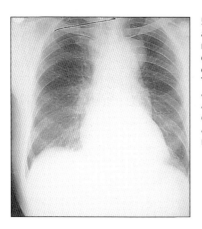

5.175 An aortic aneurysm occurring as a mediastinal mass on chest X-ray at the level of the aortic knuckle. This alone does not allow a firm diagnosis, and the differential diagnosis could include a mass in the mediastinum or lung.

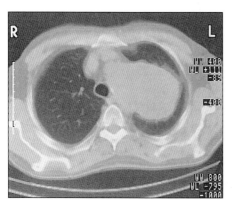

5.176 CT at the level of the aortic arch, demonstrating a large aortic aneurysm. An enhanced image is required to exclude the possibility of a dissecting aneurysm (*see* **5.179**).

Other aneurysms

Aneurysms may develop in many other situations in the arterial tree:

- Berry aneurysms in the circle of Willis result from genetic weakness at the bifurcation of vessels and probably represent developmental defects in the media and elastic fibres. The aneurysmal sac gradually enlarges, and rupture may occur with extravasation of blood into the subarachnoid space (*see* **p. 477**)
- Mycotic aneurysms may form in any part of the arterial tree, but they are found most commonly in the cerebral circulation. They are associated with damage to the arterial wall caused by sepsis, which may be embolic in nature. They are rare in developed countries.
- Polyarteritis nodosa may be associated with the formation of multiple microaneurysms (*see* **p. 127**, **183**, **275**).

- Kawasaki syndrome is probably an infectious disease caused by an unknown agent, which causes arteritis and aneurysms of the coronary arteries (*see* **p. 57**).

AORTIC DISSECTION

Dissection of the aorta often begins with an intimal tear that allows blood to dissect into the media, forming a 'false channel' which may re-enter the lumen at a point further down. About one-half of cases involve the ascending aorta, one-third the arch and the rest are found in the descending aorta. The initial tear may occur spontaneously in patients with defects in the aortic wall (as seen in Marfan's syndrome, Ehlers–Danlos syndrome and cystic medial necrosis), in patients with coarctation of the aorta and in patients with hypertension; rarely, it may be iatrogenic, after angiography or coronary artery surgery.

The clinical presentation is usually a sudden onset of severe pain in the chest, abdomen or back. Ascending aortic dissection may involve the coronary ostia and the aortic valve, which may become acutely incompetent, and the patient may present with acute left ventricular failure or with acute myocardial infarction. Dissection of the arch may involve the arteries to the brain and upper limbs with hemiplegia or an ischaemic arm. Rupture may occur into the pericardium, mediastinum, left pleural cavity or abdomen.

The diagnosis can often be made clinically by the finding of absent or diminished pulses with differences in blood pressure, and it may be confirmed by X-ray (**5.177**). Transoesophageal

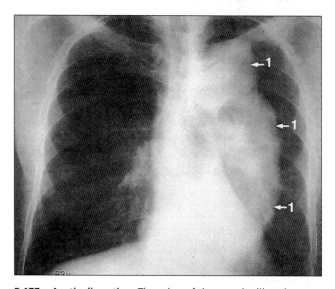

5.177 Aortic dissection. The edge of the grossly dilated descending aorta is marked (1) in this 53-year-old hypertensive man who presented with vague chest pains. Further investigation could include angiography, ultrasound, MRI or CT scan (*see* **5.179**).

echocardiography (**5.178**) is now the method of choice for diagnosing aortic root dissection, but the extent of dissecting aneurysms may also be investigated by angiography, CT (**5.179**, **5.180**) or MRI. ECG and normal serum enzyme levels exclude acute infarction. The high mortality varies with the site and length of dissection. Surgery is the only treatment and involves replacement or repair of the damaged wall if possible.

AORTIC ARCH SYNDROME

Aortic arch syndrome is a general term given to diseases of the aortic arch that interfere with blood flow in the major vessels of the arch, the innominate artery, the left common carotid artery and the left subclavian artery. A range of pathologies may produce this effect (**5.181**). The usual presentations result from cerebral ischaemia and impairment of upper arm circulation but sometimes the presenting features may relate to vascular disease elsewhere (**5.182**).

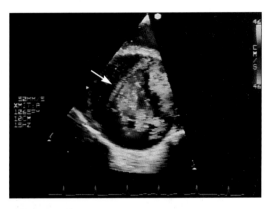

5.178 **Transoesophageal echocardiogram,** demonstrating a dissecting aneurysm of the aorta in a patient with Marfan's syndrome. This view of the ascending aorta shows a dilated aortic root with an obvious intimal flap (arrowed). The colour-flow image shows turbulent blood flow in the true lumen (blue and orange) with no flow in the dissected lumen.

CAUSES OF AORTIC ARCH SYNDROME
Atherosclerosis
Dissecting aneurysm
Takayasu's disease
Syphilis (aortitis and aneurysm)
Mycotic aneurysm
Relapsing polychondritis
Giant cell aortitis
Ankylosing spondylitis
Kawasaki syndrome

5.181 **Causes of aortic arch syndrome.**

5.179

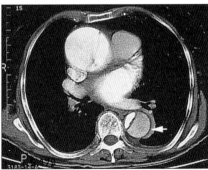

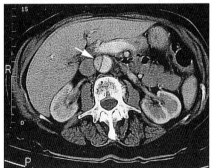

5.180

5.179 & 5.180 Dissecting aneurysm. Contrast-enhanced spiral CT demonstrates dissection of the ascending and descending aorta, extending down to the abdominal aorta below the origin of the renal arteries. In the descending aorta, the enhanced (white) part of the aneurysm represents the true lumen of the aorta through which blood is flowing. The outer, darker layer is the clot-filled 'false lumen' of the aneurysm (arrows).

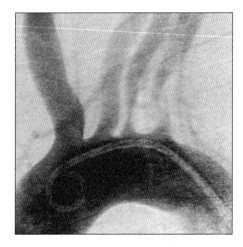

5.182 **Takayasu's disease** is a form of arteritis that mainly affects the aorta and its large branches and the pulmonary arteries, although this patient presented with unstable angina due to arteritic involvement of the coronary arteries. This digital subtraction angiogram shows the origin of four vessels from the aortic arch. From left to right in this view they are the innominate, left common carotid, an anomalous origin of the left vertebral and the left subclavian artery. The vertebral and subclavian arteries have discrete stenoses near their origins. The cause of Takayasu's disease is unknown. It may respond to systemic steroid therapy, but surgical treatment may also be necessary when major cerebral or other impairment is present.

Isolated proximal occlusion of the subclavian artery may be associated with the subclavian steal syndrome, in which the distal subclavian artery is perfused by retrograde flow through the ipsilateral vertebral artery. The 'steal' of blood via the circle of Willis may result in symptoms and signs of cerebral ischaemia when the arm is used. Aortic arch syndrome may be investigated by digital subtraction angiography (**5.183**, **5.184**) or, non-invasively, by magnetic resonance angiography (MRA).

The diagnosis is made clinically by abducting the arm to 90° and rotating it externally. This leads to disappearance of the radial pulse, a bruit over the subclavian artery and the appearance of symptoms. The scalene manoeuvre (Adson's test) consists of rotating and hyperextending the neck. This produces subclavian compression and similar symptoms and signs. X-ray of the thoracic inlet may show unilateral or bilateral cervical ribs or a rudimentary cervical rib, which is often associated with a fibrous band (**5.185**). Treatment is surgical removal of the rib(s).

5.183

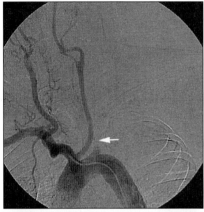

5.183 & 5.184 Subclavian steal syndrome, confirmed by digital subtraction angiography. The left subclavian artery is occluded just beyond its origin (arrow, **5.183**). A delayed film (**5.184**) shows filling of the subclavian artery (S) beyond the occlusion by reverse flow through the vertebral artery (V).

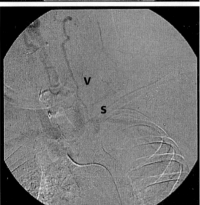

5.184

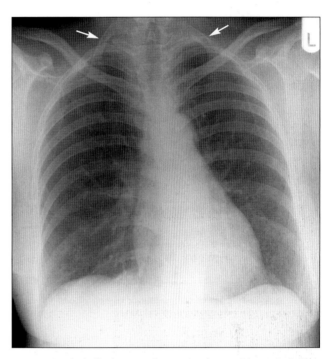

5.185 Cervical ribs (arrowed). Most patients with cervical ribs are asymptomatic, but some may develop thoracic outlet syndromes. This patient presented with bilateral Raynaud's phenomenon and has an obvious right-sided cervical rib. There is fusion of a left-sided rib with the first rib.

249

THORACIC OUTLET SYNDROMES

The neurovascular bundle that supplies the upper limb lies in the angle between the scalenus anterior muscle and the first rib. An extra rib (cervical rib), or a fibrous band equivalent to it, may compress the lower trunk of the brachial plexus (C8, T1) and the subclavian artery when the shoulder is abducted. Patients are often aware of the association between symptoms of paraesthesiae, numbness and blanching of the fingers and arm position and their immediate disappearance when the arm is returned to the side. Eventually aneurysmal dilatation of the artery occurs, which may be associated with peripheral ischaemic episodes, Raynaud's phenomenon and emboli.

VENOUS THROMBOSIS AND PULMONARY EMBOLISM

One of the most common causes of preventable death in developed countries is pulmonary embolism after deep vein thrombosis. Autopsies carried out in hospitalized patients show that up to 25% of all deaths are associated with pulmonary embolism, and it is estimated that in over one-half of these deaths venous thrombosis and pulmonary embolism were the main cause. About 1% of all hospitalized patients may die from pulmonary embolism. Most emboli originate in the deep veins of the legs; only a small number originate from the pelvis and the inferior vena cava. The types of patients who are at risk of deep vein thrombosis are shown in **5.186** and these risks are important when considering patients for prophylaxis,

RISK FACTORS FOR THROMBOEMBOLIC COMPLICATIONS

Over 40 years old

Obesity

Malignancy

Infection/inflammation

Previous thromboembolism

Family history of thromboembolism

Some haematological and biochemical abnormalities, e.g. polycythaemia, thrombophilias

Heart failure

Varicose veins

Trauma

Re-operation

Oestrogen therapy

Renal transplant recipients

Paralysis

Immobility (e.g. during long-distance flight)

Types of surgery:

  – knee surgery
  – hip fracture surgery
  – elective hip surgery
  – retropubic prostatectomy
  – general abdominal surgery
  – gynaecological surgery
  – neurosurgery

5.186   Risk factors for thromboembolic complications following surgery or during medical care.

which has now been shown to prevent deep vein thrombosis and pulmonary embolism without significant side-effects in most patients. The appropriate pharmacological prophylaxis in most patients is low dose heparin or low molecular weight heparin. This should be given by subcutaneous injection in the anterior abdominal wall (**5.187**), and may sometimes lead to

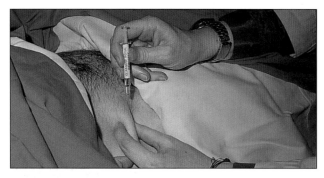

5.187   Thromboprophylaxis with subcutaneous heparin (or low molecular weight heparin) is effective in reducing the risk of deep vein thrombosis in medical and surgical settings. The injections should be given subcutaneously into the anterior abdominal wall.

multiple local haematomas (**5.188**). Prophylaxis also prevents the development of the post-phlebitic limb, which is estimated to affect about 5% of the population.

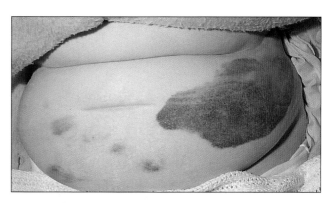

5.188   Multiple abdominal wall haematomas resulting from regular prophylactic subcutaneous heparin injections. Though relatively common, this complication is usually harmless and is not a contraindication to the continuation of prophylaxis. The appearance may, however, alarm inexperienced staff.

DEEP VEIN THROMBOSIS (DVT)

Deep vein thrombosis (DVT) is common, but its clinical history and signs are very unreliable. Up to one-half of the patient group may have no leg symptoms or signs before presenting with a pulmonary embolism and even leg symptoms are non-specific (**5.189**). A high index of suspicion is essential, especially in the at risk patients listed in **5.186**. The patient may be aware of changes in skin colour, from normal to a dusky blue or a waxy white, and this is usually associated with swelling. Signs may be present (**5.190**), but are non-specific and always require further investigation. The classic sign of unilateral oedematous leg swelling (**5.191**) is seen in less than 50% of cases of DVT. Varicose veins (**5.192**) are a common association. Superficial thrombophlebitis that migrates is often a sign of internal malignancy (**9.73**).

Massive occluding thrombosis in the femoral veins may lead to phlegmasia cerulea dolens and venous gangrene. This is heralded by acute pain in the leg, woody hard oedema and deep cyanosis from the toes to the groin (**5.193**). Multiple petechial haemorrhages develop, followed by exquisitely painful areas of gangrene of skin and subcutaneous tissue on the dorsum of the foot and skin.

The diagnosis of DVT is made by venography (**5.194**) or, for DVT above the knee, by ultrasound scanning (**5.195**). The differential diagnosis includes muscle strain, muscle haematoma, ruptured Baker's cyst (**3.26–3.28**), cellulitis, lymphatic obstruction and other causes of oedema.

Treatment of DVT is with heparin followed by warfarin for at least 3–6 months. Analgesics, support stockings, and occasionally surgery or fibrinolytic therapy may also be of value. Prevention of DVT should be considered in all hospitalized

POSSIBLE SYMPTOMS IN DEEP VEIN THROMBOSIS (DVT)

Cramping pains in the calf or thigh (usually in one leg)

Tenderness to touch or movement

Swelling and tightness

Discoloration, ranging from white to deep purple

No symptoms in the legs:

- presentation with pulmonary embolism
- sudden death
- detected in a screening test

5.189   Possible symptoms in deep vein thrombosis.

SIGNS THAT MAY INDICATE DEEP VEIN THROMBOSIS (DVT) BUT ARE NON-SPECIFIC

Swelling with some pitting oedema on the dorsum of the foot or ankle

Pain in the calf on gentle compression, in the popliteal fossa and along the line of the femoral vein

Colour changes

Increased temperature that tends to be generalized in the whole limb

Dilatation of the superficial veins, particularly around the ankles

Signs of pulmonary embolism

No apparent signs – the patient has been diagnosed by a screening test because of a high-risk situation

5.190   Signs that may indicate deep vein thrombosis (DVT), but are non-specific. All require further investigation. In one-half of patients with these signs, no DVT is detected on venography, and an alternative diagnosis must be sought.

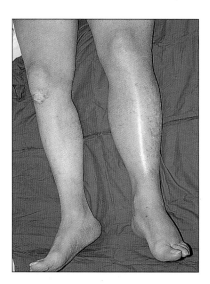

5.191   Deep vein thrombosis, presenting as an acutely swollen left leg. Note the dilatation of the superficial veins. The leg was hot to the touch, and palpation along the line of the left popliteal and femoral veins caused pain. Less than 50% of DVTs present in this way, and other conditions may mimic DVT, so further investigation is always indicated. Note the coincidental psoriatic lesion below the patient's right knee.

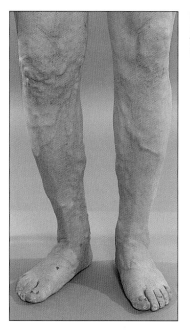

5.192   Varicose veins are a risk factor for deep vein thrombosis and may result from it.

251

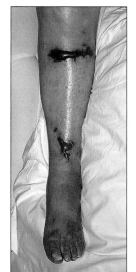

5.193   Phlegmasia cerulea dolens. The painful, swollen, blue leg results from vascular stasis caused by massive venous thrombosis, and it may lead to venous gangrene unless the resulting high tissue pressure is relieved by thrombectomy. In this patient, blood-filled blisters and gangrene of the toes have already developed. This is a relatively rare presentation of deep vein thrombosis. Most patients have few, if any, signs.

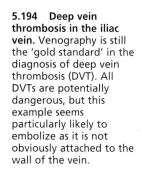

5.194   Deep vein thrombosis in the iliac vein. Venography is still the 'gold standard' in the diagnosis of deep vein thrombosis (DVT). All DVTs are potentially dangerous, but this example seems particularly likely to embolize as it is not obviously attached to the wall of the vein.

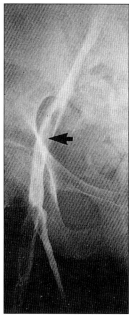

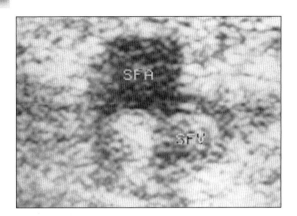

5.195   Venous duplex examination. A thrombus is seen in the femoral vein (SFV). This reduces flow through the vein and renders it relatively incompressible. This technique provides both flow dynamics and an image of the vessel under investigation. It combines pulsed Doppler waveform analysis with B-mode Doppler images of the vessel. It is now accepted as the first-line investigation for detecting significant lower and upper limb deep vein thrombosis (DVT). It can detect most clinically relevant DVTs above the knee but is poor at detecting calf vein thrombosis. SFA = femoral artery.

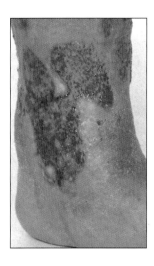

5.196   'Varicose' ulceration of the leg is usually a long-term complication of deep vein thrombosis. These ulcers can be extensive and indolent.

patients at medium to high risk and this involves the use of support stockings and low doses of heparin or related compounds (**5.187**).

DVT is uncommon in the upper limbs. When it does occur, there may be a history of recent physical activity or of rest or coma in which the arms may have been held in an unusual position or compressed. Underlying malignant disease is another important cause (**9.73**). The presenting features are similar to those in the lower limb, but there are rarely any significant sequelae. Treatment is with a short course of anticoagulants.

Thrombophilia
Patients with DVT or pulmonary embolism who do not fall into a clear at-risk category should be screened for causes of thrombophilia (*see* **p. 442**). If abnormalities are found, long-term anticoagulation is usually indicated.

Post-phlebitic syndrome
Thrombosis in the leg veins is usually centred around venous valve cusps. Resolution of the thrombus often leaves the valve leaflets damaged and incompetent; retrograde flow occurs, and this increased venous pressure distends the distal veins and makes the blood follow different pathways, especially after prolonged standing and after exercise. The long-term result is varicose veins that are under increased pressure (**5.192**). Recurrent minor haemorrhages lead to deposition of iron in the skin, which becomes brown-stained and firm from the deposition of fibrous tissue. Local anoxia and oedema lead to ulceration, often around the medial malleolus, which tends to be resistant to healing (**5.196**). Treatment should be directed at

reduction of the hydrostatic pressure by the use of support hose and healing of the ulcer by elevation of the limb and, if necessary, by plastic surgery.

PULMONARY EMBOLISM

Acute pulmonary embolism is the impaction of one or more emboli in the pulmonary circulation. It is usually the sequel of venous thrombosis in the legs, is a major cause of morbidity and causes significant avoidable mortality. The clinical presentation is often dramatic, with the sudden death of a patient who was expected to recover uneventfully from major surgery. Sometimes there are preceding symptoms, such as chest discomfort, wheeze, cough or syncopal attacks. These result from small emboli ('herald' emboli), but the symptoms are often ignored. Often there are no specific symptoms or signs, and it is the suspicious mind of the vigilant clinician that will trigger the appropriate investigations.

Symptoms that may be present in established embolism include dyspnoea, pleuritic chest pain, cough, apprehension, haemoptysis, sweating and syncope. Signs are not specific, but may include increased respiratory rate (> 20/min), pulmonary crackles, an accentuated pulmonary second sound, a rapid pulse rate (> 100 bpm), fever, phlebitis, sweating, pleural friction rub and cyanosis. A range of abnormalities is usually present in the ECG, reflecting the sudden increase in right ventricular strain (e.g. arrhythmias, axis deviation and right bundle branch block, acute cor pulmonale (S1, Q3, T3), the development of P pulmonale and T-wave abnormalities, **5.197**). The plain X-ray of the chest may be totally normal or, in a minority of cases, may show an infiltrate or consolidation, a high hemidiaphragm, pleural effusion, atelectasis or focal oligaemia (**5.198**).

The diagnosis depends on a ventilation/perfusion scan of the lungs (V/Q) using radioactive xenon gas for the ventilation part and technetium-labelled macroaggregates of human serum albumin for the perfusion part (**4.45**, **4.46**, **5.199**). The 'gold standard' test is pulmonary angiography (**5.200**), but this is

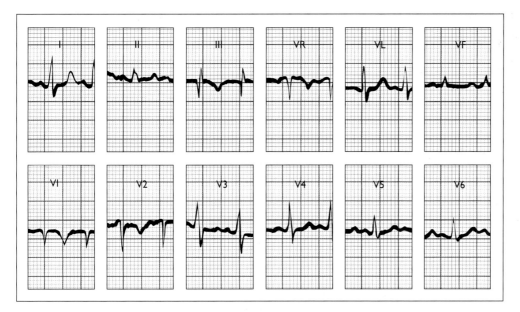

5.197 Acute pulmonary embolism. The classic changes are seen in the ECG. They include tachycardia, right-axis deviation, the appearance of an S wave in lead I and a Q wave in lead III, T-wave inversion in III and over the right ventricle, and right ventricular conduction delay. The changes are often slight and easily overlooked. More major changes may occur in massive pulmonary embolism.

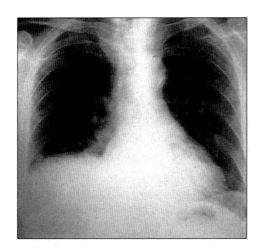

5.198 Pulmonary embolism. The chest X-ray is rarely diagnostic. In this patient it showed a raised right hemidiaphragm, some right basal shadowing and blunting of the right costophrenic angle. The diagnosis is unclear, but the combination of a history of right-sided chest pain and slight haemoptysis with these findings was an indication to proceed to lung scanning (**5.199**).

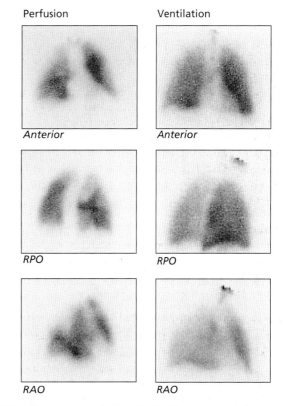

Perfusion   Ventilation

Anterior   *Anterior*

RPO   *RPO*

RAO   *RAO*

5.199 Pulmonary embolism. Ventilation and perfusion scintigrams in pulmonary embolism. There are multiple perfusion defects with normal ventilation in the same areas. This combination gives a high probability of a diagnosis of pulmonary embolism (RPO = right posterior oblique view; RAO = right anterior oblique view).

invasive and carries a small morbidity and mortality. The legs should also be examined and an ultrasound scan may define the source of the emboli. Treatment is with anticoagulant doses of heparin followed by warfarin for at least 3–6 months. Fibrinolytic agents may be used in the acute stage and emergency surgery to remove a massive embolus is occasionally life-saving. The insertion of a filter device in the vena cava (**5.201**) may prevent recurrent embolization in patients who cannot be successfully or safely treated with long-term anticoagulants.

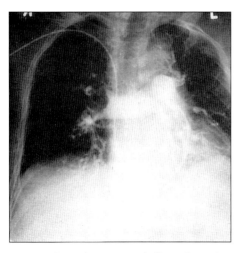

5.200 Acute massive pulmonary embolism. This pulmonary angiogram shows some filling of the left upper and lower segmental vessels only. The remaining vessels show near-total embolic occlusion. This patient responded well to streptokinase infusion.

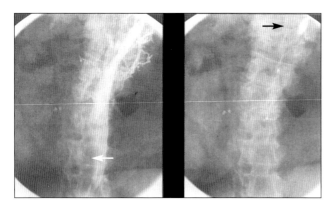

5.201 Vena caval filter. The venogram on the left showed a large intracaval thrombus (arrow). The plain film on the right shows an umbrella-shaped metal filter (arrow), which was inserted via a venous catheter. The insertion of such a device should be considered in the management of pulmonary embolus if there is a strong contraindication to anticoagulation, if there are recurrent pulmonary emboli despite adequate anticoagulation or if an ascending venogram reveals intracaval or free clot, which carry a high risk of massive pulmonary embolism.

DISORDERS OF PERIPHERAL LYMPHATICS

LYMPHANGITIS

Lymphangitis is an acute inflammation of peripheral lymphatic vessels in which a focus of infection, usually on the skin and usually caused by streptococci, drains to the regional lymph nodes and causes an acute inflammatory reaction, with redness, swelling, oedema and pain in the lymphatic vessels and nodes (*see* **p. 26**).

LYMPHOEDEMA

Oedema that results from blockage of the lymphatic drainage of a limb is termed lymphoedema. It may be secondary or primary. Secondary causes are more common and include infiltration with neoplasm, parasitic infiltration (**1.155**, **1.156**), and surgical operations or radiotherapy (**5.202**) that remove or damage lymphatics. Primary disorders result from a hereditary abnormality in the formation of the lymphatics. The most common of these is Milroy's disease but lymphoedema may also be found in ovarian dysgenesis, Noonan's syndrome and other genetic disorders.

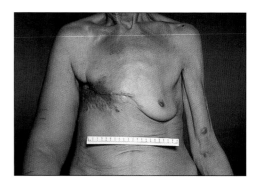

5.202 Lymphoedema of the upper limb is extremely common in women with breast carcinoma. This may be due to infiltration of lymphatics by tumour or, as in this case, it often occurs after extensive surgery where lymphatics and nodes have been dissected out and the patient has been treated by radiotherapy.

The onset of the condition varies according to the cause. Oedema is usually easily pitted, but as the disease becomes more chronic, the limb becomes hard and woody and the skin thickened and wrinkled. The diagnosis is made on isotope lymphangiography or lymphangiography (**5.203**).

Lymphoedema is a difficult condition to treat adequately, but elevation of the limb or compression bandages may help. Surgery has little to offer.

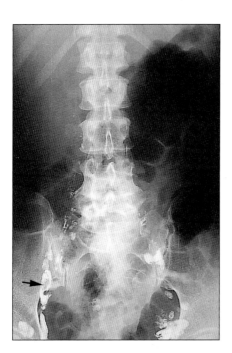

5.203 Lymphangiogram in a woman with bilateral leg oedema and carcinoma of the cervix. Invasion of lymph nodes by tumour is clearly seen, especially in the large node on the right (arrow).

6 Renal

HISTORY

A full medical history is important in any patient with suspected renal disease. Specific questions should be asked about current features and symptoms, including:

- Urine volume: high in diabetes mellitus, diabetes insipidus or with loss of renal concentration; low in advanced renal failure or urinary tract obstruction.
- Frequency of micturition or presence of nocturia, or both: high frequency associated with high urine volume or urinary infection.
- Urine appearance and colour – may be affected by a range of disorders or ingested substances; painless haematuria may be a sign of urological malignancy and requires urgent investigation.
- Pain: in loins, back, abdomen, suprapubic area? Constant or intermittent? Related to micturition? Pain may result from infection, stones, tumour or inherited renal or urinary tract disorders.
- Non-specific symptoms associated with renal failure, including; fatigue, nausea, weight loss, pallor, easy bruising and symptoms associated with heart failure (*see* **p. 206**).

Remember that the kidney has endocrine as well as excretory functions.

EXAMINATION

On general examination, there may be few, if any, abnormal findings in patients with urinary infections, renal calculi or other uncomplicated renal disorders; even some patients with acute renal failure may appear physically normal.

In acute nephritis, the patient (often a child) develops acute facial puffiness (**6.1**) and hypertension in association with haematuria, proteinuria and oliguria, whereas in the nephrotic syndrome there is usually severe oedema and ascites (**6.2**).

Chronic renal failure (CRF) is usually associated with a wide range of signs (**6.3–6.5**). Anaemia is usual in end stage renal failure and its cause is multifactorial (*see* **p. 266**).

Where renal disease is part of a multisystem disorder (diabetes mellitus, systemic lupus erythematosus (SLE), etc.), there may be other signs of the primary disease.

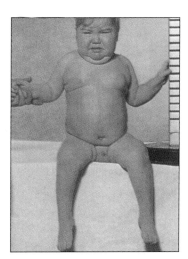

6.2 Nephrotic syndrome in a young boy. Note the severe generalized facial and body oedema. The facial oedema gives him a cushingoid appearance, but this picture was taken before he started on steroid therapy. He also had ascites.

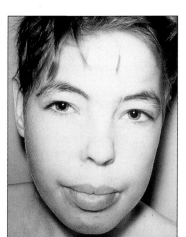

6.1 Acute nephritis. The generalized facial puffiness and the erythematous periorbital oedema are typical, and this boy also had ankle oedema and hypertension.

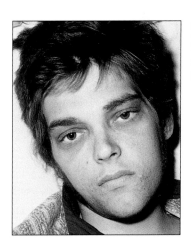

6.3 Uraemic facies. Note the pale, sallow, yellow-brown appearance of the skin and the anaemic pallor of the sclerae.

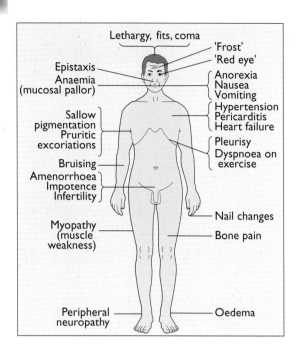

6.4   Chronic renal failure: common symptoms and signs.

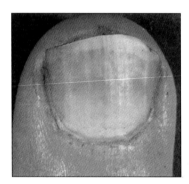

6.5   The nail in chronic renal failure. Various nail changes may be observed, including those seen here: discoloration of the distal nail, pallor of the proximal nail and lunula and pigmentation of the skin at the base of the nail.

INVESTIGATIONS

Investigations in renal disease have three main purposes:

* to establish a diagnosis
* to assess the complications of impaired renal function
* to monitor the progress of the disease or its response to therapy, or both; the ideal sequence of investigations depends upon the clinical picture, but a widely applicable approach is summarized in **6.6**.

INVESTIGATIONS ON URINE AND BLOOD

* Urine test sticks (**6.7**, **6.8**) should, as a minimum, test for pH, glucose, blood and protein, and usually also for ketones,

INVESTIGATIONS IN RENAL AND URINARY TRACT DISEASE

Initial investigations

Urine stick test
– specific gravity
– blood
– protein
– glucose
– nitrite
– pH

Urine microscopy
– red and white cells
– casts
– crystals
– epithelial cells
– parasites

Midstream urine for culture
Plasma
– urea
– creatinine
– electrolytes: sodium, potassium, chloride, bicarbonate, calcium, phosphate
– prostate-specific antigen (PSA)

Haematology
– full blood count

Investigations used commonly

24-hour urine collection
– creatinine clearance
– protein excretion

Ultrasound

Plain X-ray of renal tract
– kidney, ureters, bladder (KUB)

Intravenous urogram (IVU)

Specialized investigations

Serum complement and autoantibodies

Further radiology, including CT and MRI

Isotope scans

Specialized renal tubule function tests

Biopsy

Cytoscopy

Other tests for multisystem diseases

6.6   The investigation of patients with suspected renal disease.

bilirubin, urobilinogen and nitrites; the nitrite test is a simple screening test for the presence of infection, as many urinary pathogens convert dietary nitrates to nitrites; a positive nitrite test is an indication for urine culture.
* Urine microscopy, including phase-contrast microscopy, may identify red cells (**6.9**), white cells, casts (**6.10**), crystals, urinary tract epithelial cells or parasites.

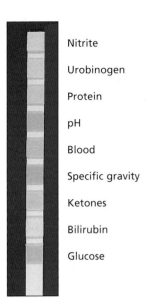

Nitrite

Urobinogen

Protein

pH

Blood

Specific gravity

Ketones

Bilirubin

Glucose

6.7 A typical urine test stick, which provides instant measurement of a range of possible abnormalities in the urine.

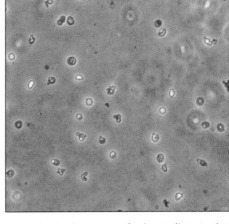

6.9 Phase-contrast microscopy of urine sediment, showing a wide range of dysmorphic red cells. In fresh urine, dysmorphic red cells imply glomerular bleeding. In lower urinary tract bleeding, the red cells appear similar to one another (isomorphic). Patients with isomorphic red cells in the urine require further detailed urological investigation, whereas patients with dysmorphic red cells require further investigation for possible renal disease.

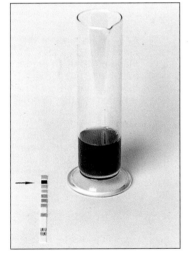

6.8 A positive result for blood (arrowed) occurred when this reddish-brown urine was tested with a standard stick.

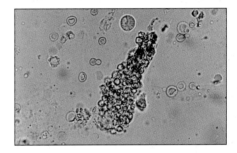

6.10 A red-cell cast, seen on direct microscopy of urine from a patient with the acute nephritic syndrome. The presence and nature of casts in the urine provide clues to the nature of the underlying renal disease: for example, red-cell casts imply bleeding at the glomerular level, whereas white-cell casts are seen most commonly in acute bacterial pyelonephritis.

- Urine culture. In women especially, urine culture samples must be collected with care to avoid contamination – usually in midstream after washing the external genitalia. Urine may be cultured on a plate or on a dip-slide impregnated with culture medium (**6.11**); if there is a suspicion of urinary tract tuberculosis, three early-morning samples may be required for concentration and culture.
- Plasma biochemistry provides an initial assessment of renal function; as most laboratories now use automated systems, the urea, creatinine, sodium, potassium, chloride and bicarbonate levels are usually accompanied by calcium, phosphate and alkaline phosphatase results and the albumin level, which allows correction of the calcium value; complement (C3, C4) values may be helpful; cholesterol elevation is found in nephrotic syndrome, and may be associated with premature vascular disease.

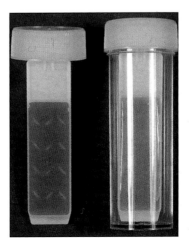

6.11 A dip-slide coated with culture medium (CLED – green; MacConkey – brown) may be used to start urine culture away from the laboratory, in general practice or in the clinic.

• Haematology profile. A fall in haemoglobin is invariable, as renal function and the production of endogenous erythropoietin decline; a normochromic normocytic anaemia may be complicated by acute episodes of haemolysis (micro-angiopathic haemolytic anaemia, MAHA) or by iron deficiency; elevation of the white cell count is a good indicator of renal tract infection, and a decline reflects the response to antibiotic therapy; thrombocytopenia is found in the consumption coagulopathies associated with haemolytic uraemic syndrome (HUS).

• Urine biochemistry is used selectively to measure 24-hour excretion of creatinine, and thus calculate the creatinine clearance; the 'selectivity' of proteinuria can also be assessed. Electrophoresis may show the presence of kappa or lambda light chains and suggest a diagnosis of multiple myeloma (*see* **p. 444**).

• Passage of a stone or gravel may reflect a metabolic abnormality and all such materials passed should be analysed (*see* **p. 287**).

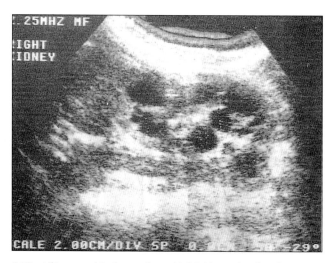

6.12 **Ultrasound** is the preferred initial investigation for kidney size, shape and position. This patient's large kidneys showed the typical appearance of polycystic kidneys. The multiple parenchymal cysts are clearly shown.

IMAGING

• Ultrasound is a low-cost, non-invasive and repeatable technique which determines kidney size, shape and position and the presence or absence of obstruction or space-occupying lesions; it is an ideal tool for screening relatives of patients with polycystic kidneys (**6.12**). Enlargement of the prostate may be further investigated by transrectal ultrasound. This allows repeated examination of patients with prostatic carcinoma to assess the presence and extent of local invasion (**6.112**); it is also used as guidance for prostatic biopsy. Ultrasound is of limited value in assessment of renal calculi and nephrocalcinosis.

• Plain X-ray of kidney, ureter and bladder (KUB) is a preliminary to specialized imaging. It is of value in detecting and following calcification in the kidney or stone in the renal tract (**6.13**) and may reveal other abnormalities.

• Intravenous urogram (IVU) requires the injection of a radio-opaque contrast medium; serial pictures reveal a nephrogram phase that shows lesions in the parenchyma and a pyelogram phase that outlines the renal collecting systems, ureters and bladder (**6.14**, **6.15**). In patients with diminished renal function, films taken many hours later may still show contrast medium. The IVU is the investigation of choice in acute renal colic.

• Renal arteriography allows precise anatomical demonstration of the branches of the renal arteries; this is of value in detecting stenosis (**6.87**), aneurysms (**6.70**) or a tumour circulation (**6.16**), although it is now rarely used in diagnosis or assessment of tumours. The quality of arteriography is enhanced by modern digital subtraction techniques (**6.17**) and in some circumstances adequate images may be obtained using an intravenous contrast medium bolus.

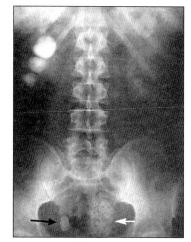

6.13 **Plain X-ray of the kidney, ureter and bladder (KUB)** is a useful initial investigation in many patients. Here it has revealed a rather unusual combination of calculi in both kidneys (more prominent on the right), in the lower right ureter (black arrow) and in a bladder diverticulum (white arrow).

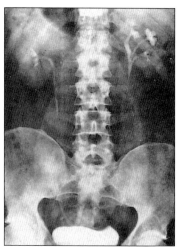

6.14 **Intravenous urogram showing a normal right kidney and ureter, but marked calyceal clubbing in the left kidney.** Note the gross dilatation of the calyces, especially in the middle and upper poles of the kidney. These changes were the result of unilateral reflux of urine and chronic infection.

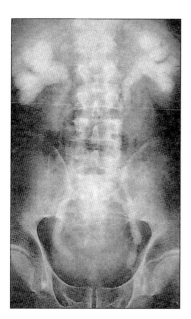

6.15 Intravenous urogram showing bilateral hydronephrosis and hydro-ureter with a large bladder. The changes are typical of an elderly patient with chronic urinary retention as a result of prostatic enlargement. Unless the bladder outflow obstruction is surgically relieved, the patient will develop progressive chronic renal failure.

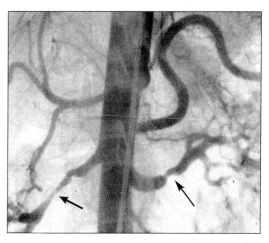

6.17 Aortogram (digital subtraction technique) showing bilateral renal artery stenosis (arrows). The appearances are typical of stenosis caused by fibro-muscular hyperplasia rather than atheroma. The stenoses were successfully treated by balloon angioplasty.

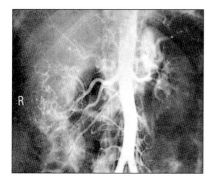

6.16 Renal arteriography (aortography). This 'flood' film, in which contrast medium is allowed to enter both kidneys simultaneously from the aorta, demonstrates a normal arterial circulation in the left kidney and an abnormal tumour circulation in the right kidney. Selective arteriography can also be performed by catheterizing individual renal arteries, and digital subtraction imaging (**6.17**) allows further detailed assessment.

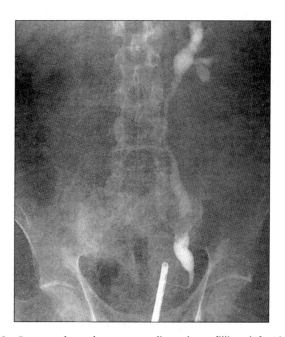

6.18 Retrograde pyelogram revealing a large filling defect in the left ureter caused by a transitional cell carcinoma. The technique is particularly useful in defining the nature and site of ureteric obstruction.

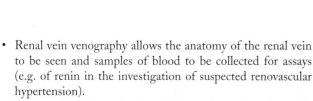

- Renal vein venography allows the anatomy of the renal vein to be seen and samples of blood to be collected for assays (e.g. of renin in the investigation of suspected renovascular hypertension).
- Retrograde pyelography is carried out in conjunction with cystoscopy; a ureteric catheter is threaded into the lower end of the ureter and contrast medium injected; retrograde pyelography can usually define the site and cause of obstruction (**6.18**).
- CT is valuable in defining retroperitoneal lesions and urinary tract obstruction; it is especially valuable in locating and staging tumours (**6.108**) and will also show abnormalities such as polycystic kidneys (**6.19**); modern spiral CT also provides excellent demonstration of the renal arteries.
- Micturating cystourethrography is used to demonstrate reflux of urine from the bladder to the ureter(s) during emptying of the bladder; the bladder is catheterized and filled with contrast medium, and films are then taken during and after micturation (**6.20**).

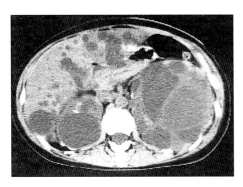

6.19 CT scan revealing bilateral congenital polycystic kidneys, larger on the patient's left (to the right of the picture). The liver also contains multiple cysts. The pancreas can be clearly seen in this view, but does not seem to contain any large cysts.

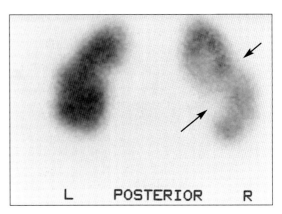

6.21 A 99m Tc-DMSA scintigram, showing defects in the right kidney. The two largest defects are arrowed, but other defects are also evident. The most common cause of this appearance is reflux nephropathy, in which recurrent pyelonephritis results in scarring. This was confirmed by micturating cystogram in this patient.

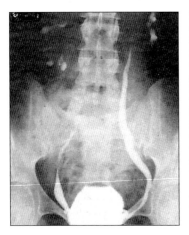

6.20 Micturating cystourethrogram, showing bilateral ureteric reflux. Reflux is categorized in three grades: grade I, in which contrast medium enters the ureter only; grade II, in which the pelvicalyceal system is filled with dye; grade III, in which dilatation of the calyces and ureter also occurs. In this patient, there is some ureteric dilatation and early calyceal clubbing, so there is grade III reflux.

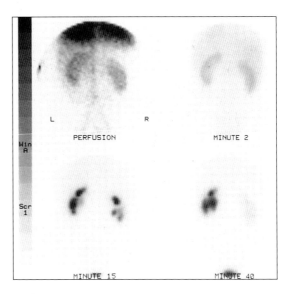

6.22 ^{99m}Tc-DTPA diuretic renogram in a patient with left-sided obstructive uropathy. The patient was given intravenous furosemide (frusemide) at 20 minutes. Note the similar perfusion scans in both kidneys, followed by accumulation of isotope in the urine in the renal collecting systems. Isotope persists in the left kidney for much longer than in the normal right kidney. The results can be quantitatively displayed as a plot of counts over the kidney against time (**6.23**).

- Radionuclide scans are of value in both static and dynamic imaging; ^{99m}Tc-DMSA provides static images of the renal parenchyma, particularly valuable in assessing the presence and extent of scarring in reflux nephropathy (**6.21**, **6.91**); ^{99m}Tc-DTPA (**6.22**, **6.23**) or ^{99m}Tc-MAG3 is used for dynamic renography, which provides information about vascularity of the kidneys and may be used to screen for renal artery stenosis. Renography is also useful in assessing suspected upper tract obstruction, and both renography and DMSA scans permit quantitation of divided renal function.
- MRI is used especially in the assessment of prostatic carcinoma, but local and distant spread of tumours, including the extent of tumour thrombus in the inferior vena cava and right atrium in renal cell carcinoma, also show up well. Magnetic resonance angiography (MRA) can provide high-quality images of the renal arteries without any contrast medium or other invasive technique (**6.24**).
- Interventional radiological techniques play a major role in urinary tract disease; these include CT and ultrasound-guided biopsy, nephrostomy, abscess drainage, ureteric stenting and percutaneous access for stone extraction; in renovascular disease, renal angioplasty is of major importance; embolization of renal tumours is practised much less widely than a few years ago, but it may still have a role in very vascular tumours as a prelude to surgery or in inoperable disease.

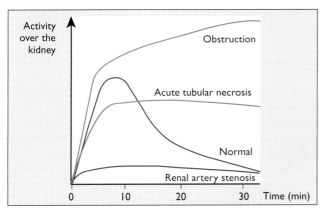

6.23 ^{99m}Tc-DTPA renogram. Activity over the kidney is measured after initial injection of the isotope and plotted against time. Typical results in normal subjects and in patients with acute tubular necrosis, obstruction and renal artery stenosis are shown here.

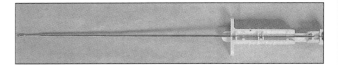

6.25 **A Trucut biopsy needle,** of the type commonly used for percutaneous renal biopsy (and for other biopsies, including liver and prostate). Renal biopsy is an important technique in the assessment of many patients with renal, especially glomerular, disease.

greater than 8 g/dl (**6.25**). Open biopsy is advisable if these criteria are not met. Contraindications to percutaneous renal biopsy include a coagulation defect that cannot be corrected, uncontrolled hypertension, acute renal or urinary tract infections (UTIs), very small kidneys, a single functioning kidney, reflux nephropathy and ureteric obstruction. Transjugular biopsy may be used in the presence of a coagulation defect.

Significant complications of renal biopsy are very rare. Haematuria follows in 5–10% of patients, and local haematomas in about 1%. Blood loss requiring transfusion and death are very rare complications.

Renal biopsy is valuable in patients with nephrotic syndrome, nephritic syndrome and unexplained renal failure. Light microscopy with special stains will often lead to a diagnosis but may be complemented by immunofluorescence and electron microscopy.

Electron microscopy of glomeruli from patients with glomerulonephritis determines the location of electron-dense deposits in relation to the glomerular basement membrane (subepithelial, intramembranous, subendothelial) or mesangium. Immunofluorescence microscopy, using cryostat sections treated with fluorescein-labelled antiserum, determines the pattern of deposition (granular, linear, mesangial) of different classes of immunoglobulin and complement within glomeruli.

Cystoscopy allows for direct vision and biopsy of bladder wall pathology (**1.170, 6.26**) and the insertion of ureteral catheters for retrograde pyelography or the direct removal of ureteric stones.

Tests for systemic disease may be needed, including investigations into diabetes mellitus or other underlying

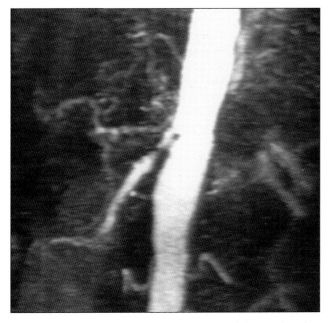

6.24 **Magnetic resonance angiography (MRA), demonstrating a 99% proximal stenosis of the main right renal artery.** This patient had a solitary right kidney after previous left nephrectomy, and the stenosis was subsequently treated by angioplasty and the insertion of a stent (*see* **6.88**). MRA has advantages over conventional angiography, as it is non-invasive and does not require the injection of contrast medium.

OTHER INVESTIGATIONS

Renal biopsy can be performed percutaneously, usually with ultrasound guidance, in patients who can cooperate and hold their breath, have normal coagulation, have two kidneys, have a reasonably controlled blood pressure and have a haemoglobin

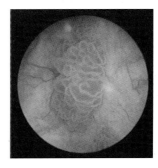

6.26 **Cystoscopy revealing a transitional cell carcinoma of the bladder.** The patient presented with painless haematuria.

disorders, a search for infection elsewhere (throat swab, ASO-titre, hepatitis B markers, syphilis serology, etc.), complement factors (C3 and C4) and an autoantibody screen. Low levels of C3 and/or C4 are usual in systemic lupus erythematosus (SLE) and common in crescentic glomerulonephritis. Antinuclear (ANF) and anti-DNA antibodies are usual in SLE. Anti-glomerular basement membrane (anti-GBM) antibodies are present in anti-glomerular basement membrane/Goodpasture's disease (**6.66**). Several anti-neutrophil cytoplasmic antibodies (ANCA) can be measured by fluorescent staining of neutrophils. Patients with microscopic polyarteritis and Wegener's granulamatosis commonly have positive ANCA, and the titre of antibody can be used to monitor disease activity.

CLINICAL PRESENTATIONS OF RENAL DISEASE

ACUTE RENAL FAILURE (ARF)

A biochemical definition of renal failure is a serum creatinine > 200 μmol/litre. Acute renal failure (ARF) is defined as a recent rapid and profound decline in renal function, whereas rapidly progressive renal failure refers to renal failure developing over weeks rather than days. These disorders, therefore, can be diagnosed only by serial observations of serum creatinine levels and urine flow rates.

Patients commonly present because of oliguria, but more than 25% of patients with acute renal failure are non-oliguric (urine volumes remain greater than 400 ml per day). There are no characteristic clinical signs, but physical features on examination may include peripheral and pulmonary oedema, pleural effusions, pericarditis, acidotic respiration and a depressed conscious level.

The causes of ARF are usually considered in three groups (pre-renal, renal or post-renal), depending on whether the main component of the initiating event is renal hypoperfusion, intrinsic renal disease or urinary outflow obstruction (**6.27**). Pre-renal failure may be prevented from evolving to established acute renal failure by correction of hypovolaemia or impaired cardiac output. Pre-renal failure is likely to be present if urinary concentrating ability (urine to plasma osmolality > 1.7) or urinary sodium retention (urinary sodium concentration > 20 mmol/litre) are demonstrated.

Established ARF that is caused by nephrotoxins (myoglobinuria, haemoglobinuria, aminoglycosides, organic solvents, contrast material), ischaemia (hypovolaemia or cardiac failure), septicaemia, surgery or obstetric complications is potentially reversible and acute tubular necrosis is usually found if the kidneys are examined morphologically.

In these forms of reversible ARF, a diuretic phase usually begins spontaneously during the second or third week after the onset of renal failure and the functional and histological abnormalities may completely resolve. ARF caused by glomerular lesions is less likely to recover without specific treatment and renal biopsy should be performed promptly in suspected cases. Post-renal failure is potentially reversible, so obstruction should be excluded in all cases of acute renal failure.

The causes of ARF can usually be identified from a full history, examination, urinalysis, urine microscopy and renal ultrasound. It is important to exclude the possibility of pre-existing chronic renal failure (CRF), because patients with CRF may present acutely.

The management of established ARF requires: careful attention to fluid and dietary intake; dialysis to correct and thereafter prevent hyperkalaemia (**6.28**), fluid overload, pulmonary oedema, pericarditis, acidosis or uncontrolled uraemia; and treatment of the underlying cause if possible (**6.29**). Dopamine increases renal blood flow and has diuretic and natriuretic effects. Immunosuppressive therapy is often needed in patients with rapidly progressive or acute renal failure

COMMON CAUSES OF ACUTE RENAL FAILURE		
Pre-renal failure	**Intrinsic renal failure**	**Post-renal failure**
Hypovolaemia	Rhabdomyolysis	Obstructive uropathy
Low cardiac output	Haemolysis	
Sepsis	Drugs or nephrotoxins	
Trauma	Glomerulonephritis	
	Interstitial nephritis	
	Multisystem diseases	
	Malignant hypertension	
	Arterial occlusion	

6.27 Common causes of acute renal failure.

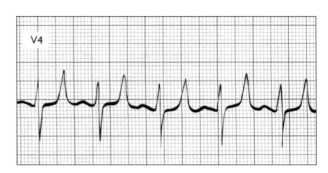

6.28 **Severe hyperkalaemia** is a common complication of acute renal failure and can be diagnosed on ECG, which shows peaked and symmetrical T waves. Hyperkalaemia is an indication for urgent dialysis.

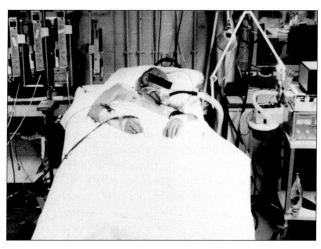

6.29 Patients with acute renal failure are often severely ill. They may require both ventilation and haemodialysis. The percentage survival of patients with acute renal failure has not improved significantly over the past decade, but this may be explained, at least in part, by an increasing proportion of patients with multi-organ failure surviving to a stage at which they develop renal failure.

caused by biopsy-proven glomerular, interstitial, vasculitic or multisystem disease.

CHRONIC RENAL FAILURE (CRF)

Chronic renal failure (CRF) is defined as a progressive decline in renal function for at least 3 months. Loss of functioning nephrons in chronic renal disease often results in an exponential rise in serum creatinine as end-stage renal failure is approached. Consequently, the decline in renal function is frequently linear when the reciprocal of serum creatinine is plotted against time (**6.30**). Progressive impairment of the excretory, homeostatic, metabolic and humoral functions of the kidneys produces a range of non-specific symptoms and signs (**6.3**, **6.30**), so CRF may be diagnosed only after biochemical investigation. The syndrome of advanced uraemia includes anaemia, osteodystrophy (*see* **p. 141**), metabolic acidosis, pruritus, nausea and vomiting, pericarditis (*see* **p. 235**) and fluid overload. When renal disease progresses insidiously, patients may not present until they develop end-stage renal failure (**6.4**, **6.31**). Long-standing pre-existing renal disease may be suspected in such patients by the presence of anaemia or evidence of hyperparathyroidism (*see* **p. 139**) and confirmed radiologically by the presence of bilateral shrunken kidneys (**6.32**). CRF may result from a range of primary diseases (**6.33**).

A number of factors may exacerbate CRF. These include infections, heart failure, acute fluid loss from diarrhoea and vomiting, hypercalcaemia, urinary tract obstruction and some drug therapy. Progression of CRF can be arrested when there is treatable urinary tract obstruction, UTI, hypertension or dehydration.

In the absence of reversible factors or effective therapy for the primary renal disease, conservative management of CRF requires restriction of dietary protein and potassium intake, maintenance of correct fluid and sodium balance, and the use of phosphate-binding agents and active metabolites of vitamin

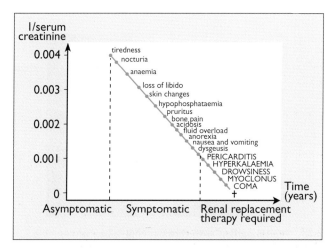

6.30 The typical progressive onset of the non-specific symptoms and signs of chronic renal failure.

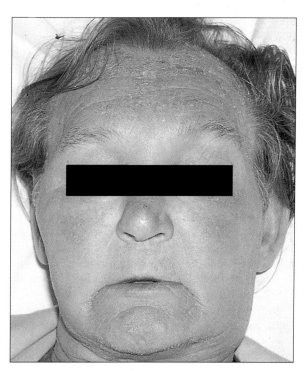

6.31 Uraemic facies. Another patient (*see* **6.3**) demonstrating sallow brown pigmentation, pallor and facial puffiness associated with long-standing renal failure.

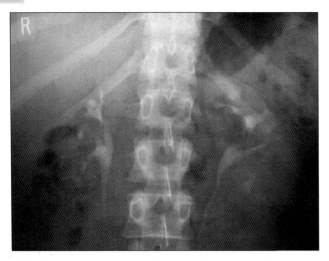

6.32   Intravenous urogram demonstrating two small contracted kidneys. The cortical scarring and calyceal dilatation and deformity, seen especially in the left upper pole, are features of reflux nephropathy (chronic pyelonephritis) (*see also* **6.96**), but shrunken kidneys without these appearances may also occur in end-stage glomerular or interstitial disease.

MAJOR CAUSES OF END-STAGE CRF	
Cause	% of patients
Glomerulonephritis	25
Diabetes mellitus	25
Hypertension	10
Pyelonephritis or reflux nephropathy	10
Polycystic kidneys	10
Interstitial nephritis	5
Obstruction	3
Miscellaneous or unknown	12

6.33   Major causes of end-stage chronic renal failure, with approximate percentage figures for prevalence in the UK and most other developed countries.

D to control hyperparathyroidism. Anaemia in CRF results mainly from inappropriately low production of erythropoietin by the diseased kidneys but other factors, such as iron or folate deficiency, chronic blood loss (resulting from frequent blood sampling, losses during haemodialysis or gastrointestinal bleeding), haemolysis, aluminium toxicity or hyperparathyroidism, may also often contribute. Renal anaemia can now be corrected by the regular administration of human recombinant erythropoietin and treatment of any coexisting causal factors, aiming at a haemoglobin level of 10–12 g/dl. Other problems associated with end-stage CRF should be sought and treated whenever possible, including myopathy,

neuropathy, infections, endocrine dysfunction and cardiovascular disorders (hypertension and hyperlipidaemia).

Renal replacement therapy

Most patients with CRF require renal replacement therapy when renal function declines to approximately 5% of the normal expected for age, usually with a creatinine clearance of 5–10 ml/min and a serum creatinine of 800–1000 µmol/l. The requirement in the UK for renal replacement therapy is approximately 70–80/million population.

The treatment options for patients with end-stage renal failure are hospital or home haemodialysis, continuous ambulatory peritoneal dialysis (CAPD) or renal transplantation.

Haemodialysis

Most patients on regular haemodialysis have an arteriovenous fistula created for vascular access (**6.34**) and require approximately 12 hours dialysis per week, usually divided into three treatment periods. This may be carried out in hospital (**6.35**) or in the patient's home. Even with this regimen, patients still need to follow dietary and fluid restriction.

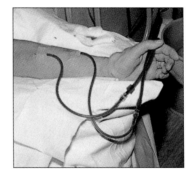

6.34   Vascular access for long-term haemodialysis is usually provided through a surgically created arteriovenous fistula. Blood leaves the patient through the distal needle to pass through the dialyser before returning to the patient through the proximal needle. Patients usually become adept at inserting their own needles.

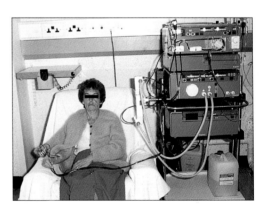

6.35   Typical patient with chronic renal failure undergoing haemodialysis in a hospital setting. In some countries, including the UK, many patients carry out this treatment on a long-term basis in a specially converted room at home.

Continuous ambulatory peritoneal dialysis

Patients on a standard CAPD regime perform exchanges of 2-litre volumes of dialysis solution through a permanent indwelling peritoneal catheter (**6.36**, **6.37**) usually four times every day, using an aseptic technique. CAPD is less restricting than haemodialysis and may be carried out at home. Patients do not usually need to restrict their dietary or fluid intake.

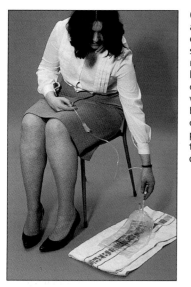

6.36 Continuous ambulatory peritoneal dialysis (CAPD) is a simpler and less restricting technique than haemodialysis, and is compatible with a virtually normal lifestyle. Bags need only be connected to the peritoneal catheter four times per day during exchanges of fluid.

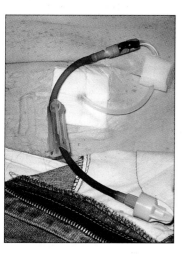

6.37 The Tenckhoff peritoneal dialysis catheter remains implanted in the CAPD patient, but it can be simply strapped to the abdominal wall when not in use for fluid exchanges.

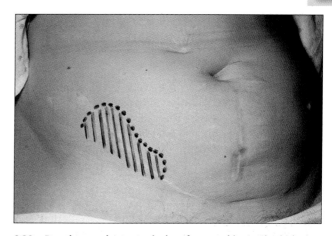

6.38 Renal transplant – typical surface markings. The kidney is usually implanted extraperitoneally in either the right or left iliac fossa, and it can be easily palpated. Percutaneous biopsy is also simple when necessary.

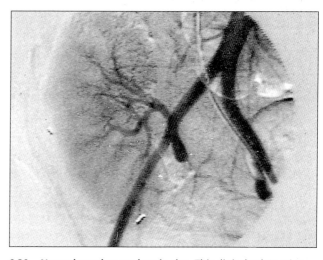

6.39 Normal renal transplant in situ. This digital subtraction angiogram shows the normal site for a renal transplant. The renal artery has been anastomosed to the right external iliac artery.

most countries by the supply of kidneys for transplantation and the cost of optimal immunosuppressive treatment.

Renal transplantation

Haemodialysis and CAPD are both associated with significant physical and psychological demands on the patient and his or her family. Almost normal renal function and much improved quality of life can result from successful renal transplantation (**6.38**, **6.39**) and recent improvements in immunosuppression protocols have increased the percentage of functioning grafts in the long term, with 80% graft survival at 3 years.

Most patients with CRF are keen to undergo transplantation, but the feasibility of this approach is limited in

ACUTE NEPHRITIC SYNDROME

In the acute nephritic syndrome (acute nephritis) there is an abrupt onset of haematuria and proteinuria accompanied by evidence of salt and water retention and reduced renal function. The clinical features are periorbital puffiness (**6.1**), ankle oedema, brown or cola-coloured urine (**6.8**) and hypertension. Sometimes the patient or his or her parents may also notice a reduction in urine volume. All patients have haematuria and proteinuria on urinalysis, but the degree of renal impairment is variable. Glomerular bleeding in patients with nephritis can be confirmed by demonstrating red-cell casts in the urinary sediment (**6.10**).

Acute nephritis may result from:

- infection: poststreptococcal glomerulonephritis, infective endocarditis or shunt nephritis
- multisystem disease: SLE, Henoch–Schönlein disease, vasculitis or Goodpasture's syndrome
- primary glomerulonephritis: mesangiocapillary glomerulonephritis, IgA nephropathy or crescentic glomerulonephritis.

Evidence of infection or extrarenal involvement should therefore be sought in all patients with acute nephritis. It is important to establish the underlying cause of the nephritic syndrome as soon as possible, as renal outcome can be improved when specific therapy is started promptly.

NEPHROTIC SYNDROME

The nephrotic syndrome is characterized by the combination of heavy proteinuria, hypoalbuminaemia and oedema (**1.147, 6.2, 6.40–6.42**) and is a common mode of presentation in a variety of glomerular diseases. Prolonged proteinuria leads to hypoalbuminaemia, decreased plasma oncotic pressure, hypovolaemia, subsequent retention of sodium and water by the kidney caused by activation of the renin–angiotensin–aldosterone axis and accumulation of fluid in the extravascular space. Hypercholesterolaemia is frequently present and may be a consequence of increased hepatic synthesis of cholesterol as well as albumin. Prolonged hypercholesterolaemia may lead to premature corneal arcus (**6.43**) and vascular disease. Serious complications of the nephrotic syndrome include bacterial infections, particularly cellulitis and peritonitis, and arterial and venous thrombotic episodes.

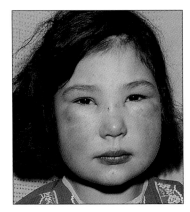

6.41 Nephrotic syndrome in childhood. Note the gross facial and periorbital oedema, which was associated with gross proteinuria.

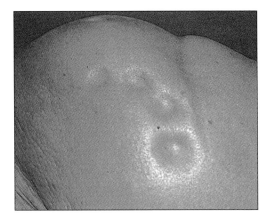

6.42 Nephrotic syndrome – gross pitting oedema of the abdominal wall, secondary to severe hypoalbuminaemia.

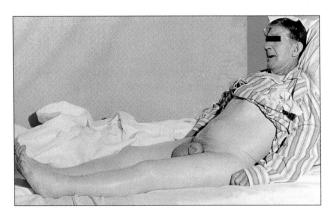

6.40 Nephrotic syndrome – a typical adult patient. He is breathless as a result of pulmonary oedema and has oedema of the ankles, calves, scrotum and penis. He has abdominal swelling as a result of oedema of the abdominal wall, and ascites.

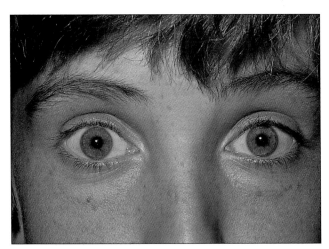

6.43 Premature corneal arcus in a 15-year-old boy with chronic nephrotic syndrome. This was associated with hyper-cholesterolaemia, and is indicative of a risk of premature vascular disease. Treatment of the hypercholesterolaemia may be indicated in these circumstances (*see* **p. 326**).

The major causes of the nephrotic syndrome are listed in **6.44**. No systemic cause is evident in 80% of cases and renal biopsy in such patients shows a variety of primary glomerular diseases (minimal change glomerulonephritis, focal and segmental glomerulosclerosis, membranous glomerulonephritis, mesangio-capillary glomerulonephritis and mesangial proliferative glomerulonephritis). Almost 20% of cases of nephrotic syndrome are caused by renal involvement from systemic disease (e.g. diabetes mellitus, amyloidosis, SLE) and the remainder are caused by drugs, neoplasia or rare hereditary disorders.

CAUSES OF NEPHROTIC SYNDROME
Glomerulonephritis
Diabetes mellitus
Amyloidosis
Systemic lupus erythematosus (SLE)
Other multisystem diseases
Drugs, gold, penicillamine, heroin, captopril
Neoplasia
Infection
Hereditary disorders

6.44   Causes of nephrotic syndrome.

The non-specific treatment of the nephrotic syndrome involves fluid and dietary sodium restriction, high protein intake and judicious use of diuretics. A mild degree of ankle oedema late in the day while on treatment is desirable, in order to avoid complications from hypovolaemia. Infusions of albumin should be reserved for patients with gross hypovolaemia or refractory oedema. In some patients, therapy to reduce hypercholesterolaemia and to prevent or treat thromboembolism may be required. Renal outcome is dependent on the underlying cause of the nephrotic syndrome. Corticosteroid treatment is of value in patients with minimal change glomerular lesions (*see* **p. 270**), and may have a role in some other forms of glomerulonephritis; however high-dose steroid therapy may produce cushingoid features (**6.45**) and its use should be carefully planned and monitored.

ASYMPTOMATIC PROTEINURIA

Screening investigations in apparently healthy patients may show persistent asymptomatic proteinuria or microscopic haematuria, or both, which may be the only evidence of underlying renal disease. The presence of urinary abnormalities in patients with hypertension strongly suggests that they are suffering from renal disease. Asymptomatic proteinuria always requires further investigation to exclude treatable causes of progressive renal disease.

GLOMERULAR DISEASES

Glomerular diseases may be classified on a three-tier basis:

- clinical syndromes
- histological appearances
- aetiology.

Glomerular disease may lead to a variety of clinical syndromes, including asymptomatic proteinuria, haematuria, acute nephritis, nephrotic syndrome and slowly or rapidly progressive renal failure. It is one of the commonest causes of end-stage CRF.

There is a degree of correlation between the histological appearance of the glomeruli (**6.46**) and the clinical presentation (**6.47**). The histological appearance often provides a valuable guide to prognosis and likely response to therapy.

In primary glomerular disease, the aetiology is usually unclear; but aetiological classification is useful in secondary glomerulopathies (**6.48**).

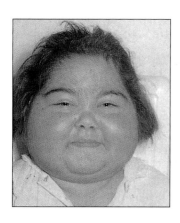

6.45   Gross cushingoid features (*see also* **p. 299**) in a 7-year-old girl with the nephrotic syndrome who was treated with cortico-steroids. Although steroid treatment is of value in children with minimal change glomerular lesions, such gross features of steroid excess should be avoided if possible by careful planning of dosage and timing of therapy.

HISTOLOGICAL TERMINOLOGY	
Diffuse:	All of the glomeruli are uniformly involved
Focal:	Some of the glomeruli are involved
Segmental:	Only part of the glomerular tufts are involved
Crescentic:	At least 70% of the glomerular tufts are compressed by crescents (proliferation of macrophages and epithelial cells of Bowman's capsule)
	Light microscopy of renal tissue also assesses pathological involvement in the interstitium, tubules and blood vessels.

6.46   Terminology used in the histological description of glomerular lesions.

HISTOLOGICAL/CLINICAL CORRELATION

Histological type	Clinical features
Minimal change glomerulonephritis	Nephrotic syndrome
Focal and segmental glomerulosclerosis	Nephrotic syndrome, progressive renal failure
Membranous glomerulonephritis	Nephrotic syndrome
Mesangiocapillary glomerulonephritis	Haematuria, proteinuria, acute nephritis, progressive renal failure
Mesangial proliferative glomerulonephritis	Haematuria, proteinuria
Diffuse endocapillary proliferative glomerulonephritis	Acute nephritis, progressive renal failure

6.47   Correlation between histology and clinical picture in primary glomerulopathy.

SYSTEMIC DISORDERS

Diabetes mellitus

Systemic lupus erythematosus (SLE)

Rheumatoid arthritis

Ankylosing spondylitis

Multiple myeloma

Amyloidosis

Vasculitis

Sarcoidosis

Neoplasia

6.48   Systemic disorders that may be associated with secondary glomerular disease.

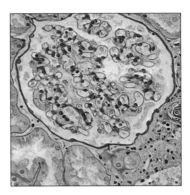

6.49   A normal glomerulus. (*PAS ×352*).

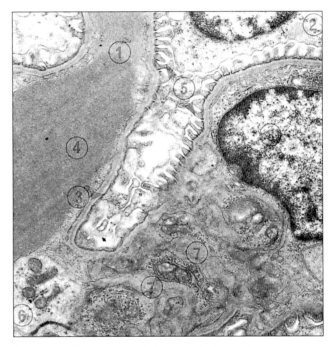

6.50   The ultrastructure of the normal glomerulus as seen on electron microscopy: 1 = capillary lumen; 2 = epithelial cell; 3 = basement membrane; 4 = red blood cell; 5 = epithelial foot processes; 6 = endothelial cell; 7 = mesangial matrix; 8 = mesangial cell.

Investigations in glomerular disease should usually include the initial investigations listed in **6.6**, together with renal ultrasound or an IVU, serum complement levels, auto-antibodies and appropriate tests for multisystem disorders. In adults, these will usually be followed by renal biopsy, with assessment of light-microscopic (**6.49**) and, often, electron-microscopic (**6.50**) and immunofluorescence-microscopic appearances.

In children, biopsy may often be postponed until after a trial of steroid therapy.

PRIMARY GLOMERULOPATHIES

Minimal change glomerulonephritis

The nephrotic syndrome (*see* **p. 268**) is the clinical presentation in almost all cases of minimal change glomerulonephritis, but occasionally asymptomatic proteinuria may be the only abnormality. Hypertension and haematuria are both rare. The disease is the underlying cause in more than 80% of children and almost 20% of adults with the nephrotic syndrome. Autoantibodies are absent and complement levels are normal; proteinuria is usually highly selective (high urinary transferrin to IgG ratio). On renal biopsy, the glomeruli are normal (**6.51**)

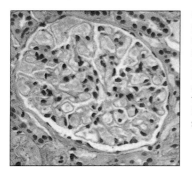

6.51 Minimal change glomerulonephritis showing a normal glomerulus on light microscopy of a renal biopsy (*MSB ×224*). The appearance is identical to that seen in **6.49**, but here the red cells are stained yellow with MSB.

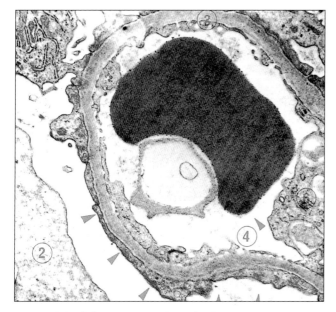

6.52 Minimal change glomerulonephritis. Electron micrograph showing fusion of the epithelial foot processes (arrowed) and absence of electron-dense deposits (magnification *×10750*): 2 = epithelial cytoplasm; 3 = basement membrane; 4 = red blood cell in capillary lumen; 6 = endothelial cell.

except for the presence of epithelial foot process fusion on electron microscopy (**6.52**), which is found with all causes of proteinuria of glomerular origin.

As remission of proteinuria can be induced in virtually all cases by a course of prednisolone, this is usually prescribed to all childhood nephrotics without first performing a renal biopsy. Renal biopsy is reserved for children with steroid-resistant or frequently relapsing nephrotic syndrome. In adults, minimal change glomerulonephritis is a less frequent cause of nephrotic syndrome and a biopsy is indicated in all cases. When relapses are frequent, or unacceptable steroid side-effects develop, an 8-week course of cyclophosphamide (2 mg/kg) may produce prolonged remission. On rare occasions, the disease is associated with lymphoma, and remission is usually induced on successful treatment of the underlying disease. Renal prognosis

in this condition is very good, even though a few patients may develop acute renal failure as a result of overuse of diuretics.

Focal and segmental glomerulosclerosis

Patients with focal and segmental glomerulosclerosis most commonly present with nephrotic syndrome; this disease is the underlying cause in almost 10% of child nephrotics. Autoantibodies are absent and complement studies are normal. Renal biopsy shows segmental areas of sclerosis, initially only in the juxtamedullary glomeruli, without evidence of cellular proliferation or necrosis (**6.53**). Immunofluorescence microscopy often shows deposition of IgM and C3 in affected glomeruli. As glomerular involvement is at first focal, early cases may be indistinguishable from minimal change glomerulonephritis, even on renal biopsy. This disease may be suspected if the nephrotic syndrome in childhood is resistant to steroid therapy or runs a relapsing and remitting course. Cyclophosphamide or cyclosporin may induce partial or complete remission of proteinuria, but in more than 50% of patients renal function declines progressively and 20–40% of patients reach end-stage renal failure after 10 years. The long-term renal prognosis may be further compromised by recurrence of the disease in about one-third of patients after renal transplantation.

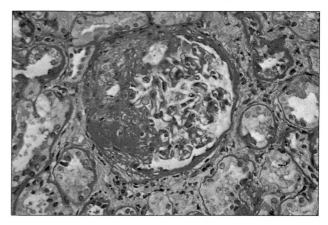

6.53 Focal and segmental glomerulosclerosis. The segmental sclerosis is clearly seen on light microscopy of a renal biopsy (*PAS ×330*).

Membranous glomerulonephritis

Membranous glomerulonephritis is a common cause of adult-onset nephrotic syndrome, but is rare in childhood. Microscopic haematuria is common and hypertension is present in about one-third of patients at presentation. Renal biopsy shows diffuse uniform thickening of the glomerular basement membrane without any associated cellular proliferation (**6.54**), and electron microscopy shows subepithelial electron-dense deposits (**6.55**). Immunofluorescence microscopy shows diffuse granular subepithelial deposition of complement and IgG in the capillary loops (**6.56**). Most cases are idiopathic, but it is important to exclude

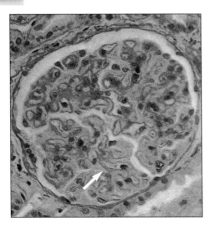

6.54 Membranous glomerulonephritis. The renal biopsy shows uniform thickening of the capillary basement membranes (arrow). Compare with **6.49** and **6.51** (*MSB ×224*).

associated infection (syphilis, hepatitis B), neoplasia, SLE or drug therapy (gold, penicillamine, captopril). Renal outcome in the secondary type depends on the underlying cause. If untreated, 20% of the idiopathic group remit spontaneously and up to 30% reach end-stage renal failure after 10 years. Corticosteroids are

of no benefit. Recent clinical studies in nephrotic patients have shown reduction in proteinuria and improvement in renal function after treatment with combined courses of prednisolone and chlorambucil. Ciclosporin may prevent further decline in renal function.

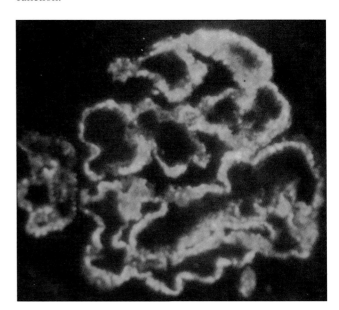

6.56 Membranous glomerulonephritis. Immunofluorescence microscopy showing diffuse granular deposition of IgG in the capillary loops (×300).

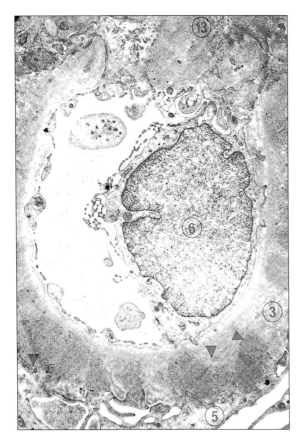

6.55 Membranous glomerulonephritis. Electron micrograph showing markedly thickened basement membrane with electron-dense deposits (arrowed) representing deposits of antigen–antibody complexes located subepithelially, that is beneath the fused epithelial cell foot processes. 3 = basement membrane; 5 = epithelial cell foot processes; 6 = endothelial cell; 13 = mesangium (magnification ×10 750).

Mesangiocapillary glomerulonephritis

The mode of presentation of mesangiocapillary glomerulonephritis is variable: 20% of patients have the acute nephritic syndrome, whereas all of the remaining patients have proteinuria; 50% have hypertension, 50% have renal failure and 30% have haematuria. The disease mainly affects school-age children and young adults and is more common in females. Its frequency is falling in the developed world. Serum C3 levels are reduced transiently in type 1 and are persistently low in type 2. These are differentiated from each other on renal biopsy. The histological feature common to both types of disease is a combination of mesangial cell proliferation and thickening of the glomerular capillary wall on light microscopy (**6.57**). In the subendothelial type (type 1) there is interposition of mesangial matrix between the endothelial cells and glomerular basement membrane, subendothelial deposits on electron microscopy (**6.58**) and granular deposition of IgG and C3 on immunofluorescence microscopy. In the dense-deposit type (type 2) there are linear dense intramembranous deposits on electron microscopy (**6.59**), and only deposition of C3 on immunofluorescence microscopy. There is no specific therapy for this form of glomerulonephritis and the renal prognosis is relatively poor: more than 50% of patients reach end-stage renal failure after 10 years. Type 2 mesangiocapillary glomerulonephritis may recur in patients after renal transplantation.

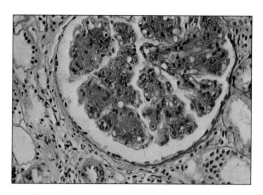

6.57 Mesangiocapillary glomerulonephritis. Light microscopy showing an increase in mesangial cells and matrix and patchy thickening of the basement membrane. This glomerulus also shows marked lobulation of the glomerular tufts (*PAS ×330*).

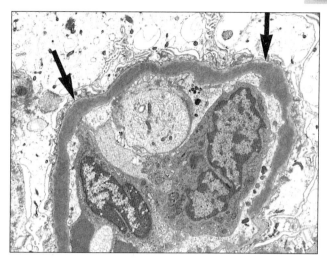

6.59 Mesangiocapillary glomerulonephritis. Electron micrograph from a patient with type 2 mesangiocapillary glomerulonephritis (dense-deposit disease) showing linear dense intramembranous deposits (arrows) (magnification *×5200*).

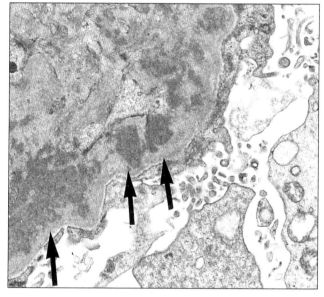

6.58 Mesangiocapillary glomerulonephritis. Electron micrograph showing subendothelial electron-dense deposits (arrowed) in a patient with type 1 mesangiocapillary glomerulonephritis (magnification *×13 200*).

These light-microscopic appearances are associated with the presence of mesangial deposits on electron microscopy (**6.61**) and commonly with mesangial deposition of IgA on immunofluorescence microscopy (**6.62**), so-called IgA nephropathy (Berger's disease). Less frequently, immunofluorescence microscopy shows mesangial deposition of either IgG or IgM. The electron and immunofluorescence microscopy appearances of IgA nephropathy are indistinguishable from those of Henoch–Schönlein nephritis. The latter is usually associated with purpura (**2.133**), abdominal pain or arthropathy, is more common in children, and is more likely to present with the nephritic syndrome and to have glomeruli containing crescents on biopsy.

There is no specific treatment for either IgA nephropathy or Henoch–Schönlein nephritis, but the overall prognosis is good. Only 5–10% of patients with IgA nephropathy reach end-stage renal failure after 10 years, and progressive renal failure is more

Mesangial proliferative glomerulonephritis

Recurrent macroscopic haematuria, often within 2 days of an upper respiratory tract infection, was the most common mode of presentation of this disorder; however, as a result of routine urinalysis many patients are now detected with microscopic haematuria or asymptomatic proteinuria, or both. Peak incidence is in young adults, and men are more commonly affected. Renal failure at presentation is uncommon. Autoantibodies and complement studies are usually normal, unless the disorder is a manifestation of SLE. Serum IgA levels may be elevated in Henoch–Schönlein disease. Renal biopsy shows increased mesangial cells and mesangial matrix (**6.60**).

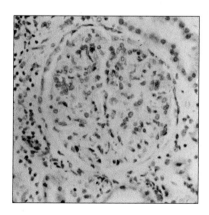

6.60 Mesangial proliferative glomerulonephritis. Light microscopy of a glomerulus from a patient with microscopic haematuria and asymptomatic proteinuria showing an increase in mesangial cells and matrix (H&E).

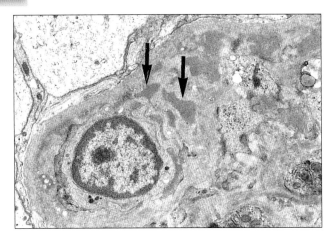

6.61 Mesangial proliferative glomerulonephritis. Electron micrograph showing electron-dense deposits distributed within the mesangium (arrows) (magnification ×13 200).

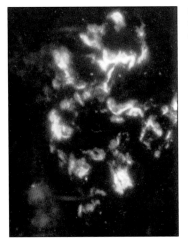

6.62 Mesangial proliferative glomerulonephritis. Immunofluorescence microscopy from the same patient as in 6.61 showing mesangial deposition of IgA, indicating that this patient has IgA nephropathy (Berger's disease).

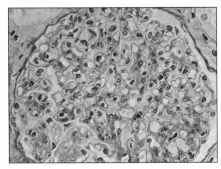

6.63 Diffuse endocapillary proliferative glomerulonephritis. The glomerulus shows increased cellularity, caused by endothelial and mesangial cell proliferation and polymorph infiltration (PAS ×330).

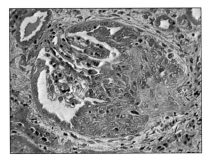

6.64 Diffuse endocapillary proliferative glomerulonephritis with a crescent. The glomerulus shows a large cellular crescent compressing the glomerular tuft (H&E ×330). Crescentic glomerulonephritis may be found in all types of acute nephritis with rapidly progressive renal failure.

Electron microscopy in the acute stage shows large subepithelial electron-dense deposits (6.65) and immunofluorescence microscopy shows granular staining of IgG and C3 within the glomeruli. The prognosis in post-streptococcal glomerulonephritis is generally good, and the

likely in patients with hypertension or nephrotic syndrome at presentation.

Diffuse endocapillary proliferative glomerulonephritis

Patients with diffuse endocapillary proliferative glomerulonephritis usually present with acute nephritis, although not all features may be evident. The condition is more frequent in children and young adults. In some patients, the onset of renal disease is associated with an extrarenal infection 10–14 days earlier, but most cases are idiopathic.

Classically, this disease is preceded by a nephritogenic group A streptococcal infection, usually of the throat or skin. However, the frequency of isolating streptococcus from the presumed site of infection, or demonstrating a rise in antibody titre to streptococcal antigens (antistreptolysin-O titre), is relatively low. Autoantibodies are negative and serum C3 levels are usually transiently decreased. Renal biopsy is characterized by hypercellularity in all of the glomeruli (6.63), not infrequently associated with crescent formation (6.64).

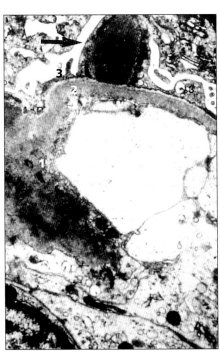

6.65 Diffuse endocapillary proliferative glomerulonephritis. The electron micrograph shows a large subepithelial electron-dense deposit (arrowed): 1 = endothelial cell; 2 = basement membrane; 3 = epithelial cell.

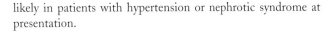

only specific treatment recommended is a 7-day course of penicillin. Complete recovery is common, and less than 5% of patients reach end-stage renal failure after 10 years; this is more likely in adult patients with persistent hypertension or nephrotic syndrome, and in patients with rapidly progressive renal failure. The long-term outcome for the larger idiopathic group is less well defined, but is generally good if there is early regression of features of renal disease.

SECONDARY GLOMERULOPATHIES

Anti-glomerular basement membrane disease

Anti-glomerular basement membrane disease (anti-GBM disease) usually presents with rapidly progressive renal failure, haematuria and proteinuria. The haematuria may be macroscopic and, if associated with haemoptysis, is termed Goodpasture's syndrome (*see* **p. 184**). The disease has a peak incidence in young adults, and is more common in men. There is often an association with recent infection or exposure to hydrocarbons at the onset or before relapses of the disease. The disease is mediated by an anti-glomerular basement membrane antibody present in the serum, and the antibody titre is used for diagnostic purposes and to assess the adequacy of treatment. Other autoantibodies and complement levels are usually normal. The diagnostic feature on renal biopsy is linear deposition of IgG and occasionally C3 along the capillary loops of the glomeruli (**6.66**). Light microscopy usually shows a focal necrotizing glomerulitis with crescent formation (**6.67**).

The prognosis is dependent on the degree of renal failure at the time of diagnosis and on whether pulmonary haemorrhage is present. Two major features of the natural history of the disease determine treatment strategies: pulmonary haemorrhage is almost invariably fatal if untreated, and recovery of renal function is rare if the patient is already dialysis-dependent when immunosuppressive therapy is begun. Consequently, immunosuppression with pulsed intravenous methylprednisolone, oral prednisolone, cyclophosphamide and plasma exchange is reserved for patients with Goodpasture's

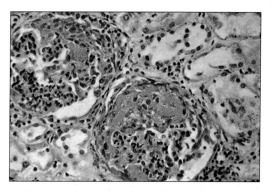

6.67   Anti-glomerular basement membrane disease. Light microscopy shows focal necrotizing glomerulitis with crescent formation (*H&E ×308*).

syndrome or patients not yet receiving dialysis. The risks of intensive immunosuppression in patients already requiring dialysis and without pulmonary haemorrhage outweigh the small chance of improvement in renal function.

Renal vasculitides

The renal vasculitides should be suspected in patients with symptoms and signs of multisystem disease in addition to renal disease. The clinical features depend to some extent on the type of vasculitis. Weight loss, anaemia, malaise, fever, high ESR and raised C-reactive protein are found in most cases. Peak incidence is in the middle-aged or elderly and patients are more often male. The more common forms of renal vasculitis can be conveniently classified according to the size of the vessels involved, the presence or absence of granulomata, and whether there is evidence of either gastrointestinal or respiratory tract disease (**6.68**). Kawasaki disease is described on **page 57**. Churg–Strauss syndrome (allergic granulomatosis, *see* **p. 183**) is relatively rare, and renal disease is usually associated with asthma and eosinophilia. Evidence of vasculitis may also be found histologically in patients with severe renal disease caused by SLE (*see* **p. 277**) or Henoch–Schönlein disease.

Polyarteritis nodosa

In polyarteritis nodosa (classic polyarteritis) there is segmental necrosis and fibrinoid change within the walls of medium-sized arteries, often associated with intraluminal thrombosis (**6.69**). Ischaemia distal to occluded vessels may produce infarcts in virtually any organ. The clinical features depend on the extent and location of the lesions (*see* **p. 127**). Mesenteric, splenic, myocardial, cerebral or renal infarction are common modes of acute presentation. Renal infarcts, often multiple, may lead to the development of loin pain, macroscopic haematuria and hypertension. The diagnosis is best confirmed by selective renal arteriography, which may show both aneurysms of the intrarenal vessels and renal infarcts (**6.70**). The prognosis without treatment is poor, and less than one-half of untreated

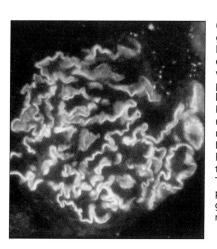

6.66   Anti-glomerular basement membrane disease in a patient with renal failure, proteinuria and haematuria. Immunofluorescence microscopy of the renal biopsy shows IgG distributed in a linear pattern along the capillary loops. The serum was positive for anti-glomerular basement membrane antibody.

CLASSIFICATION OF RENAL VASCULITIDES

	Vessel size involved		
	Medium	Small	
Granulomata absent	Polyarteritis nodosa	Microscopic polyarteritis	Gastrointestinal involvement common
	Kawasaki disease	Henoch–Schönlein disease	
		Systemic lupus erythematosus	
Granulomata present	Churg–Strauss syndrome	Wegener's granulomatosis	Respiratory involvement common

6.68 Classification of renal vasculitides.

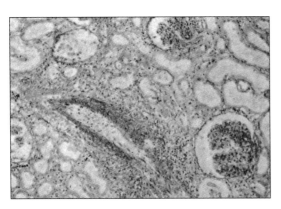

6.69   Polyarteritis nodosa. There is fibrinoid necrosis (stained red) of an interlobular artery. The glomeruli are usually normal outside the areas of renal infarction.

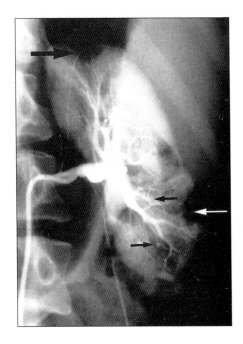

6.70 Polyarteritis nodosa. A selective left renal arteriogram shows aneurysms of the intrarenal vessels (small arrows) and subcapsular renal infarcts (large arrows).

patients survive more than 1 year. Treatment with high doses of prednisolone and cyclophosphamide produces rapid symptomatic improvement and appears to improve patient survival.

Microscopic polyarteritis

Microscopic polyarteritis (hypersensitivity angiitis) involves mainly the arterioles and capillaries. Many organs may be involved, but the kidneys, skin and lungs are most often affected. Patients with renal disease commonly present with rapidly progressive renal failure associated with microscopic haematuria and proteinuria. Serological investigations may show positive titres for rheumatoid factor and antinuclear factor in up to one-third of patients. Serum from patients with microscopic polyarteritis may also be positive for ANCA, showing a perinuclear staining pattern (p-ANCA). Renal biopsy shows diffuse proliferation and focal fibrinoid necrosis in the glomeruli (**6.71**), often associated with crescent formation. Electron and immunofluorescence microscopy usually show absence of deposits. Arteriolitis or capillaritis is seen in only a minority of renal biopsies, but may be

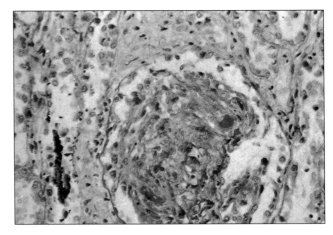

6.71   Microscopic polyarteritis. There is focal fibrinoid necrosis (red) and proliferative change in a glomerulus (*MSB ×330*).

demonstrated on biopsy of skin lesions. Prognosis is poor without treatment and is worst in patients who are already oliguric at presentation, or who have more than 70% crescent formation in the glomeruli on renal biopsy. Treatment with pulsed intravenous methylprednisolone, oral prednisolone and cyclophosphamide has significantly improved both patient and renal survival. Some centres also perform short-term daily plasma exchange in patients who are already dialysis-dependent when therapy is started.

Wegener's granulomatosis

The presence of nasal symptoms, haemoptysis, pleurisy or deafness combined with renal disease is highly suggestive of Wegener's granulomatosis (*see* **pp. 128, 182**). In many cases renal involvement is detected only during the course of investigation of either the respiratory tract or ear and nasal symptoms. Renal disease in this disorder commonly manifests itself as rapidly progressive renal failure associated with haematuria and proteinuria. Serum is usually positive for ANCA and the diagnosis can be confirmed by nasal mucosa or renal biopsy. The latter may show similar histological appearances to microscopic polyarteritis, with features of necrotizing glomerulitis, crescent formation and arteritis. Granulomata are present only in the minority of renal biopsy specimens (**6.72**), but may be found on biopsy of the nasal mucosa. Indirect immunofluorescence microscopy for ANCA shows a cytoplasmic pattern (c-ANCA) in Wegener's granulomatosis. This test may prove helpful in differentiating Wegener's granulomatosis from microscopic polyarteritis. Patient and renal survival in this condition have improved considerably since the introduction of treatment with pulsed methylprednisolone, cyclophosphamide and prednisolone. Long-term immunosuppression with cyclophosphamide or azathioprine is required, as clinical relapse is common on withdrawing cytotoxic agents.

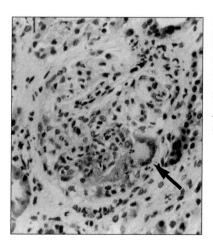

6.72 Wegener's granulomatosis. Renal biopsy showing focal necrosis in the glomerulus, associated with a small granuloma including a Langhan's type giant cell (arrowed) (*H&E ×330*).

Renal systemic lupus erythematosus

Renal involvement is evident in up to 75% of patients with other features of SLE (*see* **p. 121**), and some patients may

present with renal disease before the onset of extrarenal symptoms of SLE. The severity of renal disease varies greatly: some patients may have only asymptomatic proteinuria or microscopic haematuria, whereas others may develop nephrotic syndrome or rapidly progressive renal failure. The diagnosis is confirmed serologically by the presence of serum antinuclear factor (ANF) and often antibodies to double-stranded DNA (ds-DNA) and by a reduced concentration of C3 in the serum.

Several histological types of renal disease are evident on renal biopsy. Mesangial proliferative and membranous glomerulonephritis in SLE patients have clinical and histological features akin to idiopathic types of these disorders (*see* **pp. 273, 271**). SLE patients with nephrotic syndrome or renal failure often have a diffuse proliferative glomerulonephritis (**6.73**) with subepithelial, intramembranous and subendothelial deposits on electron microscopy (**6.74**) and peripheral deposition of IgG and complement components on immunofluorescence microscopy. Patients with this form of glomerulonephritis who have more severe renal impairment may also show evidence of crescent formation (**6.64**), vasculitis and interstitial fibrosis on renal biopsy.

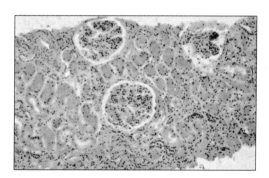

6.73 Systemic lupus erythematosus. This renal biopsy shows proliferative changes within three glomeruli (*H&E ×143*).

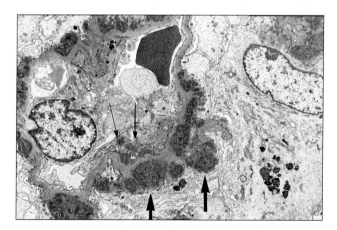

6.74 Systemic lupus erythematosus with the nephrotic syndrome. This electron micrograph shows both subendothelial deposits (small arrows) and subepithelial deposits (large arrows). (magnification ×5200).

Treatment depends on the severity of renal disease and the histological findings on renal biopsy. Patients with mesangial proliferative glomerulonephritis usually have mild renal disease, and treatment is required only for extrarenal involvement. Patients with membranous glomerulonephritis often improve with prednisolone alone, and the prognosis for renal function is good. Evolution to end-stage renal failure is relatively common in diffuse proliferative glomerulonephritis, and treatment with azathioprine or cyclophosphamide in addition to prednisolone is usually necessary. Women with SLE should be warned that renal function may worsen with use of the oral contraceptive pill or post partum.

Renal amyloidosis

The most common mode of presentation of amyloidosis in the kidney is the nephrotic syndrome associated with renal failure. Even in advanced renal failure, the kidneys may remain relatively large because of the deposition of amyloid. Clinically evident renal disease is more frequent in primary than secondary amyloidosis. Congestive cardiomyopathy, hepato-splenomegaly, peripheral neuropathy and malabsorption may result from systemic deposition of amyloid.

At the ultrastructural level, amyloid consists of protein fibrils and a glycoprotein known as amyloid P component. Two forms of fibril protein are found: amyloid light-chain (AL) proteins are found in myeloma-associated and primary amyloidosis, and amyloid A (AA) fibril proteins are found in amyloidosis secondary to chronic infections, rheumatoid arthritis or familial Mediterranean fever. Rectal or renal biopsy confirms the diagnosis. Renal biopsy sections stained with Congo Red show pink-red deposition within the glomeruli and blood vessel walls (**6.75**), which under polarized light exhibits apple-green birefringence (**6.76**). Electron microscopy of the amyloid deposits shows a characteristic arrangement of fibrils, and immunofluorescence microscopy for immunoglobulin and complement is negative. Monoclonal antibodies can be used to differentiate amyloid light-chain and amyloid A proteins.

There is no specific treatment for amyloidosis, although renal function may stabilize after chemotherapy in patients with myeloma-associated amyloidosis, or colchicine in patients

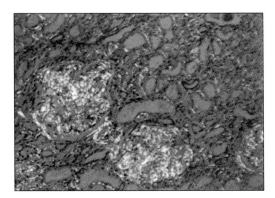

6.76 Renal amyloidosis. This Congo Red stained renal biopsy has been examined by polarized light to show the apple-green birefringence caused by amyloid deposition within the glomeruli and around the tubules (×198).

with familial Mediterranean fever. The prognosis for renal function in most cases is poor, and more than 50% of patients with biopsy-proven amyloidosis reach end-stage renal failure within 1 year.

DIABETIC NEPHROPATHY

Renal disease is evident in about 30% of patients 20 years after developing type 1 (insulin-dependent) diabetes mellitus (*see* **p. 315**) and, until recently, was a major cause of death in diabetic patients. The aetiology of diabetic nephropathy is multifactorial; both metabolic and genetic factors appear to be important, as more than 40% of patients with type 1 DM do not develop microvasculopathy in spite of the presence of long-term hyperglycaemia. Renal involvement in type 1 DM usually evolves through a number of stages:

- Stage I: at diagnosis, the glomerular filtration rate is increased, because of poor metabolic control.
- Stage II: with improved glycaemic control, renal function remains within the normal range, and urinary albumin excretion (UAE) is normal.
- Stage III: within the first 10 years after onset of diabetes, a proportion of patients develop microalbuminuria, defined as a persistent elevation in the urinary albumin excretion rate to greater than 20 μg/min but without evidence of proteinuria on urinalysis.
- Stage IV: most patients with microalbuminuria progress to overt nephropathy, which is characterized by the onset of clinical proteinuria and hypertension and is usually associated with retinopathy; the nephrotic syndrome commonly develops at this stage.
- Stage V: renal impairment from stage IV almost invariably progresses to end-stage renal failure.

The evolution of renal disease in type 2 (non-insulin-dependent) diabetes mellitus is less well defined, because of

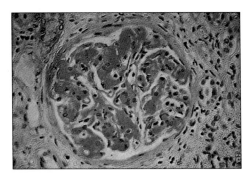

6.75 Renal amyloidosis. The glomerulus shows amyloid deposition, stained by Congo Red, in the glomerular capillaries (×330).

difficulty in ascertaining the exact time of onset of diabetes in this group.

In patients with suggestive clinical features and associated retinopathy, diabetic retinopathy is usually assumed without performing a renal biopsy. The latter is performed only if renal disease unrelated to diabetes is suspected. The most common feature on renal biopsy is diffuse glomerulosclerosis (**6.77**), which may be associated with the classic lesions of diabetic

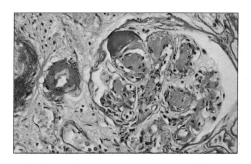

6.79   Glomerulus in diabetes showing a fibrin cap lesion (red) associated with Kimmelstiel–Wilson nodules (blue). The afferent arteriole has been infiltrated with hyaline (*MS ×330*).

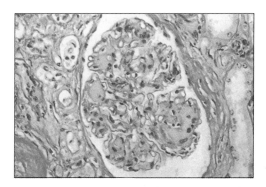

6.77   Diffuse glomerulosclerosis is the most common glomerular lesion in diabetic nephropathy. There is generalized thickening of the capillary walls throughout the glomerular lobules (*MSB ×250*).

nephropathy (**6.78**, **6.79**). Electron microscopy in diabetic nephropathy shows thickening of the glomerular membrane in all patients. It is important to exclude other renal and urinary tract disorders associated with diabetes, such as renal papillary necrosis (**6.80**), UTI, perinephric abscess or pyonephrosis and neurogenic bladder.

Progression of renal failure in patients with overt proteinuria can be retarded by achieving good control of hypertension, and good glycaemic control. The efficacy of maintenance of normal blood pressure levels and optimal glycaemic control are currently undergoing assessment in patients with micro-albuminuria. Early aggressive control of blood pressure, using angiotensin-converting enzyme (ACE) inhibitors, has demonstrated a reduction in microalbuminuria in patients with

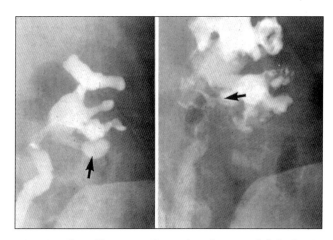

6.80   Renal papillary necrosis may be a feature of diabetic renal disease. The retrograde pyelogram on the left shows marked calyceal clubbing and distortion. One month later (right) there has been sloughing of calyceal tissue into the renal pelvis.

incipient nephropathy, and a decrease in proteinuria and improvement in renal function in patients with clinical nephropathy. These therapeutic strategies, introduced at an early stage of diabetic nephropathy, may help prevent progression of renal failure in future.

Once CRF develops, patients almost inevitably require renal replacement therapy, unless reversible factors such as UTI or obstruction are present. CAPD has been preferred to haemodialysis for most diabetic patients, as it provides steady-state control of biochemistry and fluid balance, and stable blood pressure, and avoids the need for either vascular access or heparin. Quality of life and patient survival are better with renal transplantation than with either mode of dialysis.

TUBULOINTERSTITIAL DISEASES

The generic term tubulointerstitial diseases refers to all diseases of the interstitium and tubules with little or no evidence of concomitant glomerular disease.

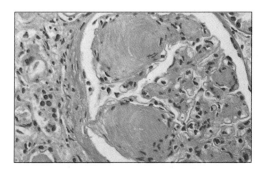

6.78   Kimmelstiel–Wilson nodules are the classic lesions of diabetic nephropathy. Their presence is virtually diagnostic of diabetes mellitus. Note the nodular intercapillary glomerulosclerosis (*MS ×250*).

ACUTE INTERSTITIAL NEPHRITIS (AIN)

Acute interstitial nephritis (AIN) frequently manifests itself as acute renal failure and may be idiopathic, associated with infection (leptospirosis, tuberculosis or pyelonephritis), or drug-induced (antibiotics, non-steroidal anti-inflammatory drugs, diuretics) or part of a systemic disease process (e.g. multiple myeloma, sarcoidosis, Sjögren's syndrome). Acute renal failure is frequently accompanied by the presence of fever, rash, eosinophilia, non-nephrotic range proteinuria and microhaematuria. On renal biopsy, there is interstitial infiltration with lymphocytes, plasma cells, polymorphs and eosinophils, interstitial oedema and variable degrees of damage to the renal tubules (**6.81**). Renal function usually recovers on withdrawal of the putative drug or treatment of the associated infection. Treatment with prednisolone may induce recovery of renal function in other cases.

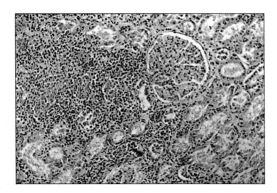

6.81 Acute interstitial nephritis. This renal biopsy shows interstitial oedema and infiltration with lymphocytes, plasma cells and polymorphs, without evidence of concomitant glomerular disease (H&E x80).

CHRONIC INTERSTITIAL NEPHRITIS (CIN)

Chronic interstitial nephritis (CIN) usually presents with CRF associated with non-nephrotic range proteinuria and evidence of tubular dysfunction. Polyuria, renal salt wasting, hypo-kalaemia and renal tubular acidosis are common, but there may be a surprising lack of symptoms even in the presence of severely impaired renal function. Renal biopsy in long-standing cases shows interstitial fibrosis, tubular atrophy and a variable degree of interstitial infiltration (**6.82**). A search for an underlying cause may reveal analgesic abuse, chronic pyelonephritis, radiation nephritis, Sjögren's syndrome, gout, sickle-cell disease or heavy metal exposure, but many cases are idiopathic. Control of fluid and electrolyte balance may require sodium, potassium or bicarbonate supplementation and subsequent renal replacement therapy for CRF.

ANALGESIC NEPHROPATHY

Analgesic nephropathy results from the long-term ingestion of large quantities of analgesic drugs, especially non-steroidal anti-inflammatory drugs (NSAIDs). Earlier cases were often related to phenacetin, with or without aspirin. An important co-factor is low fluid intake and relative dehydration. Tubulointerstitial damage occurs along with papillary necrosis. Patients may present with CRF, sterile pyuria, haematuria, renal colic resulting from ureteric obstruction by a fragment of necrotic tissue, or hypertension. Anaemia is often more severe than expected for the degree of chronic renal impairment. On IVU, the kidneys are usually bilaterally shrunken with deformed calyces, and the appearance of a 'ring sign' on the pyelogram, representing a sloughed papilla within a dilated calyx, is typical of this disorder (**6.83**). The main therapeutic

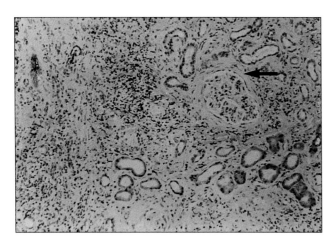

6.82 Chronic interstitial nephritis. The renal biopsy shows a diffuse lymphocytic infiltrate and fibrosis in the interstitium with focal tubular atrophy and periglomerular scarring (arrow) (*H&E ×80*).

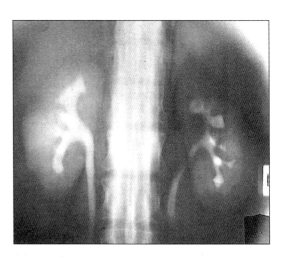

6.83 Analgesic nephropathy. This intravenous urogram shows bilaterally shrunken kidneys with typical calyceal distortions – the classic 'ring sign' plus the appearance of 'horns' and 'egg in cup'.

endeavour is in convincing the patient to stop ingesting analgesics, as continued intake invariably leads to end-stage renal failure. In addition, it is important to maintain hydration, treat infection and hypertension, and later to manage CRF.

MYELOMA KIDNEY

Myeloma kidney is the most common cause of renal failure in patients with multiple myeloma (*see* **p. 444**), and is more frequent in patients with Bence–Jones proteinuria. Renal failure in such patients is almost invariably associated with anaemia, and the diagnosis can usually be established by serum and urine electrophoresis (**10.116**), bone marrow examination (**10.117**) and skeletal survey (**10.118, 10.119**). Histologically, myeloma kidney is characterized by eosinophilic intraluminal casts, atrophic renal tubules and multinucleated giant cells within the tubule walls or interstitium (**6.84**). Renal failure in myeloma may also be caused by amyloid light-chain amyloidosis, light-chain nephropathy, acute interstitial nephritis, hypercalcaemia or hyperuricaemia, or it may follow dehydration or intravenous urography. Management of renal impairment in myeloma includes maintaining hydration, bicarbonate supplementation to improve solubility of light chains in the urine, and allopurinol to prevent hyperuricaemia after chemotherapy.

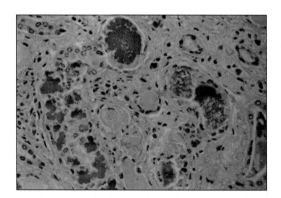

6.84   Myeloma kidney. There are prominent casts in the renal tubules, and a giant cell reaction is seen (bottom right) (*MSB ×330*).

RENAL TUBULAR DISORDERS

Most patients with renal disease have some abnormality in renal tubular function, but other manifestations of renal disease usually dominate the clinical picture. In some patients, however, renal tubular dysfunction occurs in isolation and results in clinical disorder.

There are many rare inherited and acquired disorders of renal tubular function. Their classification and management is a specialized field. The main categories of renal tubular disorders are summarized in **6.85**.

RENAL TUBULAR DISORDERS

Renal glycosuria

Aminoaciduria
   – single, e.g. cystinuria
   – multiple

Phosphate transport defects

Multiple tubular defects (Fanconi syndrome)
   – inherited
   – acquired

Renal tubular acidosis
   – type I (distal)
   – type II (proximal)
   – type IV (distal with hyperkalaemia and hyperchloraemia)

Salt-losing nephropathy

Nephrogenic diabetes insipidus

6.85   Renal tubular disorders: a simplified classification.

HYPERTENSION AND THE KIDNEY

RENAL HYPERTENSION

Renal disease is the most common cause of secondary hypertension and should be excluded in all young hypertensive patients (*see also* **p. 237**). Causes of renal-mediated hypertension can be classified into vascular diseases and parenchymal diseases (**6.86**).

The clinical features associated with hypertension depend on the underlying disease. Renal artery stenosis may be caused by atheroma or fibromuscular hyperplasia:

CAUSES OF RENAL HYPERTENSION

Vascular diseases

Atheromatous renal artery stenosis

Fibromuscular renal artery hyperplasia/stenosis

Renal infarction

Renal vasculitis

Systemic sclerosis

Parenchymal diseases

Glomerulonephritis

Chronic pyelonephritis

Polycystic kidney disease

Multisystem disease

Hydronephrosis

6.86   Causes of renal hypertension.

- Atheromatous renal artery stenosis should be suspected in patients with severe hypertension presenting in middle age or later without other evidence of renal disease; often these patients are heavy smokers and there is evidence of widespread atherosclerosis. This is now a relatively common problem in elderly patients, who may present with acute renal failure, CRF or end-stage renal failure requiring dialysis at presentation.
- Fibromuscular hyperplasia is more common in women, appears most often in the third or fourth decades, and is frequently bilateral.

A bruit may be heard over the flank, and biochemical investigation often reveals evidence of secondary hyperaldosteronism. Screening for unilateral renal artery stenosis is best performed by ultrasound, which may show unequal-sized kidneys, and the diagnosis can be confirmed non-invasively by a DTPA isotope renogram (**6.23**) or by arteriography, which will also show bilateral stenoses (**6.87**). Magnetic resonance angiography (MRA) is a non-invasive alternative (**6.24**).

Hypertension caused by fibromuscular disease is cured in more than 90% of patients after renovascular surgery. In patients with atherosclerotic disease, the failure rate after either surgery or angioplasty is much higher and corrective procedures are often restricted to patients who have severe renal failure or poorly controlled hypertension on medical therapy. The insertion of stent at angiography (**6.88**) may improve the long-term outcome.

Renal disease may ultimately develop in about one-half of patients with systemic sclerosis (*see* **p. 123**), often with the sudden onset of severe hypertension and progression to end-stage renal failure within months ('scleroderma crisis'). Renal

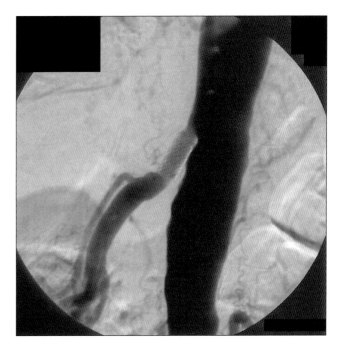

6.88 Stenting of the right renal artery to maintain patency after angioplasty. Before angioplasty, this patient had a 99% proximal stenosis of the artery in her solitary kidney, as demonstrated by MRA (*see* **6.24**). Angioplasty and the insertion of a stent near the origin of the artery restored near-normal flow to the renal artery and led to a significant improvement in renal function.

biopsy shows gross intimal thickening and reduction in the lumen of the interlobular arteries. Control of hypertension may be difficult and, if renal failure develops, recovery of renal function is unlikely.

The other causes of renal hypertension are described elsewhere in this chapter.

HYPERTENSIVE NEPHROPATHY

In hypertensive nephropathy, renal failure results from inadequately treated hypertension in the absence of primary renal disease. Long-standing moderate hypertension in itself can lead to hyaline thickening of the intrarenal arterial walls, patchy ischaemic atrophy and glomerulosclerosis. Patients with benign hypertensive nephrosclerosis usually present with CRF and mild proteinuria, without haematuria or other evidence of glomerulonephritis. Renal impairment often stabilizes if adequate, long-term control of hypertension is achieved.

Accelerated nephrosclerosis is a dramatic complication of malignant hypertension, which commonly caused progressive or acute renal failure before effective antihypertensive drugs were available. The two essential clinical features are the presence of severe hypertension and grade 4 retinopathy (**5.145**). Cardiac failure, hypertensive encephalopathy, renal

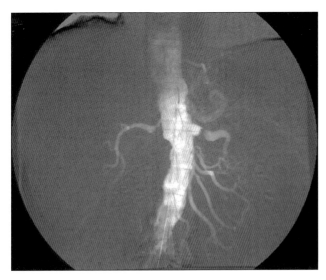

6.87 Bilateral renal artery stenosis, shown by anteriography. There are atheromatous strictures of both renal arteries with slight poststenotic dilatation. The lesions were successfully treated by angioplasty.

failure, secondary hyperaldosteronism and microangiopathic haemolytic anaemia may accompany the onset of malignant hypertension. The malignant phase may complicate essential and all forms of secondary hypertension. Renal biopsy may be required to determine whether there is underlying renal disease or whether renal failure is a direct consequence of severe hypertension. The histological features of malignant hypertension are fibrinoid necrosis of the afferent arterioles, and endarteritis of the interlobular and arcuate arteries that results in ischaemic atrophy or infarction distal to the abnormal vessels (**6.89**).

High blood pressure should be lowered gradually, to lessen the risk of a sudden drop in blood pressure either precipitating cerebral infarction or worsening renal function. In many patients, renal function may recover or at least stabilize once blood pressure is controlled and the prognosis depends on whether or not there are cardiac or cerebral complications.

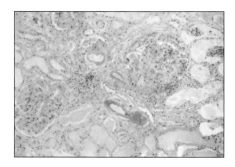

6.89 Malignant hypertension. The renal biopsy shows fibrinoid necrosis in the arterial and glomerular capillaries (red) and haemorrhage into the renal tubules (yellow) (*MSB ×132*).

FAMILIAL DISORDERS

There are many inherited disorders of renal structure and function. Some gross structural disorders, such as unilateral or bilateral duplex kidneys and ureters or a single horseshoe kidney, may predispose patients to ureteric reflux or obstruction and to recurrent UTIs, with a long-term risk of renal failure. Others, such as polycystic kidneys, may lead more directly to renal failure, by reducing the volume of functional renal tissue.

Inherited disorders may also cause both glomerular disease and tubular disorders.

Two inherited conditions are particularly important causes of CRF: adult polycystic kidney disease and Alport's syndrome.

ADULT POLYCYSTIC KIDNEY DISEASE

Autosomal dominant polycystic kidney disease (ADPKD) or adult-type polycystic kidney disease may be detected during the investigation of hypertension, loin pain or haematuria in young adults. Patients without these symptoms may not present until they develop CRF when middle-aged or older. These cases represent up to 10% of all cases coming to dialysis or transplantation. The condition is inherited as an autosomal dominant with high penetrance, and many patients are now diagnosed during screening of the proband's family. The prevalence in the UK is 1 in 2500, and the measured prevalence is rising because of increased ultrasound screening. The kidneys are almost invariably symmetrically enlarged because of the presence of multiple cysts. They may often be palpable clinically (**6.90**) and the diagnosis is best confirmed by ultrasound (**6.12**), or by CT (**6.19**, **9.57**), both of which may also demonstrate cysts in the liver and pancreas. IVU may show characteristic stretching and distortion of the calyces but is a less sensitive test than ultrasound. Cysts may also be demonstrated by radionuclide scan (**6.91**). Haemorrhage or infection in a cyst, haematuria leading to clot colic, UTI and renal calculi are not uncommon. Hypertension develops in more than 75% of patients, and renal function usually declines slowly until end-stage renal failure is reached from middle age onwards. Patients with end-stage renal failure caused by

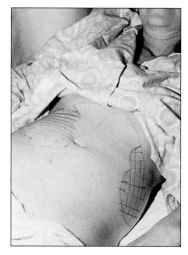

6.90 Adult polycystic kidney disease. The kidneys are huge and easily palpable as the skin markings show. Cysts are often also present in the liver and pancreas.

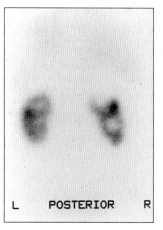

6.91 Bilateral polycystic kidneys, demonstrated by ^{99m}**Tc-DMSA scan.** The largest cysts are seen in the right kidney, especially in the upper pole.

ADPKD tend to be less anaemic than patients with renal failure resulting from other disorders. The enlargement of the kidneys does not usually lead to problems in performing peritoneal dialysis or renal transplantation.

By use of linkage analysis the ADPKD gene was located on the short arm of chromosome 16 (PKD-1); a second locus is on the long arm of chromosome 4 (PKD-2). This second defect is associated with less severe disease, and with later onset of renal cysts, hypertension and end-stage disease, although the renal and other abnormalities appear the same. A third variant (PKD-3) is so far unlinked. Genetic counselling is an important aspect of patient management, especially in families undergoing screening. Detection of carriers has now become possible with a gene probe.

In autosomal recessive polycystic kidney disease (ARPKD), the renal cysts arise from collecting tubules and the clinical features appear in childhood. There is an association with congenital hepatic fibrosis, which results from intrahepatic dilatation of bile ducts. The mutant gene locus is on chromosome 6.

ALPORT'S SYNDROME

Alport's syndrome is characterized by hereditary glomerulo-nephritis and nerve deafness (**6.92**). In about 40% of cases there are also eye abnormalities such as spherophakia, cataracts and macular and perimacular flecks. It is now appreciated that there are various pathogeneses. In some families there is diffuse leiomyomatosis involving the oesophagus, trachea and genital tracts. In the kidney the prime defect is in the glomerular basement membrane and its type IV collagen. In 80% of cases there is a dominant X-linked inheritance. Men tend to be more severely affected. It is uncommon for women to be symptomatic

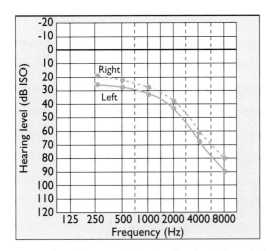

6.92 Alport's syndrome. Audiogram showing bilateral high-frequency nerve deafness. Lens abnormalities and deafness often coexist with renal failure in patients with Alport's syndrome.

before the age of 40 years, whereas most men have reached terminal renal failure by the age of 30 years. Most male patients present with recurrent or persistent haematuria in childhood, non-nephrotic range proteinuria, hypertension and CRF. Renal biopsy shows proliferative glomerulonephritis which on electron microscopy shows characteristic splitting and lamellation of the glomerular basement membrane. Renal failure is uncommon in women, but affected men usually require renal replacement therapy when adolescents or young adults.

In the 20% who are not X-linked there is a dominant or recessive autosomal trait that presents as renal disease of similar severity in both sexes.

The various genetic abnormalities have been localized to the X chromosome and chromosomes 2 and 13.

URINARY TRACT INFECTION (UTI)

ACUTE URINARY TRACT INFECTION

Urinary tract infection (UTI) is defined as the presence of microorganisms within the urinary tract with or without symptoms or signs of inflammation. Symptomatic urinary infection is a very common problem, accounting for 3–4% of consultations in general practice in the UK.

Infection affecting mainly the lower urinary tract may be asymptomatic or may lead to frequency and urgency of micturition, with local burning pain in the urethra on micturition (dysuria). The causative organism may be cultured from the urine, but a proportion of women with these symptoms have recurrent symptoms with negative cultures – probably because the causative organisms cannot be easily cultured.

The usual presentation of acute infection affecting the upper urinary tract and kidneys (acute pyelonephritis) is with pain in one or both loins, radiating round to the iliac fossa and suprapubic area. There is usually dysuria and pyrexia, often accompanied by rigors, nausea and vomiting. The main signs are tenderness in the lumbar region and on bimanual palpation of the kidneys. Examination of the urine shows white cells, red cells, proteinuria and a positive nitrate test. The blood picture shows an increased white cell count, and an elevated ESR, CRP or plasma viscosity. In acute pyelonephritis the causative organism can usually be cultured from the urine and often also in blood cultures.

Bacteriuria is considered significant if the numbers of bacteria in urine voided per urethram exceed 100 000 colony-forming units/ml in a properly collected specimen. Dip-slide urine culture (**6.11**) should be performed if delay is anticipated in a midstream urine specimen reaching the laboratory. Suprapubic aspiration may be needed to obtain a urine sample in infants, and any growth of bacteria from a suprapubic specimen of urine signifies the presence of infection.

The organisms that commonly cause UTI are listed in **6.93**, and *E. coli* is numerically most important. The organisms are thought usually to come from the patient's bowel, probably by direct spread from the anus, to colonize the urethra and then ascend to the bladder and kidney. Women are thought to be more likely to have UTIs because of the short length of the urethra. An important local defence against ascending infection is the hydrokinetic effect of passage of urine from the bladder. The clinical relevance of this is the increased incidence of UTIs in prostatic obstruction in men or in the presence of urinary stasis associated with a urinary diverticulum or urinary tract dilatation. Predisposing factors for urinary infection are listed in **6.94**.

UTI is important because of its frequency and its association with reflux nephropathy. In the female the incidence of UTI increases with age, and approximately 50% of adult women will, at some time, develop infection. In the male, there is a high incidence in the neonatal period, associated with developmental anomalies of the lower urinary tract, a low incidence in childhood and adult life, and an increase with advancing age. Investigation of the structure of the urinary tract is indicated in children of both sexes and adult men found to have a symptomatic or asymptomatic UTI. Women with recurrent infection also merit investigation (**6.94**).

UTI is usually adequately treated with a course of antibiotics, accompanied by analgesia and rehydration in severe cases, but long-term prophylaxis may be required in patients with structural abnormalities or recurrent infections.

CHRONIC PYELONEPHRITIS (REFLUX NEPHROPATHY)

Chronic interstitial nephritis that is thought to result from bacterial infection of the kidney has been termed chronic pyelonephritis. It may occur in patients with predisposing urological abnormalities (vesico-ureteric reflux, obstruction or neurogenic bladder) or in patients with apparently normal urinary tracts. The pathogenesis of pyelonephritic renal scarring in children is attributed to both parenchymal damage and impaired renal growth, which result from intrarenal reflux of infected urine. A history of recurrent UTI during childhood and evidence of vesico-ureteric reflux are therefore risk factors for the development of focal cortical scars.

During micturating cystography, reflux of contrast from the bladder may be limited to the ureter (grade I), reach the kidney but not distend the calyces (grade II) or reach the kidney and cause calyceal distension (grade III) (**6.20**, **6.95**). Vesico-

285

ORGANISMS THAT CAUSE UTI
Escherichia coli
Klebsiella spp.
Proteus mirabilis (and other spp.)
Enterobacter spp.
Streptococcus faecalis
Pseudomonas aeruginosa
Coagulase-negative *Staphylococcus* (esp. *saprophyticus*)
Staphylococcus aureus
Corynebacterium spp.
Haemophilus influenzae
Gardnerella vaginalis
The urinary tract may also be infected by *Mycobacterium tuberculosis* (see **p. 32**), by *Schistosoma haematobium* (see **p. 54**) and rarely by fungi.

6.93 **Organisms that commonly cause urinary tract infection.**

PREDISPOSING FACTORS IN UTI
Vesico-ureteric reflux
Obstructive uropathy
Calculi
Neurogenic bladder
Structural urinary tract abnormality (e.g. vesical fistula)
Pregnancy
Diabetes mellitus
Immunocompromised patient
Recent instrumentation or catheterization of urinary tract
Diaphragm use with or without spermicidal creams
Postmenopausal lack of oestrogen
Energetic sexual intercourse (especially in women)

6.94 **Predisposing factors in urinary tract infection.**

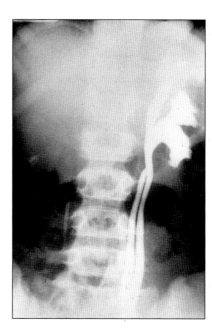

6.95 Unilateral grade III vesico-ureteric reflux with left bifid ureters, demonstrated by micturating cystogram.

ureteric reflux is present in 85% of patients with coarse scarred kidneys and 35% of children with symptomatic UTIs.

Reimplantation of the ureters to correct reflux and long-term antibiotic prophylaxis to prevent infection have been the main interventions utilized to try to prevent development of chronic pyelonephritis in children, but studies have shown no proven benefit from operative treatment of reflux when compared with antibiotic prophylaxis alone. Surgery to correct reflux is therefore now reserved for patients who have urinary infection despite antibiotic prophylaxis. Further renal scarring is unlikely after 7 years of age, so children with vesico-ureteric reflux and UTIs are often treated with prophylactic antibiotics until they reach this age and are encouraged to keep up a liberal fluid intake and practise double voiding.

Chronic pyelonephritis may be unilateral or bilateral and the characteristic appearance on IVU is clubbing of the calyces with overlying cortical scars, most commonly in the upper poles but ultimately generalized (**6.14, 6.96**). Scarring of the renal outline may also be demonstrated by DMSA isotope scan, and unilateral scarring is not uncommon (**6.21**). Chronic pyelonephritis may be detected during the investigation of patients with non-specific ill health, recurrent UTIs, hypertension or CRF. End-stage renal failure may develop in patients with bilateral renal scarring (**6.33**), even when hypertension is treated and further UTI prevented.

Renal tuberculosis is uncommon, but should be considered in all patients with sterile pyuria. The most common symptoms are fever, dysuria, haematuria, weight loss and general malaise (*see* **p. 32** for a general account of tuberculosis). At least three early-morning urine samples should be sent for culture of *Mycobacterium tuberculosis* and IVU may show calyceal changes (**6.97**), hydronephrosis, a contracted bladder or calcification at any point in the renal tract (**6.98**). Treatment with anti-tuberculous drugs should continue for at least 6 months and surgery may be required in some cases to relieve obstruction or to remove a non-functioning kidney.

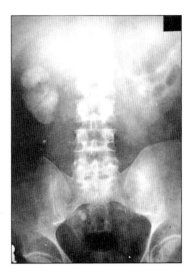

6.98 Renal tuberculosis may lead to progressive renal destruction and calcification, as here, where two-thirds of the right kidney has been destroyed and calcified.

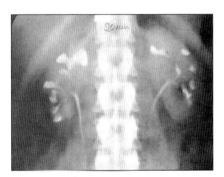

6.96 Bilateral chronic pyelonephritis. The intravenous urogram shows shrunken kidneys with gross calyceal clubbing and adjacent cortical scarring.

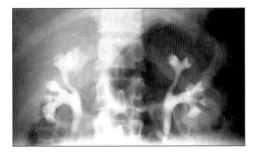

6.97 Renal tuberculosis affecting the right kidney. An initial minor lesion in the upper pole has become more invasive, and the disease has spread to affect more than one calyx, with irregularity and papillary cavitation.

OBSTRUCTIVE UROPATHY

Obstruction to the flow of urine results in increased urinary tract pressure and is a common cause of acute or chronic renal failure. Early relief of obstruction can allow renal function to recover completely, but chronic obstruction may produce cortical atrophy and permanent renal dysfunction. Obstructive uropathy should therefore be excluded promptly in all patients with acute or chronic renal failure of no established cause. Obstruction to urine flow may result from intrinsic or extrinsic mechanical blockade at any level of the urinary tract from the renal calyces to the external urethral meatus. Obstruction at or below the level of the bladder usually produces bilateral dilatation of the ureter (hydroureter) and renal pelvis and calyces (hydronephrosis), whereas obstruction may be unilateral if the site of blockage is above the level of the bladder. Mechanical causes of obstruction may be congenital (posterior urethral valves, ureterocele or pelviureteric stricture), acquired intrinsic defects (calculi, tumour, blood clot, sloughed papilla, stricture) or extrinsic defects (retroperitoneal fibrosis, fibroids, retroperitoneal or pelvic tumour). Functional impairment of urinary flow, caused by neurogenic bladder, may also cause obstruction. The most common cause of urinary obstruction in men is benign prostatic enlargement (BPE).

Patients with acute obstruction may present with loin or suprapubic pain, renal colic, oliguria or anuria. Chronic obstruction, on the other hand, may progress insidiously, but on direct questioning patients often admit to having polyuria and nocturia as a result of impaired renal concentrating ability. Hesitancy, postvoiding dribbling, urinary frequency and overflow incontinence are common in patients with obstruction at or below the level of the bladder. The possibility of obstructive uropathy should always be considered in patients with unexplained UTI or calculi. Dilatation of the urinary tract may be demonstrated by ultrasound (**6.99**) and functional obstruction confirmed by DTPA renography (**6.22**, **6.23**).

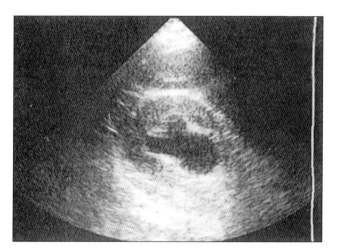

6.99 **Unilateral hydronephrosis demonstrated by ultrasound.** The normal renal outline is distorted by the fluid-filled collecting system.

Intravenous urography can be used to demonstrate obstruction anatomically and functionally, provided that the patient does not have significant renal failure (**6.15**), and retrograde pyelography may be needed in some cases (**6.100**, **6.101**).

Treatment depends on the site of obstruction and the underlying cause. The renal prognosis after relief of obstruction depends largely upon the degree of irreversible renal damage that has already occurred. Pre-renal failure may develop because of a post-obstructive diuresis, which not uncommonly occurs after relief of bilateral urinary tract obstruction. Such patients may require intravenous fluids temporarily.

RENAL CALCULI

Renal calculi are relatively common, affecting 1–5% of the population in the UK; they are more common in warm, dry countries and are composed of a mixture of chemicals, most commonly calcium oxalate alone or in combination with hydroxyapatite or calcium phosphate. Rarely, they may contain only uric acid or cystine (uric acid stones are radiolucent). About 20–40% of patients with calcium-containing stones have hypercalciuria (**6.102**) and a small number have hypercalcaemia, which should be investigated and treated (*see* **p. 139**). In the others, a search should be made for a cause of increased calcium absorption, for example vitamin D intoxication or renal tubular acidosis.

The clinical presentation of renal calculi is often dramatic, with the sudden onset of acute colicky pain resulting from impaction of the stone in the kidney, the ureter, bladder or urethra. There may also be haematuria and obstruction to urine flow. Passage of the stone produces instant relief, but if it obstructs either ureter or urethra it may cause progressive dull back pain. UTI is common (*see* **p. 284**) and may produce a pyonephrosis when combined with obstruction.

The diagnosis is usually suggested clinically and is confirmed by a plain X-ray of the abdomen (**6.13**, **6.103–6.105**), an IVU

6.100   6.101

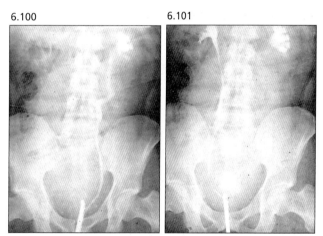

6.100, 6.101 **Retroperitoneal fibrosis.** This condition commonly affects both ureters, but it may be unilateral. In this patient, the left retrograde ureterogram (**6.100**) shows that retroperitoneal fibrosis has obstructed and distorted the left ureter and caused a left hydronephrosis; the right retrograde ureterogram and pyelogram are normal (**6.101**).

CAUSES OF HYPERCALCIURIA
Hyperparathyroidism
Immobilization
Bone metastases
Sarcoidosis
Distal renal tubular acidosis

6.102 **Causes of hypercalciuria.**

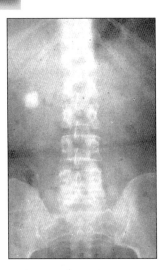

6.103 A single calculus in the renal pelvis is demonstrated on this plain (KUB) X-ray. The X-ray was performed to investigate an episode of renal colic.

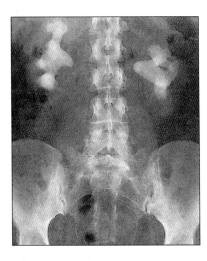

6.104 Large bilateral staghorn calculi are shown on this plain (KUB) X-ray. The patient presented with recurrent urinary infections.

6.105

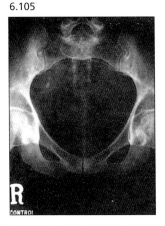

6.106

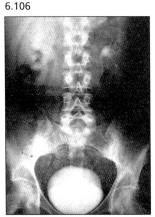

6.105, 6.106 Two small stones in the ureter are seen in **6.105**. Stones of this size may sometimes pass without symptoms or with only a transient effect, but in this patient they caused ureteric obstruction, as can be seen in the intravenous urogram (**6.106**).

(**6.106**), ultrasound or retrograde pyelography. Urine should be cultured and examined microscopically for blood. Treatment of the pain is the overriding necessity and an antispasmodic may be of value. UTI requires an appropriate antibiotic. Stones less than 5 mm in diameter will usually pass spontaneously. Surgical intervention or lithotripsy may be required for larger stones. In extracorporeal shock wave lithotripsy (ESWL), a shock wave is generated by piezoelectric crystals outside the body and focused on the renal stone(s). Such shocks are administered as short pulses up to 500–2000 times. The stone disintegrates sufficiently for the particles to be passed down the ureter. Occasionally staghorn calculi may need to be disintegrated percutaneously before ESWL, as may stones in the lower calyces. Uric acid and cystine stones tend to be harder and more difficult to break down. Ureteric stones in the upper two-thirds of the ureter may also be treated with ESWL. The success rate of ESWL is about 60–70%.

Renal and urinary tract calcification may occur in renal tuberculosis (*see* **p. 286**) and in medullary sponge kidney, a condition in which cystic change occurs in the collecting ducts in the renal papillae, with accompanying stone formation. This most commonly presents as haematuria or renal colic, or with UTI. Nephrocalcinosis, the deposition of calcium within the body of the kidneys, may also occur in conditions associated with hypercalcaemia, including sarcoidosis, hyperparathyroidism, myeloma, malignancy and Paget's disease, and in idiopathic hypercalciuria.

Bladder stones may grow to a massive size before presentation and need to be removed surgically. They may arise from stones formed in the kidneys that have migrated, from foreign bodies in the bladder (e.g. sutures) or from the same biochemical abnormalities as renal stones.

RENAL TUMOURS

Neoplasms may develop at any point in the urinary tract, but they occur most commonly in the kidney or bladder and they should be excluded in all patients presenting with painless macroscopic or microscopic haematuria. Renal cell carcinoma (hypernephroma, adenocarcinoma of kidney) is the most common renal neoplasm and is of tubular epithelial origin. Patients may present with systemic symptoms (weight loss, malaise, fever) or urinary tract symptoms (haematuria, loin pain, abdominal mass), or both. Increasingly, lesions are identified in patients undergoing CT for an unconnected reason. It is important to differentiate renal cell carcinoma from renal cysts, and from benign tumours such as renal angiomyolipomas. This is not always easy, but renal cell carcinoma may be demonstrated by ultrasound, intravenous urography (**6.107**), abdominal CT (**6.108**) or renal arteriography (**6.16**). Metastases are common and, once the diagnosis is established, patients should be investigated to evaluate whether pulmonary (**4.29**), bone (**3.158**), hepatic or cerebral (**11.57**) metastases are present. The prognosis depends largely upon the extent of tumour involvement at the time of

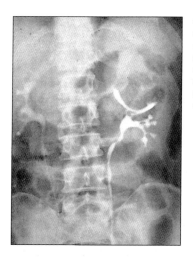

6.107   Renal cell carcinoma has caused calyceal distortion with stretching and separation of the calyces in the upper left kidney, as seen on this intravenous urogram.

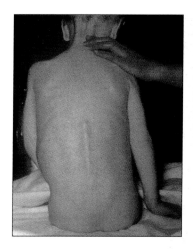

6.109   Nephroblastoma (Wilms' tumour). This 8-year-old boy had a mass in the left loin which moved on respiration and was ballotable. Its renal nature was confirmed on intravenous urogram (**6.110**) and a nephroblastoma was found at surgery.

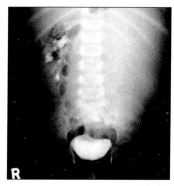

6.110   Nephroblastoma (Wilms' tumour). This intravenous urogram shows a vast mass occupying the entire left loin.

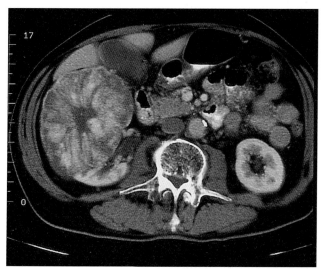

6.108   Renal cell carcinoma as seen on contrast CT. Compare the massive right renal tumour with the normal kidney seen on the left side.

diagnosis. The standard approach to treatment in patients without evidence of metastases is radical nephrectomy; in this group, the survival rate at 5 years approaches 65%. Partial nephrectomy is feasible and effective in patients with early peripheral tumours. However, many patients have metastatic disease at the time of diagnosis and have a much poorer prognosis despite treatment with chemotherapy and radiotherapy.

Nephroblastoma (Wilms tumour) is the second most common malignant tumour of the kidney and is the most common malignancy of the urinary tract in children, with a peak incidence between the ages of 2 and 4 years (**6.109, 6.110**). Aggressive treatment with nephrectomy, preoperative or postoperative radiotherapy and postoperative chemotherapy have improved the prognosis and 5-year survival now exceeds 75%.

Neoplasms of the renal pelvis, ureter and bladder, derived from transitional urothelium, are relatively common and often occur or recur at multiple sites in the lower urinary tract. There is an increased incidence of bladder cancer in workers exposed to various aromatic amines employed in chemical, rubber or dye industries. Haematuria is the most common presentation and the site and extent of involvement is usually determined by a combination of cystoscopy (**6.26**) with biopsy, and intravenous urography (**6.18**). The prognosis is dependent upon the extent of local invasion and degree of anaplasia at the time of diagnosis. Treatments include cystoscopic removal, cystectomy and local radiotherapy. Patients with urothelial tumours of the renal pelvis or ureter usually require nephroureterectomy.

Diffuse infiltration of the kidneys by neoplastic cells in lymphomas or leukaemias may result in renal enlargement or renal failure. Retroperitoneal lymphoma may also cause renal failure as a result of bilateral ureteric obstruction.

PROSTATIC DISEASE

BENIGN PROSTATIC ENLARGEMENT (BPE)

Benign prostatic enlargement (BPE) seems to be an inevitable consequence of ageing in men, though its cause is unknown.

Changes in the gland size and histology start at the age of 40 years and progress so that most men have symptoms by the age of 70 years. Patients may present with a combination of chronic symptoms associated with chronic urinary retention (**6.111**) or with acute urinary retention requiring urgent treatment in its own right. The diagnosis of BPE is suggested by the history, and rectal examination confirms the presence of an enlarged gland. It is important to exclude rarer neurological, inflammatory and neoplastic causes of lower urinary symptoms. Prostate cancer is a common associate of BPE, and its presence is suggested by irregular enlargement of the prostate, by the finding of an elevated prostate-specific antigen (PSA; *see* **6.14**) or by features suggesting secondary spread. Transrectal ultrasound (**6.112**) may be performed in BPE to investigate for possible prostate cancer.

First-line treatment for uncomplicated BPE in patients with milder symptoms is now medical. Prostatic tissue contains an enzyme, 5α-reductase, that metabolizes testosterone to dihydrotestosterone, a more potent androgen which is implicated in the hypertrophy. Finasteride is a testosterone analogue that blocks production of dihydrotestosterone. This leads to a reduction in gland size and significantly reduces symptoms. Treatment with selective α_1-blockers may also lead to symptomatic improvement, but does not arrest or reverse the underlying prostatic hypertrophy.

Surgical treatment is still required in patients with gross prostatic enlargement, with substantial urinary flow obstruction or with associated obstructive uropathy, bladder stones or recurrent UTI. Transurethral resection of the prostate (TURP) can be performed in about 95% of these cases, but open prostatectomy is still required in 5% with gross prostatic enlargement or associated pathology. Techniques such as laser ablation, electrovaporization, thermotherapy and stent insertion may provide minimally invasive treatment options in the future.

PROSTATE CANCER

Prostate cancer is the second most common type of cancer in men in the UK and is increasingly common throughout the developed world. Its incidence rises with advancing years and it occurs in one in 10 men living to the age of 70 years. The early clinical features of prostate cancer are indistinguishable from those of BPE and the gland may feel normal on digital examination. The PSA is usually elevated by the time of diagnosis (> 4 ng/ml). As the tumour grows locally it may produce bladder neck obstruction, obstruct the ureters and thus lead to rapidly progressive renal failure. In advanced disease, rectal examination shows the prostate to be large, hard and irregular. Rectal ultrasound may show the extent of the cancer (**6.112**) and is used to direct needle or aspiration biopsy. Prostatic biopsy is important in giving diagnostic and prognostic information – the prognosis being poorer with poorly differentiated tumours.

Distant spread via lymphatics and blood leads to bony metastases, which are usually sclerotic in nature (**3.157, 6.113**), and secondary deposits may also appear in other organs. Metastatic spread is likely in the presence of a very high PSA level (> 50 ng/ml).

Therapy depends on staging, and may involve surgery, local radiotherapy, orchidectomy and hormone therapy with oestrogens and anti-androgens. The PSA level is used as one method of monitoring the effects of therapy.

It has been suggested that all men between the ages of 50 and 75 years should be screened by rectal examination and PSA measurement, followed when indicated by transrectal ultrasound. The routine use of PSA in screening is still under debate, as the 'normal' range for PSA is age-dependent and a raised value can occur in other disorders such as prostatitis. A

CLINICAL FEATURES OF BENIGN PROSTATIC ENLARGEMENT (BPE)

Obstructive symptoms

Hesitancy

Weak stream

Straining to pass urine

Prolonged micturition

Feeling of incomplete bladder emptying

Chronic urinary retention

Acute urinary retention

Irritative symptoms

Urgency

Frequency

Nocturia

Urge incontinence

6.111 Clinical features of benign prostatic enlargment.

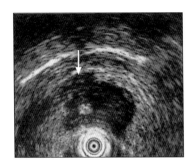

6.112 A rectal ultrasound probe can be used to define and stage carcinoma of the prostate. In this case, the right lobe of the capsule of the prostate is distorted, and anteriorly a capsular breach is evident (arrow), suggesting extracapsular spread of the tumour. Ultrasound-guided biopsy is now standard practice in the diagnosis and management of prostatic disease.

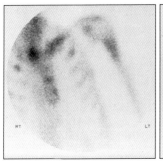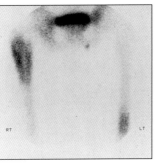

6.113 Multiple bone metastases in a patient with carcinoma of the prostate, revealed by bone scan. Areas of increased activity are present in the femora, ribs, sternum and left humerus.

rising level over a period of time may be of greatest significance. A clear plan of action (**6.114**) is essential before such a screening programme is started, and there is still a risk that screening may reveal large numbers of patients with small, clinically silent tumours for which optimal management has not been established.

INTERPRETATION OF PROSTATE-SPECIFIC ANTIGEN (PSA) AND RESULTING ACTION		
PSA level	**Interpretation**	**Action**
< 4 ng/ml	Normal	None
4–10 ng/ml	20–25% chance of cancer	Consider biopsy
> 10 ng/ml	> 50% chance of cancer	Biopsy usually indicated
Rise of > 0.75 ng/ml/year	Strong possibility of cancer	Refer urgently for evaluation

6.114 Interpretation of prostate specific antigen (PSA) and resulting action.

7 Endocrine, diabetes, metabolic and nutritional

HISTORY, EXAMINATION AND INVESTIGATION

The presentations of endocrine disease are diverse, and the findings in the history and on examination of the patient reflect this. Although multiple endocrine disorders may occur in the same patient, most have abnormalities of a single hormonal system, and the symptoms, signs and necessary investigations relate closely to those abnormalities.

A full history and examination is essential in any patient with a suspected endocrine disorder. Common presentations that should raise the possibility of endocrine disease are listed in **7.1**, and **7.2** emphasizes the common importance of aspects of the patient's previous medical and family history.

Necessary investigations depend upon the patient's clinical presentation and may include many different tests on blood and urine and imaging by radiological, nuclear or magnetic resonance (MR) techniques.

The diagnosis of endocrine diseases has been advanced by techniques that can measure low concentrations of hormones in body fluid by sensitive radiochemical or immunological means. As most hormones are produced in characteristic patterns, it is important to take appropriate samples at the relevant times. Some hormones, for example cortisol and testosterone, have a circadian rhythm, with higher levels in the morning. Others, especially the gonadotrophins, are produced intermittently. The pattern of release may vary with sex and with advancing age (growth hormone), with stress (prolactin), diet and concurrent medication. Urine collections over a 24-hour period

293

COMMON PRESENTING COMPLAINTS IN ENDOCRINE DISEASE

Body size and shape
Short stature
Tall stature
Excessive weight or weight gain
Loss of weight

Metabolic effects
Tiredness
Weakness
Increased appetite
Decreased appetite
Polydipsia or thirst
Polyuria or nocturia
Tremor
Palpitation
Anxiety

Local effects
Swelling in the neck
Nerve entrapment (e.g. carpal tunnel syndrome)
Bone or muscle pain
Protrusion of eyes
Visual loss (acuity or fields, or both)
Headache

Reproduction or sex
Loss or absence of libido
Impotence
Oligomenorrhoea or amenorrhoea
Subfertility
Galactorrhoea
Gynaecomastia
Delayed puberty
Precocious puberty

Skin
Hirsuties
Hair thinning
Pigmentation
Dry skin
Excessive sweating

7.1 Common presenting complaints in endocrine disease.

ENDOCRINE DISEASE – PAST AND FAMILY HISTORIES

Previous medical history

Previous pregnancies (ease of conception, postpartum haemorrhage)

Relevant surgery (e.g. thyroidectomy, orchidopexy)

Radiation (e.g. to neck, gonads, thyroid)

Drug exposure (e.g. chemotherapy, hormone replacement therapy, oral contraceptives)

In utero, complications of pregnancy

At birth, weight and length

In childhood, developmental milestones

Family history

Family history of: Autoimmune disease; endocrine disease; essential hypertension

Family details of: Height; weight; body habitus; hair growth; age of sexual development

7.2 Endocrine disease – past and family histories.

are of value for some hormones in measuring total output of the gland and overcoming the problems of rhythmic variations in level.

In addition to these static tests, it is often important to determine the response of a gland to stimulation and suppression:

- Stimulation tests assess the ability of the gland to increase its hormonal output; the response is diminished if the cells are structurally or functionally damaged.
- Suppression tests use the administration of purified hormone to test the negative feedback loop; hormone production is normally suppressed in these tests, but persists if there is autonomy or a functional endocrine tumour.

Although isolated endocrine abnormalities are common, many are potentially related to abnormalities of the hypo-thalamic–pituitary axis, so initial investigations may lead on to a need for further tests.

DISORDERS OF THE PITUITARY AND HYPOTHALAMUS

The pituitary gland consists of an anterior and a posterior lobe. It lies at the base of the brain, in the sella turcica, within the sphenoid bone, and has a close anatomical and physiological relationship to the hypothalamus. Its anatomical relationship to the optic chiasma is important, as pituitary tumours often affect the visual fields. The hypothalamus has a major role in integrating and coordinating pituitary function, body temperature, water, mineral and calorie balance, and sexual and reproductive behaviour. This is achieved through the hypothalamo-hypophyseal portal system. The hypothalamus controls the secretion of the anterior pituitary hormones by secreting a number of regulatory factors (releasing or inhibitory hormones).

The posterior pituitary also functionally includes various hypothalamic areas. Oxytocin is released here. Antidiuretic hormone (ADH) is secreted by the supra-optic and paraventricular nuclei; it passes down the neurohypophyseal tract to be linked with neurophysin and is stored in the posterior lobe, from which it is secreted into the general circulation.

Pituitary lesions may declare themselves by:

- local space-occupying effects
- hypopituitarism
- hypersecretion of a pituitary hormone
- an incidental radiological finding.

Both neuroradiological and endocrinological investigations are important in diagnosis and management.

Dynamic tests of pituitary hormonal reserve are summarized in **7.3**.

Space-occupying effects are caused by large tumours that commonly grow upwards, compressing the optic chiasma, which is only 1 cm above the pituitary fossa (*see also* **p. 470**).

DYNAMIC TESTS OF PITUITARY HORMONAL RESERVE		
Stimulation tests	**Hormones**	**Markers**
Insulin hypoglycaemia	ACTH, GH	GH, cortisol, blood glucose
Glucagon	ACTH, GH	GH, blood glucose
Thyrotrophin-releasing hormone (TRH)	TSH	TSH, T3, T4, prolactin, GH
Gonadotrophin-releasing hormone (GnRH)	LH, FSH	FSH, LH, spermatogenesis, ovulation
Growth hormone-releasing hormone (GHRH)	GH	GH
Corticotrophin-releasing hormone (CRH)	ACTH	ACTH, cortisol
Fluid deprivation/ desmopressin	ADH	Urine/plasma osmolality
Suppression tests	**Hormones suppressed**	
Growth hormone-release inhibitory hormone (GHRIH; somatostatin) or analogue (octreotide)	GH, TSH, insulin, glucagon, gastrin, VIP	

7.3 Dynamic tests of pituitary hormonal reserve.

The most common visual defects are a bitemporal upper quadrantic defect or a hemianopia (**11.5**). The patient may not notice the deterioration in eyesight until the central fields are affected. Expansion of the pituitary fossa is seen on a lateral skull radiograph in 90% of patients. Other important features are thinning and undercutting of the anterior and posterior clinoid processes and asymmetry of the fossa floor (**7.4**). The extent of a pituitary tumour can be demonstrated by MRI (**7.5–7.7**) or CT.

Less common effects of growth outside the pituitary fossa include:

- diplopia (cranial nerve palsies with extra-ocular muscle dysfunction, *see* **p. 450**)

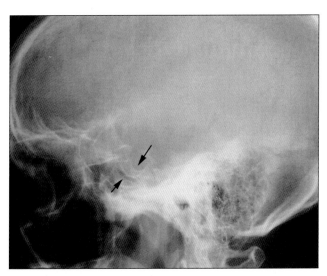

7.4 Pituitary fossa enlargement with a double floor (arrowed) on lateral X-ray. This patient had an acidophil tumour, with symptoms and signs of acromegaly.

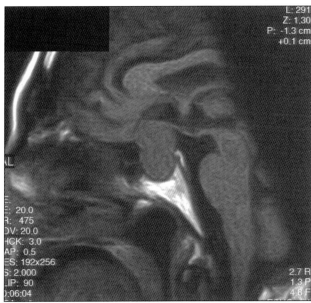

7.6

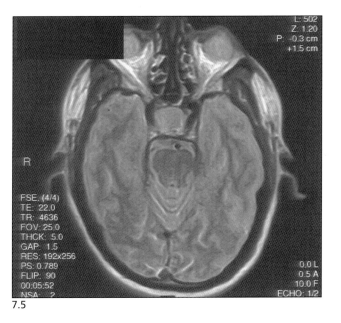

7.5

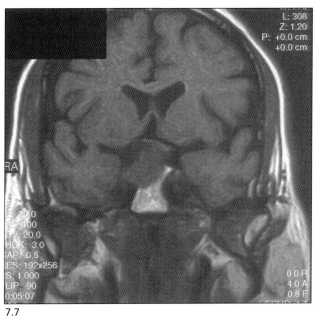

7.7

7.5, 7.6 & 7.7 Pituitary macroadenoma. A large tumour is demonstrated on axial, sagittal and coronal T1-weighted MR images. The tumour extends above the sella, distorting the optic chiasma, laterally into the right cavernous sinus and downwards, eroding the floor of the pituitary fossa asymetrically.

- pituitary apoplexy (acute enlargement of a tumour caused by haemorrhagic infarction), resulting in depressed consciousness, sudden loss of vision, other focal signs and often meningism
- personality changes, focal hemispheric neurological signs and epilepsy
- papilloedema from raised intracranial pressure is very rare, as is optic atrophy from long-standing suprasellar extension with compression of the optic pathways.

HYPOPITUITARISM

Most lesions of the pituitary cause destruction of the anterior pituitary or the hypothalamus. The pattern of deficiencies depends on the nature of the lesion and its rate of progress. The clinical picture depends on the cause, the pattern of hormone loss and local effects of the pathology within the sella. Postpartum pituitary necrosis (Sheehan's syndrome, **7.8–7.10**) was formerly the most common cause, but with improved obstetric practice this is now much less common. The main causes are pituitary tumours, that is chromophobe adenomas in adults and craniopharyngiomas in children, and iatrogenic hypopituitarism after surgical or radiotherapeutic damage. Trauma, infection and infiltration in sarcoidosis, histiocytosis X and haemochromatosis are other rare causes. Partial degrees of pituitary damage can occur, but symptoms are uncommon before at least 70% of the gland is destroyed.

The development of hypopituitarism often results in a progressive loss of function, starting with growth hormone (GH). Gonadotrophin failure – initially luteinizing hormone (LH) then follicle-stimulating hormone (FSH) – also occurs early and impotence in the male and amenorrhoea in the female are common symptoms. The clinical features in adults include fine wrinkling of the skin around the mouth with loss of facial and body hair (**7.8**), and atrophy of the genitalia in both sexes (**7.11**). In childhood, gonadotrophin failure leads to delayed puberty and short stature (**7.12**). Isolated gonadotrophin deficiency associated with anosmia is seen in Kallmann's syndrome (discussed later).

Next to be lost is adrenocorticotrophic hormone (ACTH). The features of this deficiency are asthenia, nausea, vomiting, postural hypotension, hypoglycaemia, collapse and coma, pallor of the skin and reduced sun-tanning ability. Thyroid-stimulating hormone (TSH) is eventually lost, giving rise to features similar to those seen in primary hypothyrodism, although the skin is not dry and coarse. In childhood, TSH deficiency contributes to growth retardation. Prolactin deficiency causes failure of lactation. A more common effect in hypopituitarism is hyperprolactinaemia, which occurs if a tumour prevents the prolactin inhibitor, dopamine, from reaching the pituitary by stalk compression.

Cranial diabetes insipidus (CDI) results from ADH (vasopressin) deficiency and occurs very uncommonly in anterior pituitary disease, usually after meningitis or head

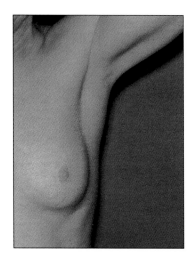

7.8   Lack of body hair in hypopituitarism. Twenty years earlier, this patient developed postpartum pituitary necrosis (Sheehan's syndrome). This resulted in many features of hypopituitarism, including a total absence of axillary and pubic hair.

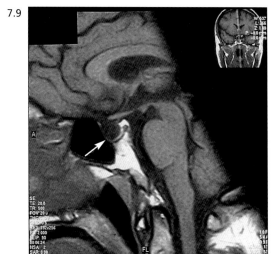

7.9

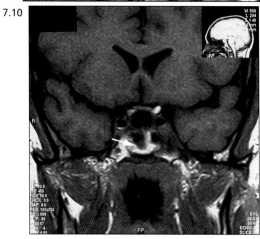

7.10

7.9 & 7.10   Empty sella (arrows) in a patient with hypopituitarism after postpartum pituitary necrosis, demonstrated by MRI. The pituitary fossa is fluid-filled, with no recognizable pituitary tissue (compare with the appearances of a pituitary adenoma in **7.6** and **7.7**).

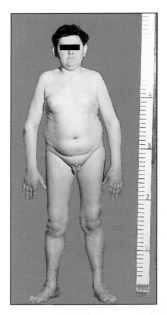

7.11 Hypopituitarism with gonadotrophin failure in a 39-year-old man. Note the extreme atrophy of the genitalia, the absence of body hair and the apparent gynaecomastia associated with obesity.

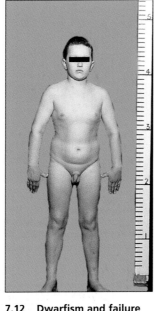

7.12 Dwarfism and failure of puberty resulted from gonadotrophin failure in this 17-year-old boy with hypopituitarism. He was well below average height at 1.4 m, and had infantile genitalia and mild gynaecomastia.

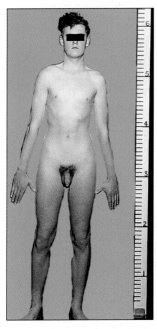

7.13 Mild gigantism resulting from the presence of increased growth hormone levels before epiphyseal fusion. The patient was 15 when this photograph was taken, and he reached a final height of 2.02 m.

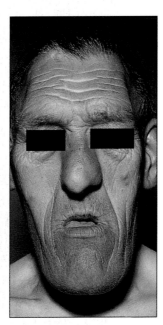

7.14 The characteristic facial features of acromegaly include thickening of the soft tissues and skin, enlargement of the nose and the supraorbital ridges, acne, thickening of the lips and prognathism.

injury. It is most frequently associated with craniopharyngioma, which may cause destruction of the posterior pituitary. There may be other hypothalamic disturbances, such as sleep disorders, hyperphagia, disturbed thermoregulation and emotional lability. The main investigation is water deprivation and measurement of urine osmolality. Treatment is with desmopressin. Nephrogenic diabetes insipidus (NDI) results from renal resistance to ADH, not from pituitary dysfunction.

Pituitary hypofunction can be confirmed by 'basal' blood samples for cortisol, thyroxine, testosterone or oestradiol, and GH and other pituitary hormones, followed by a pituitary stress test.

Treatment of panhypopituitarism is by hormone replacement. GH is replaced by biosynthetic (recombinant) GH therapy. Cortisol is normally replaced by hydrocortisone, given in the morning and evening to mimic the normal diurnal pattern. Thyroxine and either testosterone or oestrogen, usually with progestogen, are prescribed to restore libido and to prevent osteoporosis and cardiovascular disease.

DISEASES ASSOCIATED WITH HYPERSECRETION OF PITUITARY HORMONES

Acromegaly and gigantism

The excessive secretion of GH is almost invariably caused by a pituitary tumour. If this occurs before fusion of the epiphyses, it leads to gigantism (**7.13**); after fusion, it produces the features of acromegaly.

Acromegaly is an uncommon condition with a prevalence of approximately three new cases/million people per year. Some patients with multiple endocrine neoplasia (MEN type 1) may present this way. Some tumours are mixed and produce both prolactin or TSH and GH. The disease should be suspected on the finding of clinical features that include thickening of the soft tissues and skin, broadening of the nose, increased prominence of supraorbital and nuchal ridges, and prognathism, which leads to separation of the teeth (**7.14–7.16**).

Excessive sweating and acne (**7.14**) are common symptoms of acromegaly, and on examination large, spade-like hands are

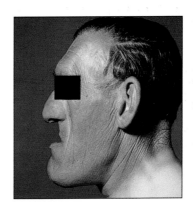

7.15 Acromegaly. Profile of the patient shown in **7.14**, showing prognathism, thickening of the soft tissues and skin, and increased prominence of the supraorbital ridge and nose.

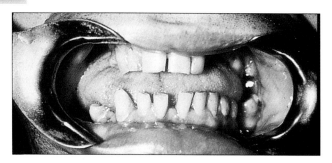

7.16 Malocclusion and separation of the teeth are commonly associated with the development of prognathism in acromegaly.

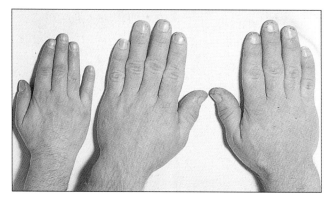

7.17 Spade-like hands are often an obvious abnormality in acromegaly. Compare the acromegalic hands on the right with the normal hand on the left. Overgrowth of the soft tissues may also cause compression of the median nerve at the wrist (carpal tunnel syndrome, *see* **p. 489**).

obvious (**7.17, 7.18**). There is enlargement of the tongue (**7.19**) and all other viscera such as liver and spleen. The voice may become hoarse, and visual field defects (bitemporal hemianopia; **11.5**) develop as the pituitary tumour enlarges. Cardiomegaly, heart failure (**7.20**) and malignancy are major causes of death.

Diagnosis is based on demonstrating that GH is not suppressed during an oral glucose tolerance test. Imaging by X-ray (**7.4**), CT or, best, by MRI (**7.6, 7.7**) defines the size and local impact of the pituitary adenoma.

Treatment is often difficult. Surgical removal of the tumour by a trans-sphenoidal or frontal route may reverse the disease, but complete removal without recurrence is difficult and external radiotherapy to the pituitary fossa is indicated postoperatively. Radiotherapy alone leads to only a slow clinical improvement, causing GH to fall over 1–10 years. Surgery with or without radiotherapy may cause hypopituitarism; this should always be assessed and treated accordingly. Medical treatment is less effective in long-term management. Somatostatin analogues, growth hormone antagonists or, in some patients, dopamine antagonists may be used to suppress the release or the effects of GH until the effect of radiotherapy is evident.

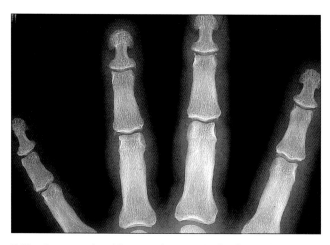

7.18 Acromegaly. This X-ray shows typical tufting of the terminal phalanges of the fingers, a common radiological associate of the clinical appearance seen in **7.17**.

Hyperprolactinaemia

Sleep, stress, nipple stimulation, coitus, pregnancy and suckling are all associated with physiological elevation of circulating prolactin levels. Hyperprolactinaemia is associated with hypogonadism, either from pathological, physiological or iatrogenic causes. Therefore, the woman who breast-feeds is often infertile and amenorrhoeic, and patients on drugs that raise prolactin (e.g. metoclopramide, haloperidol) may have infrequent periods (in women) or impotence (in men). Hyperprolactinaemia in childhood may lead to delayed onset of puberty. Pituitary tumours secreting prolactin are four times more common than GH-producing tumours, and very much more common than those producing ACTH. Some non-functioning tumours may produce moderate elevations in prolactin by pituitary stalk compression. There are no specific signs of hyperprolactinaemia except hypogonadism, although galactorrhoea (inappropriate lactation; **7.21**) should always

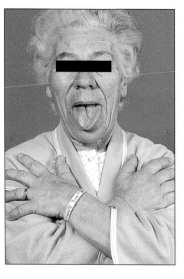

7.19 Enlargement of the tongue in acromegaly is obvious in this patient, who also shows other facial signs, and has classic changes in her hands.

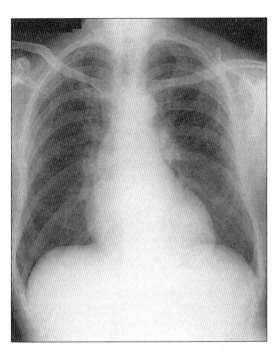

7.20 Acromegaly. The chest X-ray shows generalized cardiac enlargement (cardiothoracic ratio > 50%). Heart failure is a major cause of morbidity and mortality in acromegaly.

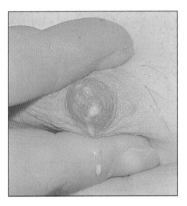

7.21 Galactorrhoea in a female patient with a prolactin-secreting pituitary tumour.

Diagnosis of a prolactinoma is made from elevated prolactin levels above 4000 mU/litre (upper limit of normal on most assays is 360 mU/litre). Smaller tumours give lower levels. CT or MRI may show the presence of an adenoma (**7.22**), and it is important to note that these may undergo considerable expansion during pregnancy.

Treatment by a long-acting dopamine agonist such as cabergoline or bromocriptine will inhibit prolactin production and produce shrinkage of 80% of tumours, thus relieving pressure symptoms particularly on the optic chiasma. Fertility is regained and, although the drug is not teratogenic, once pregnancy has been established it is usually stopped; visual fields must be monitored regularly. Patients with macroadenomas are best advised to have surgery or radiotherapy at least 3 months before attempts at conception, as these tumours may expand rapidly during pregnancy.

Cushing's syndrome

The term Cushing's syndrome describes the combination of symptoms and signs which results from persistent elevation of circulating glucocorticosteroid levels. The most common cause of Cushing's syndrome is prolonged therapy with systemic glucocorticosteroids. The term Cushing's disease is used to describe patients in whom the syndrome results from excessive ACTH production by the pituitary; this is the most common cause of spontaneous Cushing's syndrome (60%). Other causes

arouse suspicion. It should always be remembered, however, that galactorrhoea may result from other causes, especially from malignant tumours producing prolactin or oestrogen, or from drug therapy with phenothiazines, antidepressants, haloperidol, methyldopa, metoclopramide or oral contraceptives.

Prolactinomas are usually microadenomas in women and macroadenomas in men. Clinical features are related to tumour size and function. In women the clinical features relate mainly to excess production of prolactin, which causes amenorrhoea, infertility and galactorrhoea. In men excess prolactin causes loss of libido, impotence and occasionally gynaecomastia, and with larger tumours there may be headache, visual field defects and nerve palsies. Similar pressure-related features may develop in women during pregnancy.

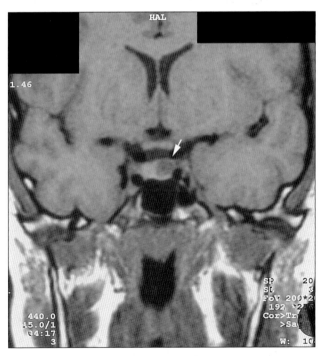

7.22 Pituitary microadenoma on a coronal MR image. This 24-year-old woman's symptoms related to hyperprolactinaemia, and she had no symptoms suggesting local pressure. Bromocriptine therapy resulted in shrinkage of the adenoma.

are ectopic ACTH production (15%), adrenal adenoma (15%) and adrenal carcinoma (10%). Cushing's disease is usually caused by a basophilic pituitary microadenoma (90%) and occurs more frequently in women.

The clinical features of the syndrome that are of greatest discriminatory importance include thinning of the skin, easy bruising and bright purple striae (**7.23–7.26**), proximal muscle weakness and myopathy (**7.26**), facial plethora (**6.45**, **7.27**), hirsuties (**7.27**, *see also* **p. 90**), acne and loss of scalp hair. Weight gain and obesity are the most common presenting features. The distribution of fat is central, involving the trunk and abdomen (**7.28**, **7.29**). This, together with the kyphosis that is often caused by osteoporosis (*see* **p. 135**), results in a 'buffalo hump', with a 'moon face' and relatively thin limbs.

Pigmentation may occur, but this is more common in ectopic ACTH production (from a malignant bronchial tumour, for example) or in Nelson's syndrome, in which ACTH levels are very high. Nelson's syndrome may follow bilateral adrenalectomy for Cushing's disease if excessive ACTH production continues (**7.30**); expansion of the pituitary fossa may occur. Pigmentation is most marked in areas exposed to sunlight and friction, and in scars. Psychiatric symptoms, hypertension, glucose intolerance, diabetes and gonadal dysfunction (oligomenorrhoea and impotence) are all common.

Adrenal tumours may secrete cortisol and cause classic Cushing's syndrome. However, the concomitant secretion of adrenal androgens may cause more virilization, particularly in the case of carcinomas. Ectopic ACTH from highly malignant tumours causes gross elevations of cortisol; patients may present

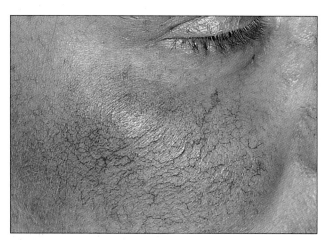

7.23   Cushing's syndrome is associated with typical thin skin and fragile blood vessels. Bruising commonly results from very minor trauma.

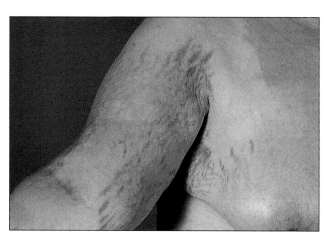

7.25   Cushing's syndrome. This patient has typical purple striae on the breast and arm, associated with thinning of the skin.

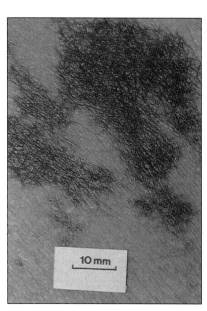

7.24   Thin, fragile skin in Cushing's syndrome and blood vessel fragility has resulted in extensive bruising.

10 mm

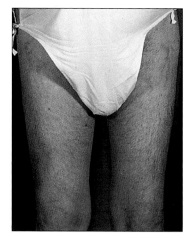

7.26   Proximal muscle wasting is common in Cushing's syndrome and leads to great difficulty in rising from the sitting position. Note the presence of striae on both thighs.

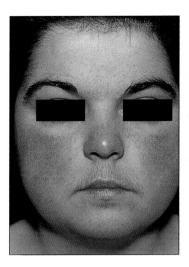

7.27 The typical facial features of Cushing's syndrome. The patient has a moon face with erythema and hirsuties. Identical appearances may result from corticosteroid therapy (*see* **6.45**).

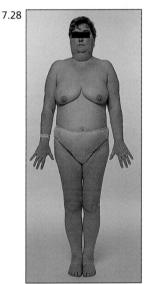

7.28

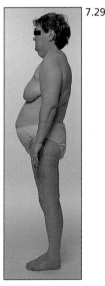

7.29

7.28 & 7.29 Cushing's syndrome results in central rather than peripheral obesity. This patient also has typical facial features and a 'buffalo hump'.

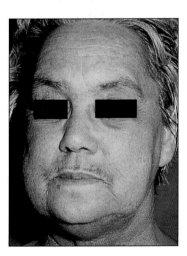

7.30 Nelson's syndrome. This woman underwent bilateral adrenalectomy for Cushing's disease, and subsequently became increasingly pigmented as a result of excessive ACTH secretion.

with fewer classic signs but with an illness of rapid onset with weight loss, profound proximal myopathy, pigmentation and a severe hypokalaemic alkalosis. Carcinoid tumours and other relatively benign sources of ectopic ACTH are clinically indistinguishable from other causes of Cushing's syndrome.

Diagnosis of Cushing's syndrome can be made by the 48–hour low-dose dexamethasone suppression test. Preliminary screening for Cushing's syndrome can be carried out by the 1 mg overnight dexamethasone suppression test, the 24-hour urinary free cortisol or assessment of a lack of circadian variation in plasma cortisol at 08:00 and 24:00 hours.

The differentiation between adrenal tumour, pituitary Cushing's disease and ectopic ACTH production needs to be made with care.

If plasma ACTH is consistently undetectable, the condition is usually caused by an adrenal tumour. Diagnosis is established by ultrasound or CT scan of the adrenals (**7.31**) and carcinomas often show local invasion. Patients with adrenal tumours also show no suppression of serum cortisol with high-dose dexamethasone, and no response to the CRH test.

Plasma cortisol and ACTH are often grossly elevated in malignant tumours. Plasma potassium is almost always subnormal in patients with ectopic ACTH, so a hypokalaemic alkalosis is a pointer to this diagnosis. The high-dose dexamethasone suppression test is valuable in about 80% of cases. Patients with pituitary-dependent Cushing's disease show significant suppression of their cortisol to less than 50% of the basal value at 48 hours, whereas those with adrenal tumours and ectopic ACTH do not show cortisol suppression. Some ectopic tumours behave as though there were a pituitary-dependent cause, but significant suppression is associated with a high probability (> 50:1) that the condition is Cushing's disease. The CRH test may provide further help in the differentiation.

301

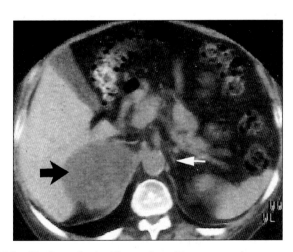

7.31 CT of a patient with an adrenal tumour causing Cushing's syndrome. The right-sided adrenal mass is extensive and is marked with a black arrow. By contrast, the left adrenal gland (white arrow) is atrophic.

Chest X-rays may reveal a bronchial carcinoma (*see* **p. 190**), and MRI of the pituitary may be helpful, as may scans of the lung fields, mediastinum, liver, pancreas and adrenals for detecting small carcinoid tumours.

The treatment of choice for adrenal tumours is surgery, but metyrapone or mitotane may be necessary to achieve a clinical remission preoperatively. In Cushing's disease, trans-sphenoidal surgery is the treatment of choice, achieving a biochemical cure in 75% of cases. Pituitary irradiation is now restricted to cases in which surgery has been unsuccessful and, as it takes several years to be effective, it needs to be combined with medical therapy. Ectopic ACTH production should be treated by eradicating the source if possible; bilateral adrenalectomy is an alternative, but is now rarely used, as the loss of feedback results in Nelson's syndrome (**7.30**) and the development of pituitary adenomas in 20% of patients.

Overproduction of other pituitary hormones

Tumours that secrete TSH and produce hyperthyroidism are rare. Most tumours that secrete gonadotrophins are large, and they often do not produce a clinical syndrome (especially in menopausal women), although testicular enlargement in men has been described. Some tumours secrete the biologically inactive alpha subunit that is common to FSH, LH and TSH. About 30% of all pituitary tumours are non-functioning.

DISORDERS OF THE ADRENAL GLANDS

The adrenal glands are made up of cortex and medulla, which have separate embryological origins and different physiological functions.

ADRENAL CORTEX

The cortex secretes glucocorticoids, mineralocorticoids and androgens.

Glucocorticoid-related disorders

- Glucocorticoid excess causes Cushing's syndrome (*see* **p. 299**).
- Primary adrenocorticoid insufficiency or Addison's disease is very uncommon and is usually caused by an autoimmune process or, more rarely, by destruction of the cells by tuberculosis, other granulomatous disease, or infiltration by metastases. It may occur in the antiphospholipid syndrome (**p. 442**).
- Acute adrenal failure follows withdrawal of suppressive doses of systemic steroids or haemorrhage into the gland in the Waterhouse–Friderichsen syndrome or during anticoagulant therapy.

The main clinical features of hypoadrenalism include tiredness, weight loss, gastrointestinal disturbances, hypo-glycaemia and depression. The loss of negative feedback on the pituitary causes massive elevation in ACTH production with associated pigmentation. This is particularly seen in skin folds, areas of friction, light-exposed areas, the buccal mucosa and often in scars (**7.32–7.36**). Aldosterone deficiency results in muscle

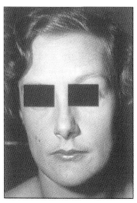

7.32 Facial appearance in Addison's disease. Note the generalized increase in pigmentation.

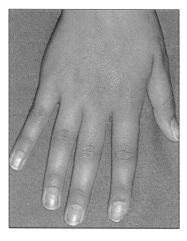

7.33 Addison's disease produces a generalized pigmentation of the hands, which – on the extensor surfaces – is often most marked over the knuckles.

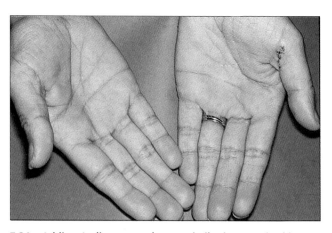

7.34 Addison's disease produces a similar increase in skin pigmentation in the skin creases of the palmar surface of the hands.

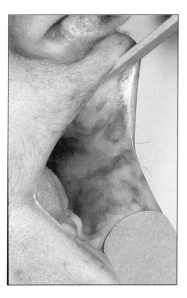

7.35 Buccal pigmentation in Addison's disease. There is a fairly general increase in mucous membrane pigmentation, and, in addition, there are some areas of much darker pigmentation. Both features are commonly seen in patients with Addison's disease.

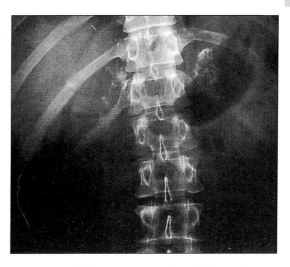

7.37 Adrenal calcification seen on plain abdominal X-ray in a patient with Addison's disease. The underlying pathology is almost certainly tuberculosis.

303

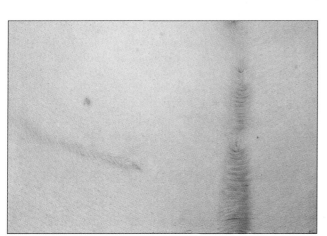

7.36 Pigmentation in scars is a common finding in patients with Addison's disease and with other causes of excessive ACTH production.

fludrocortisone, and the dose should be increased at times of physiological or pathological stress.

Synthesis of adrenal steroids is dependent on a number of enzymatically regulated stages. Congenital deficiencies exist in six specific enzymes that can lead to congenital adrenal hyperplasias. The clinical features depend on where the block occurs, as biosynthesis is diverted down alternative metabolic pathways with effects predominantly on sexual development, or on mineralocorticoid or glucocorticoid balance.

Mineralocorticoid-related disorders

Primary aldosteronism may be caused by an adrenal adenoma (Conn's syndrome), or by bilateral adrenal hyperplasia. Patients present with hypertension and hypokalaemia (< 3.5 mmol/litre) (**7.38**) and few if any symptoms. The characteristic biochemistry is a hypokalaemic alkalosis with a plasma sodium of 140–150 mmol/litre, increased plasma aldosterone, suppressed

cramps, dehydration and postural hypotension with the classic electrolyte disturbances of low serum levels of sodium and glucose and high potassium and urea. Androgen deficiency may lead to hair loss from the scalp and axillary and pubic regions in women. Associated vitiligo (*see* **p. 87**) may produce a striking contrast to the hyperpigmentation seen in other areas. The diagnosis is established by a basal ACTH level and the short Synacthen test. Other investigations may reveal the underlying cause, for example adrenal autoantibodies or adrenal calcification may be found (**7.37**).

Acute adrenal crisis in Addison's disease may be precipitated by infection or stress such as trauma or a surgical operation. Treatment in the acute crisis is intravenous hydrocortisone and 0.9% saline, with the addition of dextrose if hypoglycaemia is present. Long-term replacement is by oral hydrocortisone and

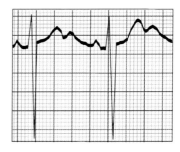

7.38 Hypokalaemia in primary aldosteronism. The ECG provides a rapid means of diagnosis. Characteristic U waves are seen after the T waves, especially in the chest leads, as here in lead V3. In extreme hypokalaemia, the T wave may become flattened and the ST segment depressed, so that there is a risk of confusing the U wave with the T wave.

plasma renin activity and an inappropriately high urinary potassium excretion. Differentiation between adenomas and hyperplasia is based on the effects of salt loading, adrenal CT (**7.39**), iodocholesterol radionuclide scanning and adrenal venous sampling. Treatment of adenomas should be surgical: 60% of patients are cured of hypertension postoperatively and a further 20% improved. In hyperplasia, the treatment of choice is spironolactone or amiloride.

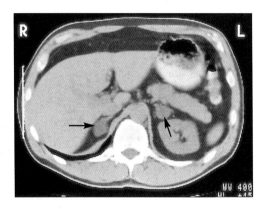

7.39 **Bilateral adrenal hyperplasia in a patient with primary aldosteronism,** revealed by CT scan. Both adrenals are clearly enlarged (arrows).

ADRENAL MEDULLA

Most phaeochromocytomas (80–90%) are found in the adrenal glands; 10% are malignant and 10% multiple. Their characteristic symptoms relate to catecholamine release. Symptoms include sustained or intermittent hypertension, tachycardia, palpitations and paroxysmal attacks of blanching and sweating. Diabetes and neuroectodermal diseases, such as neurofibromatosis, are commonly associated. Diagnosis is based on clinical suspicion and the measurement plasma levels of adrenaline (epinephrine) or noradrenaline (norepinephrine) or their urinary metabolites. The tumour may be localized by selective venous sampling of catecholamines or by scanning techniques, or both. Usually the tumours are large and can be localized by CT (appearance similar to the right adrenal in **7.31**), ultrasound (**7.40**), radioisotope scanning (**7.41**) and MRI (**7.42**, **7.43**). Treatment should be surgical removal with preoperative alpha and beta blockade.

MULTIPLE ENDOCRINE NEOPLASIA (MEN) SYNDROMES

Multiple endocrine neoplasia (MEN) syndromes are characterized by multiple endocrine hyperfunction due to hyperplasia, adenomas or carcinomas.

MEN-1 (Wermer's syndrome) is the familial occurrence of tumours of the anterior pituitary, parathyroid glands, pancreatic islets, intestinal islets and other sites. MEN 1 is associated with an increased incidence of peptic ulcer and with hyperfunction of the adrenal and thyroid. Clinical features often become apparent in middle age, most patients presenting with hypercalcaemia, peptic ulcer, hypoglycaemia or pituitary dysfunction. Because of genetic transmission by the dominant menin gene on chromosome 11, first and second degree relatives should also be investigated when the diagnosis is made.

MEN-2a (Sipple's syndrome) is characterized by medullary carcinoma of the thyroid, phaeochromocytoma, and parathyroid hyperplasia. In addition, there is an associated incidence of glial tumours and meningiomas. Clinical presentation is protean and the difficulty in diagnosis is compounded by the secretion of a range of other biologically active substances and hormones that are not produced by the normal tissues – these include ACTH, prolactin, serotonin, prostanoids, and vasoactive intestinal peptides. First and second degree family members should be screened.

MEN-2b (mucosal neuroma syndrome) is similar to MEN-2a but there may also be neuromas of the lips, tongue and buccal mucosa, and neurofibromata with café-au-lait spots on the skin. These patients tend to be tall and thin and may be mistaken for patients with Marfan's syndrome.

Management of patients with MEN must be directed to the tumour(s) causing significant clinical problems.

DISORDERS OF GROWTH AND SEXUAL DEVELOPMENT

Growth assessment is an accurate and sensitive guide to child health and growth velocity represents the dynamics of growth much better than a single measurement of stature. Abnormal height cannot be defined absolutely, but an individual is usually considered abnormally short if height is below the 3rd centile, or too tall if above the 97th centile.

SHORT STATURE

Short stature is a diagnostic challenge. A small child with normal growth velocity will be expected to achieve a normal final height, but may have growth delay following previous poor growth as a result of illness or short parents. Children with impaired growth velocity require careful examination for underlying disorders. Investigations include urinalysis, blood count, ESR or plasma viscosity, chromosome analysis, bone age and endocrine status – particularly GH, thyroxine and TSH, and sex steroids.

It is convenient to separate short children into those with normal proportions and those with abnormal proportions. Those with normal proportions form the largest group. There is a wide variety of causes of short stature:

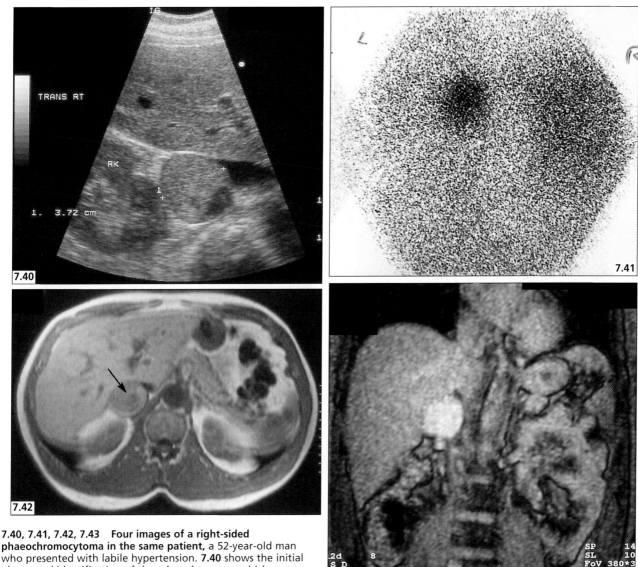

7.40, 7.41, 7.42, 7.43   Four images of a right-sided phaeochromocytoma in the same patient, a 52-year-old man who presented with labile hypertension. **7.40** shows the initial ultrasound identification of the adrenal tumour, which was found to have a maximum diameter of 3.72 cm (RK = right kidney). **7.41** is a radioisotope scan with MIBG (metaiodobenzylguanidine), which is taken up by the neuronal uptake system in the adrenal medulla and other tissues with rich sympathetic innervation, as it is structurally related to noradrenaline (norepinephrine). Some MIBG can also be seen in the liver and the bladder. **7.42** an MR image, shows the close relationship of the adrenal phaeochromocytoma (arrowed) to the right kidney. In **7.43**, a coronal turboflash MR image, the tumour is clearly seen as a bright circular abnormality, adjacent to the liver.

- Any cause of intrauterine growth retardation and low birth weight leads to short stature.
- Numerous rare congenital syndromes lead to poor growth; these include the Silver–Russell syndrome (triangular facies, clinodactyly, facial and limb length asymmetry), the Prader–Willi syndrome, Cornelia de Lange syndrome, progeria, Hallermann–Streiff syndrome, Seckel's syndrome, Ollier's disease, Aarskog's syndrome, Williams' syndrome and the mucopolysaccharidoses (*see* **p. 336**).
- Nutritional and emotional deprivation leads to short growth as does systemic disease.
- GH deficiency may be congenital or acquired; it leads to short, plump children with immature facies and genitalia, and delicate extremities (**7.44**).
- Hypothyroidism should always be considered; the earlier the onset, the more severe the delay in growth, particularly in skeletal maturity.
- Cushing's syndrome delays growth, particularly when associated with precocious puberty.

The 'fat' short child is likely to have an endocrine cause for his short stature and obesity. The underlying endocrine condition

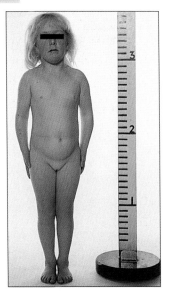

7.44 Pituitary dwarfism with growth hormone deficiency. This 10-year-old girl was 1.02 m tall, far below the 5th percentile for her age.

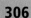

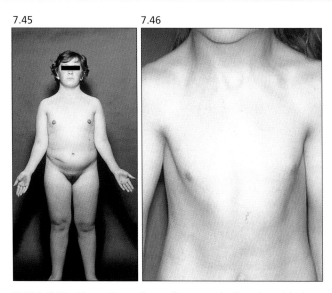

7.45   7.46

7.45 & 7.46 Turner's syndrome is a genetic disorder with the chromosome configuration 45XO. This produces a phenotypic female with gonadal dysgenesis and primary amenorrhoea, retarded growth and short stature, webbed neck, absent breast development, an increased carrying angle at the elbow (cubitus valgus), congenital heart disease (especially coarctation of the aorta) and bilateral 'streak' gonads. These patients have a normal IQ. Noonan's syndrome has broadly similar appearances, but occurs in phenotypic males.

should be treated and the growth response will be a good sign of clinical response. In GH deficiency, treatment with recombinant GH should continue throughout puberty.

Studies are under way to determine the benefits of accelerating the growth in 'short normal' children and in children with Turner's syndrome and Noonan's syndrome. Turner's syndrome (karyotype 45XO) and its many chromosomal variants (e.g. XO/XY mosaic in Noonan's syndrome) are always associated with impaired sexual development and short stature (**7.45, 7.46**). The combination of sex steroids and GH appears to increase the final height slightly.

Of the causes of short stature with abnormal proportions, achondroplasia, an autosomal dominant condition, is the most familiar with a frequency of 1 in 40 000 births (**7.47, 7.48**). There are many other forms of short limb and short trunk dwarfism.

TALL STATURE

Tall stature is a much less common problem than short stature:

- Gigantism caused by GH excess precedes acromegaly and is investigated and treated as described on **p. 297**.
- Marfan syndrome is a relatively common inherited cause of tall stature (*see* **p. 134**).
- Rarer causes include generalized lipodystrophy, Soto's syndrome and eunuchoidism.

DISORDERS OF SEXUAL DEVELOPMENT

At puberty, the growth of genitalia accelerates, secondary sexual characteristics develop and there is a general growth

spurt. These changes are induced by pulsatile secretion of gonadotrophin-releasing hormone (GnRH) which augments pituitary gonadotrophin output and promotes gonadal maturation and steroidogenesis.

Pubertal onset varies widely in different parts of the world, but in the UK the mean age of onset is 11.5 years for boys, and 10.5 years for girls with menarche occurring 2 years later. Delayed puberty in the UK for a boy is defined as a testicular volume below 4 ml by 14 years old, and for girls no breast

7.47   7.48

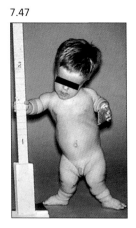

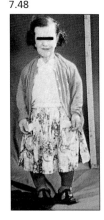

7.47 & 7.48 Achondroplasia in infancy and adult life. Note the short stature, large head, prominent forehead and disproportion between the size of the body and limbs. Around 70–80% of cases of achondroplasia represent new mutations.

development by 13.2 years of age. The most common cause is constitutional delayed puberty ('late developers').

The clinical features of hypogonadism depend on whether androgen secretion is impaired, and on the age of onset of the deficiency:

- With fetal onset, differentiation of the external genitalia along male lines is androgen dependent within the first trimester of gestation; if testosterone fails to act, pseudohermaphroditism occurs, as is seen in testicular feminization syndrome in which XY males have an X-linked deficiency of androgen receptors (**7.49**); the testes, which may be found in the labia or inguinal canals, are hyperactive, producing high levels of testosterone and oestrogens; as negative feedback is ineffective, the LH levels are high; in congenital adrenal hyperplasia caused by 21-hydroxylase

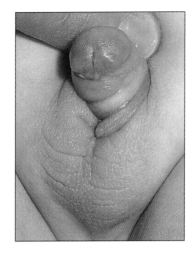

7.50 Congenital adrenal hyperplasia. A genotypically female patient presented at birth with ambiguous genitalia. The severity of the abnormalities varies considerably. In this case, there is clitoral hypertrophy and partial fusion of the labioscrotal folds.

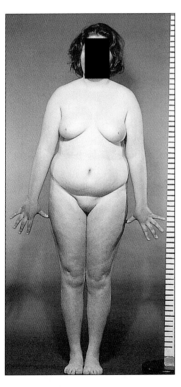

7.49 Testicular feminization syndrome. The patient is genotypically male, but phenotypically female, because of an inherited X-linked deficiency of androgen receptors. Patients should usually be brought up as females, and the testes should be removed from their ectopic position as there is an increased risk of malignancy.

measurement of testosterone or oestradiol, LH and FSH. Stimulation tests with GnRH or clomifene and pituitary stress testing may be required. Treatment depends on cause; primary gonadal failure requires either cyclical oral oestrogen and progesterone preparations or intramuscular testosterone every month. This treatment will produce secondary sexual characteristics and prevent osteoporosis, but fertility can be produced only in secondary gonadal failure by the complex administration of human chorionic gonadotrophin (HCG), FSH or pulsatile GnRH in hypothalamic lesions.

Precocious puberty in boys is generally defined as pubertal development before 10 years of age. Around 40% of cases have

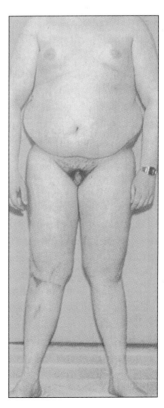

7.51 Klinefelter's syndrome. Patients are phenotypically male, but have two or more X chromosomes – most commonly 47XXY. They are eunuchoid with small, firm testes, gynaecomastia and a female distribution of body hair, and they may be unusually tall. They are infertile as a result of seminiferous tubule dysgenesis, which produces azoospermia.

deficiency, the female child presents at birth with ambiguous genitalia, clitoral hypertrophy and partial or complete fusion of the labioscrotal folds (**7.50**) caused by the excess of androgenic cortisol precursors produced.

- Prepubertal onset of androgen deficiency leads to eunuchoidism as in Kallmann's syndrome (hypogonadal hypogonadism, GnRH deficiency, anosmia, colour blindness, midline facial deformities) and Klinefelter's syndrome (**7.51**), in which there are usually high LH and low testosterone levels.

Diagnosis of hypogonadal states requires evaluation of visual fields and detection of anosmia, chromosome analysis, no detectable organic disease, but there are rare associations with hypothyroidism, hepatoblastomas and cerebral tumours that affect the hypothalamus. In girls, the definition of precocious puberty is defined as sexual maturation before the age of 8 years; 80% of girls have no detectable organic disease.

Secondary amenorrhea and infertility are common postpubertal presentations of gonadal failure. They may be caused by hypothalamic–pituitary axis disorders (*see* **p. 294–299**), and hyperprolactinaemia is common. Weight loss is the underlying cause in 20% of cases, although when severe, as in anorexia nervosa, the gonadotrophin secretion reverts to a prepubertal pattern. Ovarian failure with a premature menopause often has an autoimmune basis and is associated with other autoimmune diseases such as Addison's disease (*see* **p. 302**).

Patients with polycystic ovary syndrome (PCOS) commonly present in their mid-20s with menstrual irregularity (usually amenorrhoea or oligomenorrhoea), hyperandrogenization (hirsuties, greasy skin and acne, (**7.52**, **7.53**), infertility and often obesity. The classic triad of amenorrhoea, obesity and hirsutism (Stein–Leventhal syndrome) is at the extreme end of the spectrum of clinical presentation. The prevalence of PCOS is 7.5% in women of reproductive age, and high resolution ultrasound suggests that up to 20% of women have polycystic ovaries but no features of disease. In these patients weight gain may be associated with some of the clinical features of PCOS. By the age of 40, 40% of patients with PCOS develop impaired glucose tolerance or frank non-insulin dependent diabetes mellitus (NIDDM).

Typical laboratory findings in PCOS are a raised serum LH and slightly raised testosterone with normal FSH, prolactin and TSH. The ovaries contain multiple cysts which are easily detected by pelvic ultrasound (**7.54**). Other conditions, such as adrenal and ovarian tumours and late onset adrenal hyperplasia, present with virilization (frontal baldness, deepening of the voice, breast atrophy, clitoral hypertrophy and masculine habitus), but in these conditions the testosterone concentration is in the normal male range.

Management is of the primary problem, but in PCOS hirsutism is treated with oestrogenic oral contraceptives or antiandrogens, such as cyproterone acetate. Regular menstruation or artificially induced bleeding is necessary to prevent endometrial hyperplasia. Weight loss is important as an increased body mass index (BMI) is closely correlated with an increased rate of hirsuitism, cycle disturbance and infertility and the BMI may be improved by weight reduction. Effective treatment may take 12–18 months, during which time cosmetic treatments, shaving and electrolysis are required.

Medical therapy for infertility may involve antiandrogens or gonadotrophins. Patients may also require therapy for diabetes, obesity and hyperlipidaemia. Surgical removal of a wedge of ovarian tissue may be of value and lead to a return of ovulation. Also laparoscopic ovarian diathermy of the cysts may lead to ovulation and a fall in LH levels.

7.52

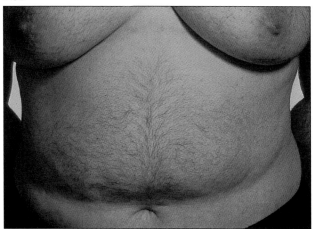

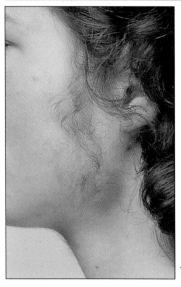

7.52 & 7.53 Hirsuties in two patients with the polycystic ovary syndrome. Male-pattern hair growth is commonly seen, and the skin may become greasy. Acne is a common complication.

7.53

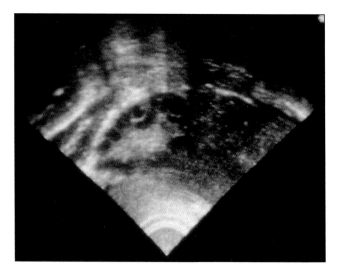

7.54 Vaginal ultrasound of the right ovary in a patient with polycystic ovary syndrome clearly shows multiple cysts.

THYROID DISORDERS

The thyroid secretes thyroxine (T4) and a small amount of triiodothyronine (T3). Approximately 85% of the biologically more active circulating triiodothyronine is converted from thyroxine in the tissues (liver, muscle and kidney). The hormones are transported in the plasma almost entirely bound to thyroxine-binding globulin (TGB), prealbumin and albumin. Production is stimulated by TSH in response to thyrotrophin-releasing hormone (TRH), and free thyroxine (FT4) has a negative feedback effect on TSH release. The thyroid parafollicular C-cells release calcitonin in response to an elevation in serum calcium. Enlargement of the thyroid gland from any cause is known as goitre.

HYPERTHYROIDISM

Hyperthyroidism (thyrotoxicosis) is caused by excess circulating thyroxine or triiodothyronine. It is a common condition with a prevalence of about 20 per 1000 in females and 2 per 1000 in males, respectively. Over 90% of cases are caused by either Graves' disease, toxic multinodular goitre or toxic solitary goitre. Graves' disease is the most common cause. The onset of the disease may be insidious. Atrial fibrillation is rare in young patients, but occurs in almost 50% of male patients over 60 years of age.

Graves' disease results from IgG antibodies against the TSH-receptor which bind and stimulate the gland via the adenylcyclase–cAMP system. These antibodies are termed thyroid-stimulating antibodies (TSAb). They may be responsible in part for thyroid enlargement in Graves' disease, but they do not appear to be responsible for the ophthalmopathy and pretibial myxoedema.

The cardinal signs of Graves' disease include a diffuse goitre, over which a vascular bruit can be heard (**7.55**), pretibial myxoedema (**7.56**), tachycardia with a bounding pulse, tremor and weight loss. Proximal myopathy may also occur. A range of eye signs occur, including exophthalmos (**7.55**, **7.57**), lid retraction (**7.58**), lid lag on downward eye movement,

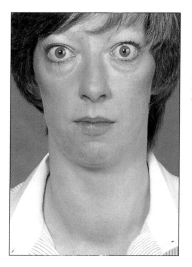

7.55 Graves' disease. This usually affects women between the ages of 20 and 40 years. This patient presented classically with a diffuse goitre over which a vascular bruit could be heard, and with eye signs.

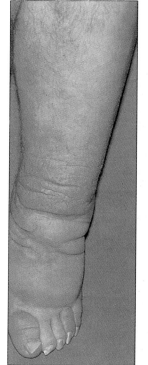

7.56 Pretibial myxoedema in Graves' disease. When this sign occurs, it may be combined with thyroid acropachy, in which there is oedema of the nail folds, producing a condition resembling clubbing.

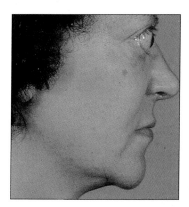

7.57 Exophthalmos (proptosis) in Graves' disease. This results from enlargement of the muscles, and fat within the orbit as a result of mucopolysaccharide infiltration.

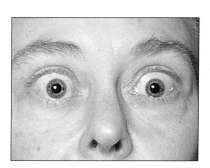

7.58 Lid retraction is a common eye sign in Graves' disease, which can be recognized when the sclera is visible between the lower margin of the upper lid and the cornea. Lid retraction is usually bilateral, but may be unilateral.

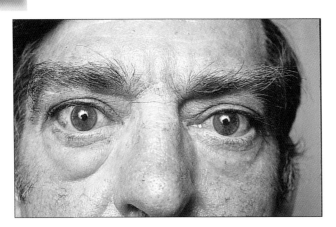

7.59 **Periorbital swelling may be associated with other eye signs,** giving an erythematous and oedematous appearance to the eyelids. Note that this patient also has chemosis, seen as reddening of the sclera.

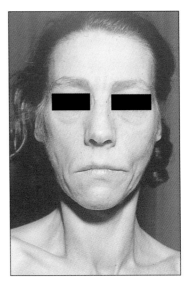

7.61 **'Masked' hyperthyroidism.** In the elderly, hyperthyroidism is commonly caused by a toxic multinodular goitre, but this does not necessarily result in significant thyroid enlargement. Because the patient does not have Graves' disease, the other signs associated with that condition are lacking. The clinical diagnosis is thus much less obvious, being suggested by a combination of tachycardia or atrial fibrillation, or both, heart failure and weight loss in a patient over the age of 60 years.

periorbital puffiness (**7.59**), grittiness, increased lacrimation, chemosis (**7.59**), conjunctival oedema and ulceration, ophthalmoplegia (**7.60**), diplopia, papilloedema and loss of visual acuity. Symptoms of ophthalmopathy may include pain, lacrimation, photophobia, blurred vision and diplopia. Rapid correction of thyrotoxicosis is necessary but may not reverse the associated ophthalmopathy. Other measures, including oral steroid or cyclosporin therapy and orbital radiotherapy, may reduce the volume of the orbital contents. Surgical decompression of the orbit, by removal of one or more orbital walls, may also be necessary. Artificial tears may be helpful while eye signs persist.

Eye signs may be absent in hyperthyroidism, especially in the elderly in whom 'masked' or 'apathetic' hyperthyroidism is common. Atrial fibrillation, heart failure and weight loss may be the only signs in this group (**7.61**).

The diagnosis is made clinically, with confirmation by detecting biochemically raised triiodothyronine and thyroxine, and undetectable TSH levels. Where a toxic multinodular goitre or a single toxic nodule (a toxic adenoma) in the thyroid is suspected clinically, a thyroid scan may provide useful information (**7.62**, **7.63**).

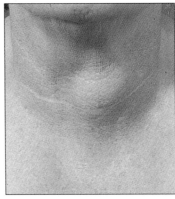

7.62 **Toxic adenoma causing hyperthyroidism.** This patient had a partial thyroidectomy 20 years previously, and a toxic nodule has now recurred. This was confirmed by isotope scanning.

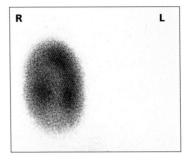

7.63 **Toxic adenoma in the right thyroid (a hot nodule), demonstrated using ^{99m}Tc-pertechnetate scanning.** The remainder of the gland does not take up significant amounts of isotope.

7.60 **Ophthalmoplegia in Graves' disease.** This is not caused by nerve palsy, but is the long-term result of swelling and infiltration of the extrinsic muscles of the eye. In this case, there is impaired upward and outward gaze in the patient's right eye. Ophthalmoplegia is usually accompanied by other eye signs. Note the presence of lid retraction. This patient also has marked corneal arcus.

Treatment options in thyrotoxicosis include:

- antithyroid drugs – carbimazole or methimazole, in decreasing dosage (titration regimen)
- antithyroid drugs in continued high dosage plus thyroxine (block and replace regimen)
- beta-blocking drugs in the initial stages of management
- subtotal thyroidectomy for relief of symptoms associated with goitre
- radioactive iodine therapy.

The choice of therapy depends upon a number of factors, especially the age and previous history of the patient. Long term follow-up and monitoring is necessary to ensure maintenance of the euthyroid state.

HYPOTHYROIDISM

Hypothyroidism (myxoedema) is the clinical syndrome that results from deficiency of the hormones triiodothyronine (T3) and thyroxine (T4). Its prevalence in the UK is about 15 per 1000 in females and 1 per 1000 in males.

Primary hypothyroidism is caused by an intrinsic disorder of the thyroid gland and is associated with raised TSH. Spontaneous atrophic hypothyroidism and thyroid failure after surgery, radioactive iodine or Hashimoto's autoimmune thyroiditis account for over 90% of cases.

Secondary hypothyroidism is much less common and is caused by pituitary disease, in which absence of TSH leads to atrophy of the gland.

Hypothyroidism affects all the systems of the body, but the wide range of clinical features means that the diagnosis will be missed if it is not positively considered. In children, the dominant features are a reduction in growth velocity and arrest of pubertal development. In adults, the presentation may vary from biochemical evidence with no clinical signs, to the insidious onset over many years of myxoedematous changes in the tissues with infiltration of mucopolysaccharides, hyaluronic acid and chondroitin sulphate (**7.64**, **7.65**). Dermal infiltration gives rise to nonpitting oedema, most marked on the skin of the eyelids and hands. This is often associated with loss of scalp (**7.66**) and eyebrow hair. Dryness of the skin, and reduced body hair are other common features and infiltration of the median nerve may lead to the carpal tunnel syndrome (*see* **p. 489**). Patients are often very sensitive to cold weather and may wear excessive clothing or use excessive bedclothes. Systemic effects including pericardial and pleural effusions, ascites, cardiac dilatation, bradycardia and hypothermia (*see* **p. 245**) may be life-threatening. There is an association with pernicious anaemia (*see* **p. 413**). Secondary hyperlipoproteinaemia is an invariable consequence of hypothyroidism and is a positive risk factor for the development of premature arterial disease, especially myocardial infarction. Treatment with thyroxine usually results in lowering of lipid levels.

Diagnosis is based on clinical suspicion – prolonged relaxation time of peripheral reflexes and a low-voltage ECG may be helpful – biochemical estimation of thyroxine and TSH and an assessment of thyroid antibodies. Antibodies to thyroid peroxidase or thyroglobulin, or both, are present in the serum of 90% of patients with Hashimoto's thyroiditis.

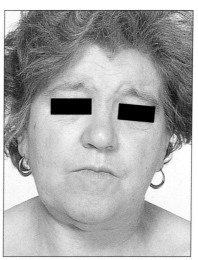

7.64 Hypothyroidism is not always clinically obvious. This patient shows some facial features, with a generalized pallor, puffiness and coarsening of the features, and coarse, uncontrollable hair. She was grossly hypothyroid on biochemical testing.

311

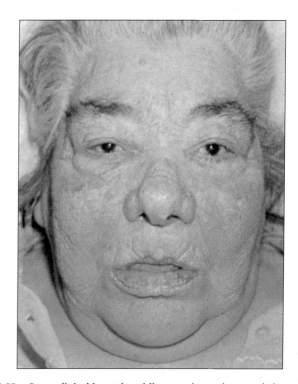

7.65 Gross clinical hypothyroidism produces characteristic non-pitting oedematous changes in the skin of the face, giving rise to a characteristic clinical appearance. Note the dry, puffy facial appearance and the coarse hair. This patient was admitted with hypothermia. Her skin was cold and she showed mental apathy.

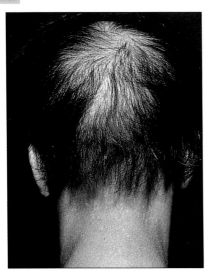

7.66 **Hair loss** is a common feature of hypothyroidism, as in this 48-year-old woman.

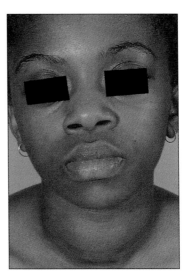

7.67 **Hashimoto's disease** is the most common cause of goitrous hypothyroidism in the world and is much more common in women than men. This teenage patient has a marked goitre but few obvious signs of hypothyroidism. She is rather unusual, as the condition is much more common in older women.

312

Hashimoto's disease is the most common form of goitrous hypothyroidism in the world. It usually manifests itself in the sixth decade, and women are affected 15 times more frequently than men. The gland characteristically feels firm and rubbery and may range in size from being scarcely palpable to many times enlarged (**7.67**).

Spontaneous atrophic hypothyroidism is the most common form of nongoitrous hypothyroidism in the UK, with a prevalence of 10 in 1000 people and an incidence that increases with age. Women are affected six times more commonly than men. This is also an autoimmune condition: many patients have TSH-receptor blocking antibodies and some have a history of Graves' disease treated successfully with drugs or radioiodine many years previously. These patients may also have other autoimmune diseases such as pernicious anaemia, diabetes mellitus, Addison's disease or vitiligo.

Drugs may induce hypothyroidism. Lithium carbonate, which like iodide inhibits the release of thyroid hormones, may result in a TSH-induced goitre; and prolonged administration of iodine, as in cough mixtures or in amiodarone given for the treatment of dysrhythmias, also occasionally induces goitrous hypothyroidism.

In certain parts of the world where there is iodine deficiency, such as the Andes, central Africa and the Himalayas, thyroid enlargement is common, affecting 5–15% of the population (endemic goitre, **7.68**). Although most patients are euthyroid and have normal or only slightly raised TSH, the greater the iodine deficiency or the greater the demands (as in pregnancy), the greater the incidence of hypothyroidism.

Dyshormonogenesis is an unusual autosomal recessive defect in hormone synthesis. The most common form results from a deficiency in peroxidase enzyme (Pendred's syndrome: goitre, hypothyroidism, deaf mutism and mental retardation). Homozygotes present with congenital hypothyroidism, which needs to be distinguished from athyrosis or hypoplasia of the thyroid, the most common causes of neonatal hypothyroidism.

Neonatal hypothyroidism (1 in 4000 live births) is screened for by TSH measurement 5–7 days after delivery. If it is undetected, cretinism results. Prompt treatment with thyroxine has been shown to result in normal development, except in the rare cases of thyroid agenesis and impaired brain development caused by intrauterine hypothyroidism.

Hypothyroidism requires treatment for life with thyroxine. In patients with ischaemic heart disease, sudden introduction of thyroxine can cause myocardial infarction and therefore thyroxine or triiodothyronine is started in low doses and the dose increased very slowly every 4–6 weeks with intensified management of anti-anginal therapy. 'Myxoedema coma' is severe hypothyroidism in an elderly patient. Its presenting

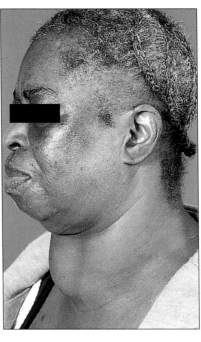

7.68 **Endemic goitre.** Large goitres like this are not unusual in areas of iodine deficiency, but they are not always associated with hypothyroidism. This African patient was euthyroid.

features may include hypothermia, cardiac failure, an altered conscious state often with convulsions, high CSF fluid pressure and protein content, hypotension, alveolar hypoventilation, intercurrent chest infection and dilutional hyponatraemia. Mortality is around 50% and careful thyroid replacement therapy with thyroxine or triiodothyronine is required.

THYROID NODULES AND THYROID CANCER

A thyroid nodule is any discrete intrathyroidal lesion and nodules may be solitary or multiple. Palpable nodules can be found in 5–10% of European and North American adults, and the incidence increases with age. In iodine deficient parts of the world, the prevalence is much greater. Clinically undiagnosed (occult) cases of thyroid cancer are found in up to 18% of routine autopsies. These are usually small (< 1 cm) papillary carcinomas without evidence of local invasion or metastases.

Thyroid nodules may be caused by involutional or degenerative changes, discrete inflammatory lesions or neoplasms. Colloid or adenomatous nodules are the most common type and consist of thyroglobulin-containing follicles.

These are often multiple and may present as a multinodular goitre (**7.69**) or a simple non-toxic goitre. They are most common in women, and require no treatment unless they are cosmetically disfiguring or cause pressure effects such as tracheal compression.

Single thyroid nodules may be benign or malignant. The chance of a nodule being benign is at least 95%, and most thyroid cancers have a mortality rate similar to skin cancer and are not immediately life threatening. Malignancy may be suspected if there is a history of previous exposure to ionizing radiation – especially external irradiation in childhood. Other suggestive features on examination include asymmetry, unusual location of the swelling, firmness, lymphadenopathy, a rapid painful increase in size, which may be caused by haemorrhage, hoarseness of the voice and fixation to skin and underlying tissues. The investigation of choice is a fine-needle aspiration (FNA), which allows immediate identification of cysts and microscopic examination of the aspirated cells (**7.70**). Ultrasonography is the most sensitive method available for delineating nodules and identifying cysts (**7.71**) but it will not distinguish benign from malignant. Radionuclide scanning may also give valuable information (**7.72**).

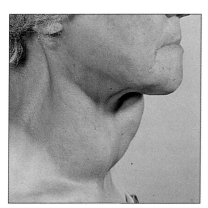

7.69 Multinodular goitre. The patient was euthyroid, but surgical treatment was ultimately required because of retrosternal extension with tracheal compression.

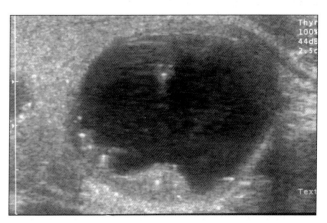

7.71 Ultrasound is the imaging technique of choice in the initial investigation of thyroid nodules. In this patient, a large cystic lesion was present. In this view, infiltrating tissue with specks of calcification can be seen in the lower part of the cyst. Biopsy confirmed papillary carcinoma of the thyroid.

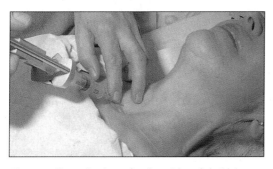

7.70 Fine-needle aspiration of a thyroid nodule is the investigation of choice in a patient with a solitary nodule of the thyroid, as it is very successful in obtaining cells for cytological examination and thus in the diagnosis of thyroid carcinoma. It can usually be performed under local anaesthesia. This patient had a recurrent nodule after previous partial thyroidectomy for thyrotoxicosis.

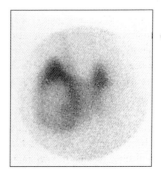

7.72 A large 'cold' nodule in the right lobe of the thyroid, demonstrated using ^{99m}Tc-pertechnetate scanning. A cold nodule could be malignant, and fine-needle or open biopsy is always indicated.

The prognosis and management of thyroid carcinomas varies according to the histological type: papillary, follicular, medullary and anaplastic.

Most thyroid carcinomas are the papillary type, which may be multifocal and spread to regional lymph nodes and to lungs and bone (**3.156**). Most occur in women aged less than 50 years with a tumour size less than 4 cm in diameter. Treatment is by total thyroidectomy; radioiodine ablation is needed postoperatively, as the metastases and any remaining thyroid take up iodine under TSH-drive after thyroidectomy. Thereafter the patients are treated with a sufficiently high dose of thyroxine to suppress TSH completely. Papillary carcinoma carries a good prognosis.

Follicular carcinoma is more aggressive. It is usually unifocal and rarely spreads to lymph nodes, but spreads via the blood to lungs and bone. Treatment is similar to that for papillary carcinoma.

Medullary carcinoma is derived from the parafollicular C cells of the thyroid. When sporadic it is usually unifocal, but when familial it is typically bilateral and multicentric and may form part of the MEN syndromes (*see* **p. 304**). In MEN-2a, it is associated with phaeochromocytoma and parathyroid adenoma. In MEN-2b, it is associated with a marfanoid habitus, phaeochromocytoma, mucosal neuromas of lips, eyelids and tongue, proximal myopathy and ganglioneuromatosis of the bowel. Medullary carcinoma metastasizes as above and is treated in the same way, but it produces calcitonin which can be used as a tumour marker.

Anaplastic carcinoma of the thyroid is very aggressive and may be inoperable at presentation.

PARATHYROID DISEASES

HYPERPARATHYROIDISM

For a discussion of hyperparathyroidism, *see* **p. 139**.

HYPOPARATHYROIDISM

Failure of parathyroid hormone (PTH) secretion is rare; the major causes are neonatal, severe magnesium depletion, postsurgical or idiopathic hypoparathyroidism. The clinical features are mainly caused by hypocalcaemia. They include tetany, which is characterized by carpal and pedal spasm (**7.73**) and paraesthesia. Idiopathic hypoparathyroidism may be sporadic or familial and is often associated with autoimmune diseases such as Addison's disease. Candidiasis, together with impaired nail and dental development, is common. Cataracts and calcification of the basal ganglia are common, but parkinsonism features are rare.

Pseudohypoparathyroidism is caused by a defect at the PTH-receptor level. In addition to the characteristic biochemical profile of hypoparathyroidism (low serum calcium, raised inorganic phosphorus and usually normal alkaline phosphatase), these patients have a raised PTH and they exhibit somatic features. They have short stature, mental retardation, a round face and short neck, abnormal dentition and shortening of some of the metatarsals and metacarpals (usually the third, fourth and fifth, **7.74**, **7.75**). A few families have these somatic features without the biochemical abnormalities; this condition is known as pseudo-pseudohypoparathyroidism.

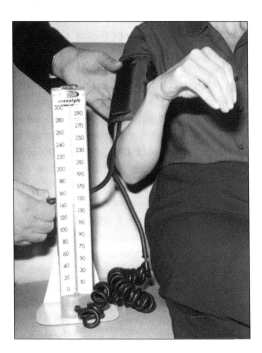

7.73 Carpal spasm (Trousseau's sign) is the most obvious manifestation of tetany in hypocalcaemia. Its onset can be provoked by inflating a sphygmomanometer cuff to just above systolic pressure for at least 2 minutes.

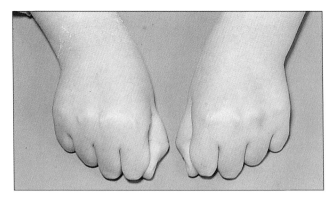

7.74 Pseudohypoparathyroidism is associated with characteristic somatic features including shortening of the metatarsals and metacarpals, in this patient especially in the fourth and fifth fingers. This shortening results in an apparent absence of the relevant knuckles on making a fist.

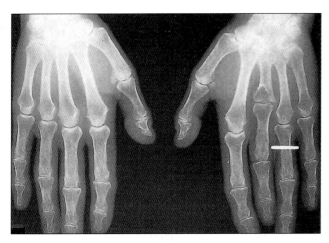

7.75   Pseudohypoparathyroidism. In this patient there is marked shortening of the third finger of the left hand, mainly as the result of shortening of the metacarpal.

Treatment of tetany is with intravenous calcium and, as oral calcium is rarely adequate alone, an active metabolite of vitamin D is prescribed to normalize the serum calcium levels.

GASTROINTESTINAL HORMONE ABNORMALITIES

A number of rare syndromes are associated with abnormalities in gastrointestinal hormones. These are summarized on **p. 373**.

DIABETES MELLITUS (DM)

Diabetes mellitus (DM) is a disease characterized by a chronically elevated blood glucose concentration, often accompanied by other clinical and biochemical abnormalities. The hyperglycaemia of diabetes results from an inadequate action of insulin, caused by low or absent insulin secretion, the presence of antagonists to the peripheral action of insulin or a combination of these factors.

The effects of the disease may be acute or chronic, involving many organs, including the eye, the kidney, peripheral nerves and large arteries. Primary diabetes mellitus is traditionally divided into either type 1 (insulin dependent, IDDM) or type 2 (non-insulin dependent, NIDDM). The classification is important because of the different genetic backgrounds, clinical presentations, metabolic effects, treatment and consequences of the two types. Diabetes may also be secondary to other disorders (**7.76**).

Diabetes is defined biochemically by the following criteria:

- a fasting venous plasma glucose level greater than 7.0 mmol/litre (140 mg/dl) on more than one occasion; or

- a 2-hour (plus one other) venous plasma glucose level in excess of 11.1 mmol/litre (200 mg/dl) in a formal 75 g oral glucose tolerance test (GTT).

IMPAIRED GLUCOSE TOLERANCE AND IMPAIRED FASTING GLUCOSE

Impaired glucose tolerance (IGT) is often classified as 'chemical', 'borderline' or 'latent' diabetes. It is defined as the finding of a fasting venous plasma glucose level below 7.0 mmol/litre, and a 2-hour sample, after an oral GTT, with levels between 7.0 and 11.1 mmol/litre. Annually, about 2–4% of these patients develop diabetes. IGT carries the same risk of atherosclerotic vascular complications (macroangiopathy) as diabetes, although the risk of retinopathy 10 years after diagnosis is negligible.

Impaired fasting glucose (IFG), in which patients have a fasting venous plasma glucose level in the range 6.0–7.0 mmol/litre but a normal oral GTT, has recently been defined and shown to be associated with an increased risk of macroangiopathy.

Management of patients with IGT and IFG should be aimed at diminishing the risk of metabolic and physical deterioration, by reducing obesity, hypertension, physical inactivity and hyperlipidaemia, and by stopping smoking. In pregnancy, IGT should be taken seriously and treated as gestational diabetes.

PRIMARY DIABETES MELLITUS

Primary DM is either type 1 or type 2. The prevalence of diabetes in industrialized countries is approximately 3–4% and about 10% have type 1. Some communities, such as the Pima Indians, have a diabetes prevalence of over 30%, mainly obese type 2 DM.

A CLASSIFICATION OF DIABETES MELLITUS

Impaired glucose tolerance (IGT) without diabetes

Impaired fasting glucose (IFG) without diabetes

Primary diabetes mellitus
  Insulin dependent type 1 (or IDDM)
  Non-insulin dependent type 2 (or NIDDM)

Malnutrition-related diabetes mellitus (MRDM)

Secondary diabetes mellitus
  Pancreatic disease
  Endocrine disorders
  Drug therapy
  Inherited disorders

7.76   A classification of diabetes mellitus.

Type 1 patients are ketosis prone and C-peptide negative. They have an absolute requirement for insulin from diagnosis. Type 1 DM is believed to be an autoimmune condition, in which environmental factors trigger the diabetogenic process via islet cell antibodies in genetically susceptible individuals. Most patients presenting under the age of 25 years have type 1.

Type 2 DM generally occurs over the age of 40 years in patients with resistance to insulin and abnormal beta cell function. An underlying genetic susceptibility is even more important than in type 1 DM and most patients are obese. The onset of the disease is insidious and biochemical evidence of diabetes may be present for several years before symptoms or complications lead to the diagnosis. These patients are not dependent on insulin for treatment but may require it temporarily for glycaemic control under stress.

MALNUTRITION-RELATED DIABETES MELLITUS

The World Health Organization has recognized malnutrition-related diabetes (MRDM) with two subtypes: fibrocalcaneous pancreatic diabetes (FCPD) and protein-deficient pancreatic disease (PDPD). MRDM has a high prevalence in certain tropical developing countries, where it manifests itself with severe symptoms but without ketosis in young people. Pancreatic calcification is common in the FCPD subtype.

SECONDARY DIABETES MELLITUS

DM may be secondary to pancreatic disease (e.g. haemochromatosis, chronic pancreatitis), other endocrine disorders (e.g. Cushing's syndrome, acromegaly, phaeochromocytoma), drug therapy (e.g. thiazides, steroids, phenothiazides), insulin-receptor abnormalities (lipodystrophy, **7.77**) and various inherited disorders (e.g. type 1 collagen diseases, Prader–Willi syndrome, and diabetes insipidus, diabetes mellitus, optic atrophy and deafness (DIDMOAD) syndrome).

PRESENTING FEATURES OF DIABETES

Patients with DM may be detected by a range of presentations which include:

- Acute: the typical presentation of the young patient with type 1 DM. Features include polyuria, polydipsia and weight loss of short duration, often associated with, or apparently precipitated by, a viral infection; if these symptoms have been neglected there may be visual disturbance or impairment of the conscious level associated with severe ketoacidosis.
- Chronic: the typical presentation of a patient with type 2 DM; the symptoms have usually been present for some

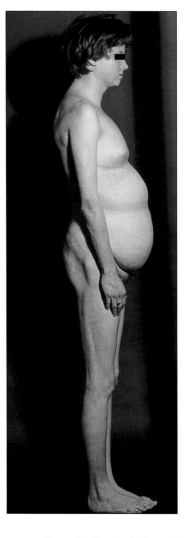

7.77 Lipodystrophy is a rare cause of secondary diabetes. The atrophy of adipose tissue occurs throughout the body, and is well seen here, especially in the gluteal region. Non-ketotic insulin resistance is combined with severe hyperlipidaemia with subcutaneous xanthomas and hepatosplenomegaly.

months and often include weight loss, thirst, excess urine volume, genital infection with *Candida albicans* and skin infections, often with *Staphylococcus aureus.*

- Coincidental discovery: routine screening for urine or blood glucose as part of a pre-employment medical, during pregnancy or in local campaigns.
- Complications: the patient may present with visual disturbance or overt retinopathy, neuropathy, nephropathy or after major thrombotic events such as premature stroke or myocardial infarction.
- Drug-related diabetes may develop in patients on long-term steroids or thiazide diuretics.
- Disease-related as in acromegaly, Cushing's syndrome, phaeochromocytoma, thyrotoxicosis, pancreatitis, haemochromatosis, cystic fibrosis, carcinoma or surgical removal of the pancreas.
- Gestational: pregnancy may unmask diabetes in a woman who is predisposed.

A full history and clinical examination are essential to detect any of the causative diseases and document the consequences.

INVESTIGATIONS

Investigations are required for screening, diagnosis, monitoring of control and the early detection of degenerative changes.

- Urine testing for glucose is still widely used, but glucose will be found in the urine only when it rises above the renal threshold (usually about 10 mmol/litre); urine tests are simple and cheap; enzyme strip tests are specific for glucose.
- Urine testing for ketone bodies is also simple; the presence of ketones suggests loss of control.
- Proteinuria is a reflection of the development of renal complications and is an early indicator of diabetic renal disease

Multiple test strips allow rapid testing for all these substances in urine (**6.7**).

- Blood glucose is the key to diagnosis in diabetes (*see* **p. 315**); The measurement of capillary blood glucose is also a key way of monitoring control in DM. The colour change on the blood test strip may be noted visually but is better recorded electronically, and meters are available for home use (**7.78–7.80**). If the patient is to read the strips visually it is important to check colour vision.
- GTT is of value if random blood glucose results are equivocal and in individuals with IFG. It defines the response to a 75 g oral glucose load. Blood and urine are monitored before and for 2.5 hours after the glucose drink; the renal threshold for glucose can be determined, as can the presence of diabetes (capillary glucose ≥11.1 mmol/litre) or IGT (capillary glucose 7.0–11.1 mmol/litre).
- Glycosylated haemoglobin (HbA_{1c}) and other proteins: measurement of these proteins reflects the degree of diabetic control in the previous 4–6 weeks and is of value in long-term management and control.
- Microalbuminuria is a very sensitive marker of early and potentially reversible renal impairment; it is the term given to the presence of 20–200 mg/litre of protein in the urine. This is below the level of detection with conventional stick methods (200 mg/litre).
- Serum electrolytes, blood gases, osmolality and anion gap are all of value in metabolic crises if there is loss of water, sodium and potassium and acidosis is developing, or if there is a hyperosmolar state.
- Lipid profile: elevations in serum cholesterol are common, and elevation of serum triglycerides is a reflection of poor glycaemic control, which usually reverts to normal when euglycaemia is achieved.

PRINCIPLES OF MANAGEMENT

The aim of management is to control symptoms, prevent acute metabolic complications of ketoacidosis and hypoglycaemia, encourage self-reliance and self-care, prevent or treat

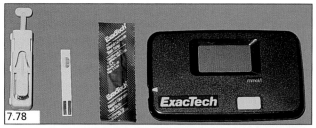

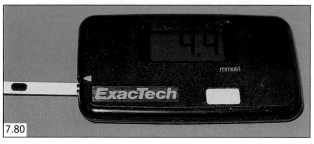

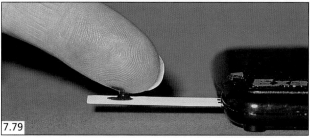

7.78–7.80 Electronic measurement of capillary blood glucose allows immediate monitoring in the clinic and at home. **7.78** shows a meter that measures blood glucose by coupling a biochemical reaction to an electronic response, together with the enzyme-containing test strip (sealed and unwrapped) and the stylet used for obtaining a finger-prick sample of blood. The test strip is inserted in the meter and a drop of blood applied to it (**7.79**). The blood glucose level appears on the meter within seconds (**7.80**). Other meters are available which measure colour changes in test sticks by reflectance methods.

complications early and prevent the increased morbidity and mortality associated with poorly managed diabetes.

In type 1 DM, glycaemic control is achieved by subcutaneous insulin administration two or more times a day, using modified insulins with differing absorption characteristics to provide an insulin profile that controls the glycaemia around meals and provides a background level for basic metabolic functions. Glycaemic control is best assessed by blood glucose and HbA_{1c} monitoring. Dietary modification is essential, and involves eliminating simple sugars and eating a low-fat, high-fibre diet with 50% of the calories from carbohydrate, 30% from fats (mainly polyunsaturated) and 20% from protein.

In type 2 DM the main form of treatment is dietary, with the emphasis on avoiding simple sugars and calorie restriction. Weight reduction is important in most patients with type 2 DM, and only if this cannot be achieved and the patients are

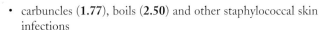
unacceptably hyperglycaemic and/or have an elevated HbA_{1c} (approximately 7% or higher) should oral hypoglycaemic agents be added. Sulphonylureas are first-line treatment in non-obese type 2 DM patients, whereas biguanides have a particular role in the obese diabetic (body mass index (BMI) > 25 kg/m^2). Hyperlipidaemia in patients with diabetes requires further investigation, and control of hyperlipidaemia should always be an aim of therapy in diabetes (*see* **p. 324**).

COMPLICATIONS OF DIABETES

The most important acute complications of DM are metabolic: diabetic ketoacidosis (**7.81**), hypoglycaemia (*see* **p. 323**), lactic acidosis and nonketotic hyperosmolar coma.

Other acute complications include acute infections and acute neuropathy.

Acute infections may be the presenting complaint in type 2 DM. They may include:

- candidal infections, presenting in the genital region as balanitis or vulvitis (**1.138**), in the finger nails (**2.62**) or as intertrigo beneath the breasts (**2.61**)

- carbuncles (**1.77**), boils (**2.50**) and other staphylococcal skin infections
- osteomyelitis, urinary infections, pneumonia, tuberculosis and other systemic bacterial infections
- in the diagnosed diabetic, finger pulp infections caused by non-sterile finger pricks (**7.82**).

Acute motor or sensory neuropathy may be seen in various guises during or after a period of poor metabolic control. The most typical are mononeuritis multiplex, often affecting the third, sixth or seventh cranial nerves (**7.83**) and diabetic amyotrophy caused by a proximal radiculopathy. Pain and skin tenderness with weakness and wasting of the upper thigh muscles is the most common presentation of amyotrophy (**7.84**). With improved glycaemic control (often with insulin), these complications may resolve.

The chronic complications of DM are summarized in **7.85**.

Insulin lipodystrophy results from frequent injections into the same injection sites, particularly in girls. Lipoatrophy (**7.86**) or lipohypertrophy may occur.

Most chronic complications result from disease of either the large blood vessels (macroangiopathy) or the small blood vessels (microangiopathy).

Macroangiopathy is responsible for a high prevalence of coronary, peripheral and cerebral artery disease in diabetics. Hypertension coexists with DM in about 50% of patients. Accelerated atherosclerosis occurs at a young age and runs an aggressive course in DM, especially in women. It accounts for most deaths, particularly in type 2 DM.

Microangiopathy is a generalized microvascular (capillary) disorder that is specific to DM and clinically most apparent in the eyes, kidneys and nerves. It is characterized by capillary basement membrane thickening, endothelial cell dysfunction, platelet aggregation, impaired fibrinolysis and a prothrombotic tendency, and results in microvascular occlusion and tissue ischaemia. The sequence of events in microangiopathy is best seen in the retina (*see* **p. 320–323**).

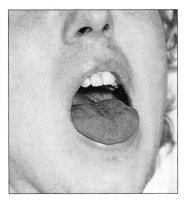

7.81 Diabetic ketoacidosis. There is evidence of marked dehydration, and the patient's eyeballs were lax to pressure. The patient was hyperventilating and confused, though not (yet) comatose. The smell of ketones on the breath allowed an instant probable diagnosis.

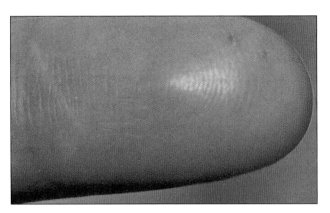

7.82 Septic finger pulp in diabetes. This young diabetic girl had been using the finger-prick method to test her own blood glucose level, but the finger became infected.

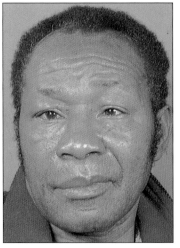

7.83 Mononeuritis multiplex in DM, affecting the right sixth and seventh facial nerves in a mild diabetic. The presenting symptoms were facial weakness and double vision. The right side of the face is palsied, as seen in this attempt to smile by the patient. He also had double vision on looking to the right, because a right sixth nerve palsy prevented lateral gaze in the right eye.

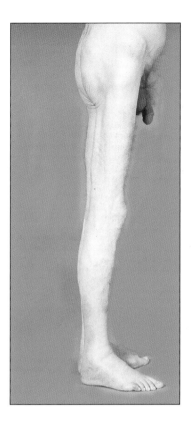

7.84 Diabetic amyotrophy, causing wasting of the thigh muscles. Adequate control of diabetes may lead to partial or total resolution of diabetic neuropathy.

Diabetic renal disease is an important cause of morbidity and mortality, especially in type 1 DM. Its diagnosis and management are discussed on **page 278**.

Chronic diabetic neuropathy may have a microvascular component in its aetiology, but intraneural metabolic derangement caused by alternative pathways of glucose metabolism is also implicated:

- sensory neuropathy usually presents in the feet as a painless trophic ulcer (**7.87**) or as a neuropathic arthropathy, that is a Charcot joint (**7.88**);
- motor neuropathy may lead to interosseous muscle wasting in the hands and feet (**7.90**)
- autonomic neuropathy may cause postural hypotension, impaired cardiovascular reflexes, gastroparesis, atonic bladder, impotence and disturbance of sweating (**7.91**).

Stiffness of the joints is a common feature of microangiopathy best demonstrated by the 'prayer sign' (**7.89**)

Care of the feet is an important part of the management of DM and patients or their relatives should be educated in the need for daily examination of the skin of the feet. The common combination of neuropathy and peripheral vascular disease often results in peripheral gangrene in the foot (**7.92**). Sometimes patients have good peripheral pulses, the ischaemic damage being secondary to small vessel occlusion. Infection of ulcers on the foot may lead to chronic sepsis with osteomyelitis

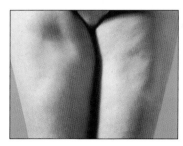

7.86 Lipoatrophy in the legs of a diabetic patient, resulting from repeated insulin injections in these sites.

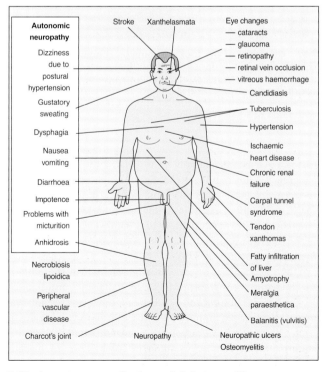

7.85 Long-term complications of diabetes mellitus.

Autonomic neuropathy
- Dizziness due to postural hypertension
- Gustatory sweating
- Dysphagia
- Nausea vomiting
- Diarrhoea
- Impotence
- Problems with micturition
- Anhidrosis

Necrobiosis lipoidica

Peripheral vascular disease

Charcot's joint

Stroke   Xanthelasmata

Eye changes
- cataracts
- glaucoma
- retinopathy
- retinal vein occlusion
- vitreous haemorrhage

Candidiasis

Tuberculosis

Hypertension

Ischaemic heart disease

Chronic renal failure

Carpal tunnel syndrome

Tendon xanthomas

Fatty infiltration of liver

Amyotrophy

Meralgia paraesthetica

Balanitis (vulvitis)

Neuropathy   Neuropathic ulcers
Osteomyelitis

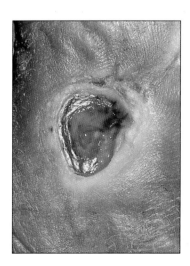

7.87 Painless trophic ulceration of the sole of the foot is a common presenting feature of sensory neuropathy in DM. Diabetic ulcers are commonly complicated by infection (*see* **3.150**) and, if peripheral vascular disease is present, gangrene may also develop.

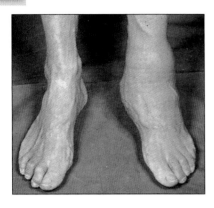

7.88 Charcot joint in diabetes. Sensory neuropathy has led to derangement of the left forefoot and ankle. Note the distortion and swelling. The derangement was painless, and there was little functional disability. On examination, the patient had loss of sensation and reflexes in the left ankle and foot.

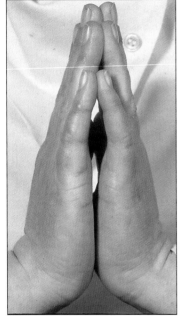

7.89 The 'prayer sign' in diabetes. Joint movement is limited, and the patient is unable to bring together the palms of the hands as in prayer. Note also the 'waxy' changes in the skin. Both these features are associated with diabetic microangiopathy.

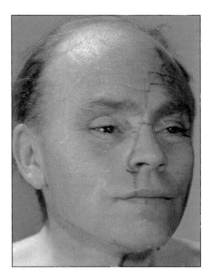

7.91 Autonomic neuropathy has led to gustatory sweating in this diabetic patient. Spicy food and cheese provokes sweating in an area on the right side of the head and trunk, as outlined with iodine in this picture. Autonomic neuropathy is an important and irreversible chronic complication of diabetes.

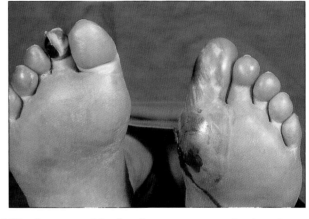

7.92 Gangrene of the foot is a common complication of chronic diabetes. In this patient 'wet' gangrene has developed in the hallux of the left foot, and dry gangrene in the second toe of the right foot. Ulceration and gangrene of the foot are commonly the result of a combination of diabetic neuropathy with large or small vessel disease, or both.

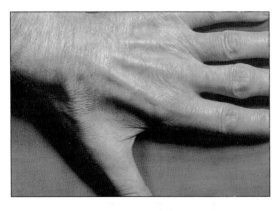

7.90 Ulnar mononeuropathy in a diabetic patient, causing wasting of the small muscles of the hand.

(**3.152**). As in other peripheral vascular diseases (*see* **p. 239**), gangrene usually requires treatment by amputation.

Dermatological manifestations of DM include acanthosis nigricans (**2.90**), necrobiosis lipoidica (**2.138**), granuloma annulare (**2.137**) and candidal and staphylococcal infections (**1.77**, **2.50**). Xanthomata are common as a result of hyperlipidaemia (*see* **p. 324**).

DM in pregnancy poses special problems, but the outlook for the fetus is greatly improved by good diabetic control. Even so, the typical baby born to a diabetic mother is overweight and prone to neonatal complications that can, however, usually be overcome by intensive care in the neonatal period. Congenital abnormalities are more common in babies born to diabetic mothers. Counselling of known diabetics before conception is helpful.

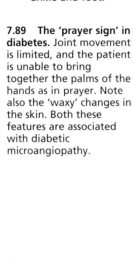

Diabetes and the eye

Diabetes mellitus is a leading cause of blindness in the developed world, and diabetes has numerous effects on the eye (**7.93**). Up to 20% of patients with type 2 DM have retinal changes at presentation, but it is essential that all patients with diabetes enter a programme of eye surveillance. Routine eye examinations should include visual acuity testing and fundoscopy after mydriatic drops.

'Senile' cataract (**7.94**) occurs at a younger age in diabetics than in other patients, and rarer conditions such as rubeosis iridis (**7.95**) may also affect the anterior parts of the eye.

Extreme hypertriglyceridaemia may be visible in the retinal vessels as lipaemia retinalis (**7.96**).

The major retinal changes in DM are a reflection of microangiopathy, and their progress gives valuable information on the likely effect of DM on other organs (especially the kidney), as well as on the retina itself.

THE OCULAR MANIFESTATIONS OF DIABETES MELLITUS	
Eyelids:	xanthelasmata caused by hyperlipidaemia (**7.108**)
Conjunctiva:	microaneurysms, venous dilatation
Extra-ocular muscles:	palsy with diplopia caused by third, fourth or sixth cranial nerve involvement (**7.83**)
Orbit:	mucormycosis – a potential complication of severe diabetic acidosis
Iris:	neovascularization of the anterior surface (rubeosis iridis, **7.95**)
Glaucoma:	neovascular glaucoma, chronic open angle glaucoma
Pupil:	poor dilatation caused by rubeosis iridis, Argyll Robertson pupil (**11.6**)
Lens:	cataract (**7.94**), refractive errors
Vitreous body:	vitreous haemorrhage (**7.103**), asteroid hyalosis
Retina:	diabetic retinopathy (**7.97–7.104**), retinal vein occlusion, lipaemia retinalis (**7.96**)
Optic nerve:	ischaemic papillitis, optic atrophy

7.93   The ocular manifestations of diabetes mellitus.

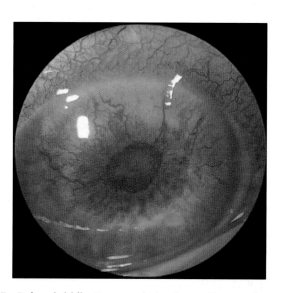

7.95   Rubeosis iridis. New vessels develop on the anterior surface of the iris in response to severe ocular ischaemia. Resulting obstruction to aqueous drainage may lead to glaucoma. Rubeosis iridis is most commonly a complication of diabetes, but may also occur in patients with carotid stenosis, long-standing retinal detachments, central retinal vein occlusion or ocular tumours.

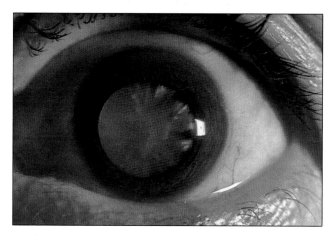

7.94   'Senile' cataract occurs at a younger age in diabetic patients than in the normal population. Reversible 'osmotic' cataracts may also form acutely in poorly controlled diabetics.

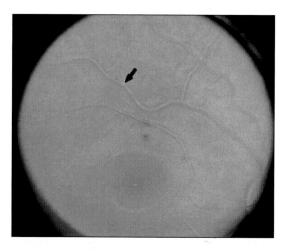

7.96   Lipaemia retinalis is a reflection of severe hypertriglyceridaemia. The retinal vessels appear white as a result of the 'milky' chylomicron-rich plasma within them. Lipaemia retinalis is commonly seen in acute uncontrolled diabetes.

The characteristic early lesions ('background' retinopathy) are microaneurysms associated with exudates and venous dilatation (**7.97**). These early changes are best visualized by fluorescein angiograms (**7.98**). They are common, occurring in 80% of patients who have had diabetes for 20 years. They do not always threaten sight and need no specific treatment, but must be monitored because exudates around the macula with associated oedema are a common cause of diabetic blindness (**7.99**). Cotton wool spots (**7.100**) are retinal infarcts and are a bad prognostic sign, as the retina responds to ischaemia by capillary proliferation. The formation of new vessels (**7.101, 7.102**) is a serious form of retinopathy as they may form on the disc (**7.102**) or in the periphery, and they tend to extend forward into the vitreous leading to haemorrhage (**7.103**) and fibrosis.

Diabetic retinopathy may be complicated by the presence of hypertension (**7.104**) or by thrombosis in the retinal veins.

Proliferative retinopathy and maculopathy can often be treated by laser photocoagulation which may prevent blindness by producing a iatrogenic choroidoretinitis (**7.103**).

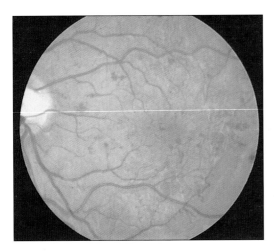

7.97   Background diabetic retinopathy. Note the presence of multiple microaneurysms ('dots') and some small areas of haemorrhage ('blots'). Despite the appearance, the patient's visual acuity is usually unaffected at this stage.

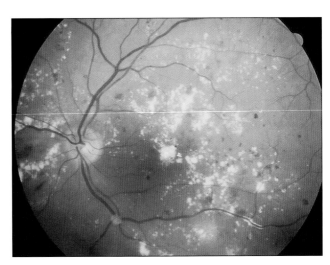

7.99   Macular involvement in diabetic retinopathy is a common cause of diabetic blindness. Note the presence of multiple exudates and the blurring caused by macular oedema – the most common cause of visual impairment in macular disease.

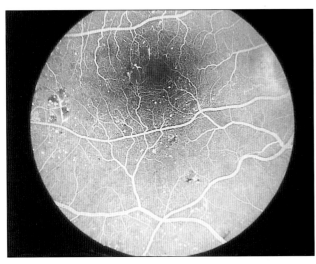

7.98   Fluorescein angiogram in background diabetic retinopathy, showing the presence of multiple microaneurysms.

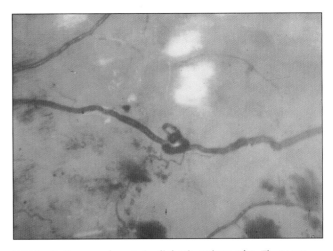

7.100   Cotton wool spots in diabetic retinopathy. These are retinal infarcts resulting from arterial occlusion. They are a bad prognostic sign because they are likely to herald capillary proliferation.

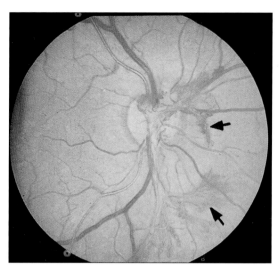

7.101 Proliferative diabetic retinopathy. Fronds of new vessels (arrowed) can be seen emerging from the disc and elsewhere.

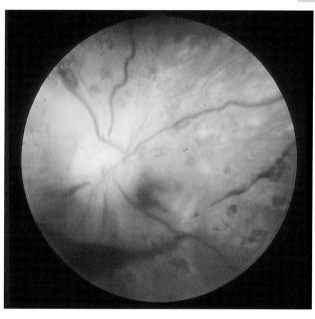

7.103 Vitreous haemorrhage resulting from proliferative retinopathy in diabetes. These haemorrhages appear as a haze or a red or black reflex through the ophthalmoscope as in the curvilinear accumulation of blood seen here. This patient's proliferative retinopathy has been treated by laser photocoagulation, which has left typical circular scars.

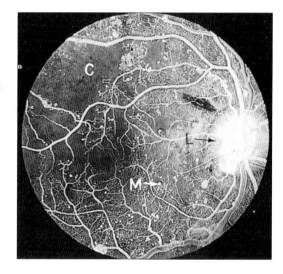

7.102 Fluorescein angiogram in diabetic retinopathy showing dark ischaemic areas in which capillaries are abnormally absent (C), microaneurysms (M) and leakage from new vessels on the optic disc (L).

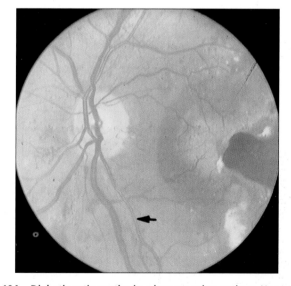

7.104 Diabetic retinopathy in a hypertensive patient. Note the presence of hypertensive vessel changes (silver-wiring, arrowed) and a macular subhyaloid haemorrhage. Hypertension adds to the risk of haemorrhage in diabetic retinopathy.

HYPOGLYCAEMIA

Hypoglycaemia is defined as a blood glucose level below the lower limit of the normal range, and may be associated with clinical features below a blood glucose level of about 3 mmol/litre.

Causes of hypoglycaemia include:

- drug-induced in diabetes (insulin and sulphonylureas), often associated with not eating
- deliberate inappropriate insulin injection
- other drugs – salicylates in children, propranolol, trimethoprim, pentamidine and quinine
- excess alcohol intake

- insulinoma (**7.105**)
- a range of other tumours
- malnutrition or starvation.

The clinical presentation of hypoglycaemia is often due to endogenous catecholamine release, which provokes anxiety, weakness, a feeling of hunger, sweating, shakiness and palpitations. There may also be confusion, irritability, reduced higher cerebral function, convulsions, coma and death, which relate directly to the effects of hypoglycaemia on the brain.

Patients whose history suggests recurrent hypoglycaemic attacks should be investigated. A low fasting blood glucose level is a pointer to possible hypoglycaemia, and this should be confirmed, usually by a supervised 72-hour fast with regular exercise (performed in hospital). Blood glucose, insulin and C-peptide levels should be measured. This will reveal almost all cases of hypoglycaemia due to insulinomas, and such a fast very rarely provokes hypoglycaemia in normal subjects.

Small insulinomas may be difficult to localize. Possible techniques include isotope scanning (**7.105**), CT, endoscopic ultrasound, pancreatic arteriography and selective venous sampling for high insulin levels.

Intravenous glucose or concentrated oral glucose (**7.106**) should be given to patients with acute symptoms and signs suggesting hypoglycaemia as soon as blood has been taken for glucose estimation. Even if the diagnosis is proved incorrect no harm will be done and prompt treatment will reduce the duration of hypoglycaemia and the risk of death or serious complications.

Insulinomas should be surgically removed when possible. Medical suppression of insulin release by diazoxide, sulphonylureas or somatostatin analogues (e.g octreotide) is possible but side-effects are frequent.

HYPERLIPIDAEMIA

Hyperlipidaemia may be classified on the basis of laboratory findings, disease entities and genetic or environmental causes. All such classifications are complex and potentially confusing.

The importance of hyperlipidaemia relates mainly to its association with atheromatous vascular disease. There is clear evidence that elevation of the level of cholesterol and triglycerides is important in the premature development of atheroma and thrombotic events, such as myocardial infarction, thrombotic stroke and peripheral gangrene. There is also evidence at population and individual patient levels that a lowering in total blood cholesterol (specifically in the LDL fraction) leads to a decrease in the risk of cardiovascular morbidity and mortality.

In many patients, lipid abnormalities are now identified in screening programmes, but a number of clinical signs may give clues, especially in patients with gross hyperlipidaemia. These include:

- premature arcus cornealis (**6.43**, **7.60**, **7.107**, **7.108**, **8.2**)

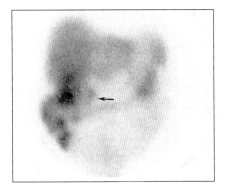

7.105 **Insulinoma demonstrated by** [123]**I-octreotide scanning.** This technique images tumours that have somatostatin receptors. The picture shows some radioactivity in the gall bladder, bowel and kidneys. The abnormal uptake in the insulinoma is arrowed. The patient had presented with symptoms suggesting hypoglycaemia, which had been confirmed by a blood glucose of 1.8 mmol/litre. Surgical removal was successful.

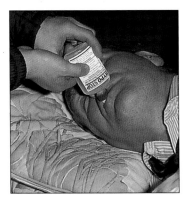

7.106 **Concentrated oral glucose gel can be administered by mouth** to patients with suspected hypoglycaemia who can swallow. This should be done with the patient in the recovery position to minimize the risk of pulmonary aspiration. The response to oral or intravenous glucose in hypoglycaemia is rapid.

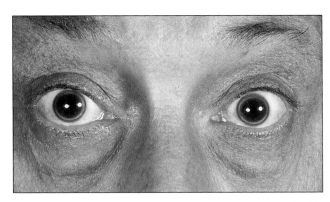

7.107 **Corneal arcus is a normal phenomenon associated with ageing (arcus senilis),** but its occurrence in patients under the age of 50 years suggests the possibility of underlying hyperlipidaemia. The ring represents deposits of phospholipid and cholesterol in the corneal stroma.

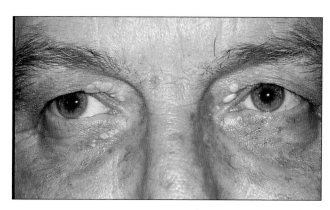

7.108 Corneal arcus and xanthelasmata in the same patient. This combination is strongly suggestive of underlying hyperlipidaemia, and the presence of xanthelasmata alone is an indication for investigation of lipid status.

- xanthelasmata (**7.108**, **9.5**, **9.35**)
- skin xanthomata (**7.109**, **7.110**, **9.6**)
- tendon xanthomata (**7.111**, **7.112**)
- lipaemia retinalis (**7.96**).

The diagnosis of hyperlipidaemia is easily made on a fasting blood sample. In Western countries, counselling and treatment can often be based on cholesterol and triglyceride levels alone, but the measurement of LDL and HDL cholesterol may be useful in some patients. It is important to identify or exclude causes of secondary hyperlipidaemia (**7.113**).

It is essential that any recommendations for dietary modification or drug therapy are made in the context of an overall assessment of the patient's cardiovascular risk profile. Other risk factors (smoking, hypertension, etc., *see* **p. 212**)

325

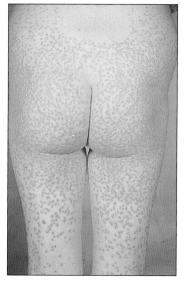

7.109 Eruptive xanthomas may be quite widespread in the skin, but they are most commonly found over the buttocks. They are strongly suggestive of underlying hyperlipidaemia.

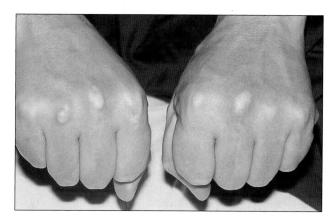

7.111 Tendon xanthomata were the first clue to the diagnosis in this patient with familial hypercholesterolaemia and premature coronary heart disease.

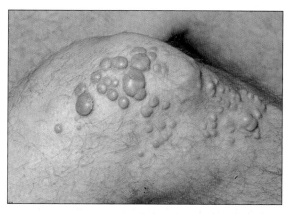

7.110 Tuberous xanthomata on the knee, occurring in a patient with familial hypercholesterolaemia. Massive xanthomata may sometimes require surgical removal.

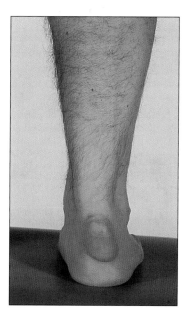

7.112 Tendon xanthomata are characteristically found over the tendons and extensor surfaces of joints. They are particularly common over the patellar and Achilles tendons. This patient had familial hypercholesterolaemia.

SECONDARY CAUSES OF RAISED CHOLESTEROL AND TRIGLYCERIDE
Raised cholesterol
Diet
Hypothyroidism
Liver disease
Nephrotic syndrome
Porphyria
Raised triglyceride
Obesity
Poorly controlled diabetes
Alcohol excess
High carbohydrate diet
Renal failure
Oestrogen therapy

7.113 Secondary causes of raised cholesterol and triglyceride.

ACTION LEVELS FOR TREATMENT OF HYPERLIPIDAEMIA

CHOLESTEROL	< 5.2 mmol/l	Satisfactory: no action
	5.2–6.5 mmol/l	Moderately elevated: diet and counselling on other risk factors; recheck in 3 months
	6.5–7.8 mmol/l	High: diet first; consider drugs only if diet fails and other risk factors are present
	> 7.8 mmol/l	Very high: diet, assess other risk factors, other family members; if diet fails use drugs (usually statins)
TRIGLYCERIDE	< 3.0 mmol/l	Satisfactory: no action
	3.0–6.0 mmol/l	High: check HDL; weight loss; diet; counsel on other risk factors; consider drugs if diet fails, especially if HDL is < 1.0 mmol/l
	> 6.0 mmol/l	Very high: check HDL; weight loss; diet; drugs are indicated to prevent coronary heart disease and pancreatitis

7.114 Action levels for treatment of hyperlipidaemia found on screening. Lipid lowering drug therapy should be started at all levels of hyperlipidaemia in all patients who have already experienced a thrombotic vascular occlusion.

should be identified and treated at the same time, and the patient's family history should be investigated so that other at-risk family members can be identified, especially if a familial disorder is suspected.

A number of international working parties have recommended levels at which treatment should be instigated for hyperlipidaemia, and a consensus view is summarized in **7.114**. Treatment of hyperlipidaemia starts with a diet low in saturated fats, and rich in fibre, complex carbohydrates and polyunsaturated or monounsaturated oils and fish. Regular consumption of 'functional' foods containing high concentrations of plant stannol can reduce LDL by an additional 10%. If this is unsuccessful over a 3–6-month period, a range of lipid-lowering drugs is available. Lipid-lowering statin drugs are effective in the primary and secondary prevention of coronary artery disease. In secondary prevention, for example, a 10% reduction in total cholesterol has been shown to reduce the risk of a further coronary event by 25%.

NUTRITIONAL DISORDERS

OBESITY

Storage of lipids in excess of daily requirements results in obesity – an excess of adipose tissue that is associated with a health risk. Obesity is defined as a 20% excess over ideal body weight and in many Western populations 30–40% of individuals are obese. The prevalence of obesity is increasing.

Most obese individuals ingest excess calories that are then stored. This may be coupled with reduced calorie expenditure resulting from a sedentary existence, or with reduced thermogenesis. In a small number of cases, obesity is secondary to diseases such as hypothyroidism, Cushing's syndrome and extremely rare disorders such as insulinoma, Fröhlich's syndrome and the Prader–Willi syndrome.

The end result of excessive calorie intake is an increase in fat deposition around the internal organs and muscles, and in subcutaneous sites such as abdomen, buttocks, breasts, thighs, face and upper arms (**7.115–7.117**). Such obesity is associated with insulin resistance and glucose intolerance, hyper-lipidaemia, hypertension and an increased incidence of thrombotic arterial and venous disease and of degenerative joint diseases. Weight reduction towards the norm is associated with improved life expectancy.

Tables of desirable weights are available for age, sex and height. A more acceptable and accurate assessment method is to use the body mass index (BMI), which is calculated as weight in kilograms divided by height in metres squared. In Caucasians, BMI values of 19–24 in women and 20–25 in men are associated with the longest life expectancy. Values over 30 (obese) and over 35 (morbidly obese) are associated with significant reduction of life expectancy. However, BMI does not differentiate between upper and lower body fat distribution.

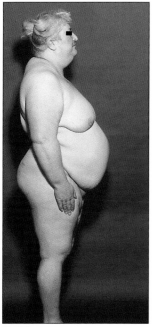 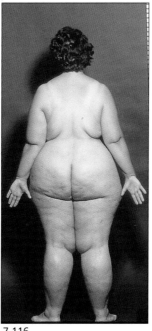

7.115   7.116

7.115 & 7.116 Simple obesity in these women has led to excessive fat deposition in the upper arms, breasts, abdomen, buttocks and thighs. This distribution is typical.

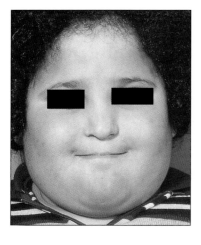

7.117 Simple obesity may lead to gross roundness and fatness of the face. It is important to differentiate this appearance from that of Cushing's syndrome (**7.27**).

SOME MEDICAL CONSEQUENCES OF OBESITY
Mechanical
Back pain
Osteoarthritis
Stress incontinence
Intertrigo
Defective wound healing
Varicose veins
Venous ulcers
Breathlessness
Sleep apnoea
Risk during anaesthesia/surgery
Metabolic
Insulin resistance
Type 2 diabetes mellitus
Hyperlipidaemia
Gallstones
Hypertension
Coronary heart disease
Stroke
Some cancers
Depression

7.118 Medical consequences of obesity.

Measurement of skin-fold thickness over the upper arm and back provides a measure of subcutaneous fat and is better for use in elderly patients who have lost muscle bulk and also in younger heavily muscled subjects. It is difficult to obtain reproducible measurements. It is probable that more information of predictive value is obtained from the waist: hip circumference ratio (WHR). Upper body obesity is defined as a WHR > 0.83 in women and WHR > 0.95 in men. The waist is measured midway between the lower rib margin and the iliac crest and the hips over the great trochanters.

Higher mortality from coronary heart disease, stroke and death from all causes is associated with higher BMI, skin-fold thickness and WHR and obesity has many other adverse medical consequences (**7.118**).

Treatment of obesity is by calorie restriction, which must be permanent and represent a real change in lifestyle. Patients should also be encouraged to exercise. Adherence to a diet providing 800–1200 calories per day results in weight loss. A waist cord may encourage the patient to maintain the lower weight.

Attempts may also be made to stop patients eating by wiring the jaws, using an inflated balloon to fill the stomach or by surgery to create a jejunoileal bypass. All these procedures may have major complications and are used only as a last resort.

Clinical studies of drugs which inhibit the intestinal absorption of fats are in progress; these compounds may prove useful in many patients in the future.

PROTEIN-ENERGY MALNUTRITION

In protein-energy malnutrition (PEM) there is a loss of adipose tissue and lean body mass, usually as a result of deficient quantitative and qualitative food intake in the developing countries, or of malabsorption or organic disease (usually malignancy) in developed countries. PEM is of insidious onset, and up to one-quarter of the world's population lives on the verge of insufficiency of protein and calorie intake.

The group most commonly affected is children. The terms 'kwashiorkor' and 'marasmus' are descriptive terms of the extent of the PEM. In marasmus, there is a deficiency in total food intake; the child is apathetic, withdrawn, and stunted in growth with spindly arms and legs. In kwashiorkor, the major deficiency is in protein intake; the child has a swollen abdomen with dependent oedema of the legs, often with skin and eye infections, a large fatty liver, and a reddish-yellow tinge to the hair. The two conditions are part of a spectrum and may coexist in the same community (**7.119**).

In the adult, weight loss is the most common feature of the disease. The person looks skeletal with significant loss of adipose tissue, skin hanging in folds, wasted limbs, ascites, dependent oedema, dry flaky skin and depigmentation (**7.120**). The blood pressure is reduced, the pulse slow, and central core temperature may be reduced. There may also be other features of vitamin or trace element deficiency.

The diagnosis is usually clinical, but investigations show anaemia that may be caused by deficiency of iron, folate, or both; biochemistry shows the extent of the protein deficiency, with low serum albumin and transferrin. There may also be impairment of renal and liver function. Immunity is also depressed, with cutaneous energy and lymphopenia. Death is often caused by infection.

Treatment is with a diet of normal calorie content and constituents. This should be implemented slowly and young children may require nasogastric feeding. Hypothermia and infections require treatment. Supplements of vitamins and minerals should also be given.

PEM is probably the most common underlying cause of death worldwide. The mortality of severe cases is 50–75%, and

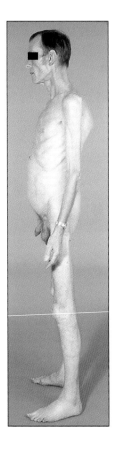

7.120 Malnutrition has resulted in severe weight loss. Underlying malignant disease, chronic infection or malabsorption is the most likely cause, but occasionally the condition may result simply from self-neglect and inadequate food intake.

there is a massive morbidity resulting from physical and mental stunting.

ANOREXIA AND BULIMIA NERVOSA

Anorexia nervosa usually occurs in white adolescent girls, with a prevalence of about 1% in this age group. It results in severe weight loss as a result of 'voluntary' starvation. There is often a history of obesity in childhood; there may have been psychological trauma with teasing at school, which has produced an intense desire to alter the body image and there may be associated psychosexual problems. Patients often deny hunger or weight loss. They become devious about avoidance of eating and may vomit up a meal surreptitiously if they have been forced to eat. The desire to lose weight may also involve the use of purgatives, diuretics and violent programmes of exercise. The clinical features include:

- onset before age 25 years in a female
- loss of > 25% of body weight – absence of body fat
- secondary amenorrhoea
- presence of lanugo hair over body
- preservation of breast tissue
- parotid enlargement
- dependent oedema caused by low serum albumin
- low blood pressure with bradycardia.

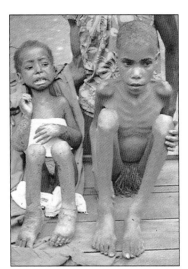

7.119 Kwashiorkor and marasmus in brothers. The younger brother, on the left, has kwashiorkor with generalized oedema, skin changes, pale reddish-yellow hair and a miserable expression. The older child, on the right, has marasmus, with generalized wasting, spindly arms and legs and an apathetic expression.

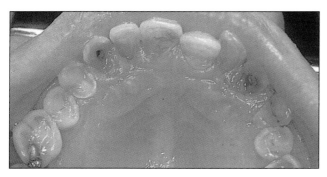

7.121   Severe tooth destruction caused by repeated regurgitation and vomiting of acid stomach contents in a patient with anorexia nervosa. This is also a common feature of bulimia.

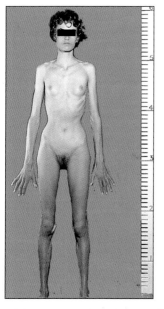

7.122   Anorexia nervosa in a 20-year-old woman. Note the low body weight and the preservation of breast tissue. Fine lanugo hair was present over the patient's back, and she had developed secondary amenorrhoea. Her blood pressure was 100/60 mmHg and her pulse 60/minute.

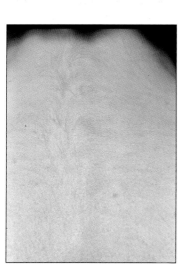

7.123   Lanugo hair in anorexia nervosa. Fine, downy body hair is characteristic of anorexia nervosa but may also occur in normal individuals.

Patients may also have diarrhoea as a result of laxative abuse or eroded teeth due to the repeated vomiting of acid stomach contents (**7.121**), or both; they may show features of depression or anxiety. The facial and bodily appearances are recognizable, but not in themselves diagnostic (**7.122, 7.123**).

There is no diagnostic laboratory test, but there may be anaemia and leucopenia, and the serum albumin may be low. There is often a disturbance of glucose tolerance. Many patients show disturbance of other endocrine functions and biochemical abnormalities may include high levels of cortisol, low potassium with metabolic alkalosis secondary to vomiting, low zinc levels and elevated triiodothyronine levels.

Bulimia nervosa is a related condition in which binge eating is associated with self-induced vomiting. It is most often seen in women in their mid-20s.

Both conditions have a mortality rate of 5–10% from the disease itself or from suicide. Osteoporosis is a long-term complication of chronic eating disorder.

Treatment of eating disorders is difficult, but includes psychological and physical support.

VITAMINS AND DISEASE

Vitamin deficiency syndromes

The syndromes which may result from isolated deficiencies of individual vitamins are listed in **7.124**. Some examples are illustrated in **7.125–7.129**.

VITAMIN DEFICIENCY SYNDROMES	
Vitamin	**Syndrome**
A	Night blindness, conjunctival lesions (**7.125**)
Niacin	Pellagra (**7.126**)
Thiamine (B_1)	Dry beri-beri (**7.128**), wet beri-beri (**7.127**), Wernicke's encephalopathy, Korsakoff's psychosis
Riboflavin (B_2)	Mucosal lesions (especially mouth and pharynx; **7.129**)
Pyridoxine (B_6)	Glossitis (**9.47**), neuropathy (*see* **p. 488**)
Folate	Macrocytic anaemia (*see* **p. 413**)
B_{12}	Macrocytic anaemia (*see* **p. 413**), neuropathy (*see* **pp. 413, 488**)
C	Scurvy (**8.25**; *see* **p. 439**)
D	Rickets, osteomalacia (*see* **p. 137**)
E	Haemolysis, neuropathy
K	Hypoprothrominaemia, bruising (**9.14**; *see* **p. 441**)

7.124   Vitamin deficiency syndromes.

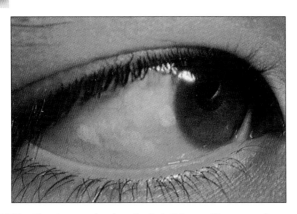

7.125 Bitot's spots in vitamin A deficiency. These may be single or, as here, multiple, and they represent areas of desquamated, keratinized conjunctival cells, together with lipid material. The patient also has dryness and inflammation of the scleral conjunctiva (xerophthalmia). This combination is typically seen in nutritional deficiency, especially when there is a lack of vitamin A.

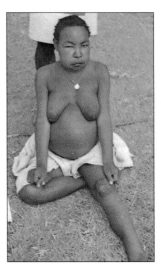

7.127 Thiamine deficiency – wet beriberi. The patient has fluid retention, with generalized oedema. Pulmonary congestion resulting from left heart failure was also present, and the patient had peripheral neuropathy.

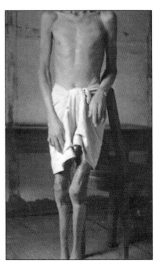

7.128 Thiamine deficiency – dry beri-beri. This patient has chronic polyneuritis, with wrist drop and foot drop. In dry beri-beri, there is also loss of tendon reflexes, joint position sense and vibration sense, tenderness in the calf muscles on pressure, anaesthesia of the skin, especially over the tibia, paraesthesia in the legs and arms, and motor weakness.

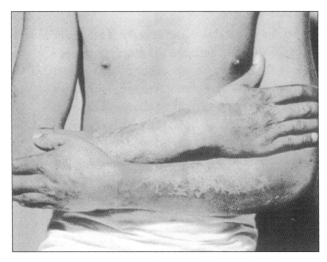

7.126 Pellagra – the result of niacin deficiency. The skin changes begin as an erythema with pruritus and burning. Bullae may form and rupture. At the slightly later stage shown here, the skin becomes hard, rough, cracked, blackish and brittle; with more severe involvement, extensive exfoliation may occur. Here only sun-exposed areas are affected, but any part of the body may become involved.

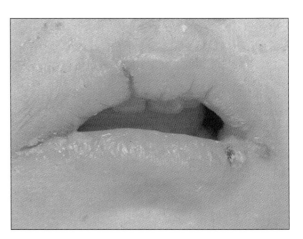

7.129 Cheilosis – one manifestation of riboflavin deficiency, though it may also occur with deficiency of iron and other vitamins. It is characterized by vertical fissuring, which is later complicated by redness, swelling and ulceration of the lips. Angular stomatitis may also be present, as here; many patients with riboflavin deficiency also have widespread seborrhoeic dermatitis involving the scrotum or perineum.

VITAMIN TOXICITY SYNDROMES	
Vitamin	**Syndrome**
A	Nausea, vomiting, headache, convulsions, periosteal proliferation, teratogenic effects
Niacin (nicotinic acid)	Vasodilatation
Pyridoxine (B$_6$)	Peripheral neuropathy
C	Increased urinary oxalate
D	Hypercalcaemia, renal failure
E	Nausea
K	Hyperbilirubinaemia

7.130   Vitamin toxicity syndrome.

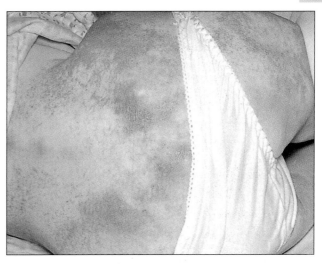

7.131   Zinc deficiency leads to a characteristic erythematous, hyperkeratotic skin rash. This 24-year-old woman had generalized malnutrition, associated with severe Crohn's disease. Note the wasting of the thigh muscles. She was managed by prolonged parenteral nutrition, and the skin rash responded well to zinc supplementation.

Vitamin toxicity syndromes

Ingestion of excessive quantities of various vitamins may also lead to acute or chronic disorders (**7.130**).

TRACE ELEMENTS IN NUTRITION

A large number of inorganic ions are essential for the maintenance of health. These include iron, iodine, copper, zinc, cobalt, selenium, chromium and tin. Deficiencies of iron and iodine are discussed on **pages 410 and 313**, respectively. Identifiable clinical syndromes have also been described in zinc and copper deficiency.

Deficiency of zinc in the diet may lead to retarded growth, retarded sexual development, hyperkeratotic dermatitis (**7.131**), loss of hair and anaemia. Supplementation of the diet with zinc produces a growth spurt and correction of anaemia.

Acrodermatitis enteropathica is an inherited disorder of zinc absorption in which patients present with chronic diarrhoea and growth retardation, weight loss, dermatitis, and perianal ulceration, often caused by candidal infections. It responds dramatically to zinc therapy.

ARTIFICIAL NUTRITIONAL SUPPORT

Artificial nutritional support improves morbidity and mortality in patients with a range of intestinal disorders and in those with swallowing difficulties.

It is indicated when a patient has:

* continuing weight loss greater than 10% of original body weight
* inability to increase normal oral intake
* active disease that cannot be controlled and will lead to either of the above criteria.

Balanced oral and parenteral feeds are available.

If intestinal function is otherwise normal, enteral feeding is suitable. In the hospital setting, enteral tube feeding must be considered for those who have swallowing difficulties due to stroke, prolonged coma or severe burns, and for those who do not eat because of nausea associated with chronic sepsis, renal failure, malignancy or brain disease. In the presence of intestinal failure (e.g. ileus, fistulae, obstruction, active Crohn's disease), the parenteral route should be used. Increasingly, these nutritional support systems may be used in the community.

Enteral nutrition can be effectively carried out by the use of a fine-bore nasoenteral feeding tube (**7.132**) or by percutaneous

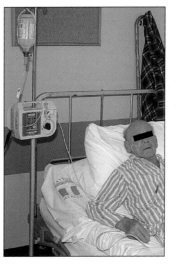

7.132   Enteral nutrition in a hospital patient with swallowing difficulties following stroke. A fine-bore polyurethane tube is passed via the nose into the stomach or duodenum, and the administration of the feed can be controlled by an automated pump. Such naso-enteral tubes are ususally well tolerated. Mucosal ulceration rarely occurs, but aspiration pneumonia is a possible complication. With practice, the tube may be reinserted at home if necessary by the patient or his family.

endoscopic gastrotomy (PEG) (**7.133, 7.134**). The PEG tube system should be used if it is predicted that nutritional support will be required for more than 3 weeks. The advantages are the increased comfort of the patient and reduction of the possibilities of aspiration.

Parenteral access has until recently concentrated on catheter placement into the central veins. However, this has been associated with a significant incidence of local venous and intracardiac thrombosis, and with generalized infection. The result is failure in about 20% of cases. In addition, there is a significant morbidity when inserting the catheter into the subclavian or internal jugular veins (e.g. pneumothorax or arterial cannulation in error). If the requirement is clearly for a prolonged period, a Hickman–Broviac line may be used. This is a silicone catheter with a Dacron cuff, which is placed in a central site via a subcutaneous tunnel (**7.135**). The cuff allows fibrous tissue to grow into it to anchor the catheter and to reduce the risk of infection. Such catheters may also be used for long-term administration of antimicrobials or chemotherapy (**4.102**). Peripheral catheters may be used for parenteral nutrition, especially when the anticipated need is relatively short term (**7.136**). Infection and local thrombosis are potential complications of all venous cannulae.

7.133

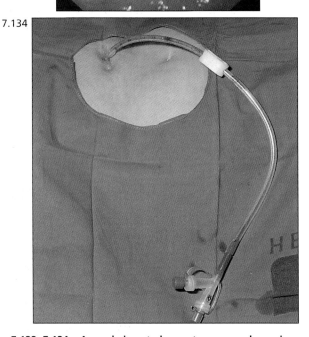

7.134

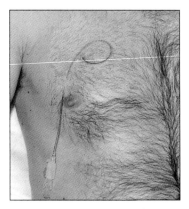

7.135 Intravenous catheter for the long-term administration of parenteral nutrition ('Hickman–Broviac line'). The line passes through a subcutaneous tunnel and has a Dacron cuff before entering the venous system. These features minimize the risks of displacement and tracking infection.

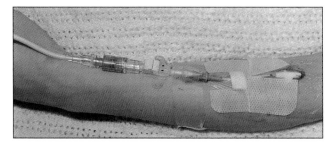

7.136 Peripheral intravenous catheter for parenteral nutrition. There has recently been a move back to appropriate peripheral intravenous cannulae for parenteral nutrition. The risk of serious complications may be lower than with central catheterization.

7.133, 7.134 A newly inserted percutaneous endoscopic gastrotomy (PEG) tube seen endoscopically in the stomach wall (**7.133**) and exteriorly (**7.134**). A cannula is inserted from the exterior abdominal wall to the stomach under endoscopic control; a guide suture is inserted through this cannula, which is then caught by an endoscopic snare and pulled up the oesophagus to the mouth. Finally, the PEG tube is attached to this suture and is pulled down via the mouth and the oesophagus to the stomach and the exterior. When the PEG tube is finally positioned, only a retaining collar and its orifice remain in the stomach. The tube is held in place on the exterior abdominal wall by a special fixation device.

INHERITED METABOLIC DISORDERS

THE PORPHYRIAS

The porphyrias are a heterogeneous group of inborn errors of metabolism in which there is an overproduction of various intermediate compounds (porphyrins) in the biosynthesis of haem. Their classification is summarized in **7.137**. The acute

THE CLASSIFICATION OF PORPHYRIAS		
	Hepatic	**Erythropoietic**
ACUTE	Acute intermittent porphyria Variegate porphyria Hereditary porphyria	
NON-ACUTE	Porphyria cutanea tarda	Congenital porphyria Erythropoietic protoporphyria

7.137 The classification of porphyrias.

hepatic porphyrias are the result of partial enzyme blocks in the biosynthetic pathway for haem.

Acute intermittent porphyria

Acute intermittent porphryia is an autosomal dominant genetic disorder of metabolism in which exposure to various drugs, including alcohol, may trigger a life-threatening crisis (a pharmacogenetic disorder). The condition results from a deficiency in porphobilinogen deaminase. It presents acutely in early adulthood with fever, tachycardia, abdominal pain and vomiting, which may be mistaken for an acute abdomen, but is caused by autonomic neuropathy. There may also be a history of acute onset of peripheral neuropathy with limb paralysis and loss of sensation, often associated with depression or anxiety. The symptoms may be mistakenly attributed to hysteria. The clues lie in a positive family history and in examination of the urine. Attacks may be precipitated by alcohol, by drugs such as anticonvulsants and oral contraceptives, by substance misuse (e.g ecstacy, amphetamines, cocaine, cannabis), by infection, by physical stress or by cyclical factors such as menstruation. Between attacks there may be no clinical features.

During the acute attacks, there may be a polymorphonuclear leucocytosis, which may be misinterpreted as an indicator of infection. There may also be hyponatraemia, hypomagnesaemia and uraemia. The best screening test is to find porphobilinogen in the urine. On standing, the urine darkens, as a result of the formation of uroporphyrin and porphobilin, and fluoresces in ultraviolet light (**7.138**). After treatment with Ehrlich's aldehyde, it develops a pink coloration. The level of delta aminolaevulinic acid in the blood is also raised.

Treatment is supportive, with avoidance of drugs known to precipitate the acute attack. Patients should wear a bracelet identifying the diagnosis.

Variegate porphyria

Variegate porphyria combines the acute features of acute intermittent porphyria with chronic skin sensitivity to sunlight and trauma. The inheritance is autosomal dominant, and the enzyme defect is in protoporphyrinogen oxidase. The clinical presentation is often similar to that of acute intermittent porphyria, but it occurs on a background of pigmentation of the skin, associated with bullae, ulceration, atrophy and hypertrichosis (**7.139**). The diagnosis is made by finding excess protoporphyrin in the urine at all times and a positive test for porphobilinogen during acute attacks. Important aspects of management include the avoidance of direct sunlight and the wearing of adequate protective clothing.

Porphyria cutanea tarda

Porphyria cutanea tarda is the most common type of porphyria and is characterized by chronic skin lesions and chronic liver disease, often associated with alcoholism and sometimes with hepatic siderosis. The enzyme defect is in uroporphyrinogen decarboxylase. The clinical features are similar to the chronic features of variegate porphyria (**7.140**). The incidence of diabetes mellitus is increased and there is an association with a

333

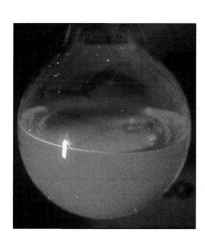

7.138 The urine in acute intermittent porphyria shows red fluorescence in ultraviolet light as a result of the presence of porphobilinogen.

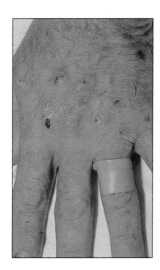

7.139 Variegate porphyria. Note the patchy but generalized pigmentation of the skin, associated with areas of ulceration and scarring. Bullae are commonly seen as precursors to ulceration, and hypertrichosis is also common in this condition, which is associated with chronic photosensitivity.

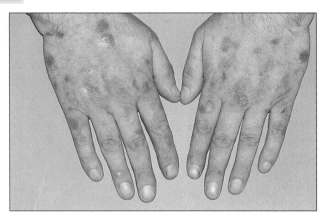

7.140 **Porphyria cutanea tarda.** Photosensitivity in this condition leads to blister formation and pigmented scarring.

range of autoimmune diseases. As the disease is caused by an inherited deficiency of uroporphyrinogen decarboxylase, there is an increased excretion of uroporphyrin in the urine, which may be pink or brown.

A similar clinical picture may be found in people poisoned with a range of polychlorinated hydrocarbons and with primary and secondary liver neoplasia.

Erythropoietic protoporphyria

Erythropoietic protoporphyria is a very rare genetic disorder of porphyrin metabolism in which the transmission is autosomal recessive. The usual clinical presentation is with solar urticaria without blistering, scarring or hyperpigmentation. Occasionally, patients may develop cirrhosis of the liver, splenomegaly, gallstones and anaemia. A characteristic feature is red pigmentation of the teeth (erythrodontia, **7.141**). The chemical defect is in the enzyme ferrochelatase, which promotes the incorporation of ferrous iron into protoporphyrin. As a result, there is excessive protoporphyrin in many tissues, especially in haemopoietic cells, liver and skin. The diagnosis is made by demonstrating the red fluorescence of protoporphyrin in red cells in a blood film.

DISORDERS OF AMINO ACID METABOLISM

Alkaptonuria

Alkaptonuria is a hereditary disorder caused by the absence of the enzyme homogentisic acid oxidase. The result of this defect is that homogentisic acid produced by degradation of phenylalanine and tyrosine cannot be further metabolized and therefore accumulates in the body. It is excreted in the urine and may manifest itself in childhood, through the brown colour that develops in nappies (diapers). This is caused by a reduction product of the colourless homogentisic acid. Homogentisic acid tends to pigment cartilage and other connective tissue, including the sclera (ochronosis) (**7.142**), and eventually causes a degenerative arthropathy (**7.143**). No prophylactic or curative treatment is available. Gene therapy may prove possible in the future.

Phenylketonuria

Phenylketonuria is an autosomal recessive disorder that produces deficiency of the enzyme (phenylalanine hydroxylase) responsible for the conversion of phenylalanine to tyrosine,

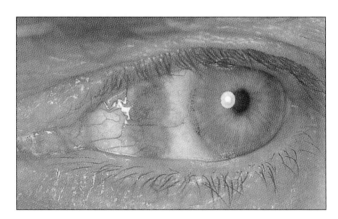

7.142 **Ochronosis – pigmentation of the sclera in alkaptonuria** – is the result of homogentisic acid accumulation in the absence of homogentisic acid oxidase.

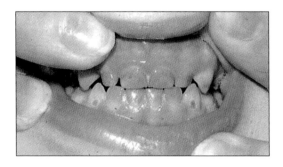

7.141 **Erythropoietic porphyria leads to erythrodontia** – reddish pigmentation of the teeth. Excessive protoporphyrin may also lead to abnormalities in the skin, liver, biliary tract, spleen and blood.

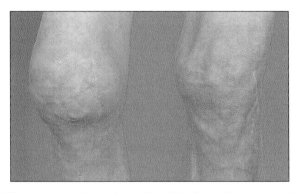

7.143 **Degenerative arthropathy of the knees in alkaptonuria.** The pathophysiology of the arthritis is unclear, and no specific treatment is available.

with resultant high levels of phenylalanine and its metabolites in the blood and body tissues. This results in progressive mental retardation and epilepsy. There is usually fair, sparse hair and eczema. Neonatal screening is routinely available (the Guthrie test), and should enable most affected individuals to be detected early and dietary restrictions to be imposed.

Homocystinurias

The homocystinurias are transmitted as autosomal recessives and are caused by at least three enzyme defects that allow the accumulation of homocystine in the body. There is progressive mental impairment with epilepsy, subluxation of the lens (**7.144**), arachnodactyly and a likelihood of arterial and venous thrombosis.

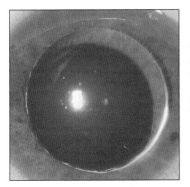

7.144 Subluxation of the lens is a common feature in homocystinuria. A similar abnormality is a feature of Marfan's syndrome, but whereas the subluxation is usually downwards in homocystinuria, it is most commonly upwards in Marfan's syndrome (**3.116**). In this case, there is complete anterior dislocation of the lens.

Cystinosis

Cystinosis is an autosomal recessive disorder in which cystine accumulates in the tissues, especially the cornea, bone marrow, liver and spleen and kidneys. A range of disorders results. In childhood, the kidney is particularly affected and renal failure may develop (Fanconi syndrome); in the adult, the cornea is particularly affected (**7.145**). There are intermediate varieties. The diagnosis is made by finding typical cystine crystals in biopsy material or in the cornea by slit-lamp examination.

LYSOSOMAL STORAGE DISEASES

Deficiencies of lysosomal enzymes may result in the accumulation of substrates or abnormal metabolites in all the tissues of the body. At least 30 separate enzyme deficiencies have been characterized and these produce different clinical syndromes of which only the most common are described here.

Lipoidoses

Gaucher's disease is an autosomal recessive disease in which deficiency of the enzyme glucosylceramidase results in the accumulation of glucocerebroside in the body. The disease is found especially in Ashkenazi Jews, and patients present in a wide variety of ways, especially with hepatosplenomegaly with neurological involvement (epilepsy and mental retardation) in children, and involvement of liver and spleen, bone marrow, bone, lung and eye in adults. The diagnosis is made by finding the characteristic Gaucher cell in biopsy tissue (e.g. bone marrow or spleen biopsy). Enzyme replacement therapy and gene therapy are now becoming feasible.

Niemann–Pick disease is an autosomal recessive disease in which a deficiency of sphingomyelinase results in accumulation of sphingomyelin in the tissues, especially in the CNS, liver and spleen and bone marrow. The clinical presentation varies according to the subtype of the disease. The common presentation in childhood is with mental retardation and hepatosplenomegaly. In type A disease, there is often a cherry-red spot in the retina (**7.146**). The diagnosis is made by finding the characteristic lipid-laden sea-blue histiocyte in biopsy material. Adults with type E disease present with hepato-splenomegaly but no neurological abnormalities.

Tay–Sachs disease (familial amaurotic idiocy) is an autosomal recessive disorder in which a deficiency of hexosaminidase A and B results in the accumulation of GM2 gangliosides in the brain and peripheral nerves. The result is mental retardation and epilepsy. There is usually a cherry-red spot on the retina (**7.146**). Programmes of antenatal detection are available.

Fabry's disease is an X-linked recessive disease that is caused deficiency of alpha-galactosidase A resulting in accumulation of a trihexoside in body tissues. Typical features

335

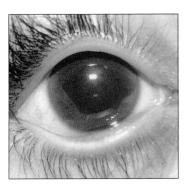

7.145 Cystinosis has led to the deposition of cystine in the cornea of this adult patient. The adult form of the disease is usually otherwise benign, though cystine also accumulates intracellularly in the reticulo-endothelial cells.

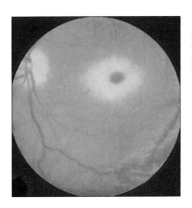

7.146 A cherry-red spot at the macula is commonly found in type A Niemann–Pick disease and in Tay–Sachs disease.

include punctate angiomatous lesions on the skin, corneal dystrophy, progressive renal failure and liability to thrombotic arterial disease. There may also be mental retardation, epilepsy and peripheral neuropathy.

Mucopolysaccharidoses

There are seven disorders in this group of metabolic defects, with very similar presentations.

Hurler's syndrome is an autosomal recessive disorder caused by a defect in the breakdown of complex carbohydrates. The glycosaminoglycans chondroitin, dermatan and heparan sulphate accumulate in subcutaneous tissues, bone, brain and liver leading to characteristic physical and mental changes. The appearances are typical with coarse facies (**7.147**), hepatosplenomegaly, corneal opacities and multiple bone abnormalities causing stunting of growth (dysostosis multiplex). There is severe mental retardation and a typical life expectancy of 10 years as a result of cardiorespiratory problems.

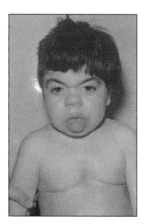

7.147 Hurler's syndrome is associated with characteristic facial features, including prominent supra-orbital ridges, thick eyebrows, a depressed nasal bridge, a broad bulbous nose, thick lips, a large protruding tongue and coarse hair. In an extreme form, the syndrome produces 'gargoylism'. Patients with other forms of mucopolysaccharidosis have a broadly similar appearance.

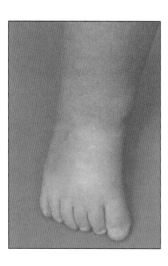

7.148 Polydactyly is a feature of the Laurence–Moon–Biedl syndrome, though it may occur in association with many other congenital abnormalities or as an isolated aberration.

LAURENCE–MOON–BIEDL SYNDROME

This is an autosomal recessive disorder that is associated with mental retardation, polydactyly (**7.148**), retinitis pigmentosa, hypogonadism and obesity.

DOWN'S SYNDROME

Down's syndrome is the result of trisomy of chromosome 21, usually due to non-disjunction and accounts for up to one-third of children with severe learning difficulties. The degree of disability ranges from mild to severe. The physical features are typical and include a small head with a flat occiput, upslanting palpebral fissures, epicanthic folds, small nose with a poorly developed bridge and small ears (**7.149–7.150**). Grey-white areas of depigmentation are seen in the iris (Brushfield spots, **7.151**); the mouth is often held open and the tongue protrudes. The hands are broad with a single transverse palmar crease (**7.152**), and the fifth finger shows clinodactyly. Congenital heart lesions are common (**7.149**). Adult stature tends to be small and there is a significant incidence of leukaemia and hypothyroidism in the older patients.

At maternal age 25 years the chance of bearing a child with Down's syndrome is 1 in 1400; at age 30 years, 1 in 800; at 40 years, 1 in 110; and at 45 years, 1 in 30. As these children tend

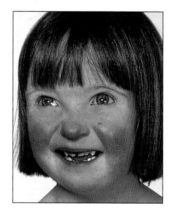

7.149 Down's syndrome is commonly associated with congenital heart disease, as in this girl who has Fallot's tetralogy (*see* **p. 229**). Her facies show the characteristic features of Down's syndrome, with prominent epicanthic folds and a small nose with a poorly developed bridge. Note that she also has a webbed neck. Her congenital heart disease has led to a prominent cyanosed facial flush.

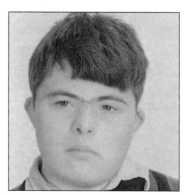

7.150 Down's syndrome in a young adult showing the characteristic adult facies. Note the prominent epicanthic folds and the small nose and ears.

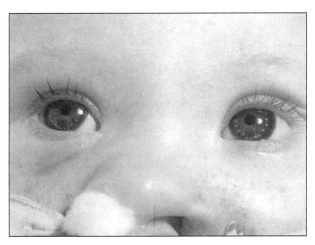

7.151 Brushfield spots are a common feature of Down's syndrome and may be seen in the newborn baby, as here. They are tiny, whitish areas of depigmentation on the iris.

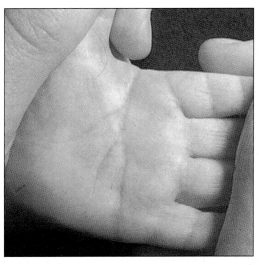

7.152 Single palmar crease is a classic feature of Down's syndrome, but it is important to remember that it can occur with other chromosomal abnormalities, and as a normal variant. It is diagnostic of Down's syndrome only when associated with the other features of the condition.

to be born to older mothers, it is important to offer amniocentesis or chorionic villous sampling to this group in early pregnancy, to identify abnormalities in chromosome 21.

Maternal blood tests have also now become available for women of all ages and have a place in screening (in combination with ultrasound). These include alphafetoprotein, unconjugated oestriol (uE3), human chorionic gonadotrophin (HCG) and neutrophil alkaline phosphatase. These tests are claimed to give a 60–80% diagnostic rate, and ultrasound scanning detects early evidence of heart defects. Such screening must be accompanied by skilled counselling on the possibility of termination of pregnancy if the fetus is found to be affected.

All neonates with Down's syndrome should be examined for heart disease and cataracts. Audiological and visual testing should be carried out regularly, and thyroid function measured at 2 year intervals. Life expectancy has increased gradually and is now often 50–60 years, but death usually results from heart disease, infection (e.g. pneumonia) or leukaemia.

Parents of a child with Down's syndrome should receive genetic counselling before further pregnancies.

8 Gastrointestinal

HISTORY

Patients with gastrointestinal (GI) disease present with a variety of symptoms (**8.1**). These may indicate a specific disease, but patients often have alimentary disease without specific symptoms, so the clinician must be alert to clinical signs.

COMMON GASTROINTESTINAL SYMPTOMS
Heartburn
Chest pain
Dysphagia
Anorexia
Abdominal pain
Vomiting
Constipation
Diarrhoea
Gastrointestinal bleeding
Anaemia
Weight loss
Jaundice
Ascites

8.1 Common gastrointestinal symptoms.

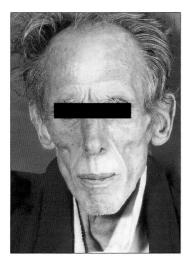

8.2 Malnutrition secondary to carcinoma of the stomach in a 61-year-old man (*see* **8.60**). Note the wasting of the facial tissues, and the pallor of his lips – an indication of probable iron deficiency anaemia.

EXAMINATION

General inspection is of particular importance. Muscle wasting, together with the more obvious depletion of fat stores, is indicative of malnutrition (**4.1**, **7.120**, **8.2**). Pallor of the mucous membranes is indicative of anaemia (**p. 405** and **8.3**, **10.2**, **10.3**) and koilonychia is found with prolonged iron deficiency (**2.103**, **10.6**, **10.18**). Finger clubbing accompanies malabsorption, small intestinal disease and cirrhosis (**2.104**, **2.105**). Palmar erythema occurs in chronic liver disease and such patients may also have jaundice, spider naevi, ascites, and, in male patients, gynaecomastia, loss of axillary hair and testicular atrophy (*see* **p. 375**). Skin rashes such as erythema nodosum (**2.45**) may accompany inflammatory bowel disease and these patients sometimes also suffer from arthritis. Inspection of the mouth and tongue may reveal evidence of candidiasis (**1.21**, **1.136**, **1.137**) or apthous ulcers (**8.4**) that may be associated with intestinal disease.

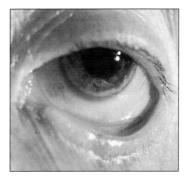

8.3 Pallor of the conjunctivae is suggestive of severe anaemia – in this case resulting from chronic gastrointestinal blood loss. Note the incidental finding of a corneal arcus.

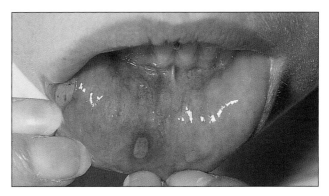

8.4 Aphthous ulcers commonly occur in isolation, but they may be an indication of an underlying intestinal disease, such as gluten enteropathy or inflammatory bowel disease.

Patients with upper gastrointestinal bleeding may present with frank haematemesis (vomiting of fresh blood), with vomiting of altered blood ('coffee ground' vomit; **1.44**), with passage of altered blood in the stool (melaena), or silently as anaemia. Those with lower intestinal bleeding may present with the passage of fresh blood or clot *per rectum* (**8.5**), with frank blood-streaking of the stool, or silently with anaemia (and occult blood in the stool on testing). The many possible causes of gastrointestinal bleeding are summarized in **8.6** and **8.7**.

The stools should be examined for colour, consistency and frank blood. In steatorrhoea, they are usually the colour and consistency of soft clay (**8.8**) and have a particularly unpleasant odour. Diarrhoea is common in gastroenteritis, and in cholera and some forms of *Escherichia coli* gastroenteritis typical 'rice water' stools are passed. Some other forms of gastroenteritis, dysentery and acute ulcerative colitis are associated with the passage of bloody diarrhoea. Parasitic worms may be seen in the stool (*see* **p. 368**).

Examination of the regional lymph nodes is important: patients with gastric carcinoma sometimes have left-sided supraclavicular lymphadenopathy (**8.9**), and posterior cervical lymphadenopathy may occur in pharyngeal carcinoma. General lymphadenopathy is a feature of Whipple's disease. Abdominal examination may reveal enlargement of the spleen or liver, or the liver may be small or craggy. Ascites (**8.10**, **9.13**), detected by shifting dullness, most commonly reflects cirrhosis or malignancy. Abdominal masses suggest colonic or other malignancy, or an inflammatory disease of the bowel such as Crohn's disease or diverticulitis.

Rectal examination provides important clues. Haemorrhoids cannot be felt but may be seen externally (**10.19**) or on proctoscopy. Perianal skin tags denote thrombosed

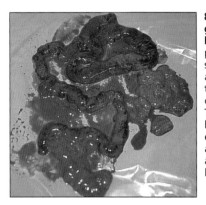

8.5 Massive lower gastrointestinal bleeding. The patient passed a large bloody stool. When teased apart, this was found to be a blood-clot cast of much of the colon. The unusual cause of bleeding here was erosion and rupture of an abdominal aortic aneurysm into the bowel.

CAUSES OF ACUTE UPPER GASTROINTESTINAL BLEEDING

		% of total
Oesophagus	Mallory–Weiss tear	5
	Reflux oesophagitis	5–10
	Carcinoma	1
	Varices	2–5
Stomach	Erosions or gastritis	5–20
	Gastric ulcer	3–5
	Carcinoma	1–2
	Other tumours	1
	Varices	2
Duodenum	Erosions	5
	Duodenal ulcer	40–50

8.6 Causes of acute upper gastrointestinal bleeding.

CAUSES OF LOWER GASTROINTESTINAL BLEEDING

Common causes
Haemorrhoids
Anal fissure
Inflammatory bowel disease
Diverticulitis
Carcinoma
Intussusception

Unusual causes
Arteriovenous fistulae
Hereditary haemorrhagic telangiectasia
Angiodysplasia
Vasculitis
Amyloidosis
Meckel's diverticulum
Blood disorders – haemophilia, thrombocytopenia
Rupture into bowel of aortic aneurysm

8.7 Causes of lower gastrointestinal bleeding.

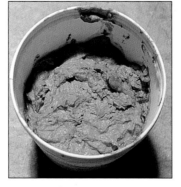

8.8 Typical steatorrhoea. The stool is pale, with the consistency of pale clay. It often floats in the lavatory (because of its high gas and fat content) and is difficult to flush away.

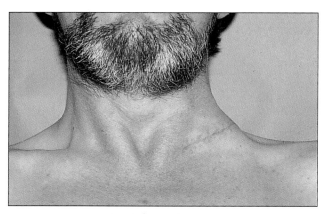

8.9 Left-sided supraclavicular lymphadenopathy (Virchow's node) may result from lymphatic spread of a gastric or pancreatic neoplasm via the thoracic duct. This may be the first sign of malignancy, as in this patient. The node mass was biopsied 1 month before this picture was taken, and has regrown since then. Histology revealed adenocarcinoma cells. The primary tumour was in the stomach.

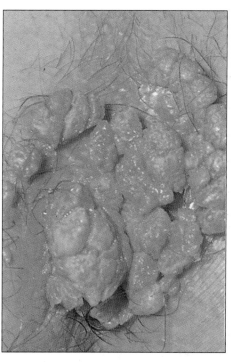

8.11 Perianal condylomata resulting from human papillomavirus infection. They are usually sexually transmitted and are most common in homosexual men (*see* **p. 59**).

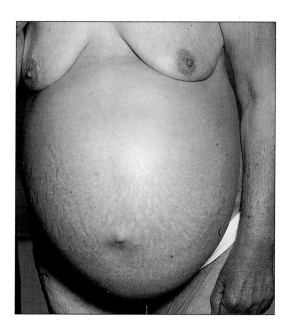

8.10 Gross ascites in a 68-year-old woman, who had no other symptoms on presentation. Note the development of stretch marks and eversion of the umbilicus. This patient had an inoperable leiomyosarcoma, but a similar clinical appearance may be seen in patients with other abdominal disorders and with cirrhosis.

haemorrhoids. In Crohn's colitis, they may be associated with fistula-in-ano. Perianal condylomata (**8.11**) may be mistaken for anal carcinoma; they are most commonly found in homosexual men.

INVESTIGATIONS

Investigations of both structure and function may be needed, including endoscopy, radiology, nuclear medicine, histopathology, tests on blood and stool, and manometry.

The video or fibreoptic endoscope allows direct inspection and biopsy of lesions as well as therapeutic intervention:

* Upper GI endoscopy may reveal oesophageal disorders (**8.12**) and allows the dilatation of oesophageal strictures, the removal of foreign bodies and the injection of oesophageal varices; gastric lesions (**8.13**) and duodenal lesions (**8.14**) are readily seen and biopsied, and haemorrhage can be arrested by the use of a laser beam or heater probe passed down the biopsy channel (**8.15**, **8.16**).
* Endoscopic cannulation of the ampulla of Vater allows retrograde radiological examination of the pancreas and biliary tree (endoscopic retrograde cholangiopancreatography, ERCP, *see* **p. 380**).
* The flexible sigmoidoscope and colonoscope are used to examine the distal and entire colon; sigmoidoscopy or colonoscopy, or both, are indicated for the diagnosis and staging of inflammatory bowel disease and for the investigation of colonic symptoms, particularly rectal bleeding. When polyps are found, they can often be removed with a diathermy snare (**8.17**).

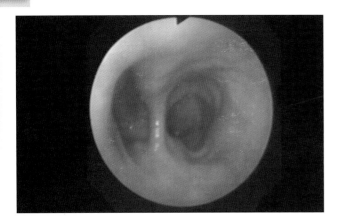

8.12   **Upper alimentary endoscopy** allows direct visualization of the mucosa and lumen of the upper gastrointestinal tract. This endoscopic view shows an oesophageal diverticulum (pouch) to the left of the picture and the oesophageal lumen to the right. The mucosa is normal. This 88-year-old woman presented with dysphagia and regurgitation of food. Diverticula can be treated by surgery, but this is only indicated if symptoms are severe.

8.15

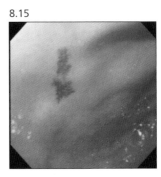

8.16

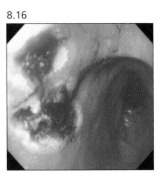

8.15 & 8.16 Gastric angiodysplasia led to recurrent GI bleeding in this patient, despite its relatively benign appearance. Argon beam (laser) treatment was carried out via the endoscope to ablate the area of angiodysplasia. The initial reaction is shown in **8.16**, and the area healed without recurrence of angiodysplasia.

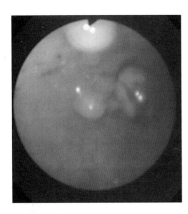

8.13   **Endoscopic view of the gastric mucosa showing several gastric polyps.** One has just been biopsied via the endoscope and is bleeding. Multiple gastric polyps are usually benign and, unlike polyps in the large bowel, most should not be regarded as premalignant lesions. Histological examination is essential, however.

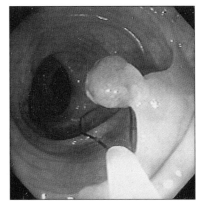

8.17   **Colonoscopic polypectomy.** A wire snare has been introduced through the colonoscope. It will be looped over the pedunculated colonic polyp, tightened around its stalk, and diathermy will then be applied via the snare to sever the stalk without bleeding.

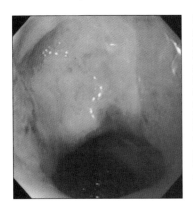

8.14   **A large duodenal ulcer, seen via a videoendoscope.** Duodenal ulcers are almost invariably benign, so histological examination is not usually required to exclude malignancy. Antral biopsies may, however, be taken to investigate the probability of underlying infection with *Helicobacter pylori*.

Radiological investigations are important. Endoscopy has reduced the need for the barium meal and the barium enema, but double-contrast techniques can still provide valuable information (**8.18**, **8.19**); and small bowel meals or enemas are still important for the identification of structural disease of the jejunum and ileum such as Crohn's disease (**8.20**). Plain abdominal radiographs are important for the recognition of toxic dilatation in colitis and to confirm clinical suspicions of intestinal obstruction (**8.21**). Angiography is helpful in the investigation of gastrointestinal bleeding of obscure cause or of suspected mesenteric ischaemia.

Ultrasound and CT are especially useful in the investigation of the liver, pancreas and biliary tract (*see* **p. 381**), but also have a useful role in generalized abdominal disease (**8.22**).

Nuclear medicine has been used extensively for structural imaging of the liver and biliary tract, and can also be applied to the assessment of intestinal function. Oesophageal dysmotility and gastric emptying can both be assessed by reference to the pattern and time of transit of swallowed isotope, measured by

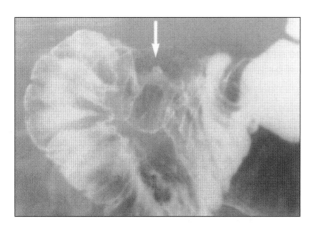

8.18 Double-contrast barium meal, showing a small duodenal ulcer crater (arrow). In expert hands, this technique has a diagnostic accuracy similar to that of endoscopy for many lesions of the stomach and duodenum; nevertheless, biopsy is not possible with radiology alone and most lesions of the stomach require biopsy.

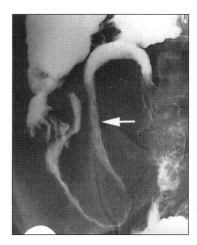

8.20 A small bowel meal demonstrates a typical feature of Crohn's disease – a long stricture of the terminal ileum. Strictures may also be caused by tuberculosis and lymphoma, but the 'cobblestone' appearance (arrow) is strongly suggestive of Crohn's disease.

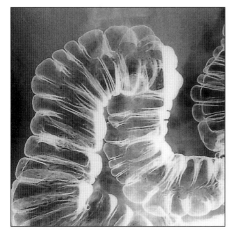

8.19 Double-contrast barium enema in a patient with familial polyposis coli. This close-up view shows multiple small, sessile colonic polyps, appearing as small, rounded, dark patches. The surface of polyps is poorly coated with barium, whereas their edges and the rest of the colonic wall retain more contrast medium. The radiological appearance of the polyps corresponds to their colonoscopic appearance (*see* **8.106**). Familial polyposis is a premalignant condition and prophylactic colectomy is indicated.

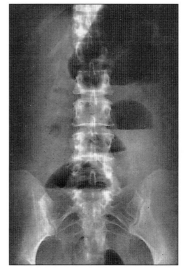

8.21 Plain abdominal X-ray, taken in the erect position, demonstrating multiple fluid levels in the bowel. In combination with a supine film, this appearance shows apparent obstruction to the gut at the distal end of the small bowel. It is important to remember that similar appearances may occur in paralytic ileus, peritonitis, gastroenteritis and coeliac disease. The films must always be interpreted in their clinical context.

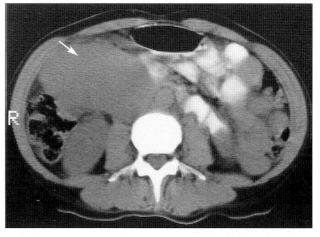

8.22 CT demonstrating a large abdominal tumour (arrowed). CT-guided biopsy showed this to be a leiomyosarcoma, which originated in the duodenum.

the gamma camera. Radiolabelled (^{99m}Tc) red blood cells (from the patient) may be used to investigate the site of chronic gastrointestinal blood loss when this is not revealed by other means (**8.23**).

The glycocholate breath test utilizes the ability of bacteria to deconjugate bile acids to investigate bacterial overgrowth in the small intestine. The patient is given ^{14}C-glycine glycocholic acid. Deconjugation leads to the rapid absorption of glycine, which is metabolized, and the measured exhaled $^{14}CO_2$

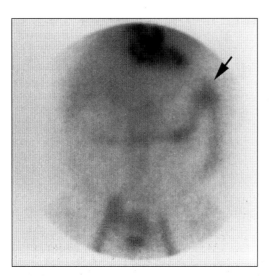

8.23   A bleeding site in the colon, revealed by scanning after intravenous administration of some of the patient's red blood cells that had been labelled with ^{99m}Tc. This 10 minute film shows two 'hot spots' in the colon, but films at other times showed that the high count at the splenic flexure (arrow) was consistent (the other 'hot spot' here is the result of retrograde flow of blood in the colonic lumen). No abnormality had been seen on colonoscopy or barium enema, but a small angioma was found on re-endoscopy and removed at subsequent surgery.

indicates the extent of deconjugation. A similar principle is applied to the measurement of fat malabsorption using the triglyceride glyceryl-^{14}C-triolein. The ^{13}C and ^{14}C breath test is helpful in the diagnosis of *Helicobacter pylori* infection.

The urease test (*see* **p. 351**) may be carried out on gastric antral biopsies to investigate the possibility of *H. pylori* infection.

The absorption of vitamin B$_{12}$ can be investigated by measuring the urinary excretion of the labelled vitamin, which is administered by mouth after saturating the body stores with an intramuscular injection (**p. 414**).

Histopathology is important for the confirmation and staging of tumours, the recognition of different types of bowel

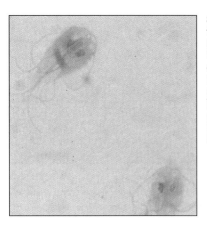

8.24   Microscopy of fresh stool or small bowel aspirate is important in the diagnosis of intestinal infections. This jejunal aspirate, from a patient with chronic diarrhoea and weight loss, showed *Giardia lamblia* trophozoites.

inflammation such as Crohn's disease, and the identification of small bowel disease such as gluten enteropathy and its response to a gluten-free diet. Biopsy samples may be obtained by endoscopy (**8.59**). *H. pylori* may be identified by appropriate staining of biopsies of the gastric antrum in many patients with peptic ulceration and gastritis (**8.49**).

Blood tests provide evidence of malabsorption (macrocytic or hypochromic microcytic anaemia), malnutrition (low transferrin, fibronectin and lymphocyte count) and liver dysfunction. Serology for *H. pylori* infection is helpful in diagnosis and management. Serum antibodies (antiendomysial, antigliadin and antireticulin) are a useful screening test for gluten-sensitive enteropathy.

Faecal occult blood testing may point to intestinal blood loss; faecal fat measurement aids the assessment of malabsorption.

Microbiological investigation is important. The need for microscopy of stool or jejunal aspirate to identify protozoa such as *Giardia* (**8.24**) is often overlooked.

Manometry is increasingly used to investigate motility disorders.

Laparoscopy has an increasing role in the investigation of intra-abdominal disease (**9.23**).

MOUTH AND TONGUE

Important information may be gained from the inspection of the mouth:

- The lips and tongue are blue in conditions associated with central cyanosis (**4.4**).
- Angular stomatitis (**7.129**, **10.2**) is common in iron deficiency and in the edentulous elderly.
- Aphthous ulcers occur anywhere in the oral cavity (**8.4**); they may be found in otherwise healthy people, especially women, but are associated with poor dental hygiene, haematinic deficiency, gluten enteropathy and inflammatory bowel disease. Large deep ulcers are sometimes found as part of Behçet's syndrome (**3.100**).
- The gums may bleed where there is periodontal disease, and in patients with acute leukaemia or scurvy (**8.25**, **10.6**).
- Hypertrophied gums are a recognized complication of prolonged treatment with phenytoin (**8.26**), ciclosporin and calcium antagonists.
- A blue line is found at the margin of the gum and teeth in lead poisoning (**8.27**).
- Yellow-brown staining of the teeth may occur if tetracycline was administered during childhood or fetal life (**8.28**).
- Candidal infection (**1.21**, **1.136**, **1.137**) is common in debilitated and immunosuppressed patients, and under ill fitting dentures.
- The tongue may be smooth and sore in patients with haematinic and B-vitamin deficiencies (**9.47**, **10.30**) and in various other conditions (**8.29**), enlarged in patients with

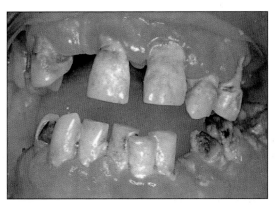

8.25 The gums in scurvy. Vitamin C deficiency characteristically leads to gingivitis. The gingival papillae are swollen and fragile, with a purplish coloration. In this patient, grossly neglected oral hygiene with resulting caries has compounded the problem.

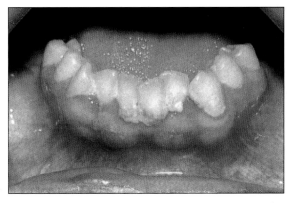

8.26 Hyperplastic gingivitis is a well established complication of phenytoin therapy (for epilepsy). Careful attention to oral hygiene may minimize the extent of this complication.

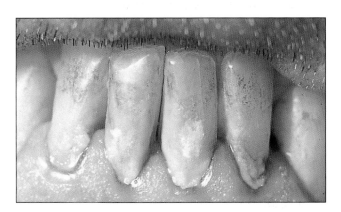

8.27 Lead poisoning produces a blue line at the margin of the gum and teeth. This patient's employment involved the dismantling of car batteries. He presented with colicky abdominal pain.

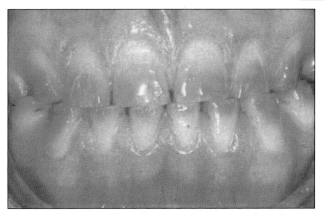

8.28 Tetracycline staining of the teeth occurs when tetracycline is administered during the period of tooth formation, either via the mother in fetal life, or to the child up to the age of 12 years. In this patient, there is generalized staining without any hypoplasia of the tooth substance. Hypoplasia often occurs, but this may frequently result from the underlying condition for which the tetracycline was administered, rather than from the tetracycline itself. There are almost always satisfactory alternatives to tetracycline therapy during pregnancy and childhood.

CAUSES OF SORE TONGUE	
Local irritation	Smoking
	Fractured tooth
	Ill-fitting dentures/crowns
	Candidiasis
	Dry mouth
Systemic disease	Folate/vitamin B_{12} deficiency
	Iron deficiency
	Collagen–vascular disorders
	Diabetes
Burning mouth syndrome – unknown cause	

8.29 Causes of sore tongue.

acromegaly (**7.19**), myxoedema and amyloidosis, and small and spastic in motor neuron disease. Inspection may reveal evidence of hereditary haemorrhagic telangiectasia (**10.102**).

- Leukoplakia (**2.127**, **8.30**) is a premalignant condition and can lead to carcinoma (**8.31**); hairy leukoplakia may occur in patients with HIV infection (**1.22**).
- Patients with conditions as varied as herpes simplex (**1.58**), lichen planus (**2.70**), Peutz–Jeghers syndrome (**2.88**) and scleroderma (**3.78**, **3.79**) may present with oral or perioral lesions.
- In the burning mouth syndrome, the patient (usually an elderly woman) complains that her mouth feels 'on fire';

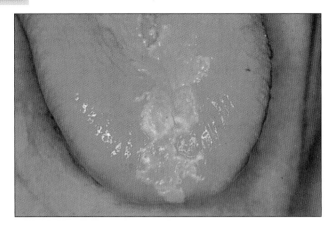

8.30 Leukoplakia of the tongue. The aetiology in this 83-year-old patient was unclear. Characteristically, leukoplakia cannot be wiped off, and it shows a non-specific histological appearance, which excludes other diagnoses. Leukoplakia sometimes has no consequences, but should always be regarded as a potentially premalignant condition.

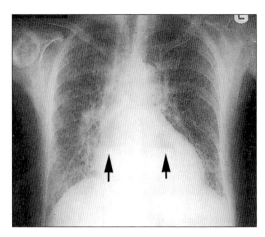

8.32 A hiatus hernia may first be revealed on chest X-ray, especially when chest pain is the presenting feature. The presence of a fluid level crossing the midline behind the heart (arrows) is virtually diagnostic of hiatus hernia or achalasia. This patient has also had a previous right mastectomy for carcinoma of the breast and has an osteolytic secondary in the head of the right humerus.

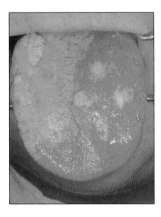

8.31 Carcinoma of the tongue. There is an extensive squamous cell carcinoma on the left side of the tongue. Note also the patch of leukoplakia on the right border of the tongue posteriorly.

which relax the sphincter. The refluxed gastric content damages the squamous oesphageal mucosa and may impair the underlying muscle function leading to delayed oesophageal clearance which exacerbates the problem.

The patient complains of heartburn and acid reflux, which is worse after meals and at night when recumbent. Other symptoms of GORD may include eructation, dysphagia, nausea and epigastric pain. The diagnosis of oesophagitis is confirmed by endoscopy (**8.34, 8.35**).

usually no abnormalities are found on examination, but underlying features may include ill-fitting dentures, anaemia, depression, diabetes mellitus and fear of cancer. Reassurance is usually appropriate.

OESOPHAGUS

PEPTIC OESOPHAGITIS

A lax oesophageal sphincter permits the reflux of corrosive gastric contents, containing acid, pepsin and sometimes bile acids, into the oesophagus. The tendency to gastro-oesophageal reflux disease (GORD) may be compounded by the intrathoracic position of the gastro-oesophageal junction in patients with a hiatus hernia (**8.32, 8.33**), by increased abdominal pressure in the obese and pregnant, and by the consumption of fatty meals, alcohol, caffeine and tobacco, all of

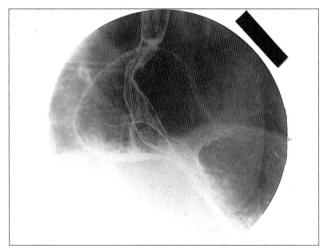

8.33 Rolling hiatus hernia on double-contrast barium meal. The fundus of the stomach has herniated into the thorax alongside the oesophagus. The constriction in the stomach marks the level of the diaphragm, and the gastro-oesophageal junction is still beneath it. By contrast, in a sliding hernia, the gastro-oesophageal junction (cardia) slides into the chest.

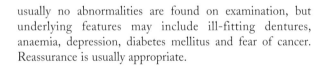

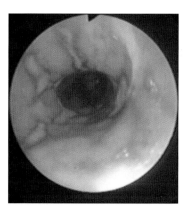

8.34 Peptic oesophagitis. This endoscopic view of moderate disease shows typical flame-like areas of shallow ulceration that are coated with yellow slough. These bleed readily when touched by the endoscope. Normal mucosa is present between these patches.

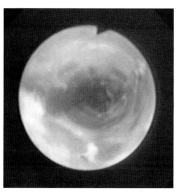

8.35 Severe peptic oesophagitis. Here the lower oesophagus is extensively ulcerated. The ulcer surface is friable. The lower oesophagus is narrowed as a result of early stricture formation.

Complications of oesophagitis include stricture formation (**8.35**, **8.36**), which causes dysphagia; oesophageal ulcer, characterized by severe pain and dysphagia; bleeding; aspiration pneumonia; and Barrett's oesophagus, in which chronic reflux leads to the replacement of the squamous epithelium by metaplastic columnar epithelium, with a risk of ulceration and carcinoma (**8.37**). Both Barrett's oesophagus and carcinoma of the gastro-oesophageal junction are increasing in incidence, and patients known to have Barrett's oesophagus should be considered for regular endoscopic surveillance.

Treatment depends on the severity of the symptoms and mucosal damage. For mild disease, advice about diet – that is, losing excess weight and avoiding late, large and fatty meals, and coffee and alcohol, stopping smoking, and avoiding sleeping flat – together with symptomatic or regular use of a protective alginate preparation, may be sufficient. More severe disease requires acid suppression with an H_2 antagonist or a proton pump inhibitor. The efficacy of such treatment can be enhanced by prokinetic drugs, such as domperidone and cisapride, which increase gastric emptying and oesophageal sphincter tone.

Oesophageal stenosis is usually amenable to endoscopic dilatation using balloons or other dilators.

Oesophageal ulceration may also be provoked by some drug therapies, especially by alendronate sodium (**8.38**)

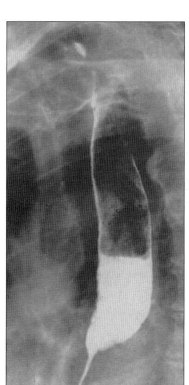

8.36 Benign oesophageal stricture, seen on barium swallow. The stricture is smooth with a tapering (or funnelling) upper end that narrows gradually from normal oesophagus. The most common cause of such a benign stricture is chronic reflux oesophagitis.

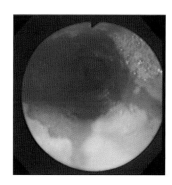

8.37 Barrett's oesophagus. In this condition, gastric (columnar) epithelium extends above the cardia into the oesophagus. The columnar epithelium is a deeper pink than the normal oesophageal squamous epithelium. In this increasingly common condition there is a greatly increased risk of dysplasia and adenocarcinoma in columnar epithelium in the oesophagus.

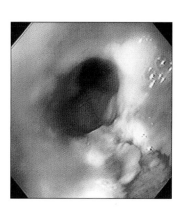

8.38 Oesophageal ulceration, provoked by the administration of alendronate sodium to a patient with a pre-existing oesophageal stricture.

INFECTIVE OESOPHAGITIS

Oesophageal candidiasis occurs in debilitated patients who have received broad-spectrum antibiotics. It is also found in patients infected with HIV. The radiological appearances of oesophageal candidiasis are shown in **1.27**, and the diagnosis should be confirmed endoscopically (**8.39**). Patients may respond to topical treatment with nystatin, but those with HIV infection require a systemically active agent such as ketoconazole.

Patients with HIV infection may also develop oesophageal infections with herpes simplex (**8.40**) and cytomegalovirus, and HIV itself may cause oesophagitis.

OESOPHAGEAL STRICTURES

Oesophageal strictures may develop as a consequence of oesophagitis (**8.35**, **8.36**), in response to the ingestion of corrosives or after radiotherapy. Such strictures are usually benign, but may require dilatation or surgery to relieve dysphagia.

The Plummer–Vinson or Patterson–Brown–Kelly syndrome is the association of iron-deficiency anaemia (with koilonychia) with angular stomatitis, glossitis and atrophy of the oesophageal mucosa in the postcricoid region, which forms an obstructing postcricoid web (**8.41** and **p. 411**). Iron therapy may reverse the process, but there is a risk of malignant change.

Oesophageal rings may also occur at or near the gastro-oesophageal junction (**8.42**). Their cause is unknown, but they are often associated with oesophageal motility disorders, and may be associated with dysphagia. Dilatation may be helpful.

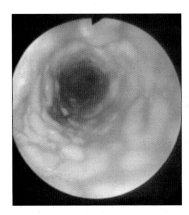

8.39 Oesophageal candidiasis in a patient with HIV infection. The multiple small white plaques of *Candida* on the background of abnormally reddened oesophageal mucosa correspond to the radiological appearance in **1.27**. Patients with oesophageal candidiasis may also present with a smaller number of plaques, or with a more or less confluent white coating of the mucosa (which must not be confused with a coating of barium if the patient has recently undergone a barium study).

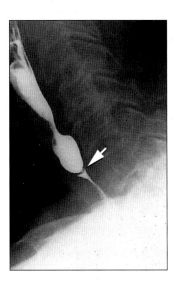

8.41 Oesophageal web in the Plummer–Vinson syndrome. The postcricoid web is arrowed on this barium swallow, and the element of oesophageal obstruction is obvious. The patient was a postmenopausal woman, and she showed other signs of severe iron-deficiency anaemia.

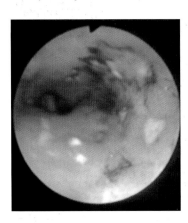

8.40 Herpes simplex ulceration of the lower oesophagus in a patient with HIV infection. Note the multiple shallow ulcers in the lower part of the oesophagus. This appearance is not diagnostic of herpes simplex infection, as a similar appearance may be seen with other causes of ulceration, including some drugs (such as potassium supplements). The presence of vesicles in the mucosa (not shown here) is virtually diagnostic of herpes simplex. Treatment with high-dose intravenous aciclovir may be helpful.

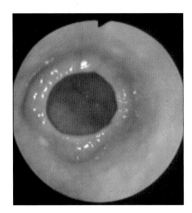

8.42 A lower oesophageal ring. This ring is at the squamocolumnar junction at the lower end of the oesophagus (a Schatzki ring). It is benign, but dilatation may be required for symptomatic relief

OESOPHAGEAL CARCINOMA

Patients with oesophageal carcinoma present with progressive dysphagia for solids, and subsequently for liquids as the lumenal stenosis progresses. Weight loss may be obvious.

The diagnosis is confirmed by the typical radiological and endoscopic features (**8.43**, **8.44**, **8.45**). CT and endoscopic ultrasound examination (**8.46**) are valuable in assessing the extent of the tumour. Surgical resection offers the only curative treatment, but is frequently not feasible. Palliation can be achieved by the endoscopic insertion of a prosthetic tube (**8.47**)

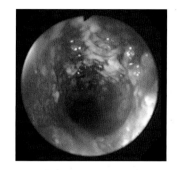

8.45 Advanced oesophageal carcinoma, which has been treated by palliative insertion of a metal stent. The carcinoma has now re-grown through the mesh of the stent.

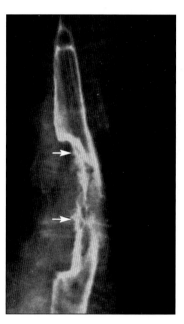

8.43 Oesophageal carcinoma. The patient had a 6-week history of dysphagia and weight loss. Note the abrupt change from normal oesophagus to the area of the tumour (cf. **8.36**). The barium spicules (arrows) represent areas of ulceration in the tumour. There is, as yet, no dilatation of the proximal oesophagus.

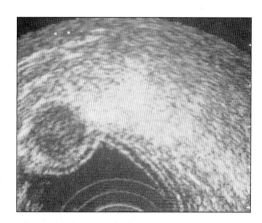

8.46 Endoscopic ultrasound of an oesophageal mass. Here the tumour (the dark circular area to the left) has well-defined margins, suggesting a lack of invasion. The lumen of the oesophagus and artefacts from the ultrasound probe are at the bottom of the picture.

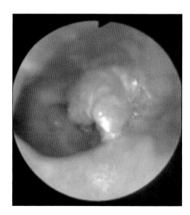

8.44 Carcinoma of the oesophagus seen endoscopically. The tumour is a pale sessile polypoid lesion to the right of the picture. Biopsy confirmed that this was a carcinoma.

8.47 Prosthetic tube used to palliate oesophageal carcinoma by allowing continued swallowing. A guide wire is introduced through the obstruction via the endoscope, the stricture is dilated, and the tube is subsequently pushed over the guide wire through the obstruction. The introducer and guide wire are then removed. This image shows a radiological view of a longer prosthesis *in situ*. Metal stents are increasingly replacing the older prosthetic tubes.

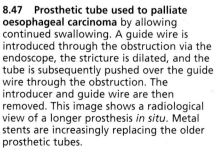

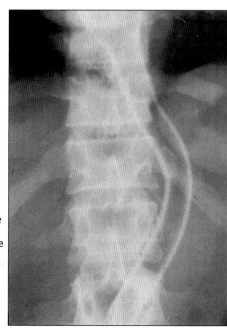

or metal stent, or by endoscopic laser therapy. Other tumours, including leiomyomas, lymphomas and Kaposi's sarcoma, may be found in the oesophagus, but are rare.

OESOPHAGEAL MOTILITY DISORDERS

Achalasia, a relatively uncommon disorder, is seen mainly in the age group 40–70 years. It is characterized by the failure of the lower oesophageal sphincter to relax and impaired peristalsis of the oesophagus. This results in dysphagia and ultimately the retention of food debris in a dilated oesophagus (**8.48**). Aspiration pneumonia is a common complication (*see* **p. 177**).

The diagnosis may be suspected from a chest X-ray that may show widening of the mediastinum, or gas/fluid levels behind the heart (**8.32**), or both. Barium swallow may show absence of peristaltic waves and later in the disease a dilated oesophagus (**8.48**). Endoscopy is essential to exclude oesophageal carcinoma.

Manometry is the investigation of choice and shows a sphincter which has a high resting tone and relaxes only partially.

Calcium antagonists or nitrates, or both, may be of some benefit, but definitive treatment is by balloon dilatation or surgical myotomy. Chagas' disease may produce a similar motility disorder (*see* **p. 51**).

Diffuse oesophageal spasm is another cause of chest pain and dysphagia, in which there are multiple high-pressure incoordinate waves. Barium examination demonstrates abnormal contractions known as tertiary waves. This disorder may complicate gastro-oesophageal reflux. Other patients may suffer severe chest pain with no demonstrable radiological abnormality but manometric studies may show that occasional peristaltic waves generate very high pressures.

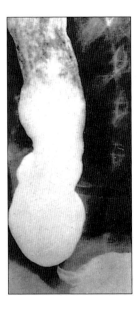

8.48   Achalasia of the oesophagus. The barium swallow shows that the dilated oesophagus narrows conically at the gastro-oesophageal junction (the cardia).

There is reduced oesophageal motility in patients with systemic sclerosis (**3.84**).

Coughing or retching, especially in alcoholic patients, may lead to an acute tear at the gastro-oesophageal junction (a Mallory–Weiss tear) with resulting upper gastrointestinal bleeding. Most patients heal spontaneously, but a few require surgery. Oesophageal varices are another cause of major lower oesophageal bleeding (*see* **p. 384**).

FOREIGN BODIES IN THE GUT

Ingestion of foreign bodies is extremely common in children, in those who are mentally disturbed and accidentally during eating (foreign bodies in food, broken teeth, dentures, etc.). Those with oesophageal strictures or carcinoma may also present with impaction of food or drug tablets in the oesophagus.

Small, blunt, non-toxic foreign bodies may often be allowed to pass through the gut, but sharp or toxic bodies must be removed, and larger bodies may become impacted in the oesophagus.

The patient is usually aware of swallowing the foreign body and of its impaction in the oesophagus. There is often pain at the site and retching or vomiting may be stimulated.

Such foreign bodies may be seen on X-ray (if radio-opaque) and may often be removed endoscopically.

STOMACH

HELICOBACTER PYLORI INFECTION

Chronic infection with the spiral Gram-negative bacterium *Helicobacter pylori* is now known to be a common underlying factor in most of the major disorders of the stomach and duodenum. The organism is found in 30–75% of the total populations that have been studied, and infection is more common in socially deprived families. It has been identified in saliva, in dental scrapings and in faeces, but is most universally found attached to gastric epithelial cells, especially in the antrum. It is thought to be transmitted by the faecal–oral and oral–oral routes.

There is evidence that some strains are not pathogenic, but there is a close association with duodenal ulcer (100% infected in some series) and gastric ulcer (80% infected) and a lesser association with duodenitis and gastritis. The organism produces large amounts of the enzyme urease, which breaks down urea into ammonia and carbon dioxide. Gastrin is secreted in excess as a result, and this leads to excess acid production, which provokes gastritis, mucosal atrophy, ulceration and intestinal dysplasia. There is also an enhanced risk of gastric cancer and mucosal-associated lymphoid tissue (MALT) lymphoma of the stomach.

Diagnosis of *H. pylori* infection may be made by:

- endoscopy and biopsy
  - part of the biopsy material is used for a rapid urease test (CLO test) that detects the enzyme urease by the colour change of an indicator induced by ammonia production; this has a 95% specificity
  - another part of the biopsy is stained to show *H. pylori* (**8.49**) and determine its resistance to antibiotics
  - a third part of the biopsy may be used to culture *H. pylori*
- serology
  - IgG antibodies against *H. pylori* may be detected using a simple serology kit test; this has an 85% specificity; repeat testing after eradication should be performed at 6 months
- ^{13}C and ^{14}C breath test
  - this involves the administration orally of labelled urea and the detection of labelled CO_2 in the breath, the implication being that active *H. pylori* infection is necessary for the urea breakdown; this test has a 95% specificity.

Treatment of proven infection is with a proton pump inhibitor such as omeprazole in combination with two antimicrobial agents (amoxicillin, clarithromycin or metronidazole, depending on local resistance patterns).

GASTRITIS

Gastritis is a common problem and its incidence is increasing. It is best defined as 'an inflammatory response to gastric mucosal injury'. There is little association between symptoms, endoscopic abnormality, histological abnormality, anatomical distribution of any abnormalities found, and the presence or absence of *H. pylori* infection or other causative factors. Endoscopy alone is not diagnostic of any particular form of gastritis, though various abnormalities may be seen including erythema, erosions and haemorrhage. Gastritis is now best classified as follows:

- Acute gastritis caused by viruses or bacteria. Vomiting is a common clinical presentation after infection with rotavirus, Norwalk agent and type-specific *Escherichia coli*. Acute infection with *H. pylori* is associated with epigastric pain, nausea, vomiting and a feeling of fullness. *H. pylori* is easy to identify on appropriately stained biopsy samples.
- Acute gastritis caused by drugs or chemicals. Aspirin (and other non-steroidal anti-inflammatory drugs, NSAIDs) and alcohol are the most common agents to cause acute gastritis; they have a synergistic effect on the gastric mucosa; aspirin inhibits local prostaglandin production and removes its cytoprotective effects, whereas alcohol produces local reduction of mucosal blood flow. The end result is acute erosions, which may bleed (**8.50**, **8.51**).
- Chronic gastritis is found in an asymptomatic form in the elderly and is often associated with *H. pylori* infection. Other causes include drugs, alcohol and gastroduodenal reflux of bile.

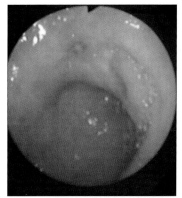

8.50 Gastric erosions. The patient had been experiencing dyspeptic symptoms for 2 months. Endoscopy revealed numerous small 'aphthous erosions', and antral biopsy revealed *Helicobacter pylori* infection. The patient responded to 'triple therapy'.

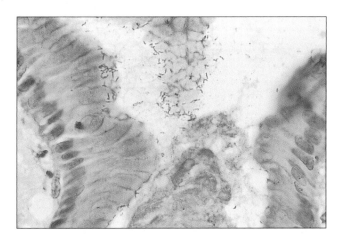

8.49 *Helicobacter pylori* infection demonstrated on gastric antral biopsy (Warthin–Starry/Alcian green stain). Numerous black-staining organisms are seen in the mucus layer on the epithelial surface and in the crypt seen bottom left. The mucus protects the organisms from attack by gastric acid and by antimicrobial therapy.

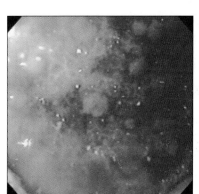

8.51 Acute gastritis in a patient on non-steroidal anti-inflammatory drug therapy. Multiple small erosions can be seen, and the mucosa bled when touched by the endoscope.

- Atrophic gastritis. A few patients have autoimmune gastritis, with a positive test for parietal cell antibodies. These patients fail to secrete acid and intrinsic factor, and may eventually develop a deficiency of vitamin B$_{12}$ (*see* **p. 413**).

Ménetrièr's disease (giant hypertrophic gastritis) is a rare, possibly premalignant condition, in which there is thickening and enlargement of the gastric mucosal folds. It may affect the entire upper gut (**8.52**), and may then be associated with protein loss (protein-losing enteropathy).

GASTRIC ULCERS

Gastric ulcers are most common in the elderly. NSAIDs are often an important factor in their genesis, and both acid and gastroduodenal bile reflux may also have a role.

Gastric ulcers present with epigastric pain or anaemia, or both. Bleeding is usually chronic, but acute haemorrhage can occur; it is a major threat in elderly patients.

Gastric ulcers cannot be distinguished on clinical grounds from duodenal ulcers or gastric cancers. Barium studies may demonstrate an ulcer and give strong clues to its benign nature (**8.53**), but definitive diagnosis requires endoscopy with brush cytology and biopsy (**8.54–8.56**).

Gastric ulcers usually respond to acid secretion inhibitors (though more slowly than duodenal ulcers), but a number of other drugs may also be used, especially when *Helicobacter pylori* infection is demonstrated. Follow-up after 6–8 weeks to confirm healing is wise.

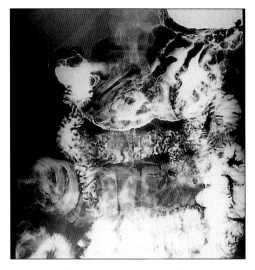

8.52   Ménétrier's disease (giant hypertrophic gastritis). The patient presented with epigastric pain and melaena. Barium meal and follow-through revealed rugal hypertrophy in the stomach and similar changes throughout the small intestine.

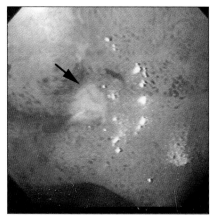

8.54   Benign gastric ulcer (arrow) seen on endoscopy. There is no sign of bleeding, and no evidence to suggest malignancy, but brush cytology or biopsy is essential to exclude this.

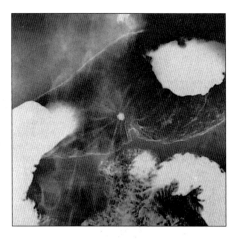

8.53   Benign gastric ulcer, as seen in a double-contrast barium meal. The ulcer heals by fibrosis and contraction, and this draws mucosal folds towards the base of the ulcer. These give rise to the streaks of barium that radiate from the ulcer crater in this view. Although these appearances are strongly suggestive of a healing benign gastric ulcer, endoscopy, brush cytology and biopsy are all wise precautions to exclude gastric carcinoma.

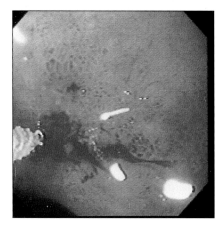

8.55   Brush cytology of the gastric ulcer seen in 8.54. In this simple technique, a small brush is passed through the operating channel of the endoscope. The brushings can be examined for malignant cells. Both malignant ulcers and gastric lymphomas may resemble benign ulcers even when viewed endoscopically, hence the need for further investigation.

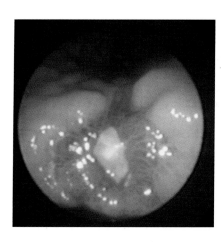

8.56 Healing benign gastric ulcer. An endoscopic view equivalent to the barium appearance in **8.53**. Despite the appearance of healing, biopsy is still advisable

GASTRIC TUMOURS

The most common gastric tumour is adenocarcinoma. There is a high incidence of this tumour (with a 2:1 male:female ratio) in some parts of the world, especially Japan, but generally it is becoming less common in developed countries. Predisposing factors may include a high salt consumption, aflatoxins, living in regions with a high nitrate content in the soil, and perhaps chronic infection with *Helicobacter pylori* interacting with other factors. Also implicated are smoking, a diet deficient in fresh fruit and vegetables and a diet deficient in selenium. There is an increased incidence in patients who have undergone gastric surgery, and those with atrophic gastritis. Factors that encourage bacterial overgrowth may favour nitrosation of luminal amines to form carcinogens.

Unfortunately, symptoms do not usually occur until the disease is advanced; then, patients complain of anorexia and weight loss. The tumour often ulcerates, leading to dyspeptic symptoms and iron-deficiency anaemia. Dyspepsia occurring for the first time in a patient over the age of 50 years is an indication for endoscopy, as is progressive iron-deficiency anaemia. Occlusion of the pylorus or cardia respectively may cause vomiting and dysphagia. Spread to the liver and lymph nodes is often present at diagnosis. Left-sided supraclavicular lymphadenopathy may be evident (**8.9**). Careful palpation of

the epigastrium may reveal a mass. Obstruction of the pylorus may lead to a demonstrable succussion splash, epigastric distension and visible peristalsis. Hepatic metastases, ascites, ovarian secondaries and secondaries in the pouch of Douglas all indicate advanced terminal disease.

Diagnosis is best confirmed at endoscopy, which reveals an ulcer or tumour mass (**8.57, 8.58**) and permits biopsy and histological examination (**8.59**). Sometimes the size of the tumour and its extension are best appreciated by a barium meal examination (**8.60, 8.61**). Liver metastases may be indentified

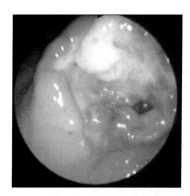

8.58 Carcinoma of the stomach. This ulcerated mass is situated between the incisura and the pylorus. The patient was an 80-year-old lady who presented with a 2-month history of dyspepsia and melaena.

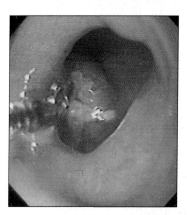

8.59 Endoscopic biopsy of an ulcerating mass in the stomach wall. The forceps are being advanced towards the lesion.

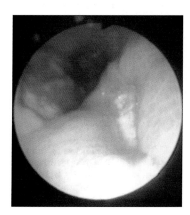

8.57 Carcinoma of the stomach. The endoscopic appearance of this ulcerating lesion is not conclusive, but malignancy was confirmed by biopsy.

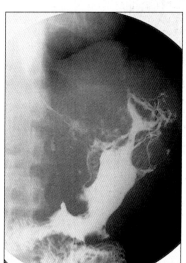

8.60 Carcinoma of the stomach. The barium meal demonstrates a large fungating mass in the gastric fundus. The patient presented with severe weight loss and iron-deficiency anaemia (**8.2**).

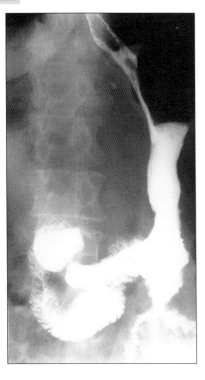

8.61 Linitis plastica of the stomach. In this form of gastric carcinoma, there is widespread submucosal invasion giving a rigid and immobile appearance on screening during the barium meal.

DUODENUM

DUODENAL ULCERATION

Duodenal ulceration is very common in the developed world, affecting about 1 per 1000 population, but the cause of duodenal ulcer diathesis remains unknown. *Helicobacter pylori* infection is present in at least 95% of cases (*see* **p. 350**) and the use of NSAIDs also plays a role in some patients. Multiple and resistant ulcers should prompt investigation for a gastrinoma (*see* **pp. 355, 373**).

Features suggestive of peptic ulceration include:

- intermittent epigastric pain related to eating
- epigastric pain causing nocturnal wakening
- relief of pain by certain bland foods and alkalis
- a close relationship of pain to cigarette smoking
- response to H_2 and proton pump inhibitors.

Many patients, however, do not have symptoms, and become aware of their ulcers only when complications occur. Suspected ulcers are best investigated by endoscopy (**8.14**, **8.63**, **8.64**), although high-quality barium meal examination can still provide useful information (**8.18**). Antral biopsy during

by ultrasound examination or CT (**9.22**), and peritoneal metastases by laparoscopy.

The only effective treatment is surgery. This can be curative in early gastric cancer when the 5-year survival is 90%, but by the time lymph node spread occurs this figure falls to 10%.

Other tumours that may be found in the stomach include benign polyps (**8.13**), leiomyoma (**8.62**), leiomyosarcoma (**8.10**), lymphoma, and Kaposi's sarcoma.

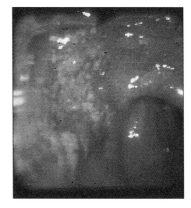

8.63 Duodenitis. Endoscopy shows superficial erosions of the duodenal mucosa on a background of inflammation, but no frank ulceration. Such 'salt and pepper' duodentitis may occur in isolation, or as a result of other inflammatory bowel diseases. It is often associated with peptic ulceration of the duodenum or stomach. If symptomatic, it usually responds to an acid secretion inhibitor.

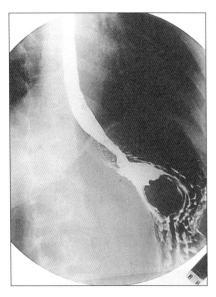

8.62 Gastric leiomyoma is a benign tumour of smooth muscle. In this patient, the barium meal shows a huge mass in the stomach. Patients with leiomyomas present with dyspeptic symptoms or with bleeding, which may be occult and lead to iron-deficiency anaemia. Surgical resection is usually possible and curative.

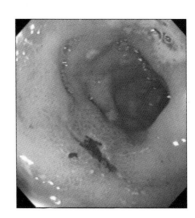

8.64 Duodenal ulceration. This endoscopic view shows two 'kissing' ulcers, with signs of recent bleeding. A background duodentitis (similar to that in **8.63**) is also present. Patients often prove to have more than one ulcer on endoscopy, but multiple ulcers should raise the suspicion of a possible gastrinoma (Zollinger–Ellison syndrome).

endoscopy is helpful to confirm the presence or absence of *Helicobacter* infection.

Complications of duodenal ulceration include haemorrhage (**8.64**), pyloric stenosis caused by scarring, and perforation, leading to acute peritonitis and pneumoperitoneum (**8.65**).

Duodenal ulcers usually respond to treatment with H_2-receptor antagonists (e.g. cimetidine, ranitidine) or proton pump inhibitors (e.g. omeprazole). Other drugs, including bismuth preparations, may be used and 'triple therapy' may be useful when *Helicobacter* is found (*see* **p. 350**). Maintenance therapy with a proton pump inhibitor or an H_2-receptor antagonist may be required to prevent relapse.

Surgical treatment is rarely needed now for the management of ulcer disease, but patients who have previously undergone surgery may present with complications, including stomal ulceration, diarrhoea, 'dumping syndrome' and nutritional deficiencies.

PEPTIC ULCERATION AT OTHER SITES

Peptic ulceration may occur in the oesophagus (*see* **p. 346**), at or near the stoma after gastric surgery, or in the ectopic gastric mucosa in a Meckel's diverticulum.

ZOLLINGER–ELLISON SYNDROME

Zollinger–Ellison syndrome results from a gastrin-producing tumour, which is often located in the pancreas, but occasionally is elsewhere in the small intestine or in the gastric antrum. The clinical features are of severe recurrent peptic ulceration (especially multiple ulceration, **8.64**), which has a high incidence of bleeding and perforation. There may also be diarrhoea with malabsorption, and there may be other endocrine neoplasms as part of the multiple endocrine neoplasia syndrome (*see* **pp. 304, 373**).

The diagnosis is made by finding a high gastrin level and a high basal secretion. The tumour may be localized by CT or MRI or by selective venous catheterization.

Treatment is with a proton-pump inhibitor to block acid secretion and surgery to remove the tumour if it has not already metastasized.

SMALL INTESTINE

MALABSORPTION

Malabsorption is the most common presenting feature of small intestinal disease and is characterized by failure to digest or absorb, or both, nutrients from the intestinal tract. Important causes are summarized in **8.66**.

Patients may present with pale offensive stools that float and are difficult to flush away (**8.8**), and they may exhibit features of nutrient deficiency (**8.2, 8.67**) in addition to those that characterize the underlying disease process.

Investigations (**8.68**) are undertaken with three objectives:

- to confirm impaired absorption, for example faecal fat collection and the Schilling test
- to identify specific deficiencies, for example anthropometric measurements, blood count, iron, transferrin, folate,

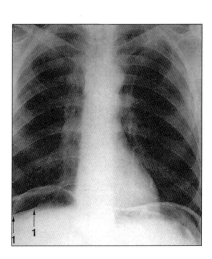

8.65 Pneumoperitoneum in a patient with a rigid abdomen caused by a perforated duodenal ulcer. The onset of his pain and rigidity was abrupt. Note the upper edge of the liver (1), and the air under both diaphragms.

CAUSES OF MALABSORPTION	
Level	**Condition**
Stomach	Post-gastrectomy dumping
	Zollinger–Ellison syndrome
	Pernicious anaemia
Hepatic/biliary tree	Biliary obstruction/cholestasis
Pancreas	Cystic fibrosis
	Pancreatitis
	Pancreatic carcinoma
Small bowel	Coeliac disease
	Crohn's disease
	Surgery and removal of small bowel
	Fistulae/blind loops
	Infection – bacterial, parasitic
	Radiation
	Lymphoma
	Drugs, e.g. neomycin, cholestyramine
	Specific enzyme defects of brush border
	Whipple's disease

8.66 Causes of malabsorption.

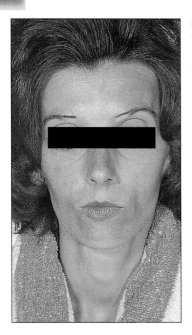

8.67   Malabsorption in coeliac disease may remain undiagnosed for many years. This woman was diagnosed at the age of 32 years, but her height was much less than all other members of her family, suggesting that her malabsorption dated from childhood. On presentation she weighed 40 kg (88 lb), she had marked steatorrhoea and she was pale and anaemic. Small bowel biopsy showed villous atrophy. A gluten-free diet relieved her steatorrhoea and reversed the changes in her jejunal mucosa. She rapidly gained weight, but should probably remain on a gluten-free diet for life.

aspiration or biopsy of the proximal small bowel to look for evidence of giardiasis (**8.24**) or gluten-sensitive enteropathy (**8.69**, **8.70**).

8.69   8.70

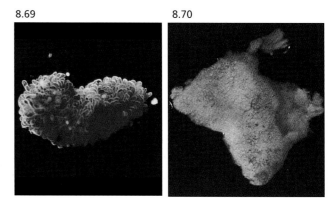

8.69 & 8.70   Distal duodenal biopsies from normal and coeliac patients, seen here under the dissecting microscope. Normal mucosa (**8.69**) shows a normal pattern and number of villi, whereas the abnormal mucosa (**8.70**) shows complete flattening – the characteristic appearance of gluten-sensitive enteropathy.

GENERAL INVESTIGATIONS OF VALUE IN MALABSORPTION	
Blood	Full blood count, film Serum B_{12} and folate ESR, plasma viscosity, C-reactive protein
Biochemistry	Calcium Zinc Albumin Faecal fat excretion Schilling test Pancreatic function tests Bile salt absorption
Bacteriology	Faecal culture Microscopy for ova, cysts or parasites Small bowel culture Glucose breath test ^{14}C xylose test
Immunology	Serum antiendomysial, antigliadin and antireticulin antibodies
Radiology	Barium meal and follow-through CT of abdomen Endoscopic retrograde cholangiopancreatography
Histology	Small bowel biopsy

8.68   General investigations of value in malabsorption.

vitamin B_{12}, prothrombin and related vitamin K-dependent clotting factors and vitamin D levels
- to establish the mechanism and cause of malabsorption; this may include a search for bacterial overgrowth, testing pancreatic exocrine function, serum antibody tests and

Gluten-sensitive enteropathy (coeliac disease)

Patients with gluten-sensitive enteropathy develop an immunological respose to gluten which damages the small intestinal mucosa, resulting in partial or subtotal villous atrophy. The prevalence of gluten-sensitive enteropathy in Europe is 1 per 300–1000 population. Gluten is a protein found predominantly in wheat, but also in rye, barley and (to a lesser extent) oats. The degradation of gluten in the intestinal lumen means that the proximal small intestine is maximally affected. Those who have more severe involvement develop steatorrhoea. The characteristic presentation is chronic diarrhoea, steatorrhoea, abdominal distension and failure to thrive in childhood. Presentation in adult life is often more obscure with megaloblastic anaemia, intermittent diarrhoea and vague abdominal symptoms.

Serum antiendomysial, antigliadin and antireticulin antibodies are present in most untreated cases. For example, IgA antiendomysial antibodies are found in nearly 100% of children and 90% of adults with gluten-sensitive enteropathy, and false-positives are very rare. Antireticulin antibodies are also very sensitive but less specific. These antibodies are a valuable screening test, but the diagnosis should usually be confirmed by endoscopic biopsy of the distal duodenum or jejunum (**8.69–8.72**).

A gluten-free diet relieves symptoms, reduces or eliminates serum antibodies and reverses the biopsy appearances in most patients. Small intestinal lymphoma and carcinoma and squamous carcinoma of the oesophagus are more common in patients with gluten-sensitive enteropathy than in the general

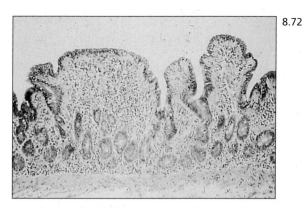

8.71 & 8.72   Microscopic sections of jejunal biopsies from normal and coeliac patients. The sections correspond to the appearance seen in **8.69** and **8.70**, respectively. The normal microscopic appearance of the jejunal mucosa is seen in **8.71**, whereas **8.72** shows the jejunum of a previously undiagnosed patient with gluten-sensitive enteropathy on a normal diet. The normal intestinal villi are absent, the mucosa is flattened and there is hyperplasia of the intestinal crypts. There is lymphocytic infiltration, and the surface mucosa is cuboidal rather than columnar.

population; some extra-gastrointestinal cancers are also more common. The effect of a gluten-free diet on the risk of these complications is unclear.

In dermatitis herpetiformis, a gluten-sensitive enteropathy is accompanied by a bullous skin eruption (**2.72**, **2.73**). Both may respond to a gluten-free diet, though treatment with dapsone may also be needed for the skin eruption.

BACTERIAL OVERGROWTH

Small intestinal bacterial overgrowth commonly accompanies the reduction of gastric acidity by drugs or surgery, and may

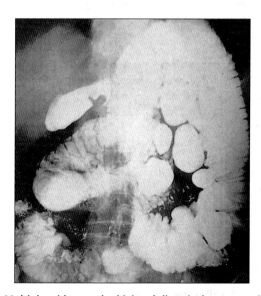

8.73   Multiple wide-mouthed jejunal diverticula are seen in this barium follow-through X-ray. The diverticula are sites of stasis; in this patient they were colonized by bacteria that created a malabsorption syndrome.

also occur in the presence of blind loops (**8.73**), motility disorders or impaired immune function. It is an important consideration in the elderly. Diagnosis is supported with a glycocholate or hydrogen breath test (*see* **p. 343**).

TUMOURS OF THE SMALL INTESTINE

Small intestinal tumours account for only 1% of gastrointestinal neoplasms. In descending order of frequency they comprise adenocarcinomas, carcinoids, lymphomas and leiomyosarcomas. Kaposi's sarcoma of the intestine may occur in patients with HIV infection.

Adenocarcinomas may complicate Crohn's disease, particularly in a bypassed segment, and coeliac disease. Almost one-half occur in the duodenum. Presentation is with pain and vomiting, anaemia and, in the case of periampullary tumours, jaundice. Diagnosis is often made by a small bowel barium study (**8.74**).

If the carcinoma involves the ampulla of Vater, the patient usually presents with obstruction of the pancreatic and biliary tracts and biochemical evidence of obstruction (high alkaline phosphatase and bilirubin) and later with clinical evidence of jaundice. There may also be steatorrhoea and positive faecal occult blood. These features may be intermittent as the tumour necroses. The diagnosis should be made endoscopically (**8.75**) and a stent may sometimes be inserted to relieve obstruction (**8.76**).

Intestinal lymphomas also occur more commonly than expected in patients with coeliac disease (**8.77**). The lymphoma is often located in the distal small intestine, whereas the proximal intestine bears the brunt of the damage from gluten. Lymphomas also occur in patients who are immunosuppressed after organ transplantation or by HIV infection. Patients develop diarrhoea and pain and lose weight.

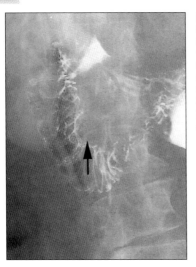

8.74 Carcinoma of the ampulla of Vater (arrowed) is shown as a filling defect in the second part of the duodenum on this double-contrast barium meal. The patient presented with anaemia.

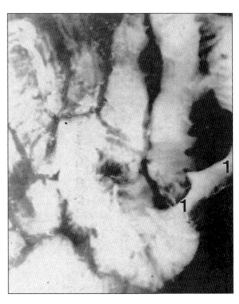

8.77 Intestinal lymphoma in a patient with coeliac disease that had been well controlled on a gluten-free diet for the past 13 years. An irregular shouldered stricture (1) is seen on barium follow-through. Radiologically, the appearance suggests lymphoma or carcinoma, and at operation a lymphoma was found. Even with surgery followed by radiotherapy or chemotherapy, the prognosis is poor.

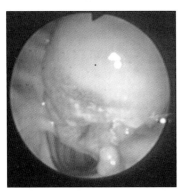

8.75 Carcinoma of the ampulla of Vater. The carcinoma is seen towards the bottom of the picture. The bulging swelling above is the grossly dilated common bile duct, which is obstructed by the carcinoma.

caused by nicotinic acid deficiency as a result of disturbed tryptophan metabolism.

Tumours and vascular malformations may present with recurrent gastrointestinal bleeding of obscure cause. As with Meckel's diverticulum, the diagnosis may be made on mesenteric angiography, or – for slow bleeding – by a technetium-labelled red cell scan (**8.23**).

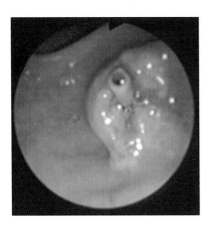

8.76 Obstruction of the ampulla of Vater relieved by insertion of a stent. This palliative procedure can often be accomplished endoscopically.

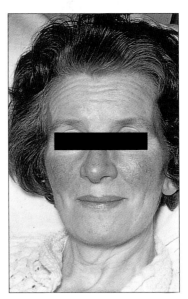

8.78 Facial flush in carcinoid. This is usually seen only when hepatic secondaries are present, although it may occur with primary tumours that drain directly into the systemic circulation (in the lung, testis or ovary). Other symptoms resulting from the release of vasoactive substances by these tumours may include abdominal pain, diarrhoea, bronchospasm and congestive cardiac failure.

Most small intestinal carcinoid tumours arise in the ileum. The clinical features are determined by local growth that can lead to intestinal obstruction, and by their secretion of humoral agents that become systemically active after metastases have developed in the liver. The characteristic syndrome of flushing (**8.78**) with diarrhoea, bronchospasm and congestive cardiac failure is well known. Patients may even develop pellagra

INFLAMMATORY BOWEL DISEASE

Inflammatory bowel disease is a term that encompasses two main conditions: Crohn's disease and ulcerative colitis.

CROHN'S DISEASE

Crohn's disease is a chronic granulomatous inflammatory disease of unknown cause, which is becoming more common.

The prevalence in the UK is about 3 per 100 000. The terminal ileum and colon are principally involved, but the disease may affect any part of the intestinal tract, often with discontinuous patches of inflammation of all the bowel wall structures ('skip' lesions). Initially, aphthoid ulcers may be seen at endoscopic examination with macroscopically normal intervening mucosa (8.79). Subsequently, more severe inflammation leads to more extensive ulceration and oedema of the mucosa (8.80–8.82) and ultimately fibrosis can cause bowel strictures (8.20, 8.83, 8.84). Inflamed bowel may adhere to surrounding structures and matted loops of bowel are a cause of internal or external fistulae (8.85) and intestinal obstruction (8.21). Involvement of the perianal area in up to 80% of patients leads to a characteristic appearance with skin tags, fissures and fistulae (8.86). Less commonly, the lips and oral cavity are affected (8.4). Biopsy of Crohn's lesions shows inflammation of all layers of the bowel wall, and giant cell granulomas are commonly found (8.87).

The clinical presentation is varied depending upon the region, extent, and manner of the intestinal involvement. Common features include diarrhoea, abdominal pain, anorexia, weight loss and pyrexia. Childhood Crohn's disease may present with growth retardation and delayed puberty. Eventually the patient may suffer from intestinal obstruction and intestinal failure, with malnutrition, often including zinc deficiency (7.131).

359

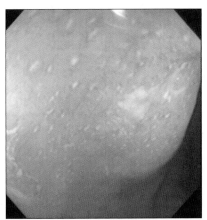

8.79 Crohn's proctitis. In this colonoscopic view, there are multiple small ulcers but the adjacent mucosa looks normal. This is a common endoscopic appearance in the rectum and colon in early Crohn's disease, though initially the ulcers may be fewer in number or even single.

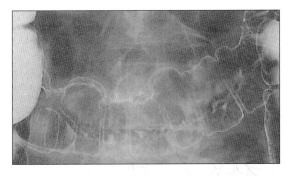

8.80 Crohn's colitis on double-contrast barium enema. Many ulcers can be seen in this view of the transverse colon, by their retention of barium, but the remaining mucosa appears normal.

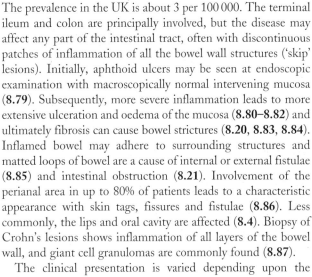

8.82 Crohn's disease in the colon. Multiple oedematous inflammatory polyps give a 'cobblestone' appearance to the mucosa. Similar changes may be seen in ulcerative colitis.

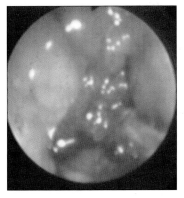

8.81 Severe ileal Crohn's disease. There is extensive boggy, inflammatory, oedema of the mucosa, leading to partial obstruction of the ileum. The 29-year-old patient had severe abdominal pain and weight loss.

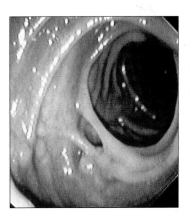

8.83 Crohn's disease in the duodenum. This videoendoscopic view shows 'bridging' lesions in the mucosa. Ulceration and healing leads to these isolated bridges of mucosa. In other parts of the bowel, such fibrosis often leads to obstruction.

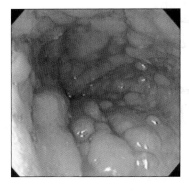

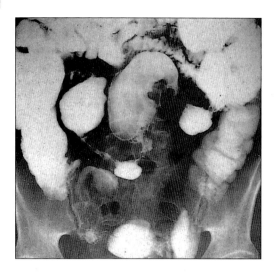

8.84 Crohn's disease of the small intestine revealed on barium follow-through X-ray. Four strictures of the small intestine are clearly seen, and the dilated segments of bowel appear between the strictures. These 'skip lesions' are characteristic of Crohn's disease, and similar appearances may be seen in the colon when there is colonic involvement.

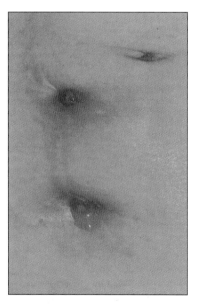

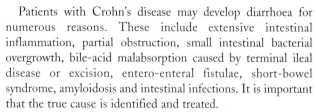

8.85 Enterocutaneous fistulae in Crohn's disease are most common, as here, in a patient who has undergone bowel resection, but they may also occur in unoperated cases. Sinography may be used to demonstrate communication with the affected bowel.

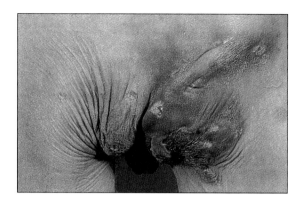

8.86 Multiple perianal fistulae resulted in the chronic, painful inflammatory reaction seen here in a patient with long-standing Crohn's disease.

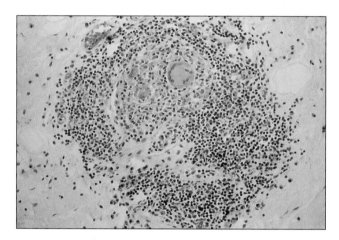

8.87 Crohn's disease histopathology. Non-caseating granulomas, as seen here in close-up, are found in most patients. The granulomas are composed mainly of lymphocytes, macrophages and plasma cells, and they characteristically contain multinucleated giant cells, as shown here. In contrast to ulcerative colitis, Crohn's disease is characterized by inflammation of all layers of the gut wall, with submucosal oedema, deep ulcers and fibrous scarring.

Patients with Crohn's disease may develop diarrhoea for numerous reasons. These include extensive intestinal inflammation, partial obstruction, small intestinal bacterial overgrowth, bile-acid malabsorption caused by terminal ileal disease or excision, entero-enteral fistulae, short-bowel syndrome, amyloidosis and intestinal infections. It is important that the true cause is identified and treated.

Extra-intestinal manifestations of Crohn's disease are similar to those experienced by patients with ulcerative colitis and may include sclerosing cholangitis (**9.51**), arthritis, uveitis, deep vein thrombosis and skin rashes such as pyoderma gangrenosum (**2.135**) and erythema nodosum (**2.45**). Most patients with Crohn's disease who develop right hypochondrial pain and jaundice do not have sclerosing cholangitis, however: the majority have gallstones.

Crohn's disease can be controlled in most patients with short-term courses of corticosteroids, and azathioprine is useful in resistant patients. Other drugs which may be helpful include 5-aminosalicylic acid, cyclosporin and interferon, and specific antibody therapy with anti-tumour necrosis factor alpha (anti-TNFα) has been used in steroid resistant or fistulating disease. Surgery is required in most patients at some stage, for example for the relief of obstruction or the correction of fistulae. Nutritional support, either enteral or parenteral, corrects malnutrition thus making a major contribution to the patient's wellbeing (*see* **p. 331**).

ULCERATIVE COLITIS

Ulcerative colitis has a stable incidence and prevalence (6 and 100 per 100 000, respectively, in the UK). It is primarily a mucosal disease that extends for a variable distance and in a continuous fashion, around the colon from the rectum, which is always involved.

Symptoms depend on the extent and severity of colonic involvement. Patients in whom the disease is confined to the rectum experience rectal bleeding and tenesmus, but the stool is formed and constipation may be a problem. Diarrhoea is the predominant symptom with more extensive disease, and severe attacks are accompanied by abdominal pain, pyrexia and tachycardia.

Endoscopy reveals the severity of the disease (**8.88–8.91**) and allows biopsy (**8.92**), which may show goblet cell depletion, crypt abscesses, distortion of the architecture with little submucosal inflammation and no granulomas (in contrast to Crohn's disease; **8.93**). Barium enema may show characteristic findings (**8.94**, **8.95**). Other important investigations include FBC, erythrocyte sedimentation rate (ESR) or C-reactive protein, serum albumin and stool microscopy and culture to exclude an infective or parasitic cause for symptoms.

The differential diagnosis of ulcerative colitis includes Crohn's disease, gastrointestinal infections, pseudomembranous colitis, ischaemic colitis, radiation-induced enteritis and drug-induced colitis.

Extra-intestinal manifestations of ulcerative colitis may include skin rashes, erythema nodosum (**2.45**) and pyoderma gangrenosum (**2.135**), hepatobiliary disease, especially sclerosing cholangitis (**9.51**) and arthritis. Inflammation involving the peripheral joints reflects the activity of the

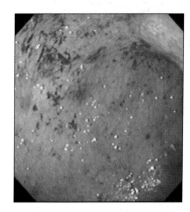

8.90 Ulcerative colitis. More severe changes than in **8.88** with multiple bleeding points. Endoscopy is hazardous in the acute phases of ulcerative colitis, due to the risk of perforation or bleeding, or both.

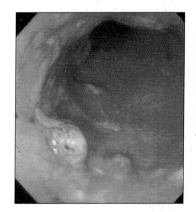

8.91 Inflammatory polyps (often known, rather confusingly, as 'pseudopolyps') are invariably found in the progression of ulcerative colitis composed of granulomatous tissue, and, like any inflammatory reaction, they are highly vascular.

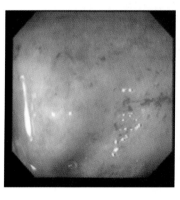

8.88 Ulcerative colitis. Relatively early changes are seen in this colonoscopic view. These include swelling of the mucosa, loss of normal haustrations and friability of the mucosa with bleeding caused by the touch of the colonoscope.

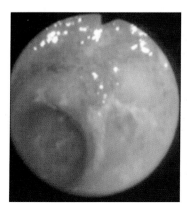

8.89 Ulcerative colitis. In this patient with chronic active disease, the loss of haustrations in the colon is obvious, and multiple ulcers are present.

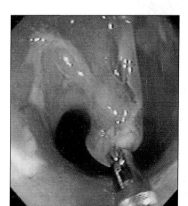

8.92 Biopsy of large inflammatory polyps in ulcerative colitis is sometimes advisable to exclude the possiblity of carcinoma, which is a major risk of chronic ulcerative colitis (*see* **8.97**).

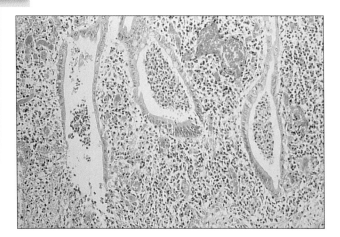

8.93 Ulcerative colitis histopathology. In contrast to Crohn's disease, the inflammatory process in ulcerative colitis is usually confined to the mucosal layer of the bowel wall and granulomas are not seen. In active disease, as here, there is an increase in the number of lymphocytes, plasma cells and neutrophils in the lamina propria (beneath the epithelium). The epithelium shows patchy or continuous ulceration, and large numbers of neutrophils migrate through the walls of the glands to form 'crypt abscesses'. Three crypt abscesses are seen in this view.

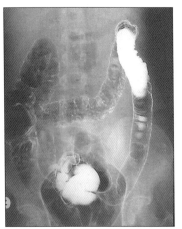

8.94 Ulcerative colitis. This double-contrast barium enema shows typical chronic changes throughout the colon. There is loss of the normal haustral pattern, giving the colon a smooth tubular appearance. Deep, penetrating ulcers can be seen, especially in the barium-filled splenic flexure, and there are many pseudopolyps, best seen in the transverse colon.

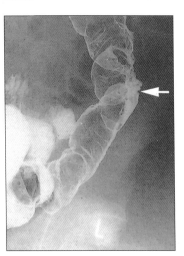

8.95 Ulcerative colitis with multiple inflammatory polyps ('pseudopolyps'). The double-contrast barium enema technique demonstrates the appearance well in the descending colon, and this correlates with the endoscopic view (**8.91**). Note the area of deep ulceration (arrow). On screening, this area showed a lack of movement that raised the suspicion of carcinomatous change.

intestinal disease, but this does not apply if patients have sacroiliitis or ankylosing spondylitis.

Complications of acute disease include colonic dilatation (**8.96**) which may lead to perforation and haemorrhage and is suggested by features of an acute abdomen. Chronic disease may also produce anaemia, and carries an increasing risk of colonic carcinoma in patients with extensive disease of more than 10 years' duration (**8.97**). Colonoscopic surveillance every

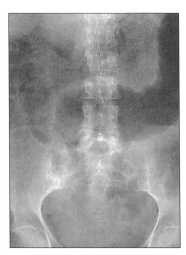

8.96 Colonic dilatation in ulcerative colitis ('toxic megacolon'). This complication of acute ulcerative colitis requires urgent intensive management, including fluid replacement and steroid therapy. The patient presents with a tender, swollen abdomen, which is tympanitic, due to the amount of gas in the colon. Fever and signs of shock are common accompaniments. It is important to auscultate the abdomen, as bowel sounds are usually absent.

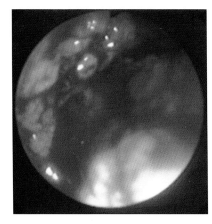

8.97 Carcinoma of the colon has developed as a complication of long-standing ulcerative colitis in this patient with a 17-year history of the disease. The blood in this view results from biopsy of the lesion. Regular colonoscopic surveillance should allow identification of this complication at an earlier stage.

2 years facilitates the detection of premalignant dysplasia in the mucosa, allowing timely surgical intervention.

Medical treatment involves the control of disease activity with short courses of corticosteroids or azathioprine, or both, the maintenance of remission with sulfasalazine or one of the preparations designed to deliver 5-aminosalicylic acid to the colon (mesalazine or olsalazine) and the correction of anaemia. Surgery is required if medical management fails, and to prevent acute and chronic complications such as perforation or carcinoma. Pan-proctocolectomy with a permanent ileostomy is usually necessary, although pouch procedures involving ileoanal anastomoses are an alternative which avoids the need for an ileostomy. Maintenance of good nutrition is essential (*see* **p. 331**)

DRUGS AND THE COLON

Inflammation of the colon may occur as an indirect consequence of antibiotic administration (pseudomembranous colitis, *see* **p. 367**), or as the result of treatment with non-steroidal anti-inflammatory analgesics. Some, such as mefenamic acid, are particularly prone to cause diarrhoea with an associated colitis.

OTHER DISORDERS AFFECTING BOTH SMALL AND LARGE INTESTINE

RADIATION ENTEROCOLITIS

Radiation enterocolitis is a sequel to radiotherapy for pelvic and abdominal malignancy. The safety margin between therapeutic effect and damage to surrounding structures is narrow and factors such as previous surgery may enhance intestinal damage by fixing loops of bowel within the field of exposure.

Early changes after exposure include increased crypt cell death and loss of villus height, and the extensive loss of intestinal function may lead to fluid and electrolyte imbalance. However, the initial clinical features of nausea, vomiting and diarrhoea, frequently with rectal bleeding, may settle.

Late complications develop from endarteritis obliterans, which leads to intestinal ischaemia. After a period that varies from a few months to many years, ischaemic strictures and fistulae may develop, and patients may suffer from subacute obstruction and chronic malabsorption (**8.98**). Sometimes, damage to the enteric nerves causes a pseudo-obstruction. The colonic symptoms can resemble idiopathic ulcerative colitis, but endoscopy reveals the typical picture of an atrophic mucosa with telangiectasia.

Medical therapy is limited in scope. Antibiotics are useful for the treatment of secondary bacterial overgrowth, colestyramine may be helpful with bile-acid malabsorption when the terminal ileum is affected, and topical steroids or mesalazine should be given to patients with proctitis. Some patients with intestinal failure need prolonged parenteral nutrition. Surgery is required for perforation, stricture and fistulae, but the morbidity of operative intervention is considerable.

ISCHAEMIC DISORDERS

Intestinal ischaemia may be acute or chronic, and it may affect the small or large intestine:

- Acute mesenteric ischaemia usually occurs in patients with generalized atheroma, but it may be embolic. Rarely, it is caused by venous occlusion in patients who are taking oral contraceptives or who have antithrombin-III deficiency; the initial presentation with diarrhoea, vomiting and vague abdominal pain is rapidly followed by increasing pain and shock; early laparotomy and resection of the affected segment offers the only prospect of survival.
- Chronic mesenteric insufficiency causes intestinal angina, a postprandial abdominal pain that usually prompts an initial search for peptic ulcer or biliary disease.
- Colonic ischaemia is more common than mesenteric ischaemia and usually affects the splenic flexure. The patient complains of abdominal pain and diarrhoea, and after a few hours the diarrhoea contains fresh blood. At this stage, the diagnosis may be suspected from plain abdominal X-ray in which 'thumb-printing' is evident (**8.99**). Infection with

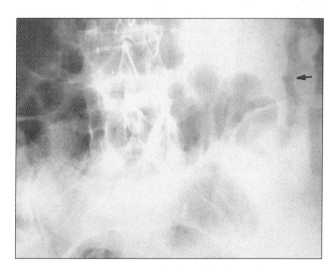

8.99 Acute ischaemic colitis. The patient was a 60-year-old woman who presented with acute bloody diarrhoea and left-sided abdominal pain. This plain X-ray of the abdomen in the supine position shows a narrowing in the bowel lumen and mucosal 'thumb-printing' (arrowed) in the descending colon. The narrowing of the colon is caused by spasm, and the thumb-printing is caused by a combination of submucosal oedema and haemorrhage. Note that the proximal large bowel is somewhat distended – the ischaemic lesion is causing partial obstruction.

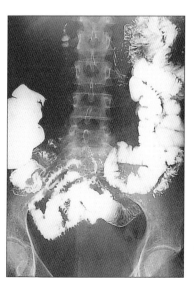

8.98 Radiation enterocolitis. This 3¼-hour barium follow-through film shows narrowing of the terminal ileum, with gross thickening of the normal mucosal folds. On screening, the ileum was seen to be matted together as an immobile mass. These changes were associated with a rapid transit time and malabsorption. This 55-year-old woman had been treated by radiotherapy for carcinoma of the cervix.

Escherichia coli 0157 may produce a similar clinical picture (*see* **pp. 36, 367**). Occasionally, the affected segment perforates, but usually the features subside. Fibrosis may lead to stenosis causing alteration of bowel habit or chronic intestinal obstruction (**8.100**).

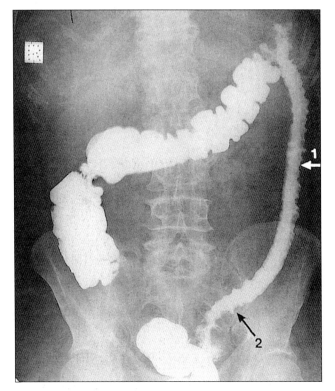

8.100   Colonic ischaemia This single-contrast barium enema shows gross ischaemic changes throughout the descending colon. There is narrowing of the lumen, accompanied by typical 'rose-thorn' ulcers (1) and some 'thumb-printing' (2) in the sigmoid colon, where a partial stricture has formed. The apparent stricture at the hepatic flexure disappeared on screening. The patient also had symptomatic coronary heart disease and peripheral vascular disease.

COLON AND RECTUM

DIVERTICULAR DISEASE

Diverticula are acquired pouches of the colonic mucosa that have herniated through the muscular layers of the colon. They are present in about one-half of the population over the age of 65 years in the developed world, and are often found by chance in barium enemas that have been carried out for other purposes. The most common sites are the sigmoid and descending colon, where they are usually multiple. The cause is unclear, but they may result from an increased pressure within the lumen in the sigmoid colon. They are most common in patients in whom dietary fibre intake is low. Many patients have no symptoms, but some have recurrent lower abdominal pain, particularly in the left iliac fossa, associated with flatulence and constipation or, sometimes, diarrhoea. Pain follows a meal and is often relieved by passing gas or by defaecation. Bleeding and localized abscess formation (diverticulitis) may occur. Diverticulitis is associated with severe localized pain in the abdomen, fever and localized guarding. Septicaemia may result, and other complications include fistulae, colonic obstruction and generalized peritonitis.

The diagnosis is made on barium enema (**8.101**, **8.102**) or colonoscopy (**8.103**). Most symptoms settle with conservative treatment, and patients should be given a high-fibre diet. Surgery may be required for complications and anaemia may require iron therapy or blood transfusion.

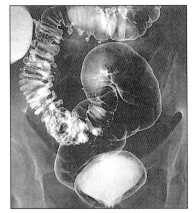

8.101   Diverticular disease of the colon. This barium enema shows typical changes, with multiple diverticula outlined by the double-contrast technique. The patient presented with a change in bowel habit and abdominal pain, and although this could be caused by the diverticular disease itself, it is important to exclude the possibility of coexistent colonic carcinoma in these circumstances. This is best done by colonoscopy.

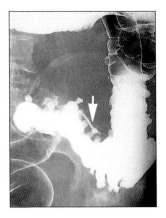

8.102   Diverticular disease of the colon with sinus formation. This patient with known diverticular disease was reinvestigated for right iliac fossa pain and tenderness. The barium enema shows the presence of multiple diverticula, and a communicating sinus is clearly seen (arrow). This appearance is diagnostic of local abscess formation.

PNEUMATOSIS OF THE COLON

Pneumatosis of the colon (also known as pneumatosis coli or pneumatosis cystoides intestinalis) is an unusual condition of unknown aetiology in which gas-filled cysts are found within the wall of the colon and, sometimes, of the small intestine.

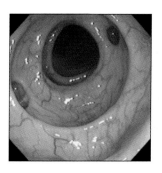

8.103　Severe diverticular disease viewed through the colonoscope. Wide-mouthed openings to diverticula are present, and these were seen throughout the sigmoid colon in this patient. Colonoscopy may be difficult and hazardous when diverticula are large enough to admit the tip of the scope.

There is an association with chronic obstructive pulmonary disease and peptic ulceration, and pneumatosis may also follow colonoscopy or a double-contrast barium enema. Pneumatosis is often found incidentally at colonoscopy or even on a plain X-ray of the abdomen (gas in wall as well as lumen). Occasionally there may be symptoms such as colicky lower-abdominal pain, diarrhoea and blood and mucus on the stools. The appearance at endoscopy is typical (**8.104**). No specific treatment is available.

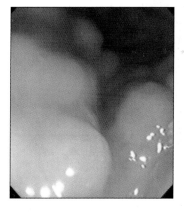

8.104　Pneumatosis of the colon. Multiple gas-filled cysts are present in the submucosa and subserosa of the colon. The cause is obscure, but it is possible that gas may track down from the pleural space in patients with chronic obstructive pulmonary disease, or that mucosal perforation during endoscopy or contrast radiography may occur. Biopsy of a cyst is often accompanied by a loud 'pop'.

LARGE BOWEL CANCER

Large bowel (colorectal) cancer is predominantly found in Western societies. In the UK, it is the second most common tumour, with a lifetime incidence of about 1 in 30 (only bronchial carcinoma is more common). High-fat, low-fibre diets have been blamed for supporting bacterial flora that result in the formation of carcinogens from intestinal contents, including bile acids, an effect compounded by a delayed transit time.

Most cancers develop from benign adenomas. There is a low risk of malignancy in single polyps that are less than 1 cm in diameter, but a much higher risk when the diameter exceeds 2 cm (**8.17**, **8.105**) or the polyps are multiple. The histological type is also important, as malignancy is much more common in villous (40%) than tubular (5%) adenomas.

Patients with familial polyposis coli (**8.19**, **8.106**) almost invariably develop bowel cancer, so they are advised to undergo prophylactic colectomy. Patients at risk include the family members with familial polyposis, those who have previously developed polyps, patients over 40 years of age with first degree relatives with colonic cancer, those with long-standing extensive ulcerative colitis, and possibly patients who have undergone cholecystectomy.

Patients with colonic cancer may present with alteration of bowel habit, rectal bleeding, abdominal pain, anaemia or symptoms of disseminated disease.

The diagnosis is usually established by a barium enema examination (**8.107**, **8.108**), which should be preceded by sigmoidoscopy. When the barium examination fails to provide conclusive information, or when polyps are found, colonoscopy is required to detect lesions missed on the barium films and to allow biopsy of suspect areas and the removal of polyps (**8.17**,

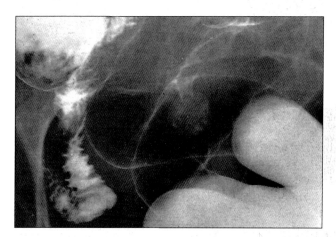

8.105　A single colonic polyp, revealed by double-contrast barium enema. Its pedunculated nature should mean that it can be successfully removed by snare diathermy performed through the colonoscope (see **8.17**). If the excision is histologically complete, no further treatment is required for this polyp; however, the patient should have a full-length colonic examination at the time of colonoscopy and any further polyps should be similarly treated. Because of the risk of recurrence of the polyp at the same or a different site, follow-up colonoscopy is usually recommended.

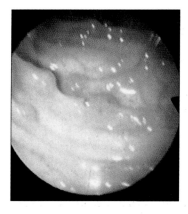

8.106　Familial polyposis coli. Multiple sessile polyps are seen in this colonoscopic view. Histologically, the lesions are adenomatous polyps, but there is a high risk of malignant change in this dominant condition, which usually presents in the second decade of life with diarrhoea, rectal bleeding and, sometimes, abdominal pain. Multiple polyps can usually also be seen on double-contrast barium enema examination (**8.19**) Prophylactic colectomy is usually advised.

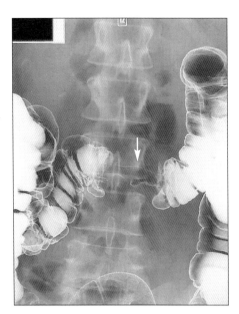

8.107 Colonic carcinoma in the transverse colon, revealed by double-contrast barium enema. This annular carcinoma has produced a characteristic apple-core appearance (arrow). This is strongly suggestive of the diagnosis, and is sufficient indication for surgery. Less obvious lesions should be confirmed by biopsy via the colonoscope. This patient presented with chronic iron-deficiency anaemia and was found to have a positive faecal occult blood test.

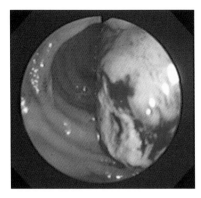

8.109 Colonic carcinoma seen through a colonoscope. This patient with an ulcerating lesion in the descending colon presented with frank bleeding.

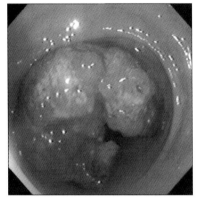

8.110 Polypoid colonic carcinoma in the descending colon. This tumour has developed by metaplastic change from a benign polyp such as that shown in **8.105**.

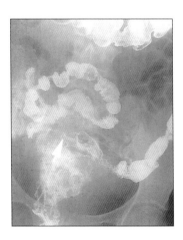

8.108 Enterocolic fistula (arrowed) in colonic carcinoma. This was an unexpected finding in a patient who presented with malabsorption and diarrhoea. A carcinoma of the sigmoid colon has formed a fistula with an adjacent loop of small intestine (identifiable by its typical mucosal pattern). Colonization of the small bowel by colonic bacteria is the cause of the malabsorption in this condition.

8.97, 8.109). Investigations are also needed to determine the effects of the disease, for example a blood count and film to look for iron deficiency, and a CT or ultrasound examination of the abdominal nodes and liver to search for metastatic disease (**9.22**).

Colonic cancer may be prevented by the identification and removal of polyps (**8.110**). The established tumour is treated by surgical resection, a right or left hemicolectomy or abdomino-perineal excision of lower rectal tumours. Rectal lesions may be palliated by laser treatment in patients unfit for surgery. The prognosis is influenced by the extent of spread and this is the basis of Dukes' classification (**8.111**). Follow-up is mandatory,

MODIFIED DUKES' CLASSIFICATION OF LARGE BOWEL CANCER		
Dukes' stage	% (at presentation)	5-year cancer-related survival (%)
A Cancer confined to bowel wall	5–10	90–100
B Extension through bowel wall, without metastases	35–40	75–85
C Spread into regional lymph nodes	30	30–40
D Distant metastases or residual disease after surgery	25	< 5

8.111 Modified Dukes' classification of large bowel cancer. A staging system should aid in prognosis in the individual patient. Dukes' classification is generally regarded as the most accurate in large bowel cancer.

and should involve at least annual barium enemas or colonoscopy plus measurement of the tumour marker, carcinoembryonic antigen (CEA).

First degree relatives of patients with large bowel cancer are at increased risk of developing the disease (1 in 6 risk if two first degree relatives are affected). Screening of relatives may be helpful, but there is no general agreement on whether such screening should be based on occult blood testing, sigmoidoscopy or colonoscopy.

GASTROINTESTINAL INFECTIONS

Infection may occur at any level in the gut. Infection of the mouth and oesophagus are important causes of local symptoms. *Helicobacter pylori* infection plays a role in the genesis of gastritis and peptic ulceration (*see* **p. 350**).

Intestinal tuberculosis is rare in the developed world but still relatively common elsewhere. It usually affects the terminal ileum, where it may produce symptoms and a barium X-ray appearance similar to those of Crohn's disease (**8.20**). Management is usually medical (*see* **p. 33**).

Gastroenteritis is a common problem throughout the world. The most common symptom is diarrhoea, and it is important to distinguish infective from other causes (**8.112**). The World Health Organization estimates that infective diarrhoea has an incidence of 1.5 billion cases per year and a mortality of 2.2 million per year – almost entirely in children in developing countries.

Secretory diarrhoea may be caused by *Vibrio cholerae* (**p. 37**), *Campylobacter jejuni* and many strains of *Escherichia coli* and *Salmonella*. Typically, there are copious fluid stools, and dehydration is the most important clinical problem.

Dysentery is a condition in which the stool contains pus, mucus and blood. This results from colonic mucosal invasion by organisms such as enteroinvasive *E. coli*, *Shigella*, *C. jejuni* and rotavirus (**8.113**). Other invasive organisms may cause a predominantly septicaemic illness. The most important example is *Salmonella typhi*: intestinal symptoms occur relatively late in the evolution of enteric fever (*see* **p. 36**). Pseudomembranous colitis is a serious infection with *Clostridium difficile* that may follow treatment with broad-spectrum antibiotics (**8.114**).

Most acute infective diarrhoea is self-limiting, but oral or intravenous fluid replacement is life-saving if diarrhoea is profuse, and antibiotic treatment is indicated for some invasive infections.

Transmission of infection is usually by the faecal–oral route, and prevention is based on hygiene in food and water preparation.

Protozoal infections are another important cause of gastrointestinal symptoms. Giardiasis is common. The organism infests the small intestine and may cause acute diarrhoea or chronic malabsorption. The cysts may be evident on stool microscopy, but small intestinal aspiration or biopsy is

COMMON CAUSES OF DIARRHOEA	
Viral	Rotavirus Norwalk agent/small round structured viruses (SRSVs) Adenoviruses
Bacterial toxin	*Escherichia coli* (enterotoxigenic) *Vibrio cholerae* *Staphylococcus aureus* *Clostridium perfringens* *Clostridium difficile* *Clostridium botulinum* *Bacillus cereus*
Bacterial invasion	*Escherichia coli* (enteroinvasive) *Shigella* *Salmonella* *Yersinia enterocolitica* *Vibrio parahaemolyticus* *Campylobacter jejuni*
Parasites	*Giardia lamblia* *Cryptosporidium parvum* *Entamoeba histolytica*
After infection	Lactase deficiency Bacterial overgrowth
Drugs	Laxatives Antacids with magnesium
Food toxins	Ciguatoxin, scombroid, puffer-fish
Chronic gastrointestinal disorders	Inflammatory bowel disease Ischaemic colitis Malabsorption Irritable bowel syndrome

8.112 Common causes of diarrhoea.

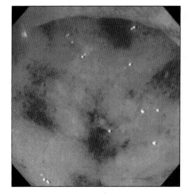

8.113 Infective colitis. This patient presented with bloody diarrhoea which ultimately proved to be the result of enteroinvasive *Escherichia coli* infection. Colonoscopy is not routinely performed in infective colitis, but was carried out here to exclude other pathology before the infective nature of the condition was confirmed. The haemorrhagic lesions are typical, and there are no structural changes in the colon.

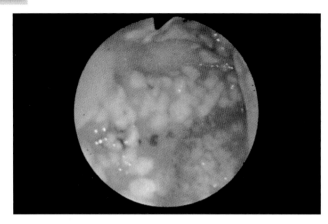

8.114 Pseudomembranous colitis may develop during, or up to 6 weeks after, treatment with antibiotics such as lincomycin, ampicillin and cephalosporins. The major symptom is diarrhoea, which may be bloody. Sigmoidoscopy or colonoscopy usually shows multiple yellow plaques and inflammatory changes and the diagnosis can be confirmed histologically. *Clostridium difficile* and its toxin are found in the stools. Patients with pseudomembranous colitis should be barrier-nursed, because there is a risk of cross infection. If the diarrhoea is severe, they may need intravenous fluid replacement, and treatment with vancomycin will eliminate the *Clostridium* infection.

sometimes needed to confirm the diagnosis (**8.24**). Eradication is achieved with metronidazole.

Entamoeba histolytica invades the colonic mucosa (**8.115**) and the patient suffers from bloody diarrhoea. The possibility of amoebiasis must always be considered in a patient with this complaint who is in, or has returned from, a developing country. An erroneous diagnosis of inflammatory bowel disease followed by corticosteroid treatment may be fatal. The management of amoebiasis and its complications is covered on **page 47**.

Cryptosporidium parvum has been widely recognized as a cause of diarrhoea in cattle, and is now known to produce a self-limiting diarrhoeal illness in man. In patients with HIV infection, it may produce a catastrophic illness with extreme dehydration, shock and death. Many other organisms may cause gastrointestinal disease in immunocompromised patients, especially those with HIV infection (*see* **p. 5**)

INTESTINAL WORM INFESTATIONS

ROUNDWORMS

Threadworm infestation with *Enterobius vermicularis* is very common worldwide. It often causes pruritus ani, especially in children, but may be asymptomatic.

Infestation with *Ascaris lumbricoides* may also be asymptomatic, but some patients develop a cough and fever during the migration of the larvae to the lung after they penetrate the intestinal mucosa. After development, the worms are coughed up, swallowed and become established in the intestinal tract. Heavy infestation can lead to distal small intestinal obstruction and, rarely, migration can cause obstruction of the bile duct (**8.116**). Piperazine and mebendazole are effective treatments (**8.117**). The whipworm, *Trichuris trichiura*, has a simple life cycle, and it does not migrate from the gut. Heavy infestation may lead to abdominal symptoms such as tenesmus and rectal bleeding as a result of mucosal penetration or occasionally to intestinal obstruction. Worms are sometimes found in the appendix at appendicectomy.

Hookworm larvae penetrate the skin and also migrate via the lungs. The adult worms such as *Ancylostoma duodenale* and

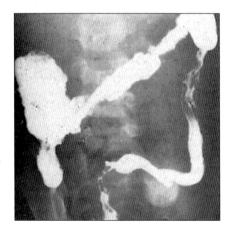

8.115 Amoebic colitis. This barium enema performed during the recovery phase of fulminating amoebic colitis shows extensive strictures and areas of mucosal damage in the colon. It is essential that these are not misdiagnosed as inflammatory bowel disease or tumours. Stool examination, colonoscopy and biopsy may all be helpful in diagnosis.

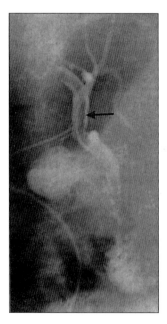

8.116 Partial common bile duct obstruction caused by a roundworm (arrow). The worm was revealed by T-tube cholangiography performed after cholecystectomy in this patient who had complained of right upper quadrant pain and dark urine. Gallstones were present, but her obstructive symptoms may well have been caused by the worm.

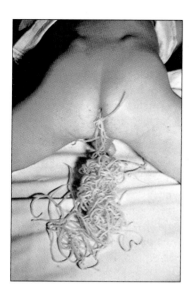

8.117 Massive *Ascaris* infection in a child has been successfully treated by anthelminthic treatment. This bolus of roundworms had caused obstructive symptoms.

liver to the bile ducts. Here they may cause biliary obstruction, hepatitis and – in the long term – portal cirrhosis.

Opisthorchis sinensis (the Chinese liver fluke) is transmitted via snails and freshwater fish, and may produce similar hepatic damage (**8.118**, **8.119**) and ultimately cholangiocarcinoma (*see* **p. 396**).

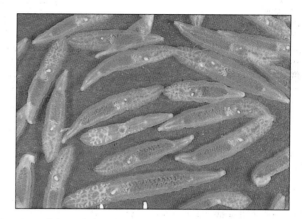

8.118 Adult *Opisthorchis sinensis*. The young worms migrate up the common bile duct to the liver. At maturity, they may reach 2 cm in length.

Necator americanus are an important cause of anaemia in many developing countries (*see* **p. 410, 10.17**).

Strongyloides stercoralis infestation resembles hookworm infestation in some respects, but the worms can have a free-living cycle in the soil. In humans, the eggs hatch into larvae in the intestine; the larvae can mature into filariform worms and cause autoinfection by direct penetration from the gut. Larva migrans may occur (**1.165**). Systemic invasion is of particular importance in immunosuppressed patients: in those with HIV, for example, hyperinfection by this route may result in severe disease of the lungs, heart, liver, kidneys and nervous system. Patients starting treatment with corticosteroids or other immunosuppressive drugs are also at risk of these complications. Thiabendazole and mebendazole are the drugs of choice in treatment.

Other roundworm infestations are covered on **pages 51–54**.

FLATWORMS

Flatworm (Trematoda) infestations include schistosomiasis (*see* **p. 54**) and paragonimiasis (*see* **p. 55**).

Fasciolopsis buski is the most important intestinal fluke. It occurs in the Far East, has an intermediate water snail host, and is transmitted via metacercariae on edible water plants such as water chestnuts. Severe infestation may result in abdominal pain, malabsorption, diarrhoea and even obstruction as a result of the attachment of flukes to the intestinal mucosa. Preventive measures involve eradication of the intermediate host and education of affected populations. Treatment with praziquantel or niclosamide is usually effective.

Fasciola hepatica and other liver flukes are also transmitted via water snails and edible water plants such as watercress. Infection occurs worldwide, mainly in sheep-rearing areas (sheep and cattle are the primary hosts). Ingested larvae migrate across the duodenal wall, and via the peritoneal cavity and the

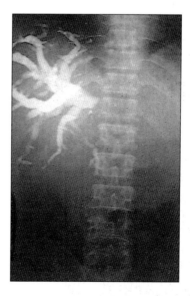

8.119 Chinese liver fluke infestation. This cholangiogram shows dilatation of the main bile ducts and disorganization of the biliary tree (secondary sclerosing cholangitis), resulting from the presence of multiple adult *Opisthorchis sinensis* (which cannot be seen on the film).

TAPEWORMS

Tapeworms include *Taenia saginata* from beef and *T. solium* from pork. Infestation occurs with the ingestion of infected and inadequately cooked meat containing viable cysts that develop in the human intestine. There may be no symptoms, but occasionally tapeworms may cause abdominal discomfort, diarrhoea or 'hunger pains'. The patient may notice proglottids in the faeces. Treatment with niclosamide or alternative drugs is effective (**8.120**).

T. solium is important because humans can be affected by the larval stage. The larvae may penetrate the intestinal wall, enter the circulation and migrate to the brain, lungs, eyes, muscle and connective tissue to cause cysticercosis. Serious neurological symptoms may result if the brain is affected, and these may worsen when the cysticerci die and calcify. Radiology, CT scanning (**8.121**) and MRI are of value in locating cysts. Treatment with praziquantel may be helpful, but surgery may be needed and neurological or ophthalmological damage may be irreversible.

Diphyllobothrium latum, the fish tapeworm, is a rare cause of vitamin B$_{12}$ deficiency, and may provoke megaloblastic anaemia in individuals who are genetically predisposed to the condition.

Humans may act as an intermediate host for the dog tapeworm (*Echinococcus granulosus*) and develop cysts – hydatid disease (*see* **p. 56**). The intestinal tract is not affected in this 'dead-end' infestation.

Various other tapeworm species may occasionally infest humans, and the larval forms of some may also invade directly, producing sparganosis (*see* **p. 56**).

IRRITABLE BOWEL SYNDROME

The irritable bowel syndrome (IBS) is probably the most common intestinal disease in clinical practice in the developed world, but it is one of the most poorly understood. It may affect up to 20% of otherwise healthy individuals, and is the underlying problem in up to 50% of referrals to specialist gastrointestinal clinics. It is a functional disease in which intestinal motility may be increased or decreased. The most common symptom is abdominal pain, and this is often accompanied by variable diarrhoea or constipation, or both. The symptoms may be exaggerated during times of stress. Patients may gain symptomatic relief from passing gas and from defaecation. Despite this, they often feel their bowels have not emptied completely and may pass small motions several or many times a day. The stool is often compressed and ribbon-like. Patients with constipation often abuse purgatives, and may present with diarrhoea for this reason. Recently agreed criteria for the diagnosis of IBS are summarized in **8.122**. Examination reveals very little except vague abdominal tenderness. Rectal examination is normal. Colonoscopy and barium enema are indicated when the patient has rectal bleeding, signs of organic disease, persistent diarrhoea or progressive symptoms, or the first presentation is above the age of 50 years. Otherwise these investigations are not required; when performed to exclude other pathology, they are normal (**8.123**). There is no specific treatment, but patients should be reassured and may benefit from a high-fibre diet, other dietary manipulation, an antispasmodic and psychological support.

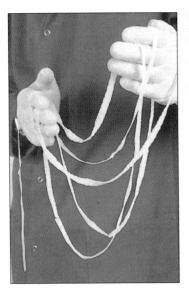

8.120 Adult *Taenia saginata* tapeworm. This is only part of a worm that was passed after treatment with niclosamide. *T. saginata* can grow to 10 m or more in length.

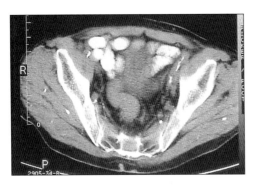

8.121 Cysticercosis. Pelvic CT scan shows numerous fusiform calcific opacities in the gluteal muscles, typical of cysticercosis. Similar opacities in the brain may have serious neurological implications.

CRITERIA FOR THE DIAGNOSIS OF IRRITABLE BOWEL SYNDROME (THE ROME CRITERIA)

At least 3 months of continuous or recurrent symptoms of:

- abdominal pain, relieved by defaecation or associated with a change in frequency and/or consistency of stool

- and/or disturbed defaecation – two or more of

    (a) altered stool frequency (> 3 movements/day or < 3/week)

    (b) altered stool form (hard, or loose and watery)

    (c) altered stool passage (straining or urgency, feeling of incomplete evacuation)

    (d) passage of mucus

- usually with bloating or feeling of abdominal distension

8.122 Criteria for the diagnosis of irritable bowel syndrome (the 'Rome' criteria).

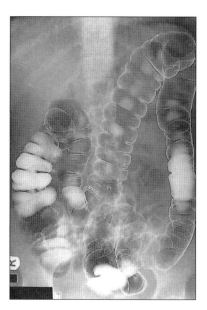

8.123 A normal barium enema, as seen in the irritable bowel syndrome (IBS). The investigation is not always necessary, but may sometimes be needed to exclude other causes of abdominal symptoms or change in bowel habit. Colonoscopy also reveals no abnormal findings in IBS.

FOOD ALLERGY AND FOOD INTOLERANCE

A number of symptoms and syndromes can be clearly related to food and food additives (**8.124**). Both gastrointestinal and remote disorders may result from food intolerance in a number of ways, most of which do not directly involve allergic or immunological reactions (**8.125**). Even if immunological abnormalities or allergic reactions have been demonstrated clearly – as, for example, in gluten-sensitive enteropathy – it is often not clear whether these are involved in the primary disease process, or whether they are simply a secondary consequence of other initiating factors. The patient will often suspect an association, but when the food is part of the everyday diet, the association may be less obvious. The possibility of food intolerance should be considered in all patients with:

- urticaria and angioedema
- atopic eczema
- migraine
- asthma
- rhinitis.

SYMPTOMS AND SYNDROMES THAT MAY BE RELATED TO FOOD

Gastrointestinal symptoms	Swelling of lips or mouth Oral ulceration Vomiting Diarrhoea Abdominal pain Bloating Constipation Pruritus ani
Secondary symptoms	Steatorrhoea and 'coeliac-like syndromes' Protein-losing enteropathy Blood loss and anaemia (rare) Eosinophilic gastroenteritis
Remote effects	Anaphylaxis Rhinitis Nasal polyps Asthma Eczema Urticaria and angioedema Dermatitis herpetiformis Transitory joint pains Migraine Hyperactivity in children (food association very rare) Henoch–Schönlein purpura (rare) Nephrotic syndrome (rare)

8.124 Symptoms and syndromes that may be related to food.

CAUSES OF FOOD INTOLERANCE

Pharmacological
- Caffeine
- Tyramine – e.g. in cheese
- Histamine – e.g. in fish and canned foods
- Histamine liberators – e.g. egg white, strawberries
- Nitrates – e.g. in preserved meat

Toxic
- Irritants of the intestinal mucosa – e.g. peppers and spices
- Poisons – e.g. from tropical sea fish; acetanilide in rape-seed oil; aflatoxin in mouldy peanuts

Idiosyncrasy
- Deficiency of enzymes e.g. lactase (cow's milk intolerance) and possibly phenolsulphotransferase (some cases of dietary migraine)

Indirect associations
- Fat intolerance caused by gall bladder disease, cystic fibrosis or steatorrhoea
- Intolerance to fried or spiced foods in peptic ulceration
- Irritable bowel syndrome (possible effects of fermentation of unabsorbed food residues)

Food allergic disease
- IgE-mediated – usually associated with other allergies
- Other immunological abnormalities – e.g. coeliac disease, cow's milk and soya protein intolerance in infants

8.125 Causes of food intolerance.

In some patients with nasal polyps and/or asthma, intolerance to aspirin may also be present.

The manifestations of food intolerance may be immediate or delayed. Symptoms such as angioedema (swelling of lips and tongue, **8.126**), urticaria (*see* **p. 75**), anaphylaxis (*see* **p. 168**),vomiting, rhinorrhoea and asthma often develop within minutes as a result of an IgE-mediated reaction or a direct pharmacological effect. In these circumstances, the provoking food is often obvious, as, for example, in most patients with the increasingly common problem of allergy to peanuts. Late reactions may develop some hours or even days after ingestion of food, possibly as a result of a delayed immune response involving circulating immune complexes. Such late reactions pose a particularly difficult diagnostic problem, because:

- there are no reliable laboratory tests for food allergy or idiosyncracy
- skin-prick testing with a few food extracts such as egg, fish, nuts and yeast gives results that correlate well with clinical symptoms, but positive results tend to persist even when clinical sensitivity has been lost
- serum IgE may be raised in an allergic response, but this does not demonstrate that the responsible antigen entered via the gut
- radioallergosorbent tests (RASTs) for specific IgE antibodies may sometimes demonstrate raised circulating antibody levels to specific foods, but for most of the food extracts used the correlation with symptoms is poor
- 'fringe' techniques, such as sublingual or cytotoxic food sensitivity tests, hair analysis, etc., are widely advertised but valueless.

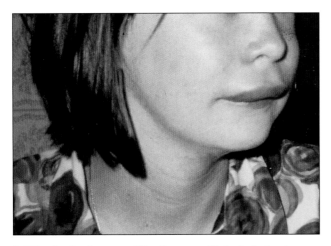

8.126 Angioedema resulting from sensitivity to tartrazine. This girl had recurrent, severe angioedema and urticaria, with episodes of life-threatening laryngeal oedema. An exclusion diet showed tartrazine (E102) to be the cause of her symptoms. This food colouring is widely used in many processed foods and drinks, so a rigorous maintenance exclusion diet is required to prevent symptoms. The mechanism of tartrazine sensitivity is unclear, and it may not have an allergic basis. Cross-sensitivity with other azo dyes, salicylates (including aspirin) and benzoates is common.

A diagnostic exclusion diet, followed by appropriate food challenge, is the mainstay of investigation, but the difficulty of adhering to and interpreting such a diet should be considered before embarking on this course. Appropriate exclusion diets are summarized in **8.127**.

Treatment involves prevention by avoidance of ingestion of provoking foods whenever possible. Problems such as urticaria, eczema, migraine, asthma and rhinitis should also be treated with appropriate therapy. Food avoidance alone is only rarely curative. Patients who are known to be at risk of anaphylaxis (for example, many patients with allergy to peanuts) should be provided with appropriate training and a syringe of adrenaline (epinephrine) for self-administration in an emergency (*see* **p. 168**).

DIAGNOSTIC EXCLUSION DIETS APPROPRIATE FOR POSSIBLY FOOD-RELATED SYMPTOMS*	
Condition	**Diagnostic diet**
Urticaria or angioedema	Tartrazine, salicylate and benzoate free
Eczema	Cow's milk and egg free
Coeliac disease	Gluten free
Dermatitis herpetiformis	Gluten free
Cow's milk sensitive enteropathy	Cow's milk free
Asthma and rhinitis	Full exclusion
Migraine	Full exclusion
Irritable bowel syndrome	Full exclusion

* *A full exclusion diet should be tried if a more specific diet is unsuccessful*

8.127 Diagnostic exclusion diets appropriate for possibly food-related symptoms.

GASTROINTESTINAL HORMONE-PRODUCING TUMOURS

The gastrointestinal tract contains the largest mass of endocrine cells in the body. The hormones produced in the gut and pancreas include gastrin, cholecystokinin (CCK), vasoactive intestinal polypeptide (VIP), somatostatin, enteroglucagon, secretin, insulin, glucagon, gastric inhibitory peptide, motilin, substance P, neurotensin, pancreatic polypeptide, enkephalin and endorphins, bombesin and other peptides.

Pancreatic endocrine tumours are rare. The Zollinger–Ellison syndrome is caused by a gastrin-secreting tumour (a gastrinoma); 85% of these arise in the pancreas (*see* **p. 355**). Appropriately two-thirds are sporadic, whereas one-third form part of the multiple endocrine neoplasia (MEN) type 1 syndrome (*see* **p. 304**). The major symptoms are caused by hyperacidity, which causes multiple duodenal and even jejunal peptic ulceration. High gastrin levels and hypertrophied gastric folds suggest the diagnosis. Treatment with a proton pump inhibitor is effective, but the tumours should ideally be removed, as 60% are malignant.

Verner–Morrison syndrome and VIPomas present with chronic profuse watery diarrhoea leading to hypokalaemia, hypochlorhydria, dehydration and flushing. Treatment of the symptoms by corticosteroids, metoclopramide, indometacin and opiates has limited effects, whereas somatostatin analogues appear to be useful, particularly if the tumour is inoperable.

The glucagonoma syndrome is usually caused by a malignant pancreatic tumour, and patients have a characteristic rash. The skin lesions (necrolytic migratory erythema) start as erythematous areas that become raised with superficial central blistering and rupture to leave crusts (**8.128**). They tend to heal from the centre leaving increased pigmentation. Diagnosis is based on clinical suspicion in patients with the rash, weight loss, glucose intolerance and often thromboembolic complications, combined with a plasma glucagon level above 300 pmol/litre. Treatment is by tumour removal and the rash may improve with oxytetracycline, steroids or zinc.

Somatostatinoma has been described in about 20 cases. Most were malignant pancreatic tumours occurring in patients with mild diabetes and gall bladder disease. Tumours secreting other gastrointestinal hormones have been described, particularly pancreatic polypeptide, but all are exceedingly rare, with the exception of insulinomas; patients with the latter present with hypoglycaemia.

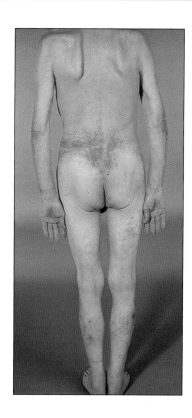

8.128 Glucagonoma syndrome is usually associated with a characteristic rash, the cause of which is obscure. The rash evolves through stages of erythema, blistering and crusting, and may ultimately be much more severe than in this patient. Note the accompanying weight loss.

9 Liver and pancreas

HISTORY

Many patients have asymptomatic liver disease which is found incidentally as hepatosplenomegaly on routine examination, positive hepatitis serology after blood donation, abnormal liver biochemistry on routine screening, or abnormal haematology (high mean cell volume or low platelets) or positive autoantibodies in patients presenting with other problems. Acute liver disease may present dramatically, however, with acute anorexia, nausea and vomiting. There may be intolerance to the sight and smell of food, to alcohol and to cigarette smoke. An intense itch may develop in the skin and this may precede the development of jaundice, which may be noticed by the family before the patient. As jaundice appears, other symptoms may disappear. The patient may now notice dark urine and pale stools. There may now be right-sided abdominal discomfort caused by an enlarged or inflamed liver, or by an obstructed biliary tree.

Complications of liver disease include liver cell failure and portal hypertension. Hepatic encephalopathy tends to develop insidiously as liver cells fail, and a history of mood change, confusion and somnolence is often obtained from the family. Portal hypertension may be associated with a history of abdominal swelling and peripheral oedema, but the patient may become aware of this only when they have difficulty in putting on their shoes or trousers. Gastrointestinal blood loss may indicate the presence of oesophageal varices or reflect a coagulation defect caused by liver disease or associated thrombocytopenia. Key symptoms in liver disease are summarized in **9.1**.

It is important in the history to ask about:

- previous jaundice and its duration – hepatitis or gallstones
- previous biliary tract surgery
- recent drug therapy – including self-administered drugs, recreational drugs, drug misuse and herbal remedies
- alcohol intake
- close contact with a jaundiced person or someone in a high-risk group
- recent blood transfusion, injections or needle stick injury
- sexual activity and proclivity
- occupation – health professional, farmer, sewer worker
- family history of liver disease
- foreign travel – timing and location
- recent eating of shellfish, salads, etc. in risk areas of the world
- hobbies – canoeing, swimming, other watersports.

EXAMINATION

The diversity of signs in liver disease (**9.1**) reflects the key role that the liver plays in homeostasis.

Jaundice is a frequent sign, and it can be detected clinically when the serum bilirubin level rises above 50 µmol/litre:

- In haemolytic states the pigment circulates attached to albumin and does not appear in the urine – it usually imparts a pale yellow colour to the skin and sclerae (**9.2**).
- In hepatocellular and obstructive jaundice the conjugated bilirubin accumulates to very high levels and may give a much darker colour to the skin and sclerae, which may become orange or greenish in colour (**9.3–9.5**).

375

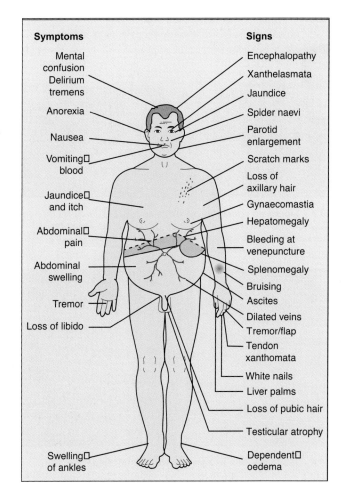

Symptoms	Signs
Mental confusion	Encephalopathy
Delirium tremens	Xanthelasmata
	Jaundice
Anorexia	Spider naevi
Nausea	Parotid enlargement
Vomiting blood	Scratch marks
Jaundice and itch	Loss of axillary hair
	Gynaecomastia
Abdominal pain	Hepatomegaly
Abdominal swelling	Bleeding at venepuncture
	Splenomegaly
Tremor	Bruising
Loss of libido	Ascites
	Dilated veins
	Tremor/flap
	Tendon xanthomata
	White nails
	Liver palms
	Loss of pubic hair
	Testicular atrophy
Swelling of ankles	Dependent oedema

9.1 **Common symptoms and signs in liver disease.**

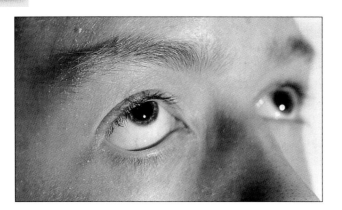

9.2 Haemolytic jaundice in a young man, who was subsequently found to have a lymphoma. The skin and sclerae have a pale lemon-yellow tinge, due to the elevation in unconjugated bilirubin.

Other yellow pigmentation of skin, which may mimic jaundice, follows mepacrine ingestion or the excessive ingestion of carotenes, but these do not colour the sclerae. Pruritus may result from retained bile salts in cholestatic disorders, and it may appear before the onset of frank jaundice. Scratch marks may be present in accessible skin areas (**9.6**).

In obstructive jaundice, the stool is pale in colour, because of the lack of bile pigments and the presence of steatorrhoea. In haemolytic jaundice, the stool is dark. The urine is dark in obstructive and hepatocellular jaundice, as a result of conjugated bile pigments; whereas in haemolytic jaundice, no bile pigment is present but there is an excess of urobilinogen, which may darken on standing.

A variety of signs may result from the failure of the liver to metabolize oestrogens:

- Spider naevi, which are usually found in the upper part of the body, above the nipple line, especially in areas exposed to sunlight (**9.7–9.9**); healthy people, especially women during pregnancy and patients on oestrogen therapy, may have one or two spider naevi, but a larger number is strongly suggestive of liver disease.
- Gynaecomastia is commonly seen in men with chronic liver disease (**9.4, 9.10**), though there are many other possible causes (**9.11**). It is important to differentiate gynaecomastia from obesity by feeling for breast tissue around the nipple.
- Palmar erythema is a red flushing on the thenar and hypothenar eminences (**9.12**). This is common but not specific to liver disease. Similar changes may also be found in the soles of the feet.

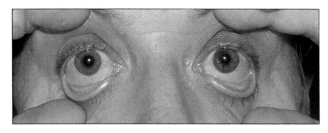

9.3 Jaundiced sclerae in a patient with hepatitis A. Mild jaundice is often most evident in the sclerae, and may be unaccompanied by obvious jaundice in the skin.

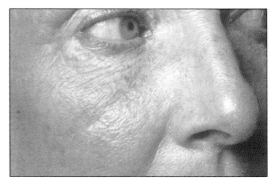

9.5 Severe cholestatic jaundice in a patient with primary biliary cirrhosis (PBC). The high level of conjugated bilirubin, maintained over a long period, gives a characteristic dark brown–orange pigmentation to the skin and sclerae. Patients with PBC usually develop large xanthelasmata and corneal arcus as a consequence of disordered lipid metabolism.

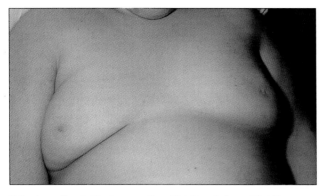

9.4 Jaundiced skin in a youth with chronic hepatitis. The jaundice results from an elevated level of conjugated bilirubin, which produces a deeper yellow colour than unconjugated bilirubin. Note the associated gynaecomastia.

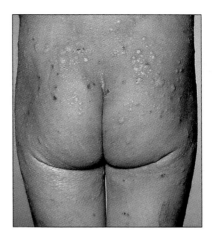

9.6 Scratch marks associated with severe pruritus, and eruptive xanthomas, in a child with intrahepatic cholestasis resulting from biliary atresia.

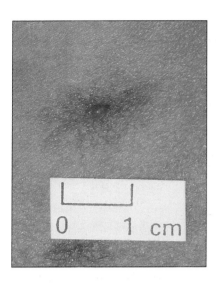

9.7 A typical spider naevus consists of a central spiral arteriole, which supplies a radiating group of small vessels. This spider naevus is of typical size, though larger and smaller examples may occur.

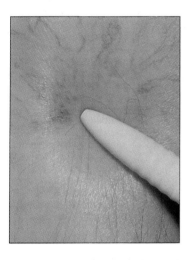

9.8 The spider naevus blanches if the central spiral arteriole is occluded by pressure, demonstrating that this is the single source of its blood supply.

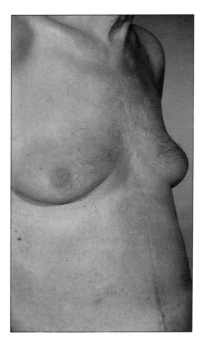

9.10 Gynaecomastia in a male patient. This patient had cirrhosis, and a hepatocellular carcinoma.

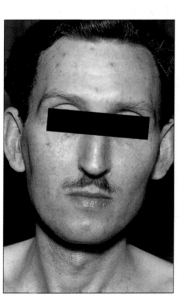

9.9 Spider naevi. This barman had alcoholic cirrhosis, accompanied by multiple spider naevi on the head and neck. The occurrence of a large number of spider naevi points strongly to underlying liver disease, though occasional spiders may be found in normal people.

CAUSES OF GYNAECOMASTIA		
Physiological	Neonatal	
	Pubertal	
	Old age	
Drugs	Oestrogenic	
	– oestrogens	
	– digitalis	
	– cannabis	
	– diamorphine (heroin)	
	Anti-androgens	
	– spironolactone	
	– cimetidine	
	– cyproterone	
	Others	
	– gonadotrophins	
	– cytotoxics	
Liver failure		
Hyperthyroidism		
Starvation and refeeding		
Human chorionic gonadotrophin-producing tumours (testis, lung)		
Oestrogen-producing tumours (testis, adrenal)		

9.11 Causes of gynaecomastia.

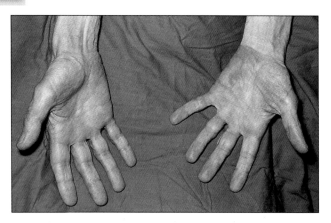

9.12   Palmar erythema is a common finding in chronic liver disease, but is also found in pregnancy, during oral contraceptive use, in rheumatoid arthritis and in thyrotoxicosis. It may also occur without apparent cause. It is usually particularly marked on the thenar and hypothenar eminences.

- Loss of body hair, including pubic and axillary hair, and testicular atrophy are also common (**9.13**).

A range of other signs develops with long-standing liver dysfunction:

- Finger clubbing (**2.104**, **2.105**) is a common feature of liver disease and may also involve the toes; it is non-specific, being also found in respiratory, cardiac, alimentary and endocrine diseases.
- White nails (**2.102**): the cause is unknown but their whiteness mirrors the severity of the liver disease. White nails are also found in other conditions in which the serum albumin is low (e.g. nephrotic syndrome, malnutrition).
- Spontaneous bruising and excessive bleeding (**9.14**) are a reflection of the failure of the liver to synthesize coagulation factors II, VII, IX and X, often compounded by the failure to absorb vitamin K, as a result of retention of bile salts.
- Xanthelasmata (**7.106**, **9.5**) develop as a result of long-standing cholestasis and hyperlipidaemia, and are a common feature of primary biliary cirrhosis; they develop in the soft tissues of the upper and lower lids. Xanthomas may also appear in other skin areas (**7.109**, **7.110**, **9.6**) and in tendons (**7.111**, **7.112**).
- Hepatomegaly (**9.15**) is frequently found in liver diseases, particularly if the liver is infiltrated with carcinoma or fat, in cirrhosis, in some chronic infections (e.g. **1.168**) and in some metabolic disorders. The liver may be abnormally firm, and localized masses or nodules may be felt. The liver may also be tender, especially if the enlargement is caused by inflammation or venous congestion. It is important to be aware of the anatomical variants of the normal liver, especially of Riedel's lobe. The upper border of the liver may be pushed down into the abdomen by an extreme degree of emphysema, giving a misleading impression of hepatomegaly.

- Ascites (**8.10**, **9.13**) is the accumulation of free fluid in the peritoneal cavity. The most common cause of ascites is the onset of liver failure, with resulting hypoalbuminaemia and portal hypertension. The differential diagnosis includes malignancy (primary or secondary), nephrotic syndrome, malnutrition causing protein deficiency, right heart failure from any cause (especially constrictive pericarditis), chronic infection such as tuberculosis and hypothyroidism. The mechanism is complex: low serum albumin, prostaglandins, atrial natriuretic factor, secondary hyperaldosteronism and venous pressure all play a role. The diagnosis is usually obvious if the condition is gross, but it should be differentiated from other causes of abdominal swelling (fat, fluid, flatus, faeces, fetus, fibroids, etc.). Peripheral oedema

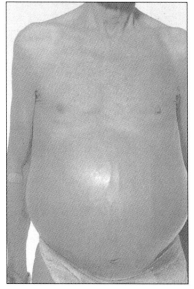

9.13   Severe ascites in a patient with hepatocellular carcinoma. The accumulation of fluid within the peritoneal cavity has led to gross abdominal distension with downward displacement and eversion of the umbilicus. Note the presence of distended veins in the abdominal wall. The flow in these veins was away from the umbilicus, and the underlying diagnosis was alcoholic cirrhosis. Note the absence of body hair in this patient – another sign of chronic liver disease.

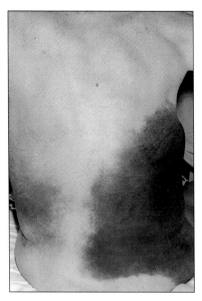

9.14   Spontaneous bruising in a patient with cirrhosis. Disturbance of coagulation mechanisms is a common problem in chronic liver disease, and the risk of excessive bleeding should always be assessed by coagulation studies before liver biopsy or other operative procedures. Similar bruising can result from uncontrolled anticoagulant therapy (see **p. 441**).

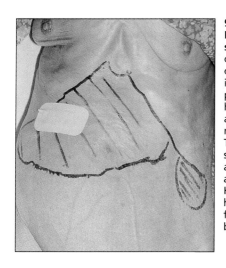

**9.15
Hepatomegaly and splenomegaly** commonly coexist in chronic liver disease in the presence of portal hypertension; hepatomegaly may also occur alone in many liver disorders. This patient shows signs of weight loss, and has dilated abdominal veins. Her hepatomegaly has just been further investigated by CT-guided biopsy.

is a common accompaniment of ascites and is gravitational. There may also be bilateral hydrothorax.

- Splenomegaly (**9.15**), often the result of a rise in portal venous pressure, may be associated with the primary liver pathology and may occur in haematological (**10.54**, **10.89**), infective (**1.146**, **1.149**, **1.168**) or metabolic disorders (**10.63**); the spleen must be differentiated from the left kidney by palpation and percussion.
- Superficial veins may often be seen on the abdominal wall surface; these may originate from the umbilicus, representing a communication from the portal to systemic circulations (caput medusae); the blood flow is from the umbilicus outwards (**9.13**). Large veins may also be found running from the inguinal region to the chest wall; the blood flow is usually upwards, implying blockage of the inferior vena cava (**9.54**).
- Weight loss is common in patients with liver dysfunction; limb size is often in stark contrast to the swollen abdomen.
- Encephalopathy is an acute or chronic neurological impairment that may result from liver cell failure associated with shunting of blood from the portal system; it is probably caused by the failure of the liver to detoxify some as yet unidentified component in the portal blood. There is progressive impairment of higher cerebral function, with eventual coma and death. Early features suggesting encephalopathy include fetor hepaticus – a sweet apple-like smell on the breath – a coarse flapping tremor and an inability to draw or write accurately. A clinical test to monitor changes in status is the patient's signature (with date) on the casesheet.

INVESTIGATIONS

Investigations are of value in defining the cause of liver disease, the extent of damage and the effects of treatment. They should be used selectively:

- **Urinalysis:** in obstructive jaundice the urine is dark orange in colour and, as obstruction deepens, it may develop a greenish tinge; it gives a positive test for bile and a negative test for urobilinogen; in haemolytic jaundice, the urine may be normal in colour but darken on standing; tests for bile are negative and tests for urobilinogen are positive; in compensated cirrhosis, there is no bile in the urine, but tests for urobilinogen are usually positive because of failure of the liver cells to cope with the normally reabsorbed amount of urobilinogen.
- **Stools:** the pallor of the stools depends on the degree of biliary obstruction and is associated with a degree of steatorrhoea as the bile salts are not excreted; the stool in haemolysis is dark in colour because of the increased levels of stercobilin; a positive faecal occult blood test is of value in detecting carcinoma of the ampulla of Vater, upper GI varices and also primary alimentary lesions that may have produced hepatic secondaries.
- **Full blood count** is of value in detecting anaemia – often iron deficient because of bleeding from oesophageal varices; macrocytosis is often found in alcoholic liver disease and with biliary obstruction and may not reflect vitamin B_{12} deficiency (B_{12} levels may be elevated if there is hepatic cell necrosis); folate levels are often low, caused by a combination of malabsorption and poor dietary intake; thrombocytopenia is often present, because of a combination of factors that may include the direct effects of alcohol on the bone marrow, secondary hypersplenism, disseminated intravascular coagulation and marrow aplasia in acute fulminant hepatitis, and folate deficiency.
- **Coagulation abnormalities** are common and often complex, as the liver makes most coagulation factors and destroys others. Correct investigation often requires expert haematological advice; tests should include the activated partial thromboplastin time (APPT), the prothrombin time (PT), the thrombin time (TT), whole blood platelet count and simple tests of fibrinolysis such as measurement of fibrinogen – fibrin degradation products (FDPs).
- **Routine biochemistry** is the keystone of diagnosis and assessment of progress. Tests should include total bilirubin, with direct and indirect values as necessary, alkaline phosphatase, the aminotransferases (especially alanine aminotransferase, ALT), γ-glutamyl transpeptidase, total proteins, albumin and γ-globulins; none of these tests is specific or diagnostic, but all are of value in combination and in following the course of the disease. Two broad patterns of liver function tests may emerge: cholestatic and hepatitic (**9.16**). Measurement of serum iron, total iron binding capacity, per cent saturation and ferritin level are of value when looking for haemochromatosis; a low serum iron and ferritin may be found in chronic blood loss states, such as after bleeding from oesophageal varices or neoplasia; serum albumin measures the synthetic capacity of the liver generally.
- **The α-fetoprotein level** is elevated in most primary hepatocellular carcinomas and is of value as a diagnostic and prognostic test.

Cholestatic

There is a marked elevation of alkaline phosphatase and γ-glutamyl transpeptidase (γ-GT) with a smaller rise in aspartate transaminase (AST) and alanine transaminase (ALT). These tests do not differentiate between intrahepatic and extrahepatic obstruction – this is best done by ultrasound. Causes of cholestasis include:

Extrahepatic

Gallstone(s) in common bile duct

Cholangiocarcinoma

Bile duct strictures

Extrinsic masses compressing ducts

Sclerosing cholangitis

Carcinoma of ampulla of Vater

Carcinoma of head of pancreas

Intrahepatic

Hepatitis

Drugs

Primary biliary cirrhosis

Hepatitic

There is a marked elevation of ALT, AST and γ-GT, but not of alkaline phosphatase. The causes are:

Virus infection – hepatitis A, B, C, D, E, cytomegalovirus, Epstein–Barr virus

Alcohol or drugs or both

Metabolic – haemochromatosis, Wilson's disease, α_1-antitrypsin deficiency

Autoimmune – chronic active hepatitis

9.16   Cholestatic versus hepatitic liver function tests.

- **Levels of viral markers** are a pointer to infection, and sequential samples provide evidence of the course of the disease.
- **Autoantibodies:** some immunological disorders are associated with liver disease; primary biliary cirrhosis is associated with the presence of anti-mitochondrial antibodies; different forms of autoimmune hepatitis are associated with different autoantibodies (*see* **p. 389**); diseases such as systemic lupus erythematosus (**p. 121**), rheumatoid arthritis (**p. 107**), dermatomyositis (**p. 125**) and CRST syndrome (**p. 124**) have specific immune abnormalities.

Imaging investigations are often useful in disorders of the liver, pancreas and biliary tract:

- **Plain X-rays** of the right upper quadrant are of little value unless lesions are calcified or contain air. About 10% of gallstones are radio-opaque (**9.17**), cysts of liver and pancreas may calcify, there may be generalized pancreatic calcification (**9.69, 9.70**), and the soft-tissue shadow of the spleen, or air in the biliary tree or under the diaphragm (**8.65**), may be seen. X-ray of the chest may show an elevated diaphragm caused by subphrenic pus or a paralysed diaphragm, or there may be a 'sympathetic' pleural effusion or empyema.
- **Cholecystogram, intravenous cholangiography and T-tube cholangiography** involve the administration of a contrast medium to outline, respectively, the gall bladder, hepatic ducts, and the hepatic ducts after surgery. These investigations have largely been superseded by other imaging techniques.
- **Endoscopic retrograde cholangiopancreatography (ERCP)** is an endoscopic technique in which the ampulla of Vater is examined (**9.18**) and cannulated, and contrast medium is injected to outline the biliary tree and pancreatic ducts (**9.19, 9.50, 9.51**); it is of value in detecting and removing stones impacted in the lower biliary tree; pancreatitis and ascending cholangitis are potential complications.
- **Magnetic resonance cholangiopancreatography (MRCP)** is a non-invasive method of imaging the biliary tree and pancreatic ducts (**9.20**), which avoids the potential comlications of ERCP.

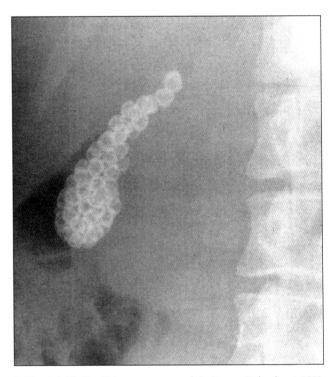

9.17   Calcified gallstones seen on plain X-ray. Only about 10% of gallstones contain enough calcium to be visible on the plain film. This patient had had remarkably few symptoms before the incidental discovery of her gallstones.

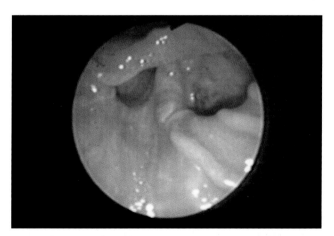

9.18 Duodenoscopy with a side-viewing endoscope is an essential preliminary to common bile duct cannulation and endoscopic retrograde cholangiopancreatography (ERCP). It may also reveal abnormalities in the duodenum or the ampulla of Vater. Here, a normal ampulla (centre of picture) is flanked by two duodenal diverticula. These abnormalities are found in 10–15% of patients endoscoped, and are usually of no clinical significance; but large duodenal diverticula may be associated with symptoms due to bacterial overgrowth (*see* **p. 357**).

- **Percutaneous transhepatic cholangiography (PTC)** involves passing a needle under anaesthesia towards the hilum of the liver in patients with obstructive jaundice under radiological control. Contrast medium can then be injected to show the site of blockage (**9.59**). PTC has been largely superseded by ERCP and MRCP but is still useful when the common bile duct cannot be cannulated or is completely obstructed.
- **Ultrasound** is a simple, easily repeatable, non-invasive test which is now widely used for imaging of the liver, bile ducts and gall bladder; it is of proven worth in gallstone disease, malignant tumours (**9.21**), cysts, abscesses, haematomas and vascular malformations (**9.62**, **9.74**); it is invaluable in controlling and directing liver biopsies. The technique is sensitive for lesions down to approximately 5 mm in diameter.
- **CT (9.22) and MRI** are of major value in detecting intrahepatic lesions, regional lymph nodes, associated tumours, abnormalities of the pancreas, and lesions in the porta hepatis; they can also be used to locate sites for biopsies.
- **Angiography and portal venography:** selective angiography of the hepatic artery may reveal vascular tumours; the portal venous system can be imaged by digital subtraction angiograms and during the venous phase of mesenteric angiography.
- **Isotope scans:** intravenous injection of ^{99m}Tc sulphur colloid results in diffuse uptake of the isotope by the reticuloendothelial (RE) cells of the liver, spleen and bone marrow; the technique may show abnormalities in the

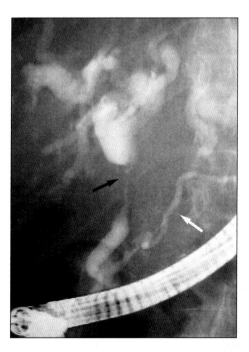

9.19 Endoscopic retrograde cholangiopancreatography (ERCP) is of great value in assessing and sometimes treating abnormalities in the biliary tree and pancreatic ducts. In this patient a cholangiocarcinoma is causing major obstruction of the common bile duct (black arrow). The biliary tree proximal to the obstruction is grossly dilated. The pancreatic duct is also filled with contrast medium (white arrow).

position of the liver and filling defects caused by space-occupying lesions, but has been largely superseded by ultrasound and CT.

- **Laparoscopy** allows direct visualization of the liver, pancreas and gall bladder, and is of value in assessing the presence and

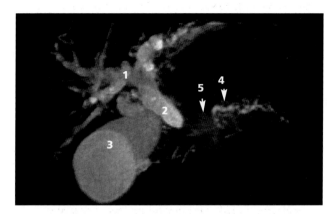

9.20 Magnetic resonance cholangiopancreatography (MRCP) is a non-invasive method of imaging the biliary tree and pancreatic ducts. In this patient, the dilated biliary tree (1), common bile duct (2) and gall bladder (3) are clearly seen, as is the dilated pancreatic duct (4). The cause was a carcinoma of the head of the pancreas (5), not shown by MRCP.

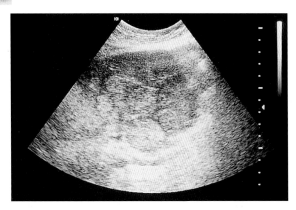

9.21   Ultrasound of liver showing multiple metastases from an unknown primary source. Ultrasound is now the routine initial imaging investigation for lesions of the liver and pancreas.

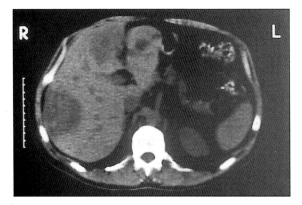

9.22   CT is of major value in the assessment of patients with many disorders of the liver and pancreas. This patient has multiple secondary tumour deposits of various sizes throughout the liver, which have contributed to marked hepatomegaly. The primary tumour was in the breast.

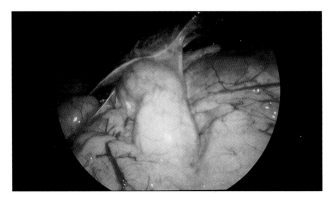

9.23   Laparoscopy is valuable in many disorders of the liver and biliary tract. This picture was taken immediately before laparoscopic cholecystectomy and shows an enlarged, turgid gall bladder. Above the gall bladder, the smooth lower border of a normal liver is clearly seen, and abnormalities in the liver can often be well visualized by this technique. Note also the loops of normal bowel to the right of the liver (left of picture) and the pylorus to its left.

Before undertaking liver biopsy, some safety precautions are necessary. These include:

- informed patient consent
- measurement of prothrombin time (PT not greater than 3 seconds over control)
- measurement of platelet count (platelet count should be above 100 x 10⁹/litre)
- there should be no evidence of dilated bile ducts nor any major degree of ascites
- the patient should be able to hold their breath for at least 20 seconds
- the patient should be cross-matched, with 2–4 units of blood immediately available for transfusion if necessary.

the extent of disease (**9.23**); biopsy under direct vision is possible, and surgery may be undertaken without laparotomy (keyhole surgery).
- **Electroencephalography (EEG)** is of value in determining the presence and severity of encephalopathy.
- **Liver biopsy** will often give the tissue diagnosis of a lesion; it may be done blind when the disease is diffuse, as in cirrhosis, or it may be performed under ultrasound or CT guidance. It is usually done percutaneously with a Menghini needle or a 'Tru-cut' needle (**6.25**), but may also be done at laparoscopy or laparotomy. Complications of needle biopsy of the liver include haemorrhage, tears in the liver capsule, bile leaks and pneumothorax. Tumour seeding may occur if a tumour is biopsied. In patients with a bleeding tendency, a transjugular catheter advanced through the hepatic vein allows multiple biopsies to be done without any bleeding outside the liver.

CLINICAL PRESENTATIONS OF LIVER DISEASE

CIRRHOSIS

Cirrhosis is a descriptive term for a liver in which there is a combination of abnormal fibrosis and nodular regeneration of liver cells (**9.24**). The balance between the two processes varies in different patients and in the same patient over time. The normal liver architecture is distorted, and the processes interfere with portal circulation, raising its pressure, opening up communications between the portal and systemic circulations and sometimes causing splenomegaly. Cirrhosis is the end result of a variety of pathological processes (**9.25**), the most common causes being viral hepatitis, alcohol and immunological and metabolic diseases.

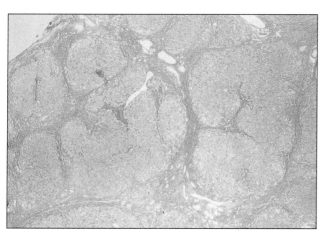

9.24 Cirrhosis. In this typical histopathological section, bands of fibrous tissue run between nodules of regenerated hepatocytes. Only some nodules contain a central vein, and the bile ducts and portal vessels run in the fibrous septa. These changes are associated with portal hypertension.

CAUSES OF CIRRHOSIS
Alcohol
Chronic viral hepatitis
Autoimmune hepatitis
Primary biliary cirrhosis
Primary and secondary sclerosing cholangitis
Cryptogenic (unknown)
Haemochromatosis
Hepatic vein obstruction
Wilson's disease
Drugs
α_1-antitrypsin deficiency
Cystic fibrosis
Galctosaemia or fructose intolerance
Veno-occlusive disease
Cardiac failure

9.25 Causes of cirrhosis.

The clinical features of cirrhosis are a result of portal hypertension and liver cell failure, and at different stages of the disorder may include any of the symptoms and signs shown in **9.1**. Initially, the liver may be normal in size or even enlarged; as cirrhosis progresses it usually becomes contracted and shrunken. Primary liver cell cancer is a potential complication of cirrhosis.

PORTAL HYPERTENSION

Portal hypertension may arise from obstruction in the portal vein before it reaches the liver (prehepatic), within the liver (intrahepatic) or between the liver and the inferior vena cava (posthepatic). A rise in pressure rapidly leads to the opening up of latent anastomoses between the systemic and portal venous systems, which are mainly to be found in the gastro-oesophageal region, in the rectum and at the umbilicus. Dilatation of these collaterals allows portal–systemic shunting and this may give rise to specific clinical problems. The spleen may be grossly enlarged.

Ascites may be gross (**9.13**). The first aim in its management is to create a net negative balance of sodium (dietary restrictions and diuretics). It is simple to monitor abdominal girth, weight, blood urea and electrolytes and 24-hour urinary sodium loss. Paracentesis is of value in excluding other diagnoses by biochemistry and cytology. It may also have a place in treatment in association with plasma expanders (e.g. albumin). Peritoneovenous shunts drain the ascitic fluid and return it into the venous system (**9.26**). Their long-term complications include infection and shunt obstruction.

Oesophageal varices lie in the submucosa of the lower oesophagus and are liable to rupture because of portal pressure and local trauma. Bleeding is also compounded by severe coagulation defects caused by liver cell failure. Haematemesis and melaena or chronic iron deficiency are the main presentations. Diagnosis is made by barium swallow or at endoscopy (**1.168, 9.27, 9.28**), and varices may also occur in the fundus of the stomach (**9.29**). Some endoscopic appearances are associated with a particularly high risk of bleeding (**9.28**). The mortality is high; after a first bleed from varices about one-half of the patients die within 6 weeks and each subsequent bleed carries a 30% mortality.

Emergency treatment of bleeding varices may be carried out by balloon tamponale with a Sengstaken–Blakemore or

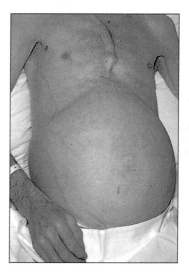

9.26 A peritoneovenous shunt in a patient with cirrhosis and severe ascites. The subcutaneous course of the valved shunt is clearly seen. Despite the presence of the shunt, which has helped to maintain his serum albumin level, this patient still has severe ascites.

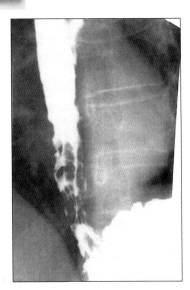

9.27 Oesophageal varices. A barium swallow, showing the typical appearance of multiple lower oesophageal varices, evident as barium-coated filling defects. In addition, gastric varices can be seen, along the lesser curvature of the stomach. These thin-walled varices are easily damaged, and bleeding is a frequent complication.

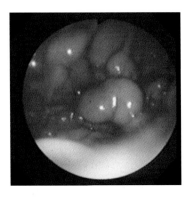

9.28 Oesophageal varices seen through the endoscope. Varices like these have been shown to have a relatively low risk of immediate bleeding, because they are covered with a thick layer of mucosa. The presence of red lines (red wale markings) or spots (cherry-red spots) is associated with a strong likelihood of bleeding.

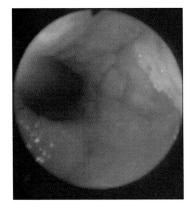

9.29 Varices may also occur in the gastric fundus in portal hypertension. In this patient the gastric varices (to the right of the picture) are above the diaphragm in a hiatus hernia. Portal hypertension may also lead to other changes in the stomach, including congestive gastropathy and 'watermelon' stomach, in which areas of erythematous and pale mucosa are intermingled.

Minnesota tube. Sclerotherapy, by direct injection (**9.30**), is of value in up to 90% of cases. There is a high complication rate (**20–25%**), mainly due to oesophageal ulceration and infection (**9.31**). Ligation of the base of the varix by application of a rubber band is also claimed to have a 90% success rate with fewer complications.

Vasopressin and its analogues (e.g terlipressin) reduces portal vein flow by provoking splanchnic vasoconstriction, but also affects other vessels. Risk to the coronary and cerebral circulation may be reduced by the simultaneous administration of glyceryl trinitrate. Somatostatin (or its synthetic analogue) has the same effects on portal vein flow but fewer side-effects. Portocaval anastomosis or the insertion of a transjugular intrahepatic portosystemic stent shunt (**9.32**) may lead to a dramatic reduction in portal vein pressure and in ascites. The most important problem is the potential for encephalopathy but this does not occur frequently. As a last resort the patient should be considered for liver transplantation.

Rectal anastomoses may become extremely large and bleed after bowel movements. Massive bleeding is extremely rare. Surgery is the treatment of choice.

Umbilical anastomoses are rarely clinically obvious. The anastomotic veins radiate from the umbilicus across the abdomen to join systemic veins, forming a 'caput medusae'. Lesser degrees of anastomosis are more common.

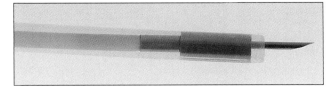

9.30 Injection sclerotherapy is commonly effective in the treatment of bleeding oesophageal varices. The needle is introduced through an endoscope, and retained within its protective sheath until it is applied to the surface of the varix. It is then used to inject sclerosant (usually ethanolamine or sodium tetradecyl sulphate) into the vein.

LIVER FAILURE

Liver failure can develop acutely in a previously normal liver (as in fulminant viral hepatitis or drug-induced hepatitis), or it may develop insidiously in a chronically damaged liver. Fluid retention is an early problem; patients present with ankle and

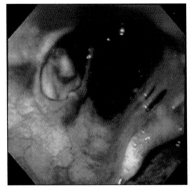

9.31 Oesophageal varices after treatment by scleropathy. The injection of a sclerosant via the endoscope results in local variceal thrombosis, followed by fibrosis and, often, mucosal ulceration. Definitive treatment (transjugular intrahepatic portosystemic stent shunt or portosystemic anastomosis) may subsequently be necessary.

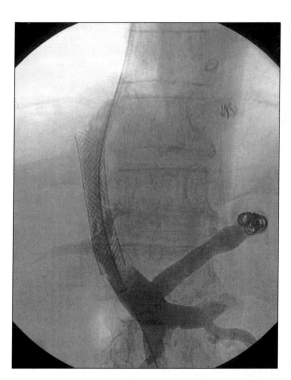

9.32   Insertion of a transjugular intrahepatic portosystemic stent shunt (TIPSS). The hepatic vein is cannulated via the jugular vein and the superior and inferior vena cava. A track is then created between the hepatic vein and the right main portal vein branch using a special needle. The track is dilated using a balloon, and an expandable metal stent is inserted to maintain the shunt. In this patient the left main gastric vein has also been embolized with metal coils to reduce the flow into the gastric and oesophageal varices

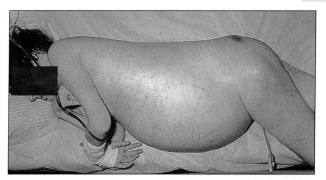

9.33   Liver failure in a patient with alcoholic cirrhosis, who presented with major haematemesis from known oesophageal varices. There is gross distension of the abdomen due to severe ascites, and visible superficial dilated veins, originating in the umbilical region. The blood flow was from the umbilicus outwards. There is also atrophy of the muscles of both upper and lower limbs. The patient was icteric, and she had fetor hepaticus. There is a large pressure sore over her left gluteal region. Close examination of her skin showed that she had purpura. Note that she is receiving a blood transfusion and that a urinary catheter is in place.

leg oedema, ascites and small pleural effusions. Bruising is seen spontaneously and after trauma, sometimes even from the pressure induced by a blood pressure cuff. This results from defective coagulation factor synthesis and from thrombocytopenia associated with splenomegaly. A bleeding tendency may also be shown by excessive bleeding at venepuncture sites. Nausea, vomiting, anorexia, drowsiness, tremor and confusion may lead on to encephalopathy: deep coma with fits and decerebrate posture (**9.33**).

Other metabolic disturbances, including hypoglycaemia, pancreatitis and renal failure, are common.

Treatment requires cooperation between a variety of specialities. Bleeding requires the intravenous administration of vitamin K, and often fresh frozen plasma. Haemodialysis may be required for renal failure. Oesophageal varices must be identified and bleeding arrested. Blood and other proteins, which contribute to the encephalopathy, must be removed from the bowel.

Death is usually caused by sepsis, gastrointestinal bleeding or cerebral oedema.

ACUTE LIVER DISEASE

ACUTE HEPATITIS

Acute hepatitis may result from a variety of causes, the most common of which are viruses and drugs (**9.34**). The clinical features at onset are usually similar, but the course and ulitmate prognosis are different. Hepatitis may be so mild that the patient does not become jaundiced but has malaise, anorexia and aversion to alcohol. In more severe cases, jaundice appears after 7–14 days (**9.35**), often accompanied by flitting arthralgia, lymphadenopathy, splenomegaly, a skin rash and hepatic discomfort. The urine is usually dark and the stools become pale. Usually the jaundice is mild and lasts only a few days with gradual recovery. In some patients, an intrahepatic cholestatic phase develops, with pruritus, deepening jaundice and increasing hepatomegaly. Occasionally the disease is progressive with deepening jaundice, peripheral oedema and ascites, bleeding, encephalopathy and death. Investigations should include:

- **Biochemistry:** the first changes are rises in the levels of ALT and alkaline phosphatase, followed by a rise in serum bilirubin; urine tests for urobilinogen are positive before jaundice occurs, and then bilirubin is found in the urine; persistence of enzyme disturbance suggests the persistence of hepatitis.
- **Haematology:** there is often leucopenia.
- **Viral markers** can be detected in the blood.

Liver biopsy is not a routine investigation in acute hepatitis, but may be carried out when there is diagnostic difficulty or severe impairment of liver function. Typically, biopsy shows swelling

CAUSES OF ACUTE HEPATITIS

Viruses	Hepatitis virus A, B, C, D, E
	Epstein–Barr virus (*see* **p. 22**)
	Cytomegalovirus (*see* **p. 21**)
	Yellow fever virus (*see* **p. 13**)
	Ebola and Marburg viruses (*see* **p. 17**)
	Other identified viruses
Bacteria	*Leptospira icterohaemorrhagiae* (*see* **p. 42**)
	Coxiella burnetii
Protozoal	*Toxoplasma gondii* (*see* **p. 48**)
Drugs	Analgesics
	– paracetamol
	– aspirin
	– non-steroidal anti-inflammatory drugs
	Cardiac drugs
	– methyldopa
	– amiodarone
	Anaesthetics
	– halothane
	Psychotropics
	– monoamine-oxidase inhibitors
	– phenothiazines
	Others
	– sodium valproate
	– oestrogens
	– methyldopa
	– rifampicin
Poisons	Carbon tetrachloride
	Amanita phalloides
Pregnancy	

9.34   Causes of acute hepatitis.

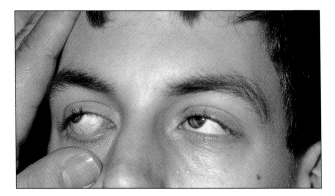

9.35   Acute viral hepatitis. This 19-year-old man presented with a 7-day history of malaise, nausea and vomiting and was found to be mildly jaundiced on examination. His hepatitis was found to be caused by Epstein–Barr virus (EBV), and he went on to develop the classic clinical features of infectious mononucleosis. This is a relatively uncommon presentation for EBV infection, but typical of the presentation of viral hepatitis of any cause.

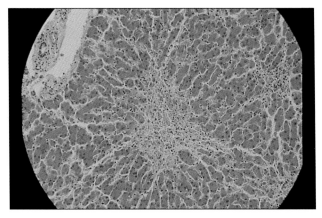

9.36   Acute viral hepatitis. The most prominent feature is centrilobular necrosis, and many of the hepatocytes outside this zone are abnormally swollen. In uncomplicated hepatitis, full regeneration of normal liver architecture will ultimately occur.

and vacuolation of hepatocytes, with focal necrosis affecting the centrilobular areas (**9.36**).

Treatment of severe hepatitis should be carried out in a specialist unit that offers elective ventilation, prophylactic antibiotics, antifungal and antiviral therapy, inotropic support, intracranial pressure monitoring, renal dialysis and liver transplantation.

VIRAL HEPATITIS

Hepatitis A virus is transmitted in water or food, and occurs especially in countries with poor water and sewerage facilities. A Western traveller to most developed countries has a 2 in 100 chance per month of contracting the infection. The incubation period is 3–6 weeks. Prodromal symptoms last 10–14 days, and the icteric phase is associated with a lessening of symptoms. Jaundice usually disappears in a week and most patients recover rapidly. In a very small number of patients, severe liver necrosis ensues, followed by coma and death. The diagnosis of hepatitis A infection is established by demonstrating a rise in specific IgM. Treatment is supportive. Immunoglobin may be given to those at risk, and protection lasts 3 months. Inactivated hepatitis A vaccine gives 95% immunity over the subsequent 10 years.

Hepatitis B virus is found in most body fluids and tissues. It is usually transmitted by sexual activity, by transfusion of blood and blood fractions, on needles (by nurses and doctors pricking fingers), tattooing (**9.37**), intravenous drug misusers (**1.6**), from

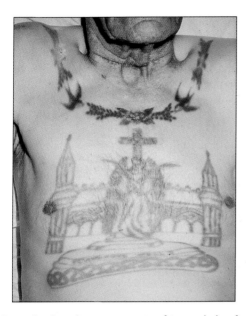

9.37 Tattooing is an important route of transmission for viral hepatitis. This patient developed acute hepatitis B after being tattooed in the Far East, and he subsequently became a long-term carrier of the hepatitis B virus. The presence of tattoos always raises the possibility of transmissible infections, including viral hepatitis and HIV.

mothers to babies and by aerosol during dental treatment. It may also be transmitted by medical and dental attendants who are carriers through open wounds. The mean incubation period is 10–16 weeks. The specific diagnosis is made by finding hepatitis B surface antigen and antibodies in serum. The symptomology and course are similar to those of the other viral hepatitides. A small percentage of people develop fulminant hepatitis and die (unless treated by liver transplantation), a small number develop chronic liver disease and a small number become carriers. Vaccination against hepatitis B is essential in health care workers, relatives of those with hepatitis B and other high-risk groups. Emergency immunoglobulin cover may be given after exposure such as needle stick injury. Lamivudine and interferon should be considered in infectious carriers.

Hepatitis C virus is transmitted by blood and blood products, and also sexually. Those who have a high incidence of infection include haemophiliacs, regular blood transfusion recipients (aplastic anaemia, sickle-cell disease, thalassaemia), renal dialysis patients, those who have recently undergone cardiopulmonary bypass, intravenous drug misusers and dentists. There is a high incidence of progression of the hepatitis to chronic disease (80%). The diagnosis is by finding viral RNA in the serum using a PCR technique or finding anti-hepatitis C virus (anti-HCV) antibodies. In the Blood Transfusion Service careful screening of donated blood by anti-hepatitis C virus antibodies has significantly reduced the incidence of cases. In selected patients interferon α with ribavirin may be of therapeutic value.

Hepatitis D (delta) is caused by a virus that is transmitted in close association with the hepatitis B virus, and this form of hepatitis only occurs in those with active hepatitis B or who are carrying hepatitis B. Hepatitis D may be clinically severe.

Hepatitis E is transmitted enterically and occurs in large epidemics. The disease is self-limiting and does not progress to chronic liver disease. Hepatitis E viral RNA can be detected in the stool and serological tests for hepatitis E antibodies are now available. Hepatitis E should be prevented by provision of a clean water supply and efficient sewage disposal.

Studies of the incubation period of acute hepatitis suggest that there are other strains of virus still to be described. Viral hepatitis may also be caused by Epstein–Barr virus (**p. 22**), cytomegalovirus (**p. 21**) and yellow fever virus (**p. 13**), and it is a component of many viral haemorrhagic fevers (**p. 17**).

ACUTE DRUG-INDUCED HEPATITIS AND CHOLESTASIS

Drugs and chemicals may cause a range of hepatic damage, including fatty change, cholestasis, granulomatous disease, acute and chronic hepatitis, cirrhosis and liver tumours. An acute hepatitis-like picture may be produced by a number of drugs (**9.34**, **9.38**). The most common of these in the UK is paracetamol, usually taken as an intentional overdose. Early features are nausea and vomiting. Most patients have few sequelae, but in some who have taken a larger dose, presented late or taken alcohol (which induces the hepatic microsomal enzymes), mild jaundice, liver tenderness and disturbance of liver biochemistry appear on the third or fourth day. Despite treatment at this stage, there is progressive deepening of jaundice, increasing liver cell failure and sometimes death (if liver transplantation is not available). The prothrombin time is a good predictor of outcome. N-acetylcysteine prevents further paracetamol-induced damage and may partially reverse the hepatic necrosis.

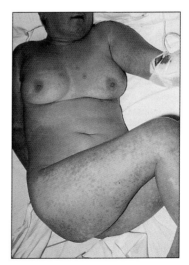

9.38 Acute drug-induced hepatitis. This patient developed severe hepatitis soon after phenytoin was added to the therapy she was receiving for epilepsy. She was clinically only mildly icteric, but her liver function was severely deranged. The hepatitis was accompanied by a morbilliform rash. She made a full recovery after withdrawal of phenytoin.

Halothane hepatitis is rare and usually follows multiple exposures to the gas for general anaesthesia. The clinical picture is of acute hepatitis that may be fatal.

Other drugs may cause acute liver damage with a predominantly cholestatic picture. These include chlorpromazine, oral contraceptives and anabolic steroids, often used for body-building (**9.39**). Poisoning with other toxins is rare. Epidemics of liver failure caused by exposure to *Amanita phalloides* occur when this fungus is mistaken for the edible mushroom.

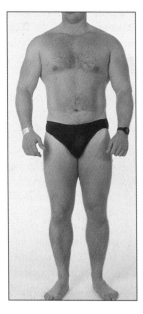

9.39 Anabolic steroid misuse is an increasingly common cause of liver dysfunction. This weight lifter was taking a cocktail of non-prescribed drugs including stanozolol, bendroflumethazide (bendrofluazide) and levothyroxine (thyroxine) (a common combination, which he believed enhanced his muscle profile), and he developed mild jaundice with elevated liver enzymes.

LIVER ABSCESS

Pyogenic infection may result from biliary tract obstruction (ascending cholangitis), from infection carried in the portal vein (portal pyaemia) or, more rarely, from the hepatic artery in the course of generalized septicaemia.

Liver abscess is now uncommon as a result of better surgical management of intra-abdominal sepsis, but intra-abdominal pus may still occur with ruptured appendix, a perforated viscus (duodenal ulcer, diverticulitis, etc.), cholecystitis and cholangitis, infiltrating carcinomas and perinephric abscess. Often, the origin of intra-abdominal sepsis is unclear.

A wide range of bowel origin Gram-negative organisms may be involved. The commonly found organisms include *Escherichia coli*, *Streptococci*, *Clostridium* (mainly *C. perfringens*), *Klebsiella* and *Bacteroides*. Early administration of antibiotics often results in failure to culture the infecting organisms.

Patients with liver abscess are usually acutely unwell, and present with a high swinging fever, rigors, malaise, nausea, vomiting and, later, liver tenderness. There may be associated features of Gram-negative septicaemia with hypotension, peripheral vasoconstriction and oliguria. There may be associated icterus, caused by related biliary pathology or by a forming abscess. In addition, there may be a right-sided pleural effusion, especially if there is pus in the subphrenic space.

Investigations usually show a leucocytosis, elevation of the ESR and disturbance of liver function tests (elevation of bilirubin, alkaline phosphatase and ALT). Blood cultures are positive in one-half to three-quarters of patients who have not been treated with antibiotics. Chest X-ray often shows elevation of the right hemidiaphragm and a reactive pleural effusion. Ultrasound (**1.139**), CT (**9.40**) or isotope scanning will localize the site and size of the abscess and treatment is usually surgical evacuation under appropriate antibiotic cover. The pus collected should be sent for culture, and the antibiotic regimen finalised. Amoebic liver abscess is a frequent complication of patients with enteric amoebic infection, but may occur in the absence of a clinical episode of dysentery (*see* **p. 47**). The organism is carried to the liver in the portal vein, usually forming multiple abscesses that coalesce and may rupture into the peritoneal cavity or into the pleural space. Amoebic abscesses may also be revealed by ultrasound (**1.139**) or CT. Diagnostic aspiration (**1.140**) produces a reddish-brown pus (anchovy or chocolate sauce), which may contain motile amoebae. Small single abscesses in the left lobe of the liver may require drainage under ultrasound guidance.

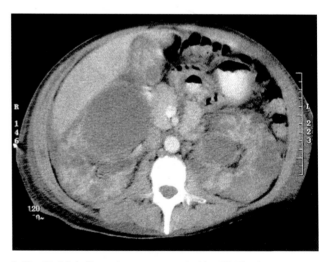

9.40 Multiple liver abscesses revealed by CT. The large abscess was drained, and the patient recovered after a prolonged course of antimicrobial therapy.

CHRONIC LIVER DISEASE

CHRONIC HEPATITIS

Chronic hepatitis is defined as any hepatitis lasting for 6 months or longer. Some cases are idiopathic, but most follow acute viral hepatitis, are autoimmune in nature, or are induced by drug therapy or alcohol.

Post-viral hepatitis

Hepatomegaly may persist after an acute attack of hepatitis and liver biopsy may show continuing periportal inflammation, with normal liver architecture (**9.41**). Enzymes may remain persistently high but other biochemistry is normal. Although there are often no long-term sequelae, progression to cirrhosis is common, and is associated with a high incidence of primary liver cell cancer. Treatment is unsatisfactory, but some patients respond to interferon. End-stage disease can only be definitively treated by liver transplantation.

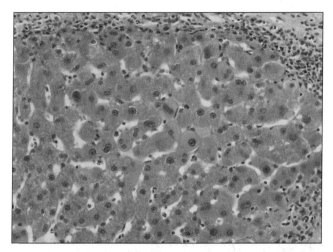

9.41 Chronic hepatitis. The liver parenchyma is normal, but there is persistent infiltration with small mononuclear inflammatory cells in the portal tracts (seen at two edges in this view). The hepatocytes are normal, even in the 'limiting plate' (the zone adjacent to the portal tract).

Autoimmune hepatitis

Autoimmune hepatitis (**9.42**) is a disease of unknown cause that is usually associated with hyperglobulinaemia, autoantibodies in the blood and the coexistence of other autoimmune disorders, for example rheumatoid arthritis, ulcerative colitis, Hashimoto's thyroiditis, peripheral neuropathy, renal tubular acidosis or keratoconjunctivitis sicca (Sjögren's syndrome). It is typically a disease of women aged 20–40 years but may occur in other patients. Four subtypes have been described, which are differentiated according to the specificity of the autoantibody produced and their clinical presentations.

- **Type I** patients often have a past history or family history of autoimmune disease. Hepatitis usually starts insidiously with fatigue, malaise and anorexia; there may be early stigmata of liver disease with vascular spiders (**9.8, 9.9**) and palmar erythema (**9.12**); occasionally, the onset may be more acute with rapid onset of jaundice, hepatomegaly, splenomegaly and ascites. Some patients also develop features of Cushing's syndrome (before being administered steroids). Biochemical tests show elevation of

aminotransferases, low serum albumin and prolongation of prothrombin time; there is hyperglobulinaemia. There are usually circulating antinuclear and smooth muscle antibodies; about 10–20% of patients have positive tests for LE cells.

- **Type 2** patients have anti-liver and kidney microsomal autoantibodies. Type 2 autoimmune hepatitis occurs mostly in younger children as an acute onset disease process that rapidly progresses to cirrhosis and hepatic decompensation. In adults, type 2 autoimmune hepatitis may be the result of hepatitis C infection.

- **Type 3 and type 4** autoimmune hepatitis are poorly defined and present a similar clinical picture to that of type 1. Type 3 autoimmune hepatitis has antibodies directed against a soluble liver antigen, but no specific antibodies have yet been found in type 4.

The diagnosis of autoimmune hepatitis is dependent on the finding of autoantibodies that are not organ-specific in a patient with characteristic liver biopsy findings (**9.43**). In

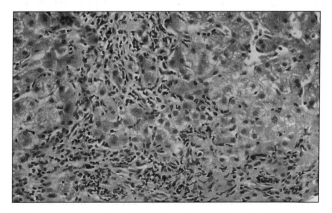

9.42 Autoimmune hepatitis. This patient developed autoimmune hepatitis as a sequel to hepatitis B infection, and ultimately developed cirrhosis, portal hypertension and liver failure.

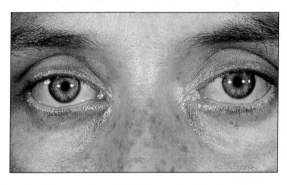

9.43 Autoimmune hepatitis. Here the inflammatory infiltrate is not confined to the portal tracts, in contrast to chronic hepatitis (see **9.41**). Small inflammatory cells can be seen in bands through the liver parenchyma, and some of the parenchymal cells are swollen and vacuolated. This form of hepatitis commonly leads to cirrhosis and liver failure.

addition, viral serology and biochemical markers may support the diagnosis of the different types. In the absence of hepatitis C infection, treatment of all four types of autoimmune hepatitis is with corticosteroids or azathioprine, or both. Steroids, used long term, have very significantly reduced the long-term mortality (from 30% to 6%). End-stage disease can only be definitively treated by liver transplantation.

Drug-induced chronic hepatitis

A wide range of drugs may cause chronic hepatitis, even after being used without adverse effects for several years. Some common drugs are methyldopa, halothane, nitrofurantoin, isoniazid, aspirin and sulphonamides. Occasionally the presentation may be florid and fulminating. In addition to the expected biochemical changes of hepatitis, there is hyperglobulinaemia, and LE cells and antinuclear and smooth muscle antibodies may be found in the serum. Treatment is to withdraw the suspected drug and follow the liver function tests. Steroids and immunosuppression are of little or no value.

ALCOHOL-INDUCED LIVER DISEASE

Excessive alcohol intake over a prolonged period may cause damage to almost every organ in the body – especially to the liver. Three separate conditions are recognized:

- alcohol-induced fatty liver, in which triglycerides accumulate in hepatocytes
- alcoholic hepatitis, in which there is neutrophil infiltration, hepatocyte damage and pericellular fibrosis
- alcoholic cirrhosis – micro- then macronodular fibrosis.

Fatty liver is common in the heavy drinker, and its only clinical feature is a large, palpable liver. Liver function tests, especially the liver enzymes (ALT and γ-GT), may be abnormal. With abstinence the liver can return to normal size and function.

Acute alcoholic hepatitis usually follows an acute bout of heavy drinking and may occur in the drinker with a fatty liver or in one who has already become cirrhotic. The usual presentation is with sudden onset jaundice that becomes rapidly deeper (**9.44**) and the liver usually enlarges. If there is pre-existing cirrhosis, there may be an exacerbation of the signs of liver failure and portal hypertension. There may be persistent leucocytosis and fever, with dark urine and pale stools.

In the chronic alcoholic, the features of cirrhosis and its consequences are usually identical to those resulting from cirrhosis of other causes, but some features are suggestive of an alcoholic origin:

- parotid enlargement (**9.45**)
- Dupuytren's contracture (**9.46**)

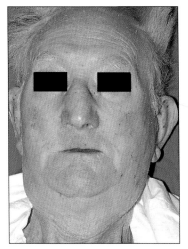

9.45 Parotid enlargement in association with cirrhosis is most common when alcohol is the cause of the cirrhosis. In addition to painful parotid enlargement, this patient had multiple vascular spiders and early acne rosacea.

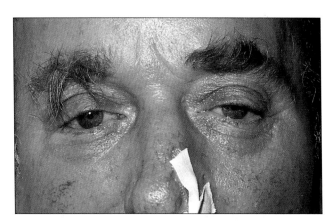

9.44 Acute alcoholic hepatitis. The patient presented with sudden onset jaundice. At first sight, the condition might be confused with acute viral hepatitis, but the patient had a history of several previous admissions after alcoholic excess. Acute alcoholic hepatitis has a significant mortality despite supportive treatment.

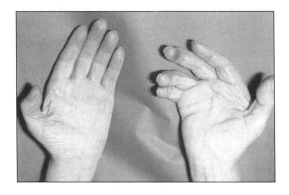

9.46 Dupuytren's contracture may be seen in association with alcoholic cirrhosis, though it may also occur as a completely independent abnormality. Contracture of the palmar fascial bands produces flexion contracture of the metacarpophalangeal and proximal interphalangeal joints, the flexor tendon apparatus and the skin itself. Surgical correction is usually possible. Note the tar staining of the fingers of this heavy smoker.

- red, sore, smooth tongue caused by associated vitamin deficiency (**9.47**)
- beri-beri (**p. 330**)
- neuropathy (**p. 488**)
- cardiomyopathy (**p. 233**)
- acne rosacea (**2.84, 9.45**)
- associated chronic pancreatitis (**p. 400**)
- associated peptic ulceration (**p. 354**)
- raised MCV and low platelet count

The diagnosis is made on the basis of the history and clinical features. Risk factors for progression of disease include high alcohol intake, hepatitis C infection, genetic factors and fatty change. The extent of liver damage can be investigated by liver biopsy (**9.48**) and monitored by blood tests. The tests which predict a poor outcome are a rising prothrombin time, a rising bilirubin, a falling serum albumin and a falling haemoglobin.

Treatment is by abstinence from alcohol and correction of associated vitamin deficiencies. Hepatic failure and portal hypertension may require treatment in their own right. Liver transplantation should be considered in those who have stopped drinking.

PRIMARY BILIARY CIRRHOSIS

Primary biliary cirrhosis is a slowly progressive disease of unknown aetiology that affects women more commonly than men (9:1) and usually occurs between the ages of 40 and 60 years. It has a prevalence of 5–15 per 100 000 population, and an incidence of 10 per million per year. Many patients are diagnosed by chance observation of disturbed liver function tests measured for some unrelated problem. Clinical presentation is often with itching of the skin caused by retention of bile salts or with increased pigmentation of skin, part of which is due to a progressive rise in bilirubin levels. Cholestatic jaundice appears later (**9.5, 9.49**). Auto-immune disorders, including Sjögren's syndrome, Raynaud's phenomenon, thyroid disorders, Addison's disease, rheumatoid arthritis, fibrosing alveolitis, dermatomyositis and scleroderma, are sometimes an associated feature. During the course of the illness, the patient becomes more icteric and pigmented, usually with marked periocular xanthelasmata (**9.5**) and hepatosplenomegaly. Patches of vitiligo may be present. The patient may complain of persistent steatorrhoea, weight loss and metabolic bone disease. The end result of the disease is liver failure, encephalopathy and bleeding from oesophageal varices. There is also an increased risk (×4) of extrahepatic malignancy, especially carcinoma of the breast.

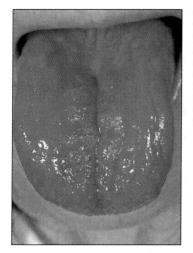

9.47 A red, sore, smooth tongue may be seen in patients with alcoholic cirrhosis as a result of associated vitamin deficiency. A similar appearance may occur in patients with nutritional deficiencies of other origins.

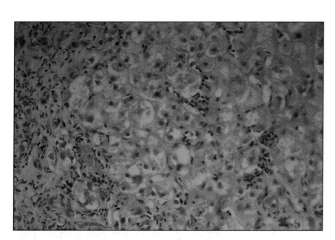

9.48 Liver biopsy in alcoholic hepatitis. There is widespread fatty change (as shown by the clear macrovesicles, which contained fat before the processing of the section). Focal necrosis of hepatocytes is indicated by the surrounding foci of neutrophils. Mallory's hyaline, shown as eosinophilic globules, has accumulated in some of the hepatocytes; this is typical but not diagnostic of alcoholic hepatitis.

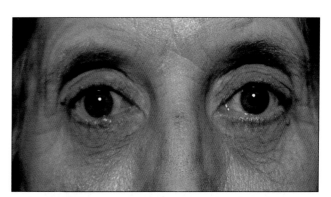

9.49 Primary biliary cirrhosis. This 55-year-old woman presented originally with severe pruritus, and jaundice developed slowly over the next 3 years. When this photograph was taken, she had deep jaundice, typical brown pigmentation, spider naevi, xanthelasmata around both eyes, enlargement of the liver and spleen, and ascites. The deepening jaundice and ascites are poor prognostic signs, and are usually followed by encephalopathy and death within weeks or months.

Serum antimitochondrial antibodies are present in over 90% of patients. Serum immunoglobulins are elevated (IgG and especially IgM) and autoantibodies against thyroid and platelets may be found, as well as antinuclear and anticentromere antibodies. Liver function tests are abnormal, with elevated bilirubin and alkaline phosphatase, and modest elevation of ALT, AST and γ-GT. Serum cholesterol is usually high. Coagulation may be abnormal, because of a combination of loss of functioning hepatocytes and malabsorption of vitamin K. Liver biopsy shows an inflammatory reaction in the portal tracts with the formation of fibrous septae and granulomas.

Ultrasound and, if necessary, ERCP should be carried out to exclude sclerosing cholangitis (**9.51**) and to ensure the patient does not have obstruction of the larger biliary ducts, as stone formation is a common association (**9.50**). These investigations may show splenomegaly and evidence of portal hypertension as the disease advances.

There is no specific treatment for the disease, but the hyperlipidaemia and the malabsorption can be treated. Persistent pruritus may respond to the use of cholestyramine. Ursodeoxycholic acid therapy leads to biochemical improvement and may slow down disease progression. Liver transplantation should be considered when plasma bilirubin reaches 100 μmol/litre.

PRIMARY SCLEROSING CHOLANGITIS

In primary sclerosing cholangitis there is fibrotic obstruction of the intra- and/or extrahepatic bile ducts. The condition may complicate inflammatory bowel disease or, less commonly, retroperitoneal fibrosis, HIV infection or autoimmune disorders and is associated with HLA types B8, DR2 and DR3. Secondary sclerosing cholangitis results from an underlying biliary tract disorder (e.g. retained stones or surgical damage).

Patients usually present with jaundice, pruritus and right upper quadrant pain. Investigations show a cholestatic picture (see **9.16**). Ultrasonography may be normal, and the diagnosis is best made by ERCP, which shows patchy dilation and stricturing of the biliary tree (**9.51**).

There is no specific treatment, but antimicrobials are needed during episodes of acute cholangitis. Occasionally a stent can be inserted at ERCP to bridge a critical stricture, but the condition is usually too widespread for this to be useful. Ultimately the condition progresses to hepatic cirrhosis (secondary biliary cirrhosis). Liver transplantation is the only effective treatment in advanced disease.

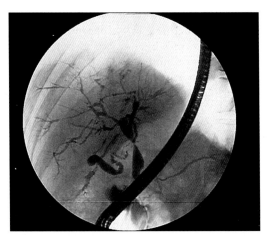

9.51 Primary sclerosing cholangitis. This endoscopic retrograde cholangiopancreatogram (ERCP; *see* **p. 380**) shows typical appearances, with patchy dilatation and stricturing of the biliary tree. The patient had ulcerative colitis (*see* **p. 361**).

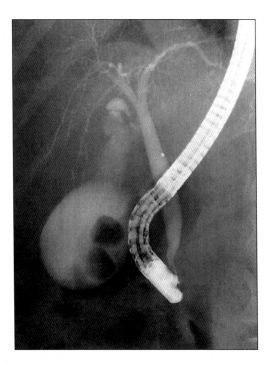

9.50 Endoscopic retrograde cholangiopancreatography (ERCP) in a patient with primary biliary cirrhosis. The intrahepatic and common bile ducts are normal, but gallstones are present in the gall bladder. Gallstones are a common association with primary biliary cirrhosis.

HEREDITARY HAEMOCHROMATOSIS

Haemochromatosis is an autosomal recessive inherited condition, with a gene frequency of 5–10%, in which excess iron is absorbed and stored in the body tissues. It typically appears in middle-aged men (male:female ratio 10:1). In women it appears much later in life, because of iron loss at menstruation and in child-bearing. The prevalence of haemochromatosis is 2–5 per 1000 population. The abnormal gene lies on the short arm of chromosome 6.

There is a wide spectrum of clinical features at presentation. Asymptomatic patients showing biochemical abnormalities alone may be found by screening families of known patients, whereas others present with the later effects, including hepatic cirrhosis, pancreatic insufficiency with diabetes mellitus (which affects at least 70% of patients) and pigmentation of the skin (bronze diabetes). Skin pigmentation is usually slatey-grey in colour (**9.52**) and results from the deposition of a combination of melanin and iron. Many patients also develop a pyrophosphate arthropathy in which chondrocalcinosis involves the articular cartilages (*see* **p. 121**). This particularly involves the first and second metacarpophalangeal joints and the knees.

Excess iron deposition is also found in the anterior pituitary, where it reduces hormone production, and in the testes. The end result is gonadal atrophy. Cardiac involvement is also common and arrhythmias and heart failure are the presenting features.

The main organ involved is the liver, which is often cirrhotic at the time of presentation, and the patient may have the additional features associated with hepatic failure and portal hypertension. Primary liver cell cancer is a common complication (one-third of patients) and is often associated with a significant decline in liver function. Osteoporosis resulting from gonadal atrophy is a long-term complication.

The diagnosis is made by finding a high serum iron with a very high saturation of iron-binding protein. Serum ferritin is also high and there may be disturbance of the profile of liver function tests. A specific gene test is positive in 80% of patients (and may be used for the screening of relatives). Excess iron is found in most tissues; on liver biopsy, iron stains show iron in the parenchyma and in the Kupffer cells (**9.53**). There is also a coarse macronodular cirrhosis.

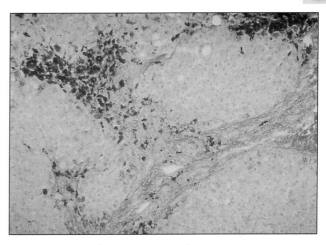

9.53   Liver biopsy in haemochromatosis, stained for iron. Excessive iron is present in the hepatic reticuloendothelial (Kupffer) cells adjacent to the sinusoids, and in parts of the liver parenchyma.

393

Treatment usually involves long-term repeated venesection. Chelating agents are rarely used, because of their expense and difficulty of administration and the success of venesection. Diabetes mellitus, other endocrine failure and joint disease may all require specific treatment.

Secondary haemochromatosis (secondary iron overload; haemosiderosis) occurs if there is excess tissue iron but no subsequent damage. This is usually seen in patients with chronic haemolytic states who have been treated with repeated blood transfusions, for example sickle-cell anaemia and thalassaemia (*see* **pp. 416-422**). The iron overload in these patients may give rise to a picture similar to primary haemochromatosis and may be treated by chelating agents.

VASCULAR DISEASE OF LIVER

The Budd–Chiari syndrome is a rare disorder that results from a large number of pathologies which ultimately obstruct the flow of blood from the hepatic veins into the inferior vena cava. These include congenital webs in the vena cava, thrombosis in the hepatic veins or adjacent vena cava as a result of thrombophilic states (**p. 442**) or use of oral contraceptives, infiltration by tumours, Behçet's disease, and trauma. The signs depend on how acutely the syndrome develops. Usually this is gradual and the patient presents with an enlarged, sometimes tender, liver. There may be associated jaundice, ascites, peripheral oedema and splenomegaly. A characteristic of the disease is the development of masses of dilated veins on the abdominal wall, the flow being upwards (**9.54**). The diagnosis may be surmised by the finding of centrilobular necrosis in the liver biopsy, and is established by CT (the caudate lobe is often enlarged) or by failure to catheterize the hepatic veins. Inferior venacavography may also be of value. The usual treatment is

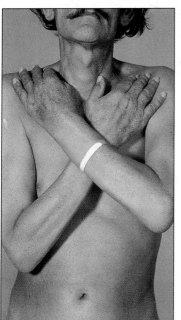

9.52   Haemochromatosis. The slatey-grey colour of this Caucasian patient's skin, most obvious in his hands, results from the deposition of a combination of melanin and iron. This patient had cirrhosis and pyrophosphate arthropathy at the time of presentation with the disease. Note also the absence of body hair, which was associated with hypogonadism.

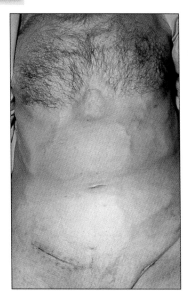

9.54 The Budd–Chiari syndrome (hepatic venous obstruction). Note the grossly dilated veins in the abdominal wall, in which the flow of blood was upwards. The patient had continued to work as a builder's labourer without symptoms, until he was admitted with coincidental appendicitis. The cause of his hepatic venous obstruction was unclear.

expressionless facies, athetoid movements and dysarthria). A Kayser–Fleischer ring may be found in the cornea in most patients over the age of 13 – this is most easily seen in blue-eyed patients as a brown ring (**9.55**). The diagnosis is made on finding an increased 24-hour urinary copper excretion and liver biopsy evidence of cirrhosis with excess copper in the liver cells. A low serum caeruloplasmin level is found in 90% of patients. Treatment is with long-term penicillamine to chelate the excess copper. Relatives of patients should be screened by caeruloplasmin level at the age of 3 (or above).

OTHER CAUSES OF CIRRHOSIS

Metabolic causes of chronic liver disease that may lead to cirrhosis include α_1-antitrypsin deficiency, glycogen storage disorders (**9.56**), galactosaemia, fructose intolerance and the Fanconi syndrome. All of these are rare disorders.

α_1-**antitrypsin deficiency** is associated with neonatal hepatitis and cirrhosis in childhood. The aetiology is unknown, but liver biopsy shows the hepatocytes to contain granules of α_1-antitrypsin. The diagnosis is made by finding a low serum α_1-antitrypsin.

Cardiac cirrhosis is a rare complication of long-standing right heart failure, seen in patients with cor pulmonale, tricuspid incompetence, cardiomyopathy and constrictive pericarditis. The clinical features are those of right heart failure (**p. 206**). Ultrasound may show dilatation of the inferior vena cava and the hepatic veins.

Drugs are rarely implicated in the generation of cirrhosis. The most common is methotrexate if used for a prolonged period, for example in chronic psoriasis.

portocaval shunting, but liver transplantation has been used in severe cases in which the inferior vena cava is normal.

Veno-occlusive disease of the liver is a small-vessel variant of the Budd–Chiari syndrome that involves the hepatic venules. It develops in people who drink medicinal teas containing alkaloids from *Senecio* and *Crotalaria* plants, and rarely after bone marrow transplantation and the use of antimitotic therapy (e.g. tioguanine).

WILSON'S DISEASE (HEPATOLENTICULAR DEGENERATION)

Wilson's disease is rare, with a prevalence of 1–30/million, and caused by a defective autosomal recessive gene on chromosome 13. There is an abnormality in the handling of copper, which accumulates in various tissues, especially the liver, basal ganglia, bones, renal tubules and cornea. The clinical presentation is usually between the ages of 5 and 30 with a combination of liver function impairment and neurological features from loss of function of the basal ganglia (parkinsonian tremor,

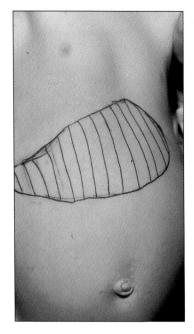

9.56 Gross hepatomegaly in glycogen storage disease. This 3-year-old child presented with a typical appearance – hepatomegaly (7 cm below the costal margin in the midclavicular line) but no enlargement of the spleen.

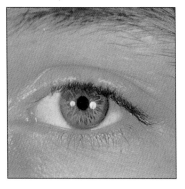

9.55 Wilson's disease. The clinical features of impaired liver function and neurological disorder are usually accompanied by Kayser–Fleischer rings in the corneae. The rings show as a rim of brown pigment, and are more clearly seen in patients with blue eyes (slit-lamp examination may be necessary in patients with brown eyes).

Hereditary haemorrhagic telangiectasia (**10.7**, **10.102**) has been associated with cirrhosis. This may be caused by hepatitis viruses transmitted in blood transfusions used for the treatment of long-term anaemia.

Ulcerative colitis and Crohn's disease are associated with a variety of liver pathologies. These include fatty infiltration of the liver, granulomas, cirrhosis, pericholangitis, primary sclerosing cholangitis (**8.51**) and carcinoma of bile ducts (*see* **p. 357**).

OTHER INFECTIONS OF THE LIVER

Schistosomiasis is a common cause of liver infection in the developing world, and is the most common cause of portal hypertension worldwide. It is usually found in patients who also have disease in the colon or bladder. Migration of ova via the portal vein to the liver causes multiple granulomas and a generalized fibrotic reaction that results in portal hypertension and splenomegaly (*see* **p. 54** and **1.168**, **1.169**).

Liver fluke infestation may lead to cholangitis, cirrhosis and cholangiocarcinoma (*see* **p. 369**).

Hydatid disease may result in multiple cysts in the liver and in many other organs (*see* **p. 56**). The cysts are often multiple and have daughter cysts. They act as space-occupying lesions and may produce pressure on the hepatic ducts. Eosinophilia is common. Many of the cysts calcify and may be seen on plain X-rays. Diagnosis is made by ultrasound or by CT (**1.175**).

FIBROPOLYCYSTIC DISEASES

There are a number of rare congenital fibropolycystic hepatobiliary diseases, including adult polycystic liver, congenital hepatic fibrosis, congenital intrahepatic biliary dilatation and choledochal cysts. There is a high association

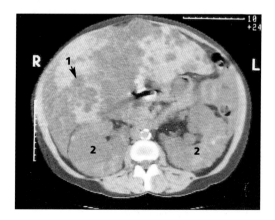

9.57 Polycystic liver disease, as seen on CT scanning. The patient has massive hepatomegaly, and a typical example of the many cysts in the liver is arrowed (1). She also had bilateral polycystic kidneys (2) (*see also* **p. 283**).

with similar renal disorders and a risk of malignant change. Diagnosis is made on ultrasonography or CT (**9.57**). Liver transplantation is a treatment option if there is serious liver decompensation.

LIVER TUMOURS

SECONDARY TUMOURS

Secondary spread from many primary carcinomas of the lung, breast, colon, stomach, kidney and pancreas frequently involves the liver. The resulting liver enlargement is often found in patients who have presented with vague symptoms, such as weight loss or anaemia. The liver is usually non-tender but firm and irregular. There may be few other signs, but a careful search for lymph node and skin metastases is required. Liver function tests may show only an elevation of alkaline phosphatase, occasionally with slight elevation of ALT or bilirubin. The diagnosis is made by ultrasound (**9.21**), CT (**9.22**) or isotope scan, which usually show multiple filling defects. Diagnostic biopsy guided by ultrasound or on laparoscopy may be of value to obtain a tissue diagnosis. Multiple metastases are usually a poor prognostic sign.

PRIMARY TUMOURS

Hepatocellular carcinoma (primary liver cancer) is one of the most common cancers in West Africa and the Far East (incidence 30/100 000), but is relatively rare in the West (incidence 1–3/100 000). It is associated with chronic carriage of hepatitis B and C viruses, cirrhosis of any cause, haemochromatosis, use of some androgenic steroids, previous exposure to thorotrast, and aflatoxin from decayed food. The lesions are often multifocal and aggressively invasive. The patient often has pre-existing hepatomegaly and there is right upper quadrant pain with localized enlargement. There may also be weight loss, ascites and occasionally features of hypoglycaemia. Jaundice usually occurs only when the tumour is hilar in site. The diagnosis is confirmed by the finding of a raised circulating level of α-fetoprotein (AFP), mild disturbance of the liver function tests and single or multiple defects on ultrasound or CT (**9.58**). Arteriography may be helpful. Histological diagnosis is made on guided ultrasound or laparoscopic biopsy. A solitary lesion may be treatable by surgical resection of a liver lobe, but the overall outlook is poor, with a median survival of 1 year. Liver transplantation is the treatment of choice for small tumours (< 5cm diameter) in a cirrhotic liver.

Cholangiocarcinoma is the second most common primary malignant tumour of the liver and may be intrahepatic or extrahepatic. Intrahepatic tumours have a similar clinical presentation to hepatocellular carcinoma; extrahepatic tumours commonly present with obstructive jaundice (**9.19**, **9.59**).

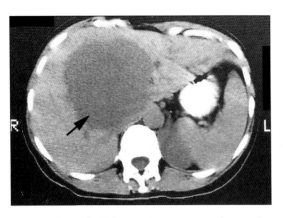

9.58   Primary hepatocellular carcinoma on CT. The massive tumour is obvious (arrow). The liver and spleen are both enlarged. This patient had a long history of chronic active hepatitis associated with hepatitis B antigen positivity, and signs of portal hypertension.

Chinese liver fluke infestation is an underlying factor in the Far East (*see* **p. 369**). Bile duct obstruction caused by extrahepatic cholangiocarcinoma can sometimes be palliatively relieved by the insertion of a stent via a side-viewing duodenoscope (**8.76**) or by a transhepatic route (**9.60**), but mean survival is 6 months.

Haemangiosarcoma is a rare, highly malignant tumour of the liver that may result from occupational exposure to vinyl chloride monomers. Hepatic enlargement, local pain and bloodstained ascites often develop rapidly.

Benign tumours of the liver include:

- liver adenomas, which may be associated with prolonged use of high-oestrogen oral contraceptives; they are highly vascular and may cause intraperitoneal bleeding
- cystadenomas, derived from bile ducts or from parenchymal cells
- haemangiomas, which may be diagonosed by hearing a vascular hum over the liver or, more commonly, as an incidental finding on ultrasound; they are usually symptomless.

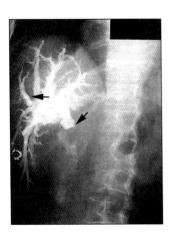

9.59   Cholangiocarcinoma causing a stricture in the common hepatic duct (right arrow), as shown by a percutaneous transhepatic cholangiogram. The patient presented with deepening jaundice. No aetiological factor was apparent. Note the needle used for the percutaneous injection (left arrow). Endoscopic retrograde cholangiopancreatography (ERCP) proved impossible in this patient because of the degree of bile duct obstruction.

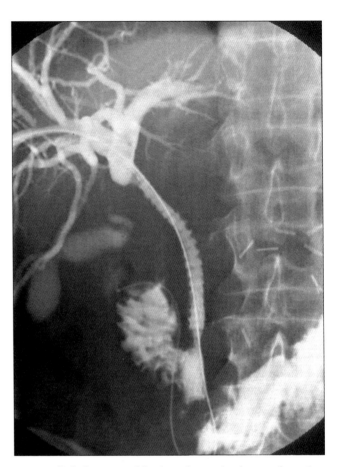

9.60   Relief of common bile duct obstruction by transhepatic insertion of a metal stent. A guide wire was inserted transhepatically, a balloon dilatation performed and the stent inserted to maintain patency.

DISEASES OF THE GALL BLADDER

GALLSTONES

Gallstones are extremely common and will affect one in three women and one in five men in the UK. Most stones are totally asymptomatic and are found by chance during other investigations or at autopsy, but they may be demonstrated on plain abdominal X-ray (**9.17**) or by ultrasound (**9.62**). There are three types of gallstones:

- **Cholesterol stones** are often solitary; they form in bile in which cholesterol is in excess relative to bile salts, and are found in about 10% of patients with stones; they are common in women who have had many children, who are overweight, who have hyperlipidaemia or who are diabetic.
- **Pigment stones** are usually multiple and green-black in colour; they account for about 10–15% of all stones and are the result of bilirubin precipitation, caused by

overproduction in chronic haemolytic states; they are later associated with recurrent ascending cholangitis.

- **Mixed stones** are by far the most common, are usually multiple and are a mixture of cholesterol, pigment, calcium carbonate and phosphate; they are found especially in people who are obese or who have lived on a diet rich in unrefined carbohydrate and high in calories.

In most patients stones form and remain in the gall bladder without causing symptoms, but they may produce a range of symptoms, including intolerance to fatty foods, with nausea, vomiting, flatulence and epigastric pain. In a minority of patients, gallstones may be associated with significant complications (**9.61**). Migration of stones may lead to additional symptoms such as colicky right hypochondrial pain, obstructive jaundice and recurrent bouts of ascending cholangitis or acute pancreatitis, or both. Chronic cholecystitis may lead to adhesion of the gall bladder to surrounding organs, for example the small bowel, colon or stomach, with subsequent erosion of a stone, which may then pass along the bowel and even cause intestinal obstruction if very large. The presence of a fistula leads to recurrent ascending infections in the biliary tree. Chronic cholecystitis may lead to carcinoma of the gall bladder.

The principal mode of therapy is cholecystectomy, by open surgery or via the laparoscope. Gallstones may be broken up by a course of extracorporeal shock-wave lithotripsy in association with dissolutation by oral bile acid (ursodeoxycholic or chenodeoxycholic acid) dissolution therapy. This is a lengthy procedure which has a 30–80% success rate after 1 year.

COMPLICATIONS OF GALLSTONE DISEASE

Acute cholestasis/cholecystitis/cholangitis

Chronic cholecystitis

Fistula formation – gallstone ileus

Impaction of stone in common bile duct

Gangrene of gall bladder, perforation or empyema

Pancreatitis

9.61   Complications of gallstone disease.

ACUTE CHOLECYSTITIS

In acute cholecystitis, there is acute inflammation of the gall bladder, caused by migration of stone(s) and impaction either in the cystic duct or in Hartmann's pouch. This leads to painful distension of the gall bladder. The swelling and inflammation may resolve, leaving the gall bladder full of mucus (hydrops or mucocele), with a risk of recurrence of pain and inflammation. Often by the time the patient seeks medical advice, little is to

be found. Occasionally, the mucus becomes infected (usually with *Escherichia coli* or other gut flora) and the inflammatory process continues with local pain and peritonitis. The gall bladder may be palpable at this time as it is distended with pus (empyema of gall bladder). There is usually an associated fever with rigors. The pain radiates to the lower rib cage at the back and to the right shoulder tip. The patient may be jaundiced if a stone has migrated into the common bile duct. The key sign is Murphy's sign, which is elicited by placing the hand under the rib cage and asking the patient to breath deeply. As the inflamed gall bladder descends and contacts the palpating hand, pain is elicited and the breath is held. In acute cholecystitis, the patient has a fever and a polymorph leucocytosis. Liver function tests are often normal. Plain X-ray may show a stone(s) (**9.17**) and sometimes also a soft-tissue shadow of a distended gall bladder. The diagnosis is made on ultrasound which shows a distended gall bladder and cystic duct and single or multiple stones (**9.62**). ^{99m}TcHIDA scans may also be of value, but oral cholecystograms have been largely replaced by ultrasound unless oral dissolution therapy for gallstones is planned, in which case it is essential to confirm that the gall bladder is functioning.

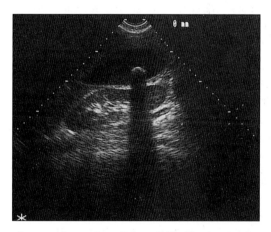

9.62   Ultrasound scanning of the gall bladder is now the preferred first investigation for gallstones. This scan shows the gall bladder containing one large stone, which casts a typical acoustic shadow, together with many much smaller stones.

Treatment consists of intravenous fluids, analgesics and a broad-spectrum antibiotic. Patients usually settle rapidly and cholecystectomy should be performed early, because recurrence of symptoms is common. Laparoscopic surgery is the treatment of choice and minimizes the recovery time for the patient.

CHRONIC CHOLECYSTITIS

Multiple episodes of acute disease lead to chronic cholecystitis, in which the wall of the gall bladder becomes thickened and fibrous, and does not usually distend when obstructed. Repeated infections also lead to the formation of mixed stones, which are small and have a greater chance of migrating into the common bile ducts and obstructing further down the system.

COMMON BILE DUCT STONES

Bile duct obstruction may result from a number of disorders (**9.63**). A common cause is obstruction by multiple mixed stones, which may lodge at the ampulla of Vater or just above. Colicky pain in the right upper quadrant is usually associated with obstructive jaundice, fever, rigors, acute nausea and vomiting. Ascending cholangitis may occur and lead to septicaemia. The features of obstructive jaundice (**9.16**) may progress over several days and the patient develops pale stools with progressive darkening of the urine. The gall bladder is not usually felt, as it cannot distend because of progressive fibrosis from previous attacks of acute cholecystitis; there may, however, be some degree of hepatomegaly.

The patient usually has a fever with a brisk polymorphonuclear leucocytosis. Liver function tests are grossly deranged with a high conjugated bilirubin and alkaline phosphatase; the ALT may also be raised if there is ascending cholangitis. Tests of coagulation become abnormal, especially the prothrombin time, which is very sensitive to vitamin K malabsorption. Plain X-ray may show a stone, but the diagnosis is usually made by ultrasound, which may show the stone and also shows the dilated bile ducts. Often the diagnosis requires an ERCP to define the position of the stone(s) more accurately (**9.64**) and also to remove them. Plain X-ray of the area may show gas in the biliary tree if infection is with a gas-producing organism (e.g. *Clostridium perfringens*), and ultrasound will also usually identify and locate stones.

Reflux of bile into the pancreatic duct, as a result of the obstruction, may produce acute pancreatitis, as may the ERCP procedure itself.

Treatment is with fluids, bed rest, control of nausea and vomiting and pain control. Elective surgery is necessary to remove the gall bladder, but ERCP is valuable to remove the impacted stones in the acute phase.

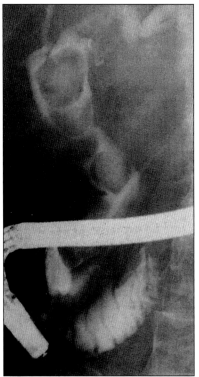

9.64 Gallstones in the common bile duct, revealed by endoscopic retrograde cholangiopancreatography (ERCP). Four stones are clearly seen, but, despite their size, there is little evidence of major biliary obstruction, as the hepatic ducts are not grossly dilated. Obstruction of the pancreatic duct by gallstones may sometimes be demonstrated by this technique in patients with acute pancreatitis, but the pancreatic duct is not seen in this view.

CAUSES OF BILE DUCT OBSTRUCTION	
Intrinsic	Gallstones
	Cholangitis
	Cholangiocarcinoma
	Carcinoma of ampulla of Vater
	Secondary tumours
	Sclerosing cholangitis
	Parasites
Extrinsic	Carcinoma of pancreatic head
	Secondary tumours
	Chronic pancreatitis or pseudocyst formation
Congenital	Biliary atresia

9.63 Causes of bile duct obstruction.

ACUTE CHOLANGITIS

Acute cholangitis is an ascending infection that results from any obstruction to the flow of bile, for example gallstones, carcinoma of the ducts and biliary stricture. The symptoms are similar to those described for stones in the common duct, but acute cholangitis is potentially fatal. Patients present with Charcot's triad of jaundice, rigors and upper abdominal pain. The common infecting organisms are *Escherichia coli*, *Klebsiella*, enterococci and a range of anaerobes. The treatment is urgent decompression of the biliary system and involves endoscopic sphincterectomy with stone removal or passing a drainage tube past the obstruction to relieve the blockage (**8.76**, **9.60**). Supportive treatment and appropriate antibiotics are essential, and surgery may be necessary.

CARCINOMA OF THE GALL BLADDER

Carcinoma of the gall bladder is an uncommon primary tumour that may be associated with the long-standing presence of gallstones and chronic cholecystitis. The presenting feature is a mass in the right upper quadrant. Jaundice occurs only when the liver is invaded. Treatment is surgical, but the outlook is poor, with a survival rate at 1 year of 20%.

PANCREATIC DISEASE

PRESENTATION AND INVESTIGATION

Clinical features of pancreatic disease may be extremely late in appearing, partly because of the deep position of the organ. Acute inflammation of the pancreas may present with epigastric pain, nausea and vomiting and occasionally hypotension. A pancreatic pseudocyst may present as a large abdominal mass. Chronic pancreatitis presents with epigastric pain, weight loss and steatorrhoea. Many patients have diabetes mellitus. There may be other features to suggest the role of alcohol in the disease process (*see* **p. 390**).

Investigations in pancreatic disease include:

- serum amylase (amylase is released from inflamed parenchymal cells)
- stimulation tests of exocrine function with measurement of bicarbonate and enzymes (trypsin and lipases)
- faecal fat estimation
- ^{14}C breath tests
- plain X-ray of the abdomen to show calcification
- ultrasound or CT
- ERCP
- exfoliative cytology by ERCP.

ACUTE PANCREATITIS

Acute pancreatitis is defined as an acute inflammatory process of the pancreas with variable involvement of adjacent tissues or remote organ systems. The causes of acute pancreatitis are shown in **9.65**. These stimuli trigger the release of pancreatic enzymes that then autodigest the pancreas. There is a wide spectrum of severity of the disease with mild to major autolytic digestion of the pancreas – often with haemorrhage.

The clinical presentation is usually with recurrent attacks of continuous epigastric pain that often radiates to the back. There is usually fever, and nausea and vomiting that does not relieve the pain. Examination shows the patient to be shocked and hypoxic (65% of acute deaths are caused by respiratory failure). Spontaneous bruising may be present as a result of inactivation of the coagulation mechanism by absorbed activated pancreatic enzymes. Bleeding may also track in the tissue planes of the body via the falciform ligament to the umbilicus (the umbilical black eye or Cullen's sign) and to the flanks (Grey Turner's sign **9.66**). The patient may be jaundiced. The abdomen is rigid, with guarding on palpation. After some days, an abdominal mass may be felt.

The diagnosis is usually confirmed by an elevated serum or urine amylase or lipase. There may also be hyperglycaemia, hypocalcaemia, hypoalbuminaemia, raised levels of liver enzymes and renal impairment. Methaemalbumin may also form, as a result of intravascular haemolysis. Elevation of bilirubin and of alkaline phosphatase may occur as the bile duct is obstructed during passage through the oedematous pancreas.

CAUSATIVE FACTORS IN ACUTE PANCREATITIS	
Gallstones and common bile duct obstruction and/or Excessive alcohol intake	80%
Trauma – following ERCP/other instrumentation – major abdominal injury, blunt trauma	5%
Viral infections, e.g. mumps, coxsackie B, Epstein–Barr virus, hepatitis A and B Parasites – *Ascaris lumbricoides* Metabolic – hypercalcaemia, hyperlipidaemia, renal failure Drug associated – corticosteroids, azathioprine, thiazide diuretics, valproate, oestrogens, ACE inhibitors Anorexia and bulimia nervosa	5%
Idiopathic	10%

9.65 Causative factors in acute pancreatitis.

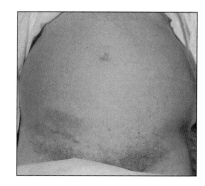

9.66 Grey Turner's sign in acute pancreatitis. This patient with severe acute pancreatitis presented with severe abdominal pain, distension and vomiting. Within 2 days of his admission, he developed characteristic discoloration in both flanks, which spread forwards to the iliac fossae. Grey Turner's sign results from the tracking of blood from the pancreatic area of the retroperitoneum.

Ultrasound and CT of the pancreas may show extreme swelling of the gland, an obstructing gallstone, a pancreatic abscess or pseudocyst formation (**9.67**). An obstructing gallstone may be shown on ERCP (**9.64**).

Various scoring systems based on the results of observations and investigations have been devised to predict outcome in actue pancreatitis. Over 70% of cases recover fully within a few days of treatment with intravenous fluids, nasogastric suction and analgesia. The rest have more severe disease and require high dependency or intensive care – especially to prevent or support the patient through renal and respiratory failure. Complications include hypovolaemic shock, adult respiratory distress syndrome, pseudocysts, abscess formation and pancreatic necrosis. Surgery is occasionally required for abscess or pseudocyst formation. The overall mortality rate in acute pancreatitis is about 10%.

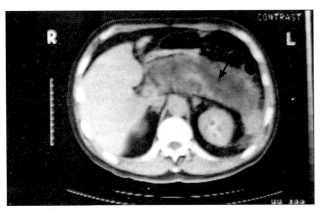

9.67 Acute pancreatitis. A pseudocyst in evolution can be seen in the pancreas (arrow) in this contrast-enhanced CT scan. Autodigestion of the pancreatic tissue gives a characteristic cystic appearance, and ultimately the cysts will coalesce to form one large pseudocyst, which may become palpable (*see* **9.71**).

CHRONIC PANCREATITIS

In chronic pancreatitis, continuing inflammation of the pancreas leads to atrophy and loss of exocrine and endocrine function. Most cases of chronic pancreatitis are associated with alcoholism, a few have had prior episodes of acute pancreatitis, often associated with gallstones and alcohol, and in a few cases no cause is evident. Worldwide there is a great range of incidence. In the UK there are about 3–10 cases per 100 000 population whereas in some countries (e.g. southern France) there is a vastly greater number. In the Third World, protein-energy malnutrition (PEM) is a common association. Other risk factors include pancreatic duct obstruction and cystic fibrosis. The most common presentation is with chronic abdominal pain, usually in the epigastrium or left upper quadrant, which radiates through the back. Weight loss is common, caused by a combination of anorexia and steatorrhoea (**9.68**). Continued alcohol consumption and

smoking may exacerbate symptoms. Calcification of the pancreas is also common, and may be associated with diabetes mellitus. Steatorrhoea may be noted clinically (**8.8**) or on faecal fat measurement. Plain X-ray may show diffuse pancreatic calcification (**9.69**), and the extent of the pancreatic disease is apparent on CT scan. Functional pancreatic tests are also of value and show a low bicarbonate and enzyme output. The serum amylase level is variable. If it remains high it is a reflection of continuing inflammation. The ESR, plasma viscosity and C-reactive protein also reflect this. Blood glucose should be measured, as should glycosylated haemoglobin and a coagulation screen.

All patients should have an ultrasound scan to exclude gallstones or a dilated biliary tree. The pancreatic structure is best seen on CT – with contrast medium. An ERCP involves

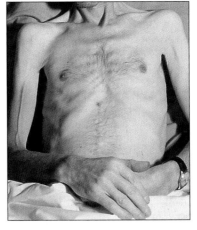

9.68 Chronic pancreatitis. The patient had a history of recurrent episodes of abdominal pain, associated with chronic pancreatitis, and leading to laparotomy on one occasion. Over the previous 2 years he developed steatorrhoea and weight loss, associated with pancreatic exocrine dysfunction.

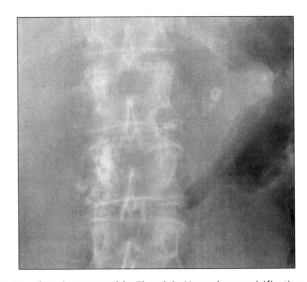

9.69 Chronic pancreatitis. The plain X-ray shows calcification throughout the pancreas, especially evident in the head. This patient was a chronic alcoholic. Pancreatic calcification is most common in malnutrition-associated chronic pancreatitis, as seen in many parts of the developing world – often in association with diabetes.

direct cannulation of the pancreatic duct for radiology (**9.70**) and sampling for pancreatic duct cytology.

Treatment of chronic pancreatitis is difficult. Pain is the major symptom that needs control, but care must be taken to avoid addiction to analgesics. Total abstinence from alcohol is essential. If the patient is extremely malnourished, admission to hospital for parenteral nutrition is of value (*see* **p. 331**). This also facilitates stopping alcohol and smoking and better analgesic control. Surgical resection and drainage may sometimes be helpful. Cholecystectomy or sphincterotomy are sometimes indicated. Malabsorption is treated with pancreatic extract taken with food and supplemented with vitamins. Diabetes mellitus may require insulin, but care should be taken to prevent hypoglycaemia as the glucagon response is absent.

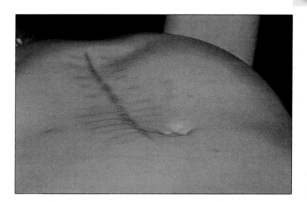

9.71   Pancreatic pseudocysts may become large enough to be visible on abdominal examination, as in this patient who underwent laparotomy at the time of presentation, and has subsequently developed an enlarging pseudocyst. Continued elevation of the serum amylase supports the diagnosis, which can be confirmed by imaging techniques (**9.67**).

CARCINOMA OF PANCREAS

Carcinoma of the pancreas affects 10–15/100 000 in the developed world (up to 100/100 000 in those over age 70). The disease appears late because of the anatomical position of the pancreas, and only 5% of carcinomas are suitable for surgical resection. The incidence of cancer is twice as high in smokers as in non-smokers and twice as great in diabetics as in non-diabetics. Over 70% occur in the head of the pancreas and patients often present with progressive obstructive jaundice caused by obstruction of the common bile duct (**9.72**). Pain may also be a feature, starting with epigastric discomfort and becoming a severe, constant pain that radiates to the back. Steatorrhoea is accompanied by severe weight loss. Secondaries

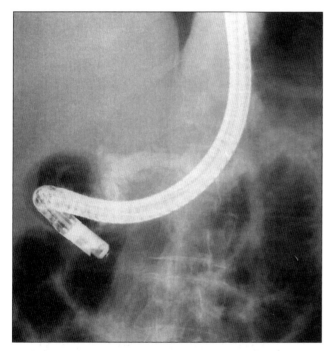

9.70   Endoscopic retrograde cholangiopancreatography (ECRP) in severe chronic pancreatitis (same patient as **9.69**). The pancreatic duct is grossly dilated and irregular. Superimposition of **9.69** and **9.70** suggests that some of the calcification reflects the presence of concretions within the duct system.

PANCREATIC PSEUDOCYSTS

Pseudocysts are a common complication of acute and chronic pancreatitis, as shown by repeated ultrasound examination. Most are small and asymptomatic and will resolve if the pancreatitis is treated. Occasionally, very large cysts appear and produce local pain and palpable swelling in the epigastrium (**9.71**). Their extent may be revealed on CT scan (**9.67**) or barium meal and they may need to be treated by repeated aspiration under ultrasound control or by marsupialization.

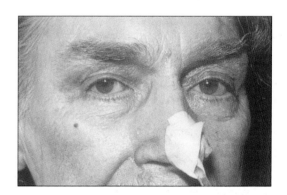

9.72   Carcinoma of the pancreas typically appears late in the course of the disease, as in this patient who is obviously jaundiced and has lost a considerable amount of weight. She presented with the painless onset of jaundice just 2 weeks before this photograph was taken, although her weight loss had occurred over several months. Pain is not always a feature of carcinoma of the pancreas – painless onset of jaundice is a common presentation of carcinoma of the head of the pancreas.

form in the liver, which may be enlarged. The gall bladder is often easily felt but non-tender (Courvoisier's sign). Ascites is often a prominent feature. There is a significantly increased incidence of superficial thrombophlebitis and deep vein thrombosis (**9.73**).

Carcinoma of the body and tail of the pancreas presents with deep epigastric pain radiating to the back, associated with weight loss. Frank diabetes or glucose intolerance is present in 30% of patients.

Liver function tests in pancreatic carcinoma usually show an obstructive pattern with a high alkaline phosphatase and bilirubin. Serum amylase and carcinoembryonic antigen (CEA) may also be elevated.

The diagnosis of pancreatic carcinoma is made by ultrasound (**9.74**), CT, ERCP or MRCP (**9.20**). ERCP (**9.75**) may show

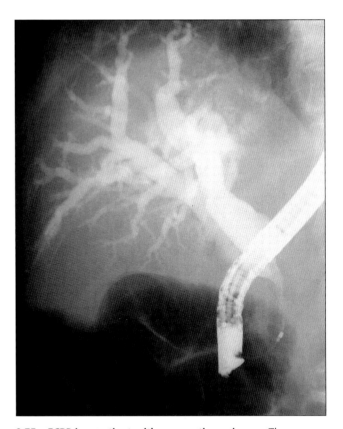

9.75   ECRP in a patient with pancreatic carcinoma. The pancreatic duct could not be cannulated, but the common bile duct has a severe distal stricture secondary to the pancreatic carcinoma, with gross dilatation of the extrahepatic and intrahepatic biliary tree.

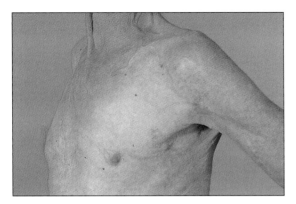

9.73   Thrombophlebitis in superficial or deep veins is relatively common in many forms of malignant disease, but it is particularly associated with carcinoma of the pancreas, and it is sometimes the presenting feature. In this patient, thrombosis in the veins of the upper arm is associated with an extensive collateral circulation in the superficial veins around the shoulder. Recurrent episodes of thrombophlebitis ('thrombophlebitis migrans') may precede the diagnosis of pancreatic carcinoma by many months, and their occurrence in an otherwise apparently fit patient should lead to a search for underlying malignancy – especially in the pancreas.

narrowing in the main duct and also allows the collection of pancreatic juice for cytology. Barium meal examination may first suggest the diagnosis (**9.76**); laparoscopy may provide supportive findings. Treatment options are limited. Surgical resection is only possible in 10–15% of patients, but endoscopically inserted stents (**8.76, 9.60**) may be valuable in relieving obstructive jaundice, and surgical bypass operations may achieve the same objective. Mean survival is 18 months following resection and 6 months in patients with non-resectable tumours.

OTHER PANCREATIC TUMOURS

A variety of other rare endocrine tumours are found in the pancreas.

Primary carcinoid (**p. 358**) can occur in the pancreas – the symptoms arise from hepatic metastases, and diagnosis rests on urinary excretion of 5-HIAA – a serotonin (5HT) metabolite. Treatment may be surgical, but recently a somatostatin analogue has been successfully used.

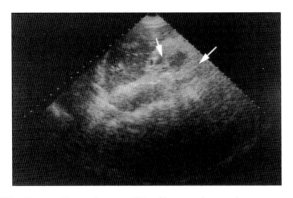

9.74   Pancreatic carcinoma. This ultrasound scan shows a mass in the head of the pancreas (arrows), containing several areas of decreased echogenicity, an appearance typical of carcinoma.

The other pancreatic tumours all arise from a single cell line – APUD (amine precursor uptake and decarboxylation) cells. They are classified by the main peptide produced, but they often produce more than one and the predominant peptide secreted can alter. Localization of these tumours may be very difficult even with selective arteriography. The major tumour types are summarized on **page 373**.

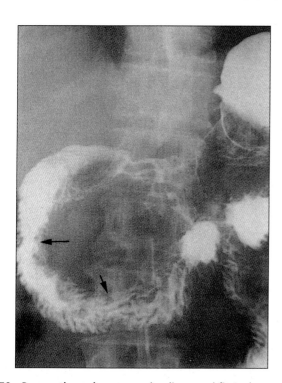

9.76 Pancreatic carcinoma may be diagnosed first when a barium meal is performed for undiagnosed gastrointestinal symptoms. In this patient, a large carcinoma in the head of the pancreas has led to a characteristic widening of the duodenal loop with compression of the second and third parts of the duodenum (arrows). This compression may lead to symptoms of intestinal obstruction, which may require palliative bypass surgery.

10 Blood

HISTORY AND EXAMINATION

Symptoms often develop late in the course of disorders of the blood and lymphoid system. In their early stages, anaemias, chronic leukaemias and other myeloproliferative disorders may be completely asymptomatic, or they may be associated with only vague symptoms, many of which are common in the general population, including fatigue, headaches, faintness, shortness of breath, palpitations, angina pectoris, intermittent claudication and recurrent minor infections.

Patients with acute leukaemia commonly present with a short history of more definite symptoms, which may include – in addition to the symptoms of anaemia – mouth ulceration, sore throat and other signs of infection, enlarged lymph nodes, bruising and bleeding, bone pain and symptoms caused by tissue infiltration. Those with thrombocytopenias present with characteristic skin changes; other major bleeding disorders also produce obvious symptoms, but more minor degrees of bleeding disorder may be subclinical and thus asymptomatic.

Thrombotic disorders usually have symptoms and signs related to arterial or venous thrombosis; however, disseminated intravascular coagulation (DIC) may cause haemostatic failure and is usually seen in severely ill patients, who are likely to have multiple symptomatology from the underlying cause of the condition.

Patients with lymphomas often present with lymphadenopathy, fever or symptoms resulting from tissue infiltration or compression by the lymphomatous process, with failure of the immune system, or with a haemorrhagic or haemolytic disorder; nevertheless, some patients remain asymptomatic and are diagnosed largely by chance.

Because of the absence of specific diagnostic symptoms in many disorders of the blood, clinical examination of the patient is of great importance. Clinical signs in haematology may result from abnormalities of red cells, white cells, platelets, plasma globulins or coagulation factors.

Excess or lack of red cells in the circulation is often obvious on examination. Polycythaemia is associated with plethora, especially of the face, which may show a bluish, cyanotic tinge because of the high levels of unsaturated haemoglobin. Comparison with a normal skin is helpful (**4.5, 10.1**).

Anaemia is often suggested by pallor of the face, lips, tongue (**10.2, 10.3**), conjunctivae (**8.3**), nailbeds and palms (**10.4**), but clinical examination is not always a good guide to the level of

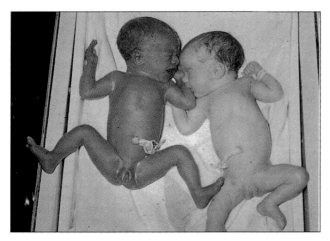

10.1 Polycythaemia and anaemia in identical newborn twins. The cause of this unusual condition was an arteriovenous fistula in the placenta; the picture is included here because it clearly exemplifies the difference in the appearance of polycythaemia (the twin on the left) from anaemia (the twin on the right). For a comparison of a polycythaemic adult with her normal sister *see* **4.5**.

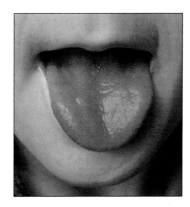

10.2 Iron deficiency anaemia commonly leads to pallor of the face, lips and tongue, and – when chronic – to atrophic glossitis and angular stomatitis. All these are seen in this young woman whose iron deficiency anaemia resulted from excessive menstrual bleeding. She responded to oral iron supplementation.

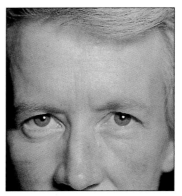

10.3 Severe anaemia commonly leads to generalized pallor, which is particularly obvious in the face. This patient had iron deficiency anaemia. Her haemoglobin was 5.0 g/dl.

405

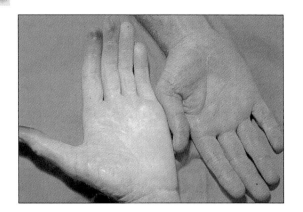

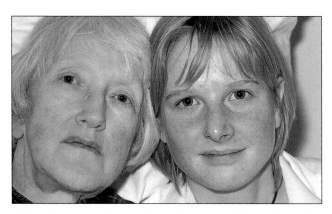

10.4   Pallor of the hand in anaemia is obvious in this patient, especially when compared with the physician's hand on the right. The patient's haemoglobin was 7 g/dl. The hand also shows that he was a heavy smoker. His anaemia resulted from chronic blood loss from a carcinoma in the oesophagus – a site where the risk of carcinoma is increased in smokers.

10.5   Clinical examination is not always a reliable guide to the haemoglobin level. Here a normal individual (right) is compared with a patient with severe anaemia (left). The patient had pernicious anaemia (her hair had been grey since the age of 30 years), with a haemoglobin of 5.0 g/dl when the picture was taken, but she does not look exceptionally pale.

haemoglobin (**10.5**, **10.6**). Examination of the mouth, lips and tongue may give a clue to the aetiology of the anaemia: for example, iron deficiency is associated with atrophy of mucosa, especially on the tongue and often with the presence of angular stomatitis (**7.129**, **10.2**). Lack of vitamin B_{12} and other B vitamins produces a tongue that is red and 'beefy' (**9.47**, **10.30**). The finger nails may show evidence of tissue iron deficiency with 'spooning' (koilonychia, **2.103**, **10.6**, **10.18**).

Excessive breakdown of red cells results in changes in urine colour; if the red cell destruction has occurred in the intravascular compartment, the urine passed is black to brown in colour ('blackwater', **1.145**); in extravascular haemolysis, it becomes dark and orange on standing because of the presence of excess urobilinogen, which is converted to urobilin.

Haemolysis leads to excessive production of indirect bilirubin which usually imparts a pale lemon-yellow colour to the skin and conjunctivae, such as is seen in pernicious anaemia (**9.2**, **10.28**, **10.30**), or a deeper yellow to orange colour in more active haemolytic anaemias (**10.38**).

General examination may also show the cause of anaemia, as in the perioral black-brown pigmentation in Peutz–Jeghers syndrome (**2.88**), the telangiectasia in hereditary haemorrhagic telangiectasia (**10.7**, **10.102**), or the skin purpura or ecchymosis of a bleeding disorder (**2.133**, **7.24**, **9.14**). The associated neurological features of a vitamin B_{12} deficiency anaemia include combined deficiencies in the posterior and lateral column function of the cord.

If anaemia develops quickly, it can lead to rapid cardiac decompensation and patients present with acute left ventricular failure (*see* **p. 206**). However, if it develops insidiously, there are compensatory mechanisms with tachycardia, tachypnoea and gradual onset of heart failure.

Bone and soft-tissue changes may result from extreme erythroid hyperplasia in chronic anaemia such as thalassaemia.

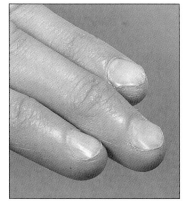

10.6   Pallor of the nailbeds is said to be characteristic of anaemia, but is often difficult to assess. This patient with menorrhagia had a haemoglobin of 9.0 g/dl, but her nailbeds were not grossly pale. She also has early koilonychia. Suspected anaemia should always be confirmed by the measurement of haemoglobin and other values in the blood.

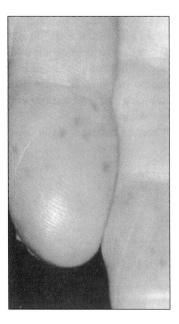

10.7   Hereditary haemorrhagic telangiectasia (HHT) is a condition in which occult blood loss in the gut may lead to severe iron deficiency anaemia. Patients commonly present with lesions on or close to mucous membranes (**10.102**), but the telangiectasia may occur anywhere on the body, as in this patient whose fingers were affected. The lesions are dilated capillaries, and they blanch if pressure is applied with a glass slide.

Deficient production of mature normal white cells leads to neutropenia (below 1.5×10^9/litre), which increases the chances of infection – patients often present with bacterial, viral, fungal or protozoal invasion of the skin, gums, throat or lungs. In conditions with malignant white cell production, the skin, liver, spleen, lymph nodes, tongue, testes and ovaries may be infiltrated and enlarge. High white and red cell turnover may be associated with elevation of the serum uric acid, and occasionally with acute and chronic gout (*see* **p. 120**).

Increased production of collagen in the marrow cavity in myelofibrosis or myelosclerosis leads to haemopoiesis elsewhere, especially in the liver and spleen, which become massively enlarged. Similar enlargement of the liver, spleen and lymph nodes (**10.8**, **10.9**) may be found in lymphomas and chronic leukaemias.

Reduction of platelet number below about 40×10^9/litre, or defects in platelet function, result in purpura and haemorrhages into the skin (**10.10**) and mucous membranes and may be associated with overt external or internal bleeding. Platelet number increases to over 1000×10^9/litre result in a likelihood of thrombosis, usually in the periphery, with gangrene of the

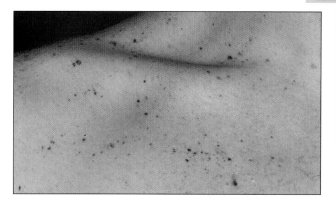

10.10   Purpura – in this case thrombocytopenic purpura (TP). The patient was a 15-year-old boy whose antiepileptic treatment regimen had recently been modified to include sodium valproate. This is just one of a number of drugs that may induce TP (*see* p. **438** and **10.99**), but the disorder is almost always reversible if the drug therapy is stopped.

407

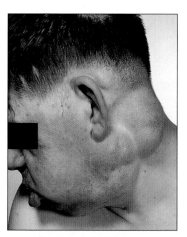

10.8   Gross enlargement of the cervical lymph nodes in a patient with Hodgkin's disease. The cervical lymph nodes are a common presenting site for lymphomas of all types and for leukaemia – especially chronic lymphatic leukaemia. This patient was severely mentally retarded, but he lived in the community and presented late in the course of the disease. It is unusual to see such advanced disease on presentation.

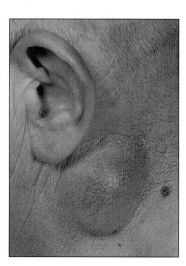

10.9   Enlargement of the postauricular lymph node in a patient with non-Hodgkin's lymphoma. Biopsy is required for confirmation of the diagnosis.

fingers or toes, and also occlusion in the cerebral or coronary arteries.

INVESTIGATIONS

The full blood count (FBC) (**10.11**) is easily measured using automated counters and is a routine investigation (**10.12**, **10.13**). Microscopic examination (**10.14**) is indicated if the FBC shows an abnormality or if a haematological disorder is suspected for other reasons. This may reveal changes characteristic of particular systemic diseases, for example atypical lymphocytes in infectious mononucleosis (**1.72**), malaria parasites (**1.148**), trypanosomes (**1.12**) or other parasites (**1.157**), or of haematological disorders, for example the misshapen red cells of hereditary elliptocytosis (**10.42**), or leukaemic cells (**10.71**, **10.72**, **10.74-10.76**). More commonly, a general abnormality is suggested, for example anaemia or infection, and this may require more detailed investigation.

In the investigation of anaemia, the reticulocyte count (**10.15**) provides an assessment of effective red cell production. The 'normal' proportion of reticulocytes is about 1%. In anaemic patients, hypoxia stimulates increased production of erythropoietin by the kidneys, and the reticulocyte count should thus markedly increase. The absence of an appropriate increase suggests anaemia caused by disordered red cell production (either because of inadequate numbers of red cell precursors, i.e. hypoplasia, or as a result of their premature death within the marrow, i.e. ineffective erythropoiesis) rather than increased red cell destruction (haemolysis) or blood loss.

Red cell size and colour are important. Decreased production related to impaired haemoglobin synthesis, whether of haem (e.g. in iron deficiency) or globin (in thalassaemias), tends to give rise to hypochromic, poorly haemoglobinized, often small (microcytic) red cells. In contrast, the larger, well

NORMAL VALUES FOR THE FULL BLOOD COUNT

	Men	Women	Units
Haemoglobin*	13.5–17.5	11.5–15.5	g/dl
Red cells	4.5–6.0	3.8–5.2	$\times 10^{12}$/litre
PCV (haematocrit)	0.40–0.52	0.37–0.47	%
MCV (mean cell volume)*		80–96	fl
MCH (mean cell haemoglobin)		27–32	pg
MCHC (mean cell haemoglobin concentration)		31–36	g/dl
Reticulocytes**		25–85	$\times 10^9$/litre
WBC (white blood cells)*		4–11	$\times 10^9$/litre
Neutrophils		2.0–7.5	$\times 10^9$/litre
Lymphocytes		1.5–4.0	$\times 10^9$/litre
Monocytes		0.2–0.8	$\times 10^9$/litre
Eosinophils		0.04–0.4	$\times 10^9$/litre
Basophils		< 0.1	$\times 10^9$/litre
Platelets		150–400	$\times 10^9$/litre

* In the neonate haemoglobin and MCV are normally higher, and in children below 12 years of age lower, than these adult values. Children also have higher lymphocyte counts

** Reticulocytes are often expressed as a percentage of total red cells (normal range 0.2–2.0% of red cells), but are best reported as absolute number since the red cell count may vary considerably

10.11 Normal values for the full blood count (FBC). The normal range varies to some extent between different laboratories.

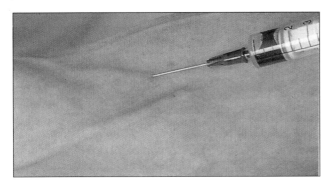

10.12 Venous blood sampling is a routine procedure, but it is important that it is carried out correctly for haematological and biochemical investigations to be accurate. In particular, it is essential that blood is not drawn up rapidly through a narrow-gauge needle, as this may cause artefactual haemolysis. The minimum possible degree of venous occlusion should be used for sampling, as stasis can affect the results of both biochemical and haematological investigations. It is essential that the blood sample is immediately transferred into the appropriate container for the investigation required, and that the blood is processed rapidly.

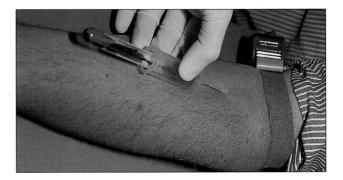

10.13 Venous blood sampling using a vacuum tube. This method is now commonly used in many countries. It allows blood to be drawn into several containers on a single occasion without the risk of creation of a potentially infective aerosol, and without a significant risk of spillage.

haemoglobinized (macrocytic) cells are associated with disordered nuclear maturation (e.g. in megaloblastic anaemias). In many anaemias secondary to systemic disorders, the red cells are of normal size and haemoglobin content (normocytic, normochromic). The red cell mean cell volume (MCV) and mean cell haemoglobin (MCH) can thus be helpful, with the reticulocyte count, in the initial classification of the cause of anaemia.

A bone marrow examination may be indicated if the cause of anaemia is obscure or if an abnormality of production of one or more of the blood cell lines is suspected, or if there is other evidence of a malignancy that commonly involves the bone marrow (e.g. lymphoma). Marrow smears from a needle aspirate of sternal or posterior ilium marrow cavities are taken

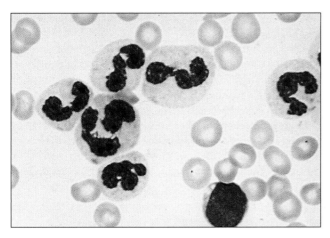

10.14 A blood film can often aid the interpretation of the full blood count. This patient had an elevated white cell count, and the film showed that most of the cells were neutrophils. Some of the neutrophils contain small blue-staining areas in the cytoplasm. These are known as Dohle bodies. They are a non-specific finding, but are common in patients with infections.

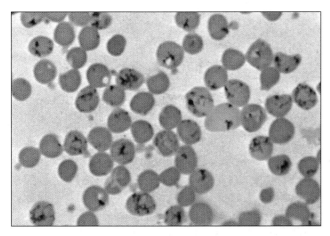

10.15 The reticulocyte count showed gross reticulocytosis in this patient. Up to 80% of the red cells in the peripheral blood film are reticulocytes, as shown by supravital staining for RNA. This patient had haemolytic anaemia caused by congenital pyruvate kinase (PK) deficiency.

for detailed morphological studies of haemopoietic cells (**10.16**). A marrow aspirate can also provide cells for cytogenetic studies, detailed immunological studies of cellular antigens (cell-marker studies) or molecular analysis of DNA, all of which may help in defining the precise cell type of abnormal cells (e.g. in leukaemia or lymphoma). Histology of a trephine biopsy often adds information and is needed if marrow is scanty. It provides less information about individual cells, but retains the marrow architectural relationships, gives a better guide to overall cellularity and may identify focal lesions (e.g. tumour infiltration) that are absent in the aspirate.

Biochemical studies are of value in further defining the causes of anaemia:

- Serum iron with total iron binding capacity (TIBC) gives information about iron transport and is complemented by the ferritin level, which more accurately reflects total body iron stores.
- Serum levels of vitamin B_{12} and folate, and the red cell folate level, give a clue to the presence or absence of essential components for red cell haemoglobin synthesis; low levels of vitamin B_{12} necessitate a two-stage Schilling test, which may indicate whether malabsorption of B_{12} is caused by lack of intrinsic factor or by intestinal disease.
- Excessive breakdown of haemoglobin can be monitored by measurement of indirect bilirubin, urobilinogen in the urine and stercobilinogen; occasionally, in intravascular breakdown, haemoglobin will appear in the urine and there is depletion of haptoglobins and appearance of methaemalbumin.

The cause of haemolysis may become obvious from examination of the blood film (e.g. parasites), from the presence of antibodies coating the red cells, or from the presence of abnormal haemoglobins on electrophoresis or abnormal enzymes within the red cells.

Abnormalities of blood coagulation and related systems require the expertise of highly specialized laboratories and physicians. Initial bedside investigations including the whole blood clotting time, bleeding time and capillary resistance test (Hess test) are still sometimes helpful, but laboratory studies are usually needed.

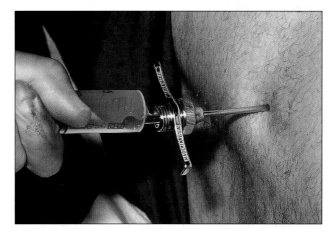

10.16 Bone marrow aspiration is now most commonly carried out from the posterior iliac crest, though satisfactory samples may be obtained from the sternum. Local anaesthetic is injected in the skin and down to the level of the periosteum, and a needle is pushed through the outer layer of the ilium into the marrow cavity. Marrow can then be aspirated into the syringe. A relatively small amount of marrow is required for investigation. A trephine bone biopsy adds further information, especially when little or no marrow is aspirable; this may also be performed using the Jamshidi needle shown here.

The basic screening tests should include a platelet count, the activated partial thromboplastin time (APTT), the prothrombin time (PT), the thrombin time and a test for fibrin degradation products (the D-dimer test). These indicate which part of the coagulation cascade is likely to be defective. Acquired haemostatic deficiencies (e.g. DIC, hepatic disease) may be the result of multiple deficiency in the coagulation and platelet system. Examination of the quality of the fibrin clot is worthwhile and it may also be incubated to see if there is active fibrinolysis present. These tests also may form the basis of control of anticoagulant therapy, but generally purpose-designed tests are more accurate (e.g the international normalized ratio, INR). It is probable that the biggest group of patients with haemostatic defects are those on oral anticoagulant therapy or prophylaxis.

ANAEMIAS

Anaemia is defined as a condition in which the blood has a deficient concentration of haemoglobin, which reduces its ability to transport oxygen. The most common form of anaemia worldwide, which affects over 500 million people, is that caused by iron deficiency. In hospital practice, secondary 'anaemia of chronic disease' predominates.

IRON-DEFICIENCY ANAEMIA

Iron deficiency commonly arises from a combination of reduced dietary intake of iron with a physiological increase in iron requirement. Occult blood loss, usually into the gut, and more rarely malabsorption (e.g. in coeliac disease or after gastrectomy) can also give rise to negative iron balance. The most common form of blood loss worldwide is hookworm infection (**10.17** and *see* **p. 368**).

It is important to take a detailed dietary history extending over the past year or so, and enquiry should be made about intake of meats, liver, green vegetables, eggs and milk. Strict vegetarians may eat iron in a non-absorbable form.

A history of obvious blood loss should be sought, as in women who have had multiple pregnancies or in whom there has been excess loss at menstruation. Obvious blood loss may also occur in patients with haemorrhoids. If bleeding occurs higher up in the alimentary tract, the red colour of haemoglobin is converted to give the stool the black colour of acid haematin (melaena). Occult alimentary bleeding may occur in patients taking aspirin or related non-steroidal anti-inflammatory drugs (**3.9**, **8.51**), with duodenal or gastric ulceration and from carcinomas and polyps in the bowel. Right-sided colonic carcinoma is particularly likely to manifest itself as unexplained anaemia. A history of previous alimentary surgery is important, especially if this has involved the removal of part of the acid-secreting portion of the stomach or the

creation of a bypass. Evidence of malabsorption should also be sought (*see* **p. 355**).

The patient should be examined for the signs of anaemia (**10.2**–**10.6**), especially for those that point to iron deficiency, such as koilonychia (**2.103**, **10.6**, **10.18**) and angular stomatitis (**10.2**), and for pointers to possible underlying blood loss such as telangiectasia (**10.7**) and haemorrhoids (**10.19**).

In iron deficiency, iron stores are mobilized first (reflected by a falling serum ferritin concentration) and only when these have been exhausted does the iron supply to the tissues, assessed by the serum iron and transferrin saturation, begin to decline,

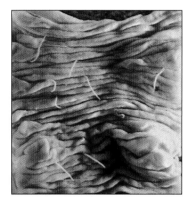

10.17 Hookworm infection is the most common cause of iron-deficiency anaemia worldwide. The worms are seen attached by their buccal capsules to the villi of the small intestine, where they feed by sucking blood (up to 0.2 ml per day per worm). In gross hookworm infection, severe iron-deficiency anaemia may result.

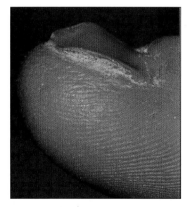

10.18 Koilonychia or 'spooning' of the nails is a result of a non-haemopoietic effect of iron deficiency. For views of koilonychia *see* **2.89**, **10.6**.

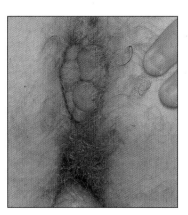

10.19 Haemorrhoids are a common cause of rectal bleeding. Interoexternal piles – as seen here – commonly bleed on defaecation, and over time this blood loss can lead to iron deficiency.

eventually giving rise to frank anaemia. Iron is essential for maturation and function of all cells and non-haemopoietic effects of deficiency include koilonychia and oral changes. The underlying cause of the negative iron balance must always be sought, paying particular attention to possible gastrointestinal blood loss. Investigations should include:

- FBC and film. This shows a reduction in red cell numbers and haematocrit. The red cell size (MCV) is reduced (< 75 fl) and may be as low as 60 fl. The cells have a reduced MCH that is below 25 pg. The film confirms that the cells are microcytic, hypochromic and have variations in size and shape (**3.9**, **10.20**). There may be early forms present. The

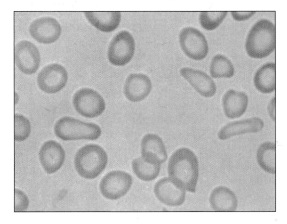

10.20   Blood film in iron deficiency showing hypochromia, anisocytosis and poikilocytosis. All the red cells show marked hypochromic central pallor. A few also show distortions in shape, but this is not a marked feature of simple iron deficiency.

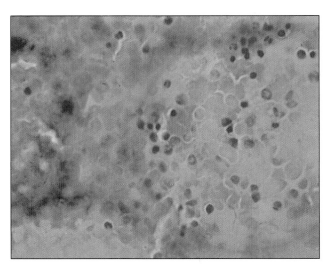

10.21   Bone marrow smear in iron-deficiency anaemia, stained for free iron by the Prussian Blue method. Iron stores are completely absent in this marrow. Free iron would stain bright blue (*see* **10.23**).

platelet count may be raised, and white cells are usually normal. If the cause of anaemia is hookworm infection, eosinophilia is often present.

- Faecal occult blood measurement is of value, but the results must be interpreted with caution because of the possibility of false-positive and false-negative results.
- Serum ferritin is low, reflecting reduction of tissue iron; a low serum iron and a high transferrin with a low percentage saturation is a reflection of deficient transport.
- Bone marrow aspiration shows a hyperplastic marrow dominated by active red cell series proliferation; staining with Prussian Blue shows reduced or absent iron staining (**10.21**).
- Endoscopy of the upper and lower alimentary tract may define bleeding lesions (**8.44**, **8.45**, **8.50**, **8.51**, **8.57**, **8.58**, **8.89**, **8.90**).
- Barium series of the upper and lower alimentary tract may show associated changes of iron deficiency, for example the Plummer–Vinson or Paterson–Brown–Kelly syndrome (**8.41**) or a lesion that may have bled (**8.94**, **8.85**).
- Occasionally, mesenteric arteriography or nuclear medicine studies may help to reveal obscure sites of blood loss in the gut (**8.23**).

Treatment is usually with simple oral iron salts (ferrous sulphate or fumarate), and any adverse effects (e.g. constipation) may be ameliorated by reducing the dose or by changing to a preparation that contains less available iron in each tablet (e.g. ferrous gluconate). Failure of response is most commonly caused by lack of compliance, but should lead to re-assessment of the diagnosis as other causes of hypochromic anaemia include alpha- or beta-thalassaemia trait and sideroblastic anaemias, which may be associated with excessive iron absorption and thus with a risk of damage from iron overload with prolonged oral iron therapy.

SIDEROBLASTIC ANAEMIA

Sideroblastic anaemias are a rare group of hypochromic anaemias in which the serum iron levels are high and the transferrin is saturated. A variety of acquired and inherited defects in porphyrin biosynthesis lead to diminished synthesis of haem. The key diagnostic feature is the presence of the ringed sideroblast in the marrow aspirate. This is a normoblast, containing iron granules in the mitochondria that have a perinuclear distribution (**10.22**, **10.23**). Acquired causes include alcoholism, drugs such as isoniazid, lead poisoning, myelodysplasia and myeloproliferative disease. Patients should abstain from alcohol and possibly causative drugs should be withdrawn. Lead poisoning may require treatment with chelating agents. Transfusion should be used as infrequently as possible in these patients, because of the dangers of iron overload. Some patients may respond to large doses of vitamin B$_6$ or rarely to androgens.

411

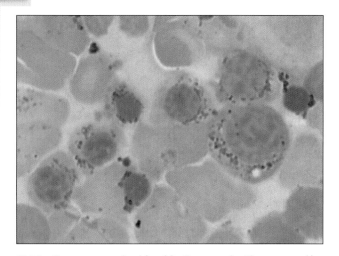

10.22 Bone marrow in sideroblastic anaemia. The marrow has been stained for free iron, thus revealing ringed sideroblasts. These are erythroblasts with free iron granules arranged as a nearly continuous ring around the nucleus. This iron is chiefly concentrated in mitochondria.

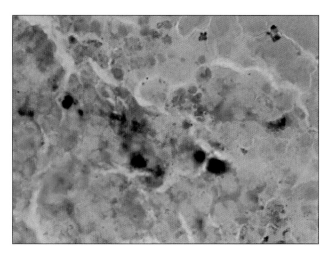

10.23 Bone marrow smear in sideroblastic anaemia. In this case, the bone marrow has been stained with Prussian Blue (the same method as used in **10.21**) revealing increased (blue) iron stores. Normal subjects have stainable free iron amounts midway between the appearance seen here and that in **10.21**.

ANAEMIA OF CHRONIC DISEASE

The main differential diagnosis for early iron-deficiency anaemia is the anaemia associated with many chronic disorders, for example chronic arthritis, chronic infections, renal and liver failure, neoplasia and endocrine disorders (**10.24**). This anaemia, at least initially, is normocytic and normochromic and is multifactorial in origin, with a slight reduction in red cell survival, inappropriately low production of erythropoietin, and a disturbance of iron delivery to the developing erythroblasts, which in time can give rise to a degree of hypochromia and

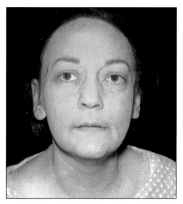

10.24 Anaemia of chronic disease, manifest as severe pallor in a diabetic patient with severe uraemia. Her haemoglobin was 6.5 g/dl, but the blood film demonstrated that the anaemia remained normochromic and normocytic.

microcytosis of the red cells (**10.25**). In contrast to uncomplicated iron deficiency, the iron stores in this form of anaemia tend to be normal or increased (high serum ferritin); increased storage by macrophages of the iron released from destroyed red cells results in impaired release of iron to circulating transferrin and thus reduced delivery of iron to the bone marrow (low serum iron and low transferrin).

Iron-deficiency anaemia and the anaemia of chronic disease may coexist (e.g. in a patient with active rheumatoid arthritis who also has occult gastrointestinal blood loss induced by non-steroidal anti-inflammatory drugs). Under such circumstances, a bone marrow examination will determine whether iron stores are reduced (*see* **10.21**, **10.23**).

The anaemia of chronic disease improves only with treatment of the underlying disease and does not respond to iron therapy or other haematinics. Though a response to recombinant human erythropoietin (rEPO) has been seen in

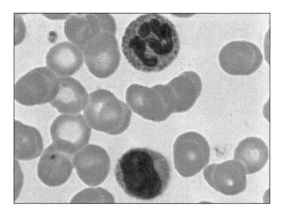

10.25 Anaemia of chronic disease. The anaemia is normocytic, but some hypochromia is obvious. In addition, there is prominent rouleaux formation – red cells are grouped together in piles or stacks. In a properly prepared smear, rouleaux formation suggests the same range of abnormalities that are revealed by a high erythrocyte sedimentation rate, so rouleaux formation may be found in any chronic inflammatory process or malignancy and, especially, in multiple myeloma and other monoclonal gammopathies.

some patients, this is by no means established, in contrast to the proven value of this growth factor in the hypoplastic anaemia associated with chronic renal failure.

MACROCYTIC ANAEMIA

Macrocytic red cells are seen in association with liver disease, as a result of regular alcohol intake or in haemolysis. They may also occur in hypothyroidism and in haemolytic anaemias in which there is an increase in reticulocytes (which are larger than mature red cells). Macrocytosis also occurs as a result of an underlying nuclear maturation defect affecting blood cell precursors in the bone marrow and giving rise to a megaloblastic marrow. This is commonly caused by either vitamin B_{12} or folic acid deficiency, though cytotoxic chemotherapy and other intrinsic marrow disorders may give rise to a similar picture. Folic acid is required for the synthesis of the pyrimidines and purines of DNA, and vitamin B_{12} maintains the intracellular folate in an active form.

Causes of B_{12} deficiency are summarized in **10.26**; causes of folate deficiency are summarized in **10.27**.

Deficiencies in folate or B_{12} give rise to an anaemia of insidious onset, which is often very severe at the time of presentation. – usually with non-specific features of anaemia such as lethargy, tiredness and weight loss. Clinically the combination of pallor with mild icterus related to intramedullary premature death of erythroblasts typically gives rise to a lemon-yellow skin colour (**10.28**). Prematurely grey hair may occur in pernicious anaemia (**10.5, 10.29**). Glossitis may occur (**9.47, 10.30**). Bruising and purpura may suggest coexistent thrombocytopenia, and fundal haemorrhages may occur, as in any severe anaemia. There may be hepatosplenomegaly and signs of heart failure.

Subacute combined degeneration of the cord in vitamin B_{12} deficiency presents with symmetrical paraesthesiae of hands and feet, and impairment of proprioception and vibration sense

leads to ataxia. Higher cerebral function is also frequently impaired and dementia may occasionally result.

Neurological signs, particularly posterior column signs, may point to deficiency of vitamin B_{12}, and a personal or family history of other autoimmune disorders (e.g. thyroid disease, diabetes, Addison's disease, rheumatoid arthritis or vitiligo,

---

CAUSES OF FOLATE DEFICIENCY

Decreased intake

Nutritional deficiency
   Lack of fresh fruit and vegetables
   Alcoholism
   Milk-fed premature infants

Malabsorption
   Coeliac disease
   Tropical sprue
   Post-gastrectomy
   Crohn's disease
   Drugs – phenytoin, methotrexate

Increased requirement

Physiological
   Pregnancy
   Lactation
   Prematurity
   Growth in childhood

Pathological
   Haemolytic states
   Myeloproliferative disorders
   Severe inflammatory states
   Dialysis

Impaired folate utilization

Cytotoxic drugs – methotrexate
Trimethoprim
Anticonvulsants – phenytoin, phenobarbitone
Alcohol

10.27 Causes of folate deficiency.

CAUSES OF VITAMIN B$_{12}$ DEFICIENCY

Nutritional deficiency
   Vegan or strict vegetarian diet
   Alcoholism
   Severe protein-calorie malnutrition

Competition in gut by microflora or fish tapeworm

Malabsorption
   Intrinsic factor deficiency (pernicious anaemia)
   Diseased terminal ileum
   Surgical removal of terminal ileum
   Pancreatic failure
   Drugs – biguanides, potassium supplements

10.26 Causes of vitamin B$_{12}$ deficiency.

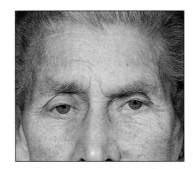

10.28 Pernicious anaemia often gives rise to characteristic pallor with a lemon-yellow tinge. The pallor relates directly to the haemoglobin level, whereas the mild jaundice is the result of the premature breakdown of erythroblasts (ineffective erythropoesis), and is associated with elevated plasma indirect bilirubin and urinary urobilinogen. Typically, patients with pernicious anaemia have blue eyes and (often prematurely) grey hair.

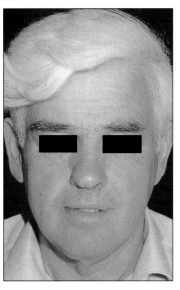

10.29 Prematurely grey hair in a 45-year-old man with pernicious anaemia. The patient developed grey hair at the age of 25 years and had two close relatives who died from gastric carcinoma.

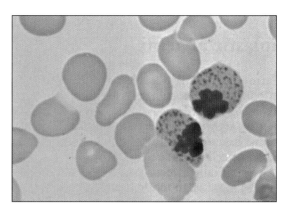

10.31 Peripheral blood in macrocytic anaemia caused by B_{12} deficiency. Note the presence of two late megaloblasts with nuclear rosette formation and basophil stippling. The red cells show macrocytosis, anisocytosis and poikilocytosis.

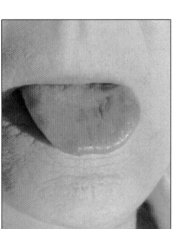

10.30 Pernicious anaemia. This patient shows similar skin coloration to that seen in **10.28**. In addition, she has a 'raw beef' tongue. The surface is smooth, with an absence of filiform papillae. Similar changes may be seen as a result of deficiency in other B-group vitamins.

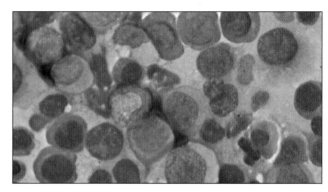

10.32 Marrow smear in pernicious anaemia. Erythroblasts predominate, and erythropoiesis is megaloblastic.

2.89) may suggest B_{12} deficiency resulting from intrinsic factor deficiency (pernicious anaemia). Pernicious anaemia affects 1% of individuals over the age of 60 years. There is a strong association between pernicious anaemia and carcinoma of the stomach; this is an indication for GI investigation in the presence of GI symptoms or a family history of gastric carcinoma.

Defective maturation of all proliferating cell lines means that a pancytopenia with reduction in neutrophils and platelets may be present. There may be nucleated megaloblasts in the circulation (**10.31**), but bone marrow examination is usually needed to confirm a megaloblastic basis for the macrocytosis of the circulating red cells (**10.32**). Serum B_{12} and folate assays and red cell folate assay help to identify the underlying deficiency.

In vitamin B_{12} deficiency, it is essential to demonstrate that impaired absorption of the vitamin is corrected by the addition of oral intrinsic factor before making a diagnosis of classic pernicious anaemia, as other gut pathology (e.g. Crohn's ileitis)

may also impair vitamin B_{12} absorption from the terminal ileum. This can be done using the Schilling test, in which urinary B_{12} is measured after oral administration, or by whole-body counting of orally administered radiolabelled B_{12}.

In pernicious anaemia, virtually all patients have circulating gastric parietal cell antibodies; 50% also have antibodies to intrinsic factor (which are more specific), and a small percentage have a range of other circulating autoantibodies.

Treatment is with oral replacement of folate and vitamin B_{12} if the cause is dietary. In classic pernicious anaemia, after gastrectomy, and with other uncorrectable gut pathologies, regular injections of hydroxocobalamin are required. Treatment results in a rapid rise in the reticulocyte count, which can be monitored (**10.33**) and precedes the rise in haemoglobin levels. There may also be a need for supplemental iron therapy. Hydroxocobalamin therapy may reverse early neurological changes in pernicious anaemia; the later changes may be arrested. Folate treatment should not be given in megaloblastic anaemia until B_{12} deficiency is ruled out, as folate administration may precipitate neurological changes in patients with B_{12} deficiency.

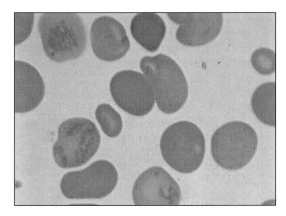

10.33 The 'reticulocyte response' to treatment of megaloblastic anaemia caused by B$_{12}$ or folate deficiency can be very dramatic. This peripheral blood film has been stained for reticulocytes, and it shows a strong response 5 days after the start of hydroxocobalamin therapy in a patient with pernicious anaemia. The rapid increase in erythropoiesis on treatment may put the patient at risk of developing iron deficiency.

SOME DRUGS THAT MAY CAUSE MARROW APLASIA	
Antimitotics	methotrexate, cytosine arabinoside, busulphan, cyclophosphamide, 6-mercaptopurine
Antibiotics	chloramphenicol, methicillin, penicillin, tetracyclines, sulphonamides
Anti-rheumatics	gold salts, penicillamine, indomethacin, colchicine
Anticonvulsants	phenytoin, carbamazepine
Anti-diabetic	chlorpropamide, tolbutamide
Anti-thyroid	carbimazole, thiouracil, potassium per-chlorate
Tranquillizers	chlorpromazine, chlordiazepoxide, meprobamate, promazine

10.34   Some drugs that may cause marrow aplasia.

Neural tube defects in the fetus (spina bifida, anencephaly and encephalocele) are more common when the mother's plasma and red cell folate levels are low (even though they may be within the normal range); and dietary supplementation with folate (or the consumption of good dietary sources of folate) from before conception to at least the end of the first trimester can greatly reduce this risk. Supplementation with folate may also reduce the risk of coronary heart disease in patients with elevated homocystine levels.

APLASTIC ANAEMIA

Marrow aplasia is a rare condition in which there is a peripheral pancytopenia resulting from failure of the stem cells of the bone marrow to continue to produce all cell lines. The marrow architecture remains normal, but fat replaces the normal haemopoietic cells. Rarely, only one cell line may be initially affected – as in agranulocytosis – but this usually progresses to total aplasia.

Aplasia is the end result of a variety of processes that include autoimmunity, drugs, toxins, viral infections and radiation. Rarely, there may be a genetic component, and in many cases a cause is not found. In clinical practice the most common causes are drugs (**10.34**), some of which may damage one cell line more than another. Often the drug therapy is being given as part of a treatment regimen for neoplasia or immunosuppression. In these cases the aplasia is usually reversible. There is also an association of aplastic anaemia with the later development of acute lymphocytic leukaemia in childhood, and in adults exposed to benzene or radiation there is a significant incidence of acute myeloid leukaemia after many years.

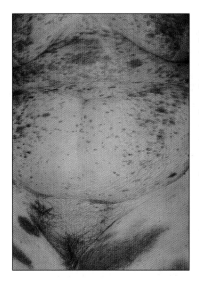

10.35   Aplastic anaemia developed when this 76-year-old woman was treated with co-trimoxazole for a urinary tract infection. Thrombocytopenia is responsible for her widespread purpura and ecchymoses, and she also had a severe throat infection as a result of her low white cell count.

Clinical symptoms and presentation in aplastic anaemia relate to the lack of functional cells in the peripheral blood. There is an insidious onset of the symptoms of anaemia, with recurrent infections as the white cell count falls, and bleeding from multiple sites as a result of thrombocytopenia. Clinical examination usually shows purpura and ecchymoses (**10.35**), and there may also be internal bleeding, especially from the gums and alimentary tract and into the eye. There may be infection in the mouth (**10.36**), or skin.

The diagnosis is suggested on finding pancytopenia in the peripheral blood, but it must be differentiated from hypersplenism (*see* **p. 426**). Bone marrow aspiration may yield little available marrow and a trephine bone biopsy may be required for histological section (**10.37**). Treatment should be initially directed at the cause. Androgens and corticosteroids are of value in some patients. Supportive treatment with red cell, platelet and white cell transfusions may be necessary. Bone

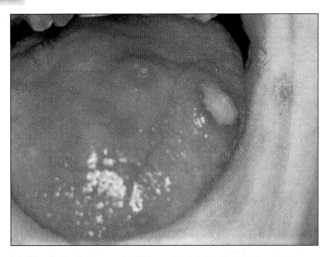

10.36 Aplastic anaemia. This patient initially developed agranulocytosis, manifesting as severe, intractable mouth ulcers and respiratory tract infections. The cause was unclear, but he progressed to develop pancytopenia and true aplastic anaemia.

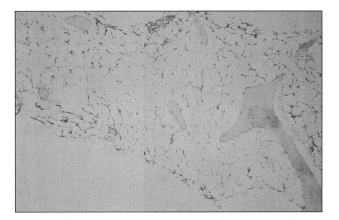

10.37 Aplastic anaemia can be confirmed by trephine biopsy of iliac crest marrow. This low-power view of a trephine biopsy from a young woman with drug-induced severe aplastic anaemia, showed loss of virtually all haemopoietic cells, with only a few residual lymphocytes and no inflammatory response. This marrow picture usually carries a grave prognosis.

marrow transplantation is successful in about 70% of patients with aplastic anaemia, but a matched donor is not always available. Anti-lymphocyte globulin (ALG) or other immunosuppressive therapy is sometimes helpful if marrow transplant is not possible. Recently, growth factors produced by recombinant DNA technology have been shown to be of value.

HAEMOLYTIC ANAEMIAS

Haemolysis is suggested by evidence of both increased red cell production (reticulocytosis) and increased red cell destruction. The destruction may be intravascular (giving rise acutely to

haemoglobinuria, or chronically to haemosiderinuria) with a reduced concentration of serum haptoglobin (haemoglobin-binding protein), or extravascular (mediated by macrophages) and associated with increased unconjugated bilirubin in the blood. Clinically, the combination of pallor, jaundice (**9.2**, **10.38**) and splenomegaly should suggest haemolysis, and, in chronic cases, there may be symptoms or signs of pigment gallstones, or signs of iron overload (secondary haemochromatosis; **10.39**). A blood film may sometimes show red cell abnormalities that are diagnostic of particular causes of haemolysis, but it may show only a non-specific polychromasia associated with the reticulocytosis.

Haemolysis may result from intrinsic, nearly always inherited, defects of the red cell, or from acquired disorders, usually related to extracorpuscular changes:

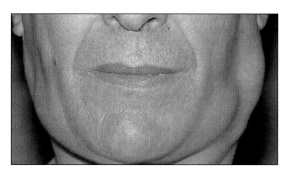

10.38 Haemolytic anaemia may lead to a characteristic lemon-yellow jaundice, as in this man who developed warm autoimmune haemolysis in association with chronic lymphocytic leukaemia (*see* **p. 429**). Such patients have no bilirubin in the urine but excess urobilinogen ('acholuric jaundice'). Note his 'bull neck' appearance, which results from gross cervical lymphadenopathy.

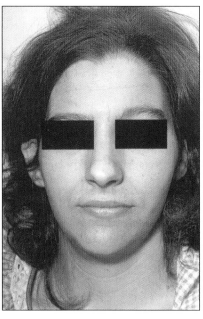

10.39 Secondary haemochromatosis (haemosiderosis), giving a characteristic skin pigmentation, may be a long-term consequence of the iron overload associated with chronic haemolytic anaemia. This 19-year-old patient had thalassaemia intermedia (*see* **p. 422**). Note the combination of pigmentation and pallor.

- Intrinsic disorders include those of the cell membrane (e.g. hereditary spherocytosis, hereditary elliptocytosis), of haemoglobin synthesis (e.g. sickle-cell disease) and of cell metabolism (e.g. pyruvate kinase or glucose-6-phosphate dehydrogenase deficiencies).
- Extrinsic causes of haemolysis include chronic renal failure and liver disease, but the shortening of red cell survival in these conditions is usually only modest. Excepting these, the most common acquired haemolytic anaemias are immune in origin: isoimmune, as in haemolytic disease of the newborn or haemolytic blood transfusion reactions; autoimmune with antibodies directed against red cell antigens and giving rise to positive direct antiglobulin (Coombs') test; or drug-induced, in which the effect may result from autoantibodies or neoantigens involving the drug as a hapten. Non-antibody-mediated haemolytic anaemia may also be acquired, as in paroxysmal nocturnal haemoglobinuria and in some drug-induced haemolyses.
- Fragmentation haemolysis may be seen in association with DIC (microangiopathic haemolysis, **10.115**), in patients with artificial heart valves and in malaria.
- Hypersplenism with haemolysis may be a feature of a variety of disorders associated with splenomegaly.

Red cell membrane defects
A variety of defects have been described in the red cell membrane. The most common and important is hereditary spherocytosis, which is found in 1–2 per 10 000 of the population, and is usually transmitted as an autosomal dominant. The biochemical defect is in the production of the protein spectrin; the result is the production of spherical red cells that have an altered permeability and a significantly shortened half-life. Clinically there is a wide spectrum of severity, even within families, but the picture usually includes

haemolytic anaemia, acholuric jaundice and splenomegaly (**10.40**). Most patients can lead a normal life, even when slightly anaemic. However, at times (e.g. in acute infections) an acute haemolytic crisis may occur, which requires blood transfusion. Aplastic crises may also occur during parvovirus and other infections in these patients, especially in young children (*see* **p. 17**). The erythroid hyperplasia leads to an increased need for folic acid, which should be given prophylactically. The chronic haemolytic state is associated with pigment gallstones in most adults and patients may occasionally present with a confusing mixed haemolytic and obstructive jaundice. Other cells require spectrin for normal function and associated abnormalities have been described in neurological and cardiac cell function.

The diagnosis is confirmed by finding evidence of chronic haemolysis and a typical blood film with microspherocytosis of red cells and reticulocytosis (**10.41**). The red cells are osmotically fragile and this provides a useful screening test.

417

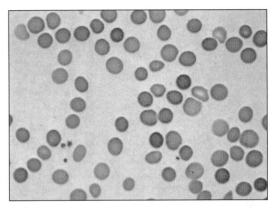

10.41 Hereditary spherocytosis. This low-power view of a peripheral blood film shows that approximately one-half of the red cells are small and very deeply stained. These cells have the characteristic appearance of spherocytes, though the other cells in the film are within the normal range. Often, only a proportion of the red cells are affected in spherocytosis. Supravital staining revealed a reticulocyte count of 60% in this patient.

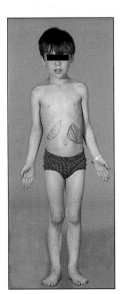

10.40 Hereditary spherocytosis. This 9-year-old boy shows typical mild pallor. He has marked splenomegaly and mild hepatomegaly.

Assay of spectrin is possible in some laboratories. It is important to screen family members for the condition. The treatment of choice is splenectomy, which should be preceded by appropriate vaccination and followed by long-term prophylactic antibiotic therapy (*see* **p. 426**). It is important at surgery to ensure that there are no accessory splenunculae as these will hypertrophy if not removed and haemolysis will continue.

Hereditary elliptocytosis is caused by a variety of molecular defects and is usually asymptomatic. The diagnosis is made on the typical appearances of the blood film (**10.42**), but only a few patients have significant anaemia or any evidence of haemolysis.

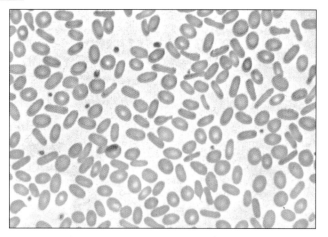

10.42   Hereditary elliptocytosis. This inherited anomaly of red cells leads to their assuming an oval or cigar shape. As in hereditary spherocytosis, some normal red cells are also usually present – in this case, about 50%. Pseudo-elliptocytosis may occur as a result of bad technique when a blood smear is prepared; however, when this occurs, the 'elliptocytes' are usually found only at one end of the smear, and the long axes of the cells are roughly parallel.

Enzyme deficiencies in red cells

Many enzyme defects have been described, but only two are common: glucose-6-phosphate dehydrogenase (G6PD) deficiency and pyruvate kinase deficiency:

- **G6PD deficiency** results in inability of the red cell to resist oxidants that may result from infections or from drug administration. As a result, haemoglobin is oxidized to methaemoglobin, which is functionless in terms of oxygen carriage, is relatively insoluble and precipitates in the red cells as Heinz bodies (**10.43**). The red cells are then vulnerable to destruction in the spleen. A large number of variants of enzyme activ-

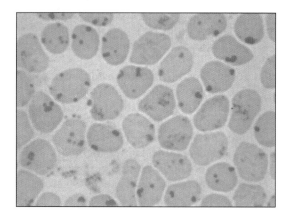

10.43   Glucose-6-phosphate dehydrogenase deficiency leads to the formation of Heinz bodies in the erythrocytes. Here the bodies have been stained with methyl violet. They represent precipitates of denatured haemoglobin, resulting from the lack of reducing enzymes.

ity have now been identified, accounting for a wide spectrum of disease activity. The disorder usually presents with acute intravascular haemolysis – jaundice, haemoglobinuria, anaemia and methaemoglobinaemia. A large number of drugs and foods have been implicated in precipitating the acute episodes. Offending substances should be avoided or withdrawn. Blood transfusion may be life-saving during acute attacks.

- **Pyruvate kinase deficiency** is inherited as an autosomal recessive, and it is only the homozygotes that haemolyse. The enzyme-deficient cells have a significantly shortened life span, and the haemolysis is chronic and not related to infections, drugs or foods. Splenomegaly is usually found. The definitive diagnosis is made by measurement of enzyme activity, and homozygous patients are usually clinically anaemic with a reticulocytosis (**10.15**). Secondary haemochromatosis may occur (**10.39**).

Sickle-cell syndromes

A single amino acid substitution (valine for glutamic acid) at position 6 of the beta-chain of globin results in a haemoglobin with abnormal physical and chemical properties. Haemoglobin S (HbS) can be found in the homozygous state (Hb SS, sickle-cell disease), in the heterozygous state (Hb AS, sickle-cell trait), or in association with all the other globin chain variants, including haemoglobin C, D and E, or with beta-thalassaemia. The abnormal gene has a worldwide distribution, but is most common in those of African origin. It may confer a biological advantage against infection with falciparum malaria.

Disease results from polymerization of HbS molecules within the red cells. Polymerization occurs only when HbS is in the deoxy form, and the subsequent crystallization results in cells that become rigid and sickle shaped and are unable to deform to pass through capillaries. This physical alteration is reversible when the molecules are again oxygenated, unless the red cell membrane is severely damaged.

People who are homozygous for HbS (sickle-cell disease) suffer from chronic haemolysis, which is usually adequately compensated. Their haemoglobin level runs at 5–10 g/dl, with a reticulocyte count of 10–30%. There is usually mild jaundice resulting from elevation of the unconjugated bilirubin fraction. Acute haemolytic crises may be precipitated by infections, pregnancy, drugs, surgery and anaesthesia all of which may also precipitate acute vascular occlusion in the microcirculation with tissue death. Sickle-cell crises are associated with fever, malaise and pain, which may be severe, and can occur in most parts of the body. Organs affected include bone (**10.44–10.46**), muscle, brain, eye (**10.47**), lung, spleen, liver, kidney and skin. Infection often occurs in the infarcted tissue, and chronic infection frequently complicates bone and joint ischaemia (**3.153, 10.48**). Pigment gallstones are common as a result of the chronic haemolysis. The disease carries a high mortality in young children, and death usually results from renal failure, overwhelming infection or vascular occlusion. Such patients should be managed in the same way as splenectomized patients with immunization and antibiotic prophylaxis (*see* **p. 426**).

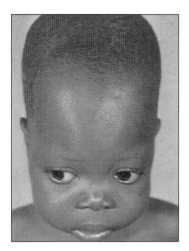

10.44 Bossing of the skull caused by hyperplasia of the bone marrow in sickle-cell disease. Similar appearances are more commonly seen in thalassaemia and other severe congenital haemolytic anaemias.

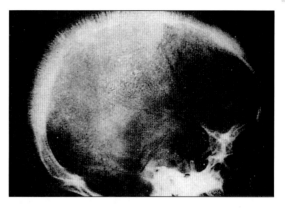

10.45 A 'hair on end' appearance of the skull on X-ray is commonly associated with frontal bossing. As with bossing, this appearance is most common in thalassaemia and other severe congenital haemolytic anaemias.

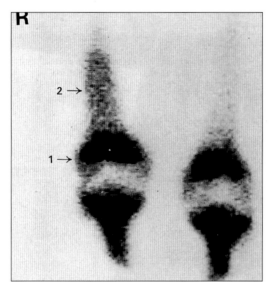

10.46 A bone scan in a patient with sickle-cell disease. There is increased activity in both epiphyseal growth plates (1) and an area of abnormal isotope uptake in the lower right femur (2). This abnormality reflects recurrent episodes of avascular necrosis with repair, but this process also renders the bone especially susceptible to osteomyelitis caused by *Salmonella* or other organisms.

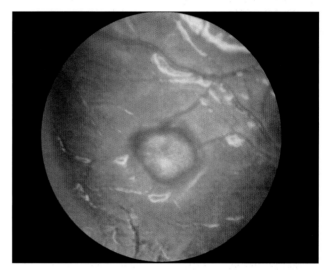

10.47 Sickle-cell retinopathy. Intermittent occlusion of small blood vessels by inflexible sickle-shaped cells commonly leads to characteristic 'salmon-patch' haemorrhages in the retina. These may evolve into pigmented retinal scars. The retinal vessels are also tortuous. At a later stage, proliferative retinopathy may also occur. Similar changes may be seen in other severe haemolytic anaemias, including thalassaemia.

The diagnosis is confirmed by a positive sickling test (**10.49, 10.50**) and by haemoglobin electrophoresis (**10.51**). Prenatal and cord-blood screening programmes should aid early diagnosis, and subsequent medical supervision may prevent long-term sequelae.

Management should be aimed at the prevention of infections and other situations that cause acute haemolytic and vascular crises. Acute crises require adequate oxygenation, rehydration, antibiotics and adequate pain control. Anaemia may be treated by blood transfusion but, in the long term, this may result in secondary haemochromatosis (**10.39**).

People heterozygous for HbS (sickle-cell trait) are usually asymptomatic unless exposed to lowered oxygen tensions (as in

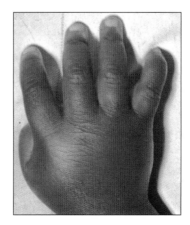

10.48 Severe dactylitis (inflammation of the fingers) is a common presentation of sickle-cell disease in children, and similar changes may occur in the feet. The painful swelling of the fingers commonly results from destructive changes in the small bones resulting from multiple infarctions, and sometimes complicated by osteomyelitis.

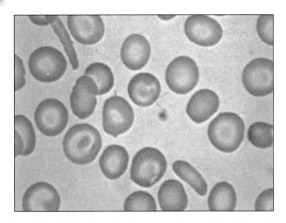

10.49   A fresh blood smear from a patient with sickle-cell disease shows few elongated or sickled cells, but anisocytosis, poikilocytosis and target cells are all seen.

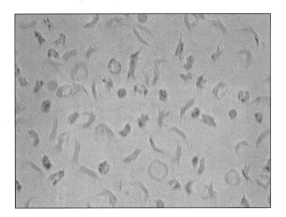

10.50   Sickle cells can be formed by exposing red cells from a patient with sickle-cell disease to the reducing action of sodium metabisulphite under a sealed coverslip. As the reduced HbS crystallizes within the cells, they all come to assume the distorted, elongated sickle shape.

unpressurized aircraft, at high altitude, or sometimes during anaesthesia). Renal microinfarcts occur in heterozygotes, however, and patients may complain of haematuria and eventually develop renal impairment.

Thalassaemia

Thalassaemia is the name given to a group of haemoglobinopathies that result from genetic mutations affecting synthesis of normal globins. The two major types are alpha- and beta-thalassaemia, which are caused by defective synthesis of the alpha- and beta-globin polypeptides. This results in failure of normal haemoglobin synthesis and the production of abnormal red cells that are hypochromic and microcytic.

Thalassaemia trait

The most common abnormality is thalassaemia trait (or thalassaemia minor), which is the heterozygous form of alpha-

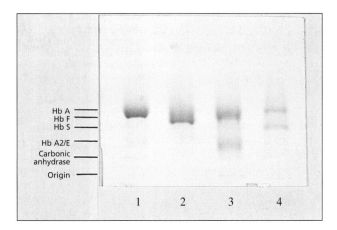

10.51   Haemoglobin electrophoresis. Haemoglobins containing variant globin chains may have different electrophoretic mobility. Cellulose acetate electrophoresis at alkaline pH is commonly used as an initial screen. Lane 1, normal adult (predominantly HbA, $\alpha2\ \beta2$); lane 2, neonatal cord blood (predominantly HbF, $\alpha2\ \gamma2$), lane 3, heterozygous HbE (containing both HbA and HbE, $\alpha2\ \beta E2$); lane 4, HbS heterozygote (sickle-cell trait containing both HbA and HbS, $\alpha\ \beta S2$).

or beta-thalassaemia. This is usually associated with very mild defects in the red cells with microcytosis (MCV 55–75) and hypochromia (MCH 20–22) and sometimes with a chronic very mild anaemia with a haematocrit of about 0.30 and a slightly raised red cell count (**10.52**). The condition is common in certain parts of the world and affects up to 20% of people from parts of Africa, Asia and the Mediterranean. There are many variants of thalassaemia minor associated with a range of other minor abnormal haemoglobins. Thalassaemia trait probably confers protection against falciparum malaria and this selective advantage accounts for the high gene frequency in areas where malaria is or was endemic.

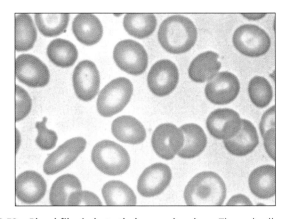

10.52   Blood film in beta-thalassaemia minor. The red cells are hypochromic, there are prominent target cells, and the film shows anisocytosis and poikilocytosis. Several thin, flat cells (leptocytes) and elliptocytes are also present. Some patients with thalassaemia minor show little more than microcytosis and hypochromia.

No treatment is required for thalassaemia minor, but it is important to exclude iron deficiency that may compound the anaemia; routine measurement of ferritin and serum iron is necessary. Detection of the condition before reproductive age allows appropriate genetic counselling.

Severe beta-thalassaemia (Cooley's anaemia)

People homozygous for beta-thalassaemia (in whom both genes are defective) have a marked defect in beta-globin synthesis, whereas alpha-globin synthesis continues normally. This results in the accumulation in red cells of excessive alpha-globin chains, which are relatively insoluble when uncombined with beta-globin chains and thus form large intracellular inclusions. The red cells have a high incidence of failure of maturation within the marrow (ineffective haemopoiesis), and those that are released have a short life span because of splenic trapping. The resultant severe anaemia stimulates production of excess erythropoietin which in turn stimulates further erythroblast proliferation, extension of marrow production to most bones and increased absorption of iron. The process is so active that osteoporosis and pathological fractures may occur, and some bones may become extremely hyperplastic (**10.44**, **10.45**, **10.53**). Compression of the cord may result from vertebral growth, and alteration of the facies may result from overgrowth of the bones of the face ('chipmunk facies'). Retinal changes may occur, as in sickle-cell disease (**10.47**). In severe anaemia (thalassaemia major), there is an absolute need for repeated blood transfusion (which results in iron overload) to maintain oxygenation. In less severe forms (thalassaemia intermedia), the patient is able to maintain a reasonable haemoglobin level (6–8 g/dl) without recourse to blood transfusion, and these patients survive into adult life.

In thalassaemia major, the clinical picture emerges in the first year of life with severe anaemia, failure to thrive and retardation of growth. Examination shows evidence of both spleen and liver enlargement (**10.54**). Laboratory tests show typical red cell appearances (**10.55**), and examination of the parents' blood shows the presence of thalassaemia trait. The diagnosis is confirmed by haemoglobin electrophoresis (**10.51**) and demonstration of defective beta-globin synthesis by the reticulocytes.

There is a high morbidity and mortality unless the infants are regularly transfused with blood to suppress their own haemopoiesis. This can reduce the disease manifestations and allow normal growth and bone development. Repeated transfusion produces problems of iron overload with secondary

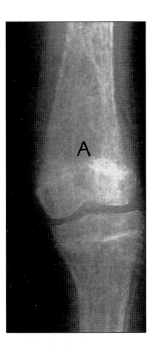

10.53   Thalassaemia major is usually associated with widespread bone changes resulting from marrow hyperplasia. The distal femur in this patient is expanded, giving a 'flask shaped' appearance. The bones are generally osteopenic (A), with a sparse, coarse, dense trabecular pattern. This appearance is not in itself diagnostic of thalassaemia: similar appearances may occur in other haemolytic anaemias, especially sickle-cell disease.

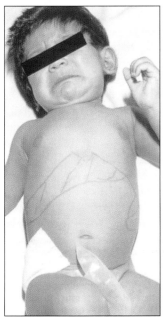

10.54   Beta-thalassaemia major. Hepatosplenomegaly is usual, as in this young patient.

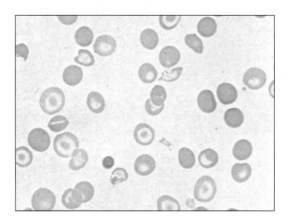

10.55   Severe beta-thalassaemia. The blood film shows much more severe changes than those seen in **10.52**, with hypochromia, target cells, macrocytes, spherocytes, schistocytes – including helmet cells – and small cell fragments.

haemochromatosis, and also a risk of viral infections (especially with hepatitis viruses and HIV). Cardiac disease is also common, with heart failure, myocarditis and pericarditis.

Iron overload can be treated with desferrioxamine, but it must be given by subcutaneous infusion, is difficult to administer to large numbers of patients and is expensive. Vitamin C may also be given to enhance iron chelation. Splenectomy should be considered, in an attempt to increase the life span of red cells. It is important to immunize the child against infection before splenectomy and to administer long-term antibiotic prophylaxis (*see* **p. 426**). Bone marrow transplantation should be considered in selected cases.

Thalassaemia intermedia

Some patients with thalassaemia are able to maintain their haemoglobin levels adequately without recourse to blood transfusion. However, iron accumulation occurs because of increased intestinal absorption and eventually causes secondary haemochromatosis (**10.45**) with all the effects already described. Osteoporosis, bone overgrowth and arthritis are frequent and produce disfiguring skeletal abnormalities.

Alpha-thalassaemia

Various gene mutations or deletions may lead to defects in the synthesis of alpha-globin chains, and a spectrum of red cell abnormalities in which the red cells are hypochromic, microcytic and easily fragmented. The defective alpha chains may be accompanied by the production of abnormal beta chain polymers, which are unstable and lead to rapid haemolysis.

From one to four genes may be involved, resulting in:

- no detectable disease (one- or two-gene defect)
- moderately severe haemolysis (three-gene defect – haemoglobin H disease)
- fetal death – hydrops fetalis (**10.56**) (four-gene defect).

In haemoglobin H disease, splenomegaly is frequent, and the spleen may require removal if there is evidence of hypersplenism. Folic acid and occasional blood transfusion may be required.

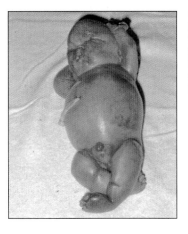

10.56 Hydrops fetalis in severe alpha-thalassaemia. The most severe form of the disease is incompatible with life, and the fetus usually dies in utero.

Acquired haemolytic anaemias

The most common type of acquired haemolytic anaemia results from the presence of autoantibodies, which attach to the red cells and reduce their survival by enhancing their phagocytosis by reticuloendothelial cells. This condition is diagnosed by finding a positive Coombs' test. The antibodies may be 'warm antibodies', most active at 37°C (usually IgG), or 'cold antibodies', most active at lower temperatures (usually IgM). Both types of anaemia may be idiopathic, but underlying causes may be found.

- **Warm autoimmune haemolysis** may be associated with lymphoma, chronic lymphatic leukaemia (**10.38**), systemic lupus erythematosus, HIV infection or hypogammaglobulinaemia. It gives rise to red cell spherocytosis, which can be morphologically indistinguishable from that of congenital spherocytosis (**10.41**); treatment with prednisolone may produce a remission, but splenectomy needs to be considered if this is ineffective or requires an unacceptably high steroid dose.
- **Cold autoimmune haemolysis** (**10.57**, **10.88**) may be transient in association with infectious mononucleosis (*see*

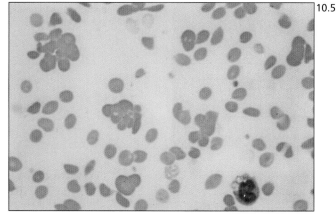

10.5

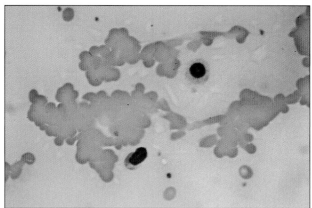

10.5

10.57, 10.58 Cold autoimmune haemolysis. A blood film from the patient viewed at 37°C (**10.57**) shows slight clumping of the red cells. By contrast, in a film made at room temperature (**10.58**), extreme agglutination of the cells has occurred.

p. 22) or mycoplasma pneumonia (*see* **pp. 43**, **175**), may be seen in malaria (*see* **p. 48**), and may occur with a monoclonal IgM paraprotein in idiopathic cold haemagglutinin disease (CHAD) and with lymphoma; avoidance of the cold is the main line of treatment to avoid precipitating intravascular haemolysis or exacerbating the Raynaud's phenomenon that is common in this disorder (*see* **p. 243**). Cold antibodies often do not cause haemolysis; they may then be suspected from the presence of a strikingly raised ESR or plasma viscosity.

Drug-induced immune haemolysis

Drugs may induce haemolysis in three ways:

- Acute intravascular haemolysis may occur when a drug stimulates antibody formation and the resulting immune complex is absorbed on to the red cell where it fixes complement; haemolysis occurs on a second exposure; drugs such as chlorpropamide and quinine are involved.
- Slow-onset haemolysis may occur when a drug becomes attached to the red cell membrane and acts as a hapten; IgG antibody against the drug attaches to the cell and leads to extravascular destruction of the coated cell; this type of reaction is seen with penicillins and cephalosporins.
- Autoimmune haemolysis may be seen after some months of therapy with methyldopa, L-dopa, mefenamic acid and flufenamic acid; the mechanism is not well understood.

Stopping the drug usually leads to rapid resolution, but a short course of prednisolone may be necessary in the autoimmune haemolysis caused by methyldopa.

Haemolytic disease of the newborn

In haemolytic disease of the newborn, maternal IgG antibodies to fetal red cell antigens cross the placenta and affect the fetal red cells, leading to isoimmune haemolysis. Antibodies are usually against the rhesus-group antigens, usually Rh(D), and they develop if the mother is Rh(D) negative, but they may also be against ABO and other rarer blood groups. Sensitization in a Rh(D)-negative mother occurs after a first pregnancy with a Rh(D)-positive fetus, usually as a result of leakage of fetal red cells into the maternal circulation at parturition; it may also result from a previous blood transfusion. Subsequent pregnancies may be affected with increasing severity, depending on the antibody levels that result. Severe haemolytic anaemia may appear in the fetus at the end of the first trimester or in the second trimester, and may result in fetal death (hydrops fetalis, **10.56**). In less severe cases, icterus may be apparent at birth and may lead to kernicterus, the deposition of indirect bilirubin in the basal ganglia of the neonate brain.

All mothers should have their blood tested for anti-Rh(D) antibodies at the initial visit to the antenatal clinic. A rising titre of antibody is an indication for fetal blood transfusion and careful fetal monitoring. Early delivery may be required, in which case prematurity with its complications must be weighed against the risks of anaemia.

If the presentation is at birth, the cord blood sample will show anaemia with a positive Coombs' test, an elevated indirect bilirubin and normoblasts and a high reticulocyte count on the blood film. Exchange transfusion is urgently indicated.

The incidence of this disease has fallen dramatically as a result of the administration within 72 hours of delivery of human anti-D IgG to all Rh(D)-negative mothers who have their first Rh(D)-positive child and who are not already sensitized. This attaches to fetal red cells in the maternal circulation and neutralizes their sensitizing effect. Occasional cases of haemolytic disease of the newborn still occur because of ABO blood group antibodies or because of Rh(D) sensitization at earlier stages in pregnancy.

Non-immune haemolytic anaemia

Paroxysmal nocturnal haemoglobinuria (PNH) is a clonal change in red cells in which the red cell lacks a factor that destroys the complement that normally accumulates on red cells. This results in an intermittent type of acute intravascular haemolysis. PNH may complicate aplastic anaemia. Acute attacks of intravascular haemolysis are precipitated by infection, surgery and anaesthesia and the patient passes dark red-brown urine, often first thing in the morning. There is an association with acute thrombotic episodes caused by platelet and white cell activation and there may be a sequel of acute myeloid leukaemia or aplastic anaemia.

MYELOPROLIFERATIVE DISORDERS

POLYCYTHAEMIA

Polycythaemia refers to a group of disorders in which there is elevation of the haemoglobin, packed cell volume and red cell count (**10.59**). In true polycythaemia there is an absolute increase in the red cell mass, whereas in apparent or relative polycythaemias the red cell mass is normal and the rise in packed cell volume is secondary to a reduced plasma volume. The clinical significance of these disorders is their significant association with thrombotic disorders, for example myocardial infarction, stroke, peripheral vascular disease and deep vein thrombosis. This results from the increase in whole blood viscosity, which leads to reduced blood flow.

Primary proliferative polycythaemia (polycythaemia rubra vera) is like myelofibrosis and essential thrombocythaemia, a myeloproliferative disorder.

Often, the diagnosis is reached by chance, with the finding of an elevated haemoglobin on a routine blood sample, or the chance finding of splenomegaly on clinical examination; it may be recognized only after an acute thrombotic event. The major clinical clues are facial plethora (**10.60**), conjunctival suffusion and splenomegaly, present in 70% of patients. Other associated features are acne rosacea (*see* **p. 86**), urticaria, leg ulcers, retinal changes (**10.61**) and loss of vision because of retinal

POLYCYTHAEMIAS

True

Primary proliferative polycythaemia

Secondary

(a) Hypoxic	Altitude Chronic lung disease Cyanotic congenital heart disease Smoking	
(b) Excess erythropoietin	Polycystic kidneys Renal carcinoma Renal cysts Chronic glomerulonephritis Chronic liver disease Hepatocellular carcinoma Ovarian carcinoma Bronchial carcinoma	
(c) Overtransfusion		

Apparent

Acute fluid loss

'Gaisbock's syndrome'

10.59 Polycythaemias.

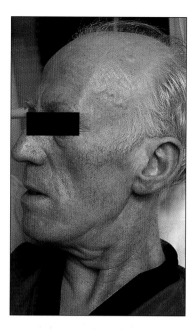

10.60 Primary proliferative polycythaemia (polycythaemia rubra vera). The patient has a generalized plethoric appearance, most obvious on, but not confined to, the face. Note that he also has a prominent temporal artery, which raises the possibility of temporal arteritis (see **p. 128**). His ESR could not be used as a guide to the diagnosis of temporal arteritis, as it should be very low in polycythaemia. Plasma viscosity or C-reactive protein would be a better guide.

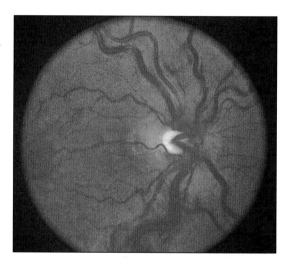

10.61 The fundus in polycythaemia of any cause usually shows engorged and tortuous vessels. Other causes of blood hyperviscosity, including multiple myeloma, may lead to a similar retinal appearance (see **p. 444**). Thrombosis in the retinal vessels and retinal haemorrhages may occur in patients with hyperviscosity of any cause.

haemorrhage. The liver is enlarged in up to 50% of patients, and hypertension is present in about 20%. Evidence should be sought of previous stroke, peripheral vascular disease or deep vein thrombosis. Itch is found in about 15% of patients, and there may be signs of chronic excoriation. The condition is also associated with peptic ulcer and acute gout (see **p. 120**).

The diagnosis is suspected from the FBC and confirmed by the measurement of red cell mass. There may be associated elevation of the white cell count and platelets. The bone marrow shows gross erythroid hyperplasia with normoblastic erythropoiesis. There may be associated iron deficiency, seen on staining the marrow with Prussian Blue. The leucocyte alkaline phosphatase score is high, which is the opposite of that found in chronic myeloid leukaemia. The uric acid levels are characteristically elevated. About 60% of untreated patients die of thrombotic events, about 20% progress to myelofibrosis and a small number (< 10%) progress to acute myeloid leukaemia. Treatment is required to lower the haemoglobin and this is done with repeated venesection or with ^{32}P. Because radiophosphorus is associated with an increase in the risk of leukaemia, its use is best reserved for elderly patients. Allopurinol should be routinely administered to patients with hyperuricaemia to prevent gout.

Secondary polycythaemia (**4.5**) is not associated with such a large risk of thrombotic events. Treatment should be directed at the cause, but often this is not amenable to change. A reduction in haematocrit may be achieved by continuous oxygen therapy. Patients must stop smoking.

MYELOFIBROSIS

In myelofibrosis increased fibrous tissue is formed within the marrow cavity, normal haemopoiesis is disturbed and there is extramedullary haemopoiesis in spleen and liver. It is in the same group of myeloproliferative disorders as polycythaemia, chronic myeloid leukaemia and essential thrombocythaemia and it may be a consequence of these disorders, the fibrous tissue being reactive to the other events in the bone marrow.

In many patients the disease is asymptomatic and the diagnosis is made by finding hepatosplenomegaly on routine clinical or blood examination for some other reason. Some patients present with anaemia or with progressive abdominal swelling (caused by the hepatosplenomegaly) and some with splenic infarction as the enlarging spleen outgrows its blood supply. Portal hypertension may also develop, with ascites and even bleeding from oesophageal varices. Purpura and bleeding may result from thrombocytopenia caused by hypersplenism, and also from coagulation abnormalities caused by liver disease. Gout may occur, as a result of hyperuricaemia.

In a typical patient there is usually evidence of weight loss, with thin spindly legs and arms that contrast with the obvious abdominal distension. The spleen is usually grossly, and the liver moderately, enlarged (as in other conditions, *see* **1.146**, **1.149**). There may be some ascites. Lymph nodes may also be large but non-tender. Bruises and purpura may be present.

Characteristic changes in routine blood tests include a low haemoglobin, which may partly result from blood loss and resulting iron deficiency, folate deficiency and dilution from an increased plasma volume. Normoblasts may be present in great numbers in peripheral blood (this may interfere with automated white cell counters) showing a leucoerythroblastic state (**10.62**).

The platelet count and white cell count may be low. The leucocyte alkaline phosphatase is high, as in primary proliferative polycythaemia, and this allows differentiation from chronic myeloid leukaemia. Attempts to aspirate bone marrow often result in a 'dry tap' because of the amount of fibrous tissue. Trephine biopsy shows a hypercellular marrow with an increase in fibrous tissue, a decrease in fat and haemopoietic tissue, but often an excess of megakaryocytes. It is important to remember other causes of marrow fibrosis, including carcinomatous infiltration (especially from breast and prostate), previous radiation exposure, infections such as tuberculosis and osteomyelitis, and Paget's disease. Using iron-52 it is possible to identify the sites of active erythropoiesis, which will include the liver, spleen and lymph nodes (extramedullary haemopoiesis). X-ray of bones will show an increase in bone density, particularly in the vertebrae.

Treatment is supportive and symptomatic. Iron and folate deficiency should be corrected and gout treated with allopurinol. Blood transfusion may be necessary for severe anaemia. In some situations splenectomy should be considered to reduce haemolysis, remove an infarcted spleen, or when there is severe abdominal discomfort or swelling. Unfortunately, this may often lead to rapid enlargement of the liver. Splenic size may also be controlled with radiotherapy.

Death usually occurs from progressive marrow failure, with bleeding from thrombocytopenia, leucopenia and overwhelming infection, and persistent anaemia. Transformation to acute myeloid leukaemia sometimes occurs.

425

10.62 Leucoerythroblastic peripheral blood film in myelofibrosis. A leucoerythroblastic state is characterized by the presence of abnormally immature white cells and nucleated red cells, and the appearance commonly reflects severe marrow dysfunction. The appearance is not in itself diagnostic of myelofibrosis: it may be seen in chronic infection, malignancy, metabolic disorders that affect bone and in acute severe haemolytic anaemia. This blood picture is usually an indication for marrow aspiration and trephine biopsy.

ESSENTIAL THROMBOCYTHAEMIA

Essential thrombocythaemia (essential thrombocytosis) is part of the myeloproliferative spectrum in which there is proliferation of the megakaryocyte series with the production of excessive numbers of platelets, which may be functionally impaired. Patients present with some of the features of the associated disorders (polycythaemia, chronic myeloid leukaemia and myelofibrosis), including spontaneous bruising, epistaxis and gastrointestinal, vaginal or respiratory tract bleeding. Thrombotic occlusion of arteries, leading to myocardial infarction, stroke, gangrene or intestinal infarction, is common.

Clinical examination may show evidence of bleeding or of thrombosis. The spleen and liver are often felt, although in the later stages splenic atrophy is common.

The diagnosis is made on the finding of platelet counts of $1000–2000 \times 10^9$/litre. The red cell and white cell counts may also be high. The bleeding time may be prolonged and platelet function studies are often abnormal. Megakaryocytes are increased in the marrow. Straight X-ray of the abdomen may show an atrophic calcified spleen.

Treatment is aimed at reduction of the platelet count, using hydroxyurea, busulfan, ^{32}P or platelet phaeresis.

HYPERSPLENISM

Any pathological condition that causes splenomegaly (**10.63**) may result in peripheral blood cytopenia caused by:

CAUSES OF SPLENOMEGALY

Infections
    Viral: Infectious mononucleosis
                     Hepatitis
    Bacterial: Septicaemia
                     Bacterial endocarditis
                     Tuberculosis
                     Typhoid
    Protozoal: Malaria
                     Visceral leishmaniasis
    Helminths: Schistosomiasis

Sarcoidosis

Connective tissue disorders
    Rheumatoid arthritis
    Systemic lupus erythematosus

Metabolic disorders
    Glycogen storage disease
    Gaucher's disease
    Mucopolysaccharidoses

Vascular disorders
    Portal hypertension
    Chronic congestive cardiac failure
    Hepatic or portal vein thrombosis

Haematological disorders
    Haemolytic anaemias
    Myeloproliferative disorders
    Lymphoproliferative disorders

10.63   **Causes of splenomegaly.**

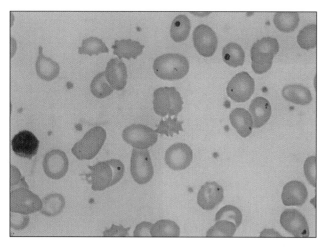

10.64   **Peripheral blood film in an asplenic patient** whose spleen was removed after trauma in a road traffic accident. Howell–Jolly bodies and punctate basophilia are seen in the red cells, which also show anisocytosis, poikilocytosis and abnormal burr forms. There is also thrombocytosis.

- Pooling of cells within the spleen and their subsequent destruction
- Increased plasma volume with dilution of cell numbers.

The diagnosis is usually obvious from the findings of peripheral cytopenia, a hypercellular marrow and splenomegaly. The diagnosis may be confirmed by ^{51}Cr-red cell labelling with surface counting over the spleen.

Splenectomy results in a rapid reversal of these abnormalities. Acutely, there is a transient thrombocytosis and neutrophil leucocytosis. In the long term in the red cells there may be nuclear remnants (Howell–Jolly bodies; **10.64**), siderocytes, target cells and occasional normoblasts.

IMMUNITY AND THE ASPLENIC PATIENT

The normal spleen has the role of removing opsonized encapsulated bacteria and red cells parasitized by malaria parasites from the blood. Individuals who have had their spleens removed surgically (usually for trauma) or who have splenic hypofunction caused by disease (e.g. coeliac disease, lymphoma, systemic lupus erythematosus, sickle-cell disease or thalassaemia) have a 12-fold greater risk of severe infection. This risk persists throughout life although it is greatest in the early years after splenectomy.

Infections are usually fulminant, with pneumonia, meningitis, multiple organ failure and death. The most common infections are with *Streptococcus pneumoniae*, *Haemophilus influenzae* type b and *Neisseria meningitidis*. Malaria also presents a significant risk for the traveller.

Patients should be made aware of the risk of infection and of the early symptoms of bacteraemia, such as malaise and fever, which may be misinterpreted as no more than mild influenza.

It is essential that patients at risk are given pneumococcal vaccine before splenectomy (if elective) and this should be repeated every 5 years to maintain lifelong immunity. In young children (< 4 years) consideration should be given to *H. influenzae* type b (Hib) vaccination if this has not already been given. Meningococcal vaccine should also be given.

Antibiotic prophylaxis with penicillin or ampicillin (or erythromycin) is also indicated for at least 2 years after splenectomy, and this should be continued until at least the age of 16 years in children.

In the long term patients should be supplied with a course of antibiotics for self-administration if 'flu-like' symptoms appear. All patients should carry a card or wear a bracelet identifying their asplenic state.

LEUKAEMIAS

The leukaemias result from the clonal proliferation of cells derived from a single early haemopoietic progenitor cell that has undergone somatic mutation. In the acute leukaemias, this results in the accumulation of early myeloid or lymphoid precursors ('blast' cells) in the bone marrow, blood and other tissues; marrow failure rapidly follows as normal blood cell production ceases. In the chronic leukaemias, either the malignant clone allows differentiation to functional end cells (as in chronic myeloid leukaemia), or the malignant proliferation progresses more slowly (as in chronic lymphocytic leukaemia).

ACUTE LEUKAEMIA

Acute leukaemias have an incidence of 3–4 cases per 100 000 of the population. Acute lymphoblastic leukaemia (ALL) is found mainly in young children (peak incidence 3–5 years). In adults, acute myeloblastic leukaemia (AML) is more common. The aetiology of acute leukaemia is unknown, but may include viruses, chemicals and radiation; it is sometimes a sequel to the administration of chemotherapy or radiotherapy for previous cancers. Acute leukaemia presents with infection, bleeding or anaemia – all the result of bone marrow failure – and occasionally with bone pain. There may also be organ infiltration with lymphadenopathy, splenomegaly or CNS involvement. The peripheral blood may contain blast cells, or occasionally the leukaemic infiltration is discovered on bone marrow examination carried out to determine the cause of a pancytopenia. No clinical features absolutely distinguish between AML and ALL.

The clinical presentation is often with pallor and tiredness resulting from anaemia. Other signs of anaemia include dyspnoea, tachycardia and occasionally pulmonary oedema. The cause of the anaemia is usually infiltration of the marrow.

Fever is also usually present and is often related to infection, especially when the white cell count falls below 1×10^9/litre (**10.65–10.67**). Bleeding is usually due to thrombocytopenia and skin purpura is a frequent finding, especially when the platelet count falls below 20×10^9/litre. There may also be a qualitative platelet defect and occasionally DIC. The skin and gums are common sites of bleeding, but bleeding may occur from any site.

Leukaemic infiltration is common in the terminal stages of the disease, and multiple small purple papular lesions can often be found in the skin (**10.66, 10.68, 10.69**). There may also be gingival infiltration (**10.67**), often with involvement of the tongue and tonsils. The eye may also be affected and infiltrates may be visible in the retina and choroid (**10.70**). The testes may be involved, usually causing painless swelling. Involvement of

427

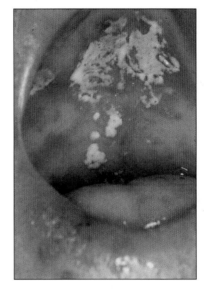

10.66 Oral candidiasis is a common complication of acute leukaemia, as in other conditions associated with immunodeficiency. This patient also has multiple petechiae on the palate, tongue and lips; some small nodules of leukaemic infiltrate can also be seen near the lower lip.

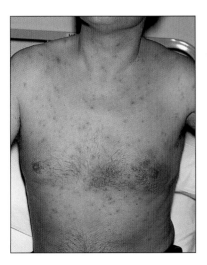

10.65 Shingles and chickenpox in an adult patient with acute myeloblastic leukaemia. Varicella zoster infection is a common complication of acute leukaemia, and it often presents with shingles alone, or more rarely combined with disseminated chickenpox (*see* **1.24, 1.64, 10.91**).

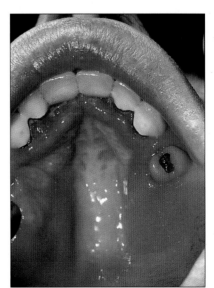

10.67 Infiltration of the gums is a common feature of acute leukaemia, and may be very marked. Secondary infection often exacerbates the swelling, and bleeding is a common complication.

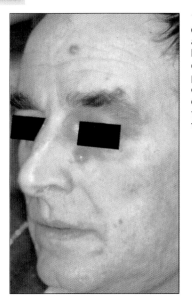

10.68 Leukaemic skin deposits in a patient with acute myeloblastic leukaemia. Similar small deposits may occur in patients with lymphomas or carcinomas; if the deposits are an isolated finding, biopsy is essential for diagnosis.

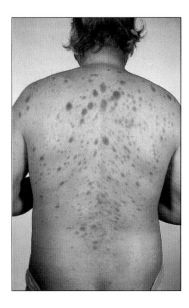

10.69 Extensive leukaemic infiltration of the skin may sometimes occur – most commonly, as here, in patients with acute myeloblastic leukaemia.

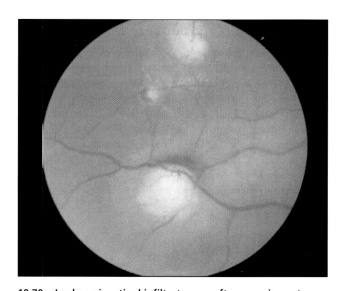

10.70 Leukaemic retinal infiltrates are often seen in acute leukaemia, as in this patient with acute lymphoblastic leukaemia. Retinal haemorrhage is often also seen but is probably a consequence of the thrombocytopenia that accompanies the leukaemia, rather than a manifestation of the leukaemic process itself. Similar haemorrhages are seen in patients with thrombocytopenic purpura.

10.71

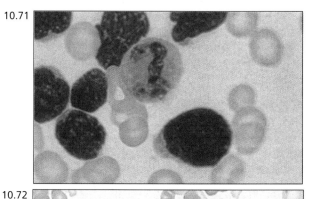

10.72

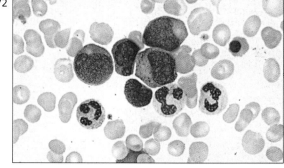

10.71, 10.72 Peripheral blood films often provide initial diagnostic information in acute leukaemia. 10.71 shows a film containing many lymphoblasts, whereas **10.72** shows a film with a group of myeloblasts. Detailed typing of the leukaemia is dependent on cytochemical and cell-marker studies on peripheral blood and marrow aspirates. Classification of the leukaemia has important therapeutic implications, and a detailed diagnosis cannot be made on blood film alone.

the testes or ovaries and of the meninges (found on CSF examination) may be an important source of cells that cause relapse and this requires special consideration in treatment planning. Liver, spleen and bone marrow involvement is common. Bone and joint involvement is rare at presentation, but becomes more common as the disease advances. Bone pain is often present at the sites of major marrow production, especially over the sternum. Periosteal elevation may be seen on X-ray, and bone infarction may occur.

The distinction of the types of leukaemia depends upon the morphology of the blasts and on detailed cytochemical and monoclonal antibody cell marker studies (**10.71, 10.72**).

Management should be carried out in specialized units. Chemotherapy may include combinations of steroids, vincristine, asparaginase, methotrexate, daunorubicin and cytosine arabinoside, and other combinations are currently under trial. Treatment with intensive cytotoxic chemotherapy exacerbates immunosuppression in the short term and isolation nursing and supportive therapy with broad-spectrum antibiotics sometimes including antifungal agents, and blood products, particularly red cells and platelets, are almost invariably required. In addition fluids are often needed to correct dehydration, and allopurinol to correct hyperuricaemia. In childhood ALL, around two-thirds of patients will enter long-term remission, and the inclusion of prophylactic treatment to the CNS largely prevents meningeal relapse. Similarly, testicular and ovarian radiotherapy may be of value. In adults with either AML or ALL, the outlook is much less good with chemotherapy alone; if the patient is less than approximately 40 years old and has an HLA-compatible sibling, allogeneic bone marrow transplantation would now be recommended after achieving a first remission.

CHRONIC LEUKAEMIAS

In chronic leukaemias, there is an accumulation of abnormal white cells in the marrow with resultant disruption of normal marrow function and progressive infiltration into other tissues. Chronic leukaemias differ from the acute forms in that the time course is longer and the onset is more insidious, the cells are more mature and the treatments required are less intense. The classification depends on the cell type involved.

Chronic lymphocytic leukaemia (CLL)

Chronic lymphocytic leukaemia CLL) is the most common leukaemia in Europe and the USA and accounts for 30% of leukaemic deaths. It is a disease predominantly of the elderly, with a mean age at diagnosis of 60 years. In CLL, there is neoplastic proliferation of moderately mature lymphocytes, primarily in the marrow and blood, but also in the lymph nodes, spleen and liver. It is the result of a monoclonal transformation, usually of B lymphocytes (only 5% show a T-cell phenotype). The monoclonal nature of the disorder is confirmed by the finding of surface and cytoplasmic (and sometimes serum) immunoglobulins restricted to one light or heavy chain class.

CLL may present with lymphadenopathy, or increased numbers of small lymphocytes may be found coincidentally when a blood count is carried out for another reason (in about 25% of cases). Weight loss, night sweats, anorexia and lymph node enlargement in the superficial lymph nodes (**10.38**, **10.73**), mediastinum and mesenteric nodes are common. On examination of the patient, there is usually moderate splenomegaly and sometimes hepatomegaly. Jaundice may develop as a result of lymphocytic infiltration of the liver or haemolysis (**10.38**). Later in the disease there may be extreme weight loss, pressure effects caused by lymph node involvement

and skin infiltration that may be compounded by local infections with bacteria, viruses or fungi. Shingles is common (**p. 20**). Generalized infections are also common, as immunosuppression is related to a combination of hypogammaglobulinaemia, lymphocyte dysfunction and, in more advanced disease, neutropenia. Related disorders with a different phenotype and prognosis have been recognized, including hairy-cell leukaemia and prolymphocytic leukaemia, both typically associated with more pronounced splenomegaly and less lymphadenopathy than CLL.

The diagnosis depends on finding a persistent lymphocytosis of >15 × 10^9/litre lymphocytes, with a total white cell count that can range up to 200 × 10^9/litre (85–95% of the white cells are lymphocytes; neutrophil count reduced). Peripheral blood films show typical CLL lymphocytes (**10.74**, **10.75**) with characteristic staining. Anaemia becomes more marked as the disease advances and is usually normochromic and normocytic. There is

429

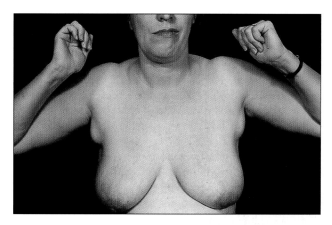

10.73 Chronic lymphocytic leukaemia commonly presents with widespread lymph node enlargement. Often these are first noted in the neck (see **10.38**), but in this patient the presenting feature was bilateral axillary lymphadenopathy.

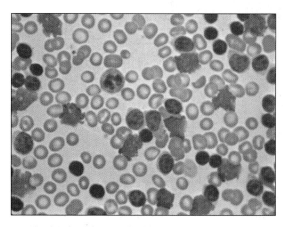

10.74 Chronic lymphocytic leukaemia. The intact white cells on the peripheral blood film are nearly all lymphocytes. A few precursor cells can be seen, and there are numerous smeared disrupted cells – a typical finding in this disease.

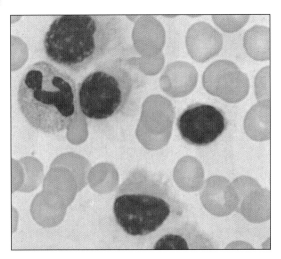

10.75 Hairy-cell leukaemia. The peripheral blood film shows cells containing a typical eccentric nucleus and fine surface projections or hairs. The distinction between chronic lymphocytic leukaemia and hairy-cell leukaemia has therapeutic importance.

often a haemolytic component because of the presence of warm antibodies (**10.38** and *see* **p. 422**). Marrow aspirate or trephine biopsy shows a reduction in normal marrow elements with a lymphocytic infiltrate (**10.76**). Serum immunoglobulin measurement and electrophoresis reveals hypogammaglobulinaemia and a monoclonal paraprotein spike. Lymph node histology shows a similar picture to that in well-differentiated lymphocytic lymphoma (*see* **p. 435**). X-ray of the chest may show marked mediastinal enlargement caused by bilateral lymphadenopathy.

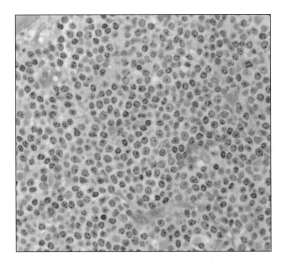

10.76 Chronic lymphocytic leukaemia. This high-power view of a trephine biopsy of bone marrow shows overwhelming, diffuse, uniform infiltration by lymphocytes – a picture found typically at advanced stages of the disease and commonly associated with marked anaemia and thrombocytopenia.

Combinations of these clinical and laboratory criteria form the basis of a variety of staging techniques that may be used to plan treatment or as prognostic indicators. Poor prognostic factors include the following:

- lymphocyte counts > 50×10^9/litre
- lymphocyte doubling time of <1 year
- prolymphocyte count > 15×10^9/litre
- extensive lymph node involvement
- splenomegaly > 10 cm
- diffuse pattern of bone marrow infiltrate
- poor response to treatment.

Complete remission is defined as the disappearance of the abnormal lymphocytes from blood and marrow, and the normalization of blood counts, immunoglobulins and light chains. A partial response is defined as a 50% reduction in lymphocytosis and a 50% reduction in adenopathy and splenomegaly, with haemoglobin >11 g/dl and platelets >100 × 10^9/litre.

Asymptomatic CLL usually requires no treatment, but more advanced cases with bone marrow failure, tissue infiltration or severe lymphadenopathy are treated with single alkylating agents (e.g. chlorambucil or cyclophosphamide), one of the base analogues (e.g. fludarabine) or local radiotherapy. Chemotherapy with a single agent can induce partial remission in 50–60% of cases and complete remission in 10–15%. Addition of corticosteroids increases the number of partial remissions to 70–80%, but also increases the chances of infectious complications. Resistant or advanced cases may require the use of vincristine, melphalan and doxorubicin. All these agents may be associated with side effects such as nausea, vomiting, anorexia and weight loss. Myelosuppression is inevitable, but improves when therapy is stopped or the dosage reduced. There is a significant incidence of acute myeloid leukaemia (10%) after 5–10 years of treatment. In the case of the prolymphocytic leukaemic variant, the very high white cell number may rarely require reduction by leucophoresis for chemotherapy to be effective. In hairy-cell leukaemia alpha interferon is of value.

All patients require general supportive measures, often including the supportive treatment of anaemia with blood or red cell transfusions, treatment of thrombocytopenia with platelet concentrates and treatment of infections with antibiotics and gammaglobulin. Prevention of hyperuricaemia with allopurinol may be required, and the patient must be adequately hydrated throughout treatment. About 50% of patients with CLL die from unrelated causes, mainly cardiovascular disease and other malignancy.

Chronic myeloid leukaemia (CML)

Chronic myeloid leukaemia (CML) accounts for 15% of leukaemias and is a disorder predominantly of middle life (median age at diagnosis is 45 years). The malignant clone of haemopoietic cells that spill into the peripheral blood is marked by the presence of the Philadelphia chromosome in about 95%

of cases. In the minority of cases in which this is absent, there may be differences in the course of the disease and in the response to treatment. The most common cell type involved is the granulocyte series, but rare cases of eosinophilic, basophilic and neutrophilic leukaemia occur.

The clinical course of chronic myeloid leukaemia is insidious with overgrowth of cells, predominantly those of the myeloid series but also those of the erythroid and megakaryocytic series. This often results in a leucoerythoblastic picture (10.62) that may terminate after several years in an acute leukaemia relatively resistant to therapy, or in myelofibrosis.

Clinical features on presentation include those caused by anaemia, weight loss, abdominal distension from massive splenomegaly and bone tenderness from periosteal infiltration. Purpura and bleeding from other sites as a result of thrombocytopenia may occur. Hyperviscosity syndromes may result in retinal haemorrhages, priapism and neurological deficit. Gouty arthropathy is rare despite the presence of hyperuricaemia.

The diagnosis is suspected when a white cell count in excess of 50 × 10⁹/litre is found that is composed of myelocytes,

metamyelocytes and blast cells in the peripheral blood film (10.77). There is also usually a normochromic normocytic anaemia, with a haemoglobin in the region of 9 g/dl. There may also be thrombocytosis with giant platelets and other fragments of megakaryocytes.

Bone marrow aspirate (10.78) or trephine biopsy shows a generalized increase in cellularity, with loss of fat spaces caused by the myeloid hyperplasia. The leucocyte alkaline phosphatase is greatly reduced in CML, and this allows its differentiation from the neutrophils resulting from infection and from other myeloproliferative disorders. The Philadelphia chromosome (10.79) and related DNA abnormalities are found in the myeloid cells in 95% of cases, and the percentage of cells showing these abnormalities may act as a guide to treatment response and prognosis.

Treatment is by control of the hyperproliferation using busulfan or hydroxyurea, but after a median of 2–3 years the disease becomes more difficult to control, with increasing marrow fibrosis or a sudden transformation to acute leukaemia, or both.

In patients with a hyperviscosity syndrome caused by the presence of excess white cells, leucophoresis is of value. During initial treatment, a high fluid intake and allopurinol are important in the control of hyperuricaemia. Splenectomy may be of value in selected patients.

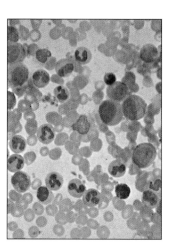

10.77 Chronic myeloid leukaemia. This low-power view of peripheral blood shows granulocytes at all stages of maturation. A peripheral blood smear with as many leucocytes of different stages of maturity as shown here is virtually diagnostic of chronic myeloid leukaemia.

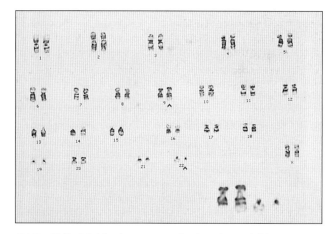

10.79 Philadelphia chromosome in chronic myeloid leukaemia. The Philadelphia chromosome is number 22 from which the long arms are deleted (22q-) and is found in 95% of patients with chronic myeloid leukaemia. It is part of a reciprocal translocation usually involving chromosome 9 (9q+). In this karyotype, the arrows indicate the truncated Philadelphia chromosome 22 and the extended chromosome 9 in a Giemsa-banded metaphase from bone marrow cells of a patient with chronic myeloid leukaemia: the inset (lower right) shows the affected chromosomes and their normal partners in more detail. The reciprocal translocation results in the formation of a chimeric gene, formed from part of the chromosome 22 and the c-abl gene from chromosome 9; this transcribes a novel mRNA to produce a protein with enhanced tyrosine kinase activity thought to be the metabolic basis of this leukaemia.

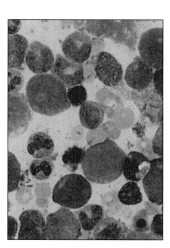

10.78 Bone marrow smear in chronic myeloid leukaemia (low-power view). There is a preponderance of neutrophil granulocytes, with all stages of development represented. Some erythroblasts and a pro-erythroblast can also be seen.

Allogeneic bone marrow transplantation is of value in the chronic phase for younger patients who have a compatible donor, and this represents the best chance for cure.

MYELODYSPLASTIC SYNDROMES

The myelodysplastic syndromes (**10.80**) are a heterogeneous group of disorders, characterized by the liability to develop acute myeloid leukaemia, which present with multiple

MYELODYSPLASTIC SYNDROMES

This classification, devised by a French, American and British (FAB) co-operative group, is based on findings in the peripheral blood and the bone marrow

Classification	% marrow blasts	% peripheral blood blasts	Ringed sideroblasts
Refractory anaemia (RA)	< 5	< 1	0
Refractory anaemia with ringed sidero-blasts (RAB)	< 5	< 1	+
Refractory anaemia with excess blasts (RAEB)	5–20	< 5	+/–
RAEB in transition (RAEB-t)	20–30	> 5	+/–
Chronic myelomono-cytic leukaemia	< 20	< 5	+/–

10.80 Myelodysplastic syndromes.

cytopenias in the presence of a hypercellular marrow. The range of abnormalities includes refractory anaemia – which may be associated with excessive marrow iron or with ringed sideroblasts in the marrow – and chronic myelomonocytic leukaemia. These disorders occur particularly in the elderly, and clinical presentation is often caused by failure of the marrow, with signs of bleeding (**10.81**) or with infection. Up to 20% of patients have splenomegaly.

Laboratory investigation usually shows that all three cell lines are involved. The prognosis is generally poor because of the patient's age, increasing anaemia, infection resulting from granulocytopenia and bleeding from thrombocytopenia. The median survival is of the order of 30 months.

Treatment consists of supportive care, with correction of anaemia with blood transfusion, and appropriate treatment of infections and bleeding.

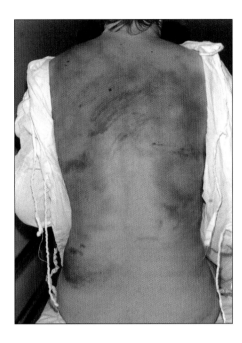

10.81 Excessive bruising after trauma in a patient with a myelodysplastic syndrome. This lady was beaten in a domestic assault but her bruising was excessive for the described severity of the attack. She proved to be seriously anaemic (Hb 5.7 g/dl), and marrow findings showed that she had refractory anaemia, RAB type (*see* **10.80**).

LYMPHOMA

The lymphomas are a group of malignant disorders originating in one of the lymph nodes or other lymphatic tissues of the body and disrupting the normal lymphoid architecture. The disorders are divided into Hodgkin's disease (in which the origin of the abnormal Reed–Sternberg cell is still a matter of debate), and the non-Hodgkin's lymphomas (which can be shown to be of clonal B- or T-cell origin).

HODGKIN'S DISEASE

Hodgkin's disease occurs more frequently in men than in women and has bimodal peaks of increased incidence in the late 20's and around 60 years of age. Its incidence in the UK is approximately 4/100 000 population. The tumour is unusual in that the putative malignant cell (the Reed–Sternberg cell) forms a tiny proportion of the cells in the tumour, the remaining tissue being thought to be 'reactive'. In 70% of cases patients present with isolated painless swelling of a lymph node in the neck, axilla or groin, which spreads to adjacent groups of lymph nodes (**10.8, 10.82**).

In advanced cases there may be hepatosplenomegaly. Skin lesions may develop at a late stage (**10.83**).

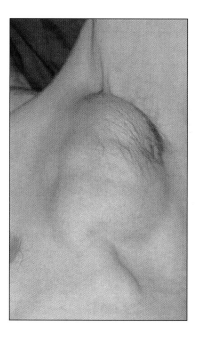

10.82   Gross, painless, rubbery lymph node enlargement is the common presenting feature of Hodgkin's disease. This patient had generalized lymphadenopathy, but his left axillary nodes were particularly prominent.

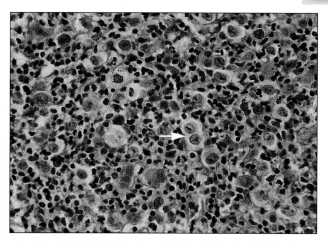

10.84   The histopathological appearance of Hodgkin's disease varies, but the presence of Reed–Sternberg cells is usually essential for the diagnosis. Here, a typical bi-nucleate 'owl-eye' Reed–Sternberg cell is seen in a tumour of mixed cellularity (H&E staining). The histological subtype of Hodgkin's disease is an important factor in prognosis and, in general, lymphocyte-depleted Hodgkin's lymphomas have the worst prognosis.

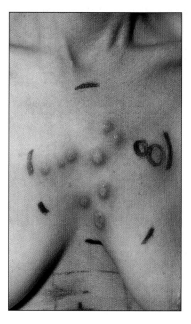

10.83   Skin deposits of tumour may occur in advanced Hodgkin's disease. This patient had multiple skin nodules, and their nature was confirmed by biopsy. Palliative radiotherapy is about to be started.

The extent of the disease (**10.85**) and its prognosis is determined by staging procedures (**10.86**), and prognosis is also affected by the histological appearance on biopsy.

Systemic symptoms (B-stage), including fever with sweats, especially at night (Pel–Ebstein pattern), and weight loss are characteristic of more advanced disease.

Hodgkin's disease is associated with impaired cell-mediated immunity and an increased risk of infections, including herpes zoster (*see* **p. 20, 10.91**).

ANN ARBOR STAGING IN HODGKIN'S DISEASE AND NON-HODGKIN'S LYMPHOMA

Stage I   Involvement of lymph nodes in a single region (I) or infiltration of a single extralymphatic site (IE)

Stage II   Involvement of lymph nodes in two distinct regions on the same side of the diaphragm (II) which may also include spleen (IIs), localized extra-lymphatic involvement (IIE) or both (IIsE)

Stage III   Involvement of lymph nodes on both sides of the diaphragm (III) which may include the spleen (IIIs), localized extralymphatic involvement (IIIE) or both (IIIsE)

Stage IV   Diffuse or disseminated involvement of extralym-phatic sites (e.g. bone marrow, liver and lung)

In addition, the suffix letters A and B are used to denote the absence (A) or presence (B) of any of the additional systemic features of fever, night sweats and loss of 10% body weight in the previous 6 months.

10.85   Ann Arbor staging in Hodgkin's disease and non-Hodgkin's lymphoma.

Investigations show a variety of non-specific features, usually including a normochromic normocytic anaemia and elevation of the ESR (especially in the presence of 'B' grading). Lymphopenia is present in about one-third of cases, and there may also be neutrophilia, eosinophilia and monocytosis. There may rarely be autoimmune thrombocytopenia or haemolytic anaemia. The diagnosis is made on lymph node or tissue biopsy, which should be conventionally fixed and stained (**10.84**) and also examined immunohistochemically.

RECOMMENDED STAGING PROCEDURES IN HODGKIN'S DISEASE

Required evaluation procedures

Adequate surgical biopsy (**10.84**)
Detailed history with emphasis on the presence or absence of B symptoms
Complete physical examination with special attention directed to the evaluation of lymphadenopathy, liver and spleen size, and the detection of bony tenderness
Laboratory studies: FBC and platelet count, liver and kidney function, serum alkaline phosphatase
Chest X-ray PA and lateral (**10.87**)
Bilateral lower extremity lymphangiogram (**10.88**)
Abdominal CT (**10.89**)
Bone marrow aspirate and biopsy

Required evaluation procedures under certain conditions

Chest tomography or chest CT (**10.90**)
Bone scan
Staging laparotomy including splenectomy

Useful ancillary procedures

Skeletal radiographs
Gallium scan

10.86   Recommended staging procedures in Hodgkin's disease.

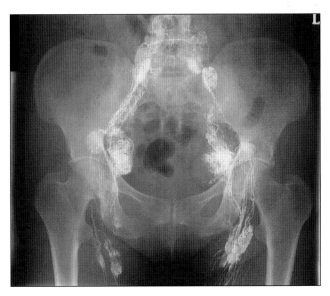

10.88   A lymphangiogram in Hodgkin's disease, performed by cannulating lymphatics in the feet. Grossly abnormal and enlarged inguinal, iliac and para-aortic lymph nodes can be seen.

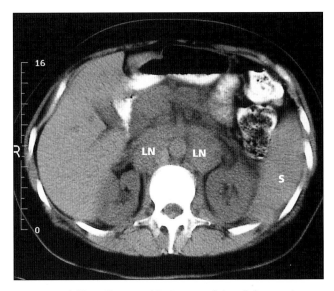

10.89   Hodgkin's disease. This CT scan of the abdomen shows enlargement of the spleen (S) and bilateral para-aortic lymph node enlargement (LN) at the level of the superior mesenteric artery.

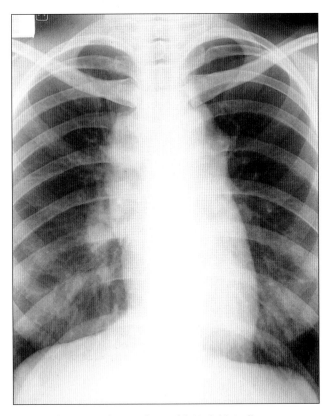

10.87   Chest X-ray in a patient with Hodgkin's disease, showing bilaterally enlarged mediastinal lymph nodes.

Treatment of localized disease is by radiotherapy, especially where the disease is above the diaphragm, when the cervical, axillary, mediastinal and para-aortic nodes can be irradiated. The prospects for cure are 80–90% over 5 years.

For more advanced disease (stage IIIB and IV) treatment is with a combination of chemotherapeutic agents that include chlormethine (mustine), vincristine (Oncovin), procarbazine and prednisolone (MOPP), and sometimes also chlorambucil,

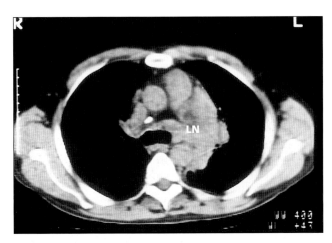

10.90 Thoracic CT in Hodgkin's disease, demonstrating enlarged mediastinal lymph nodes (LN).

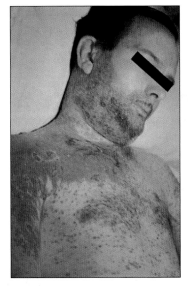

10.91 Widespread herpes zoster infection in a 38-year-old man with advanced Hodgkin's disease. Note that he has also developed a generalized chickenpox rash over the unaffected segments.

natural history and outcome from Hodgkin's disease. Their incidence in the UK is approximately 14/100 000 population and is rising. The median age at diagnosis is 64 years, but they may occur in younger patients, especially in association with advanced HIV infection.

Non-Hodgkin's lymphoma may present in exactly the same way as Hodgkin's disease, with the diagnosis being made at lymph node biopsy (**1.33**, **10.9**, **10.92**). However, the range of presentations and course of disease is highly variable, and extranodal tissue involvement, including the bone marrow and organs as varied as the tongue and the testis (**10.93**), is much more common. The Ann Arbor staging system (**10.85**) is also widely used for non-Hodgkin's lymphomas, although its prognostic value is less clear in non-Hodgkin's lymphomas (which commonly spread via the bloodstream) than in Hodgkin's disease (which spreads mainly contiguously via the lymphatic system).

Histological classification of the non-Hodgkin's lymphomas has been improved by immunophenotyping. In general, tumours showing a diffuse (rather than follicular) pattern and larger 'blastic' cells (rather than small lymphoid cells), as shown

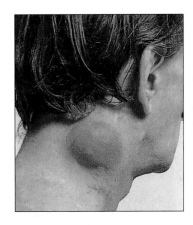

10.92 Non-Hodgkin's lymphoma may present in a similar way to Hodgkin's disease, as in this patient who developed lymphoma as a component of AIDS (the lymphoma of AIDS is usually of non-Hodgkin's type). Despite the redness of the skin over the enlarged lymph node in this patient, the lesion was completely painless.

vinblastine, doxorubicin and bleomycin. Such combinations must be given in specialized units and can give an 80% remission rate. Cure can be expected in 30–40% of patients. If relapse occurs, different drugs are required and may be given in combination with radiotherapy.

Cytotoxic therapy compounds the existing defect in cell-mediated immunity and makes infective complications likely, for example disseminated tuberculosis, herpes zoster, and other bacterial, viral, fungal and protozoal infections.

NON-HODGKIN'S LYMPHOMAS

Non-Hodgkin's lymphomas are a heterogeneous group of neoplasms of the immune system that differ in cell type,

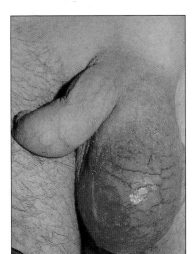

10.93 Lymphoma of the testis is the most common testicular neoplasm in the elderly. Patients usually present with swelling of the testis and cord up into the abdomen, as here. The condition is commonly associated with lymphoma in the para-aortic nodes and elsewhere, and the prognosis is poor.

in **10.94**), have a more aggressive course and are regarded as 'high-grade' rather than 'low-grade' lymphomas. Ironically, high-grade lymphomas, which include B-lymphoblastic (Burkitt's) lymphoma (**p. 22**), are curable in a proportion of cases with intensive cytotoxic chemotherapy combined with radiotherapy to 'bulky' areas of disease, whereas the low-grade lymphomas, although compatible with longer survival, are not currently curable, though they may be controlled by intermittent chemotherapy or by local radiotherapy. Combination chemotherapy is usual, following the CHOP regimen (cyclophosphamide, doxorubicin, vincristine (Oncovin) and prednisolone) or the BACOP regimen (bleomycin, doxorubicin (Adriamycin), cyclophosphamide, vincristine and prednisolone). Combination chemotherapy usually produces significant marrow suppression, and the BACOP regimen uses non-myelotoxic agents during those periods. Splenectomy may be required if there is hypersplenism (*see* **p. 426**).

Prognosis for individual patients depends upon histological grade, staging and age (prognosis is poorer in older patients). Complete remission following treatment is more likely in high-grade lymphomas, but the prognosis for those with high-grade lymphomas which do not remit is worse than for those with low-grade lymphomas (which rarely remit).

The majority of non-Hodgkin's lymphomas are B-cell in origin and they often present with some of the features of CLL (*see* **p. 429**). Tumours of small lymphocytes or lymphoplasmacytoid cells may be associated with the production of paraproteins, and an IgM paraprotein may give rise to hyperviscosity problems (Waldenström's macroglobulinaemia, *see* **p. 446**).

The rarer T-cell lymphomas tend to be more aggressive. They include mycosis fungoides, a chronic skin lymphoma that progresses from psoriasiform lesions and skin plaques (**2.123**), sometimes associated with generalized erythroderma, to more generalized lymph node involvement and the appearance of typical convoluted lymphocytes (Sézary cells) in the blood. When the disease is localized to the skin it may run a benign course and be amenable to local therapy with ultraviolet light or radiotherapy or to local or generalized nitrogen mustard. Once it has spread to local lymph nodes the prognosis is bleak, with a median survival time of only 2 years despite intensive combination therapy.

PLATELET DEFECTS

Defects in either the number or the function of platelets may produce easy bruising, epistaxis and intestinal bleeding. Purpura is usually seen only when there is a fall in circulating platelets to around $10–20 \times 10^9$/litre from the normal of $200–300 \times 10^9$/litre. Bleeding may occur at a level of up to 50×10^9/litre if there has been major surgery or extensive trauma. The causes of thrombocytopenia are numerous and are summarized in **10.95**.

There is usually a history of spontaneous bruising and bleeding, especially recurrent bilateral nose bleeds, mucous membrane bleeding in the mouth, persistent menorrhagia and

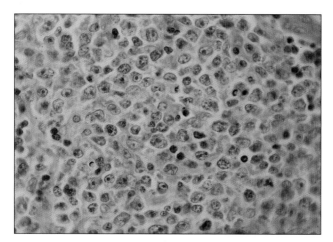

10.94 **Non-Hodgkin's lymphoma – centroblastic type** (H&E staining). The spectrum of histological appearance in non-Hodgkin's lymphomas ranges from small-cell lymphocytic ('low-grade') to large-cell immunoblastic (centroblastic; high grade). This lymph node biopsy has a centroblastic appearance and only a small number of benign, small lymphocytes are seen. In general, tumours composed of larger cells run a more aggressive course than those composed of small cells, especially if they are diffuse rather than follicular.

CAUSES OF THROMBOCYTOPENIA	
Infections	Viral infections
	Malaria
	Other infections
Immune	Acute/chronic ITP
Marrow disorders	Hypoplasia
	Infiltration
	– leukaemia
	– carcinoma
	– myelofibrosis
	– myeloma
	B_{12}/folate deficiency
Haemolytic anaemias	Microangiopathic
Hypersplenism	Lymphoma
	Congestion
	Storage
Excess consumption	Massive blood transfusion
	Disseminated intravascular coagulation
	Trauma and burns – especially with infection
	Extracorporeal circulation – especially cardiopulmonary bypass

10.95 Causes of thrombocytopenia.

intestinal bleeds. It is important to ask about recent drug therapy. Careful examination is required to identify or exclude a basic disease process such as infection, malignancy, liver disease or a connective tissue disorder. The age of the purpuric lesions may give a clue to the duration of the disease. Evidence of splenic enlargement should be sought. Investigations include FBC, platelet count, coagulation screen, bone marrow aspirate and bleeding time.

IDIOPATHIC THROMBOCYTOPENIC PURPURA (ITP)

Idiopathic thrombocytopenic purpura (ITP) is an autoimmune disorder characterized by the accelerated removal of platelets coated with antibody by cells of the reticulo-endothelial system. These antibodies may be found in lymphoproliferative disorders or after infections; rarely, they may be associated with drug therapy. The likelihood of haemorrhage is related to the degree of thrombocytopenia or interference with normal function. Clinically, ITP can be classified as acute or chronic.

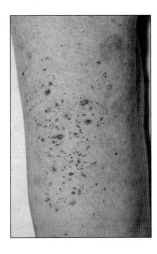

10.96 Acute idiopathic thrombocytopenic purpura (ITP) commonly manifests itself with purpuric lesions of this kind, though they may often be more widespread by the time the patient seeks medical attention. It is important to remember that purpura of identical appearance may result from many other causes.

In acute ITP, purpura (**10.10, 10.96, 10.97**), bruises and bleeding appear abruptly, usually in children or young adults. There is often a history of an upper respiratory tract infection in the preceding 2 weeks. Occasionally, there may have been an obvious viral disease such as measles, mumps or infectious mononucleosis. The blood film is usually normal, but may show some atypical lymphocytes. The platelet count is significantly reduced and some platelets may be larger than normal. Bone marrow examination shows an increase in megakaryocytes (**10.98**). Most children have a spontaneous remission in a week or so and few have any serious haemorrhage. If frank bleeding occurs, steroids should be given in a short course. Failure to remit spontaneously or with steroids should lead to re-evaluation for an alternative cause or to consideration of splenectomy, or both.

Chronic ITP is a disease of adults that affects women more often than men. The usual presentation is with progressive purpura, ecchymoses and mucocutaneous bleeding. There may be a history of multiple episodes over many years, or of a concomitant systemic illness, especially an autoimmune disease or lymphoproliferation. Examination shows purpura (**10.96**) and ecchymoses (**10.97**), and lesions may also be found in the mouth and eye (**10.70**). The spleen is palpable in only 5% of patients.

The peripheral blood is usually normal unless blood loss has produced anaemia. The platelet count may vary over the years from normal to very low; the level correlates well with episodes of bleeding. Bone marrow aspirate shows normal erythroid and myeloid cell lines with a normal or increased number of megakaryocytes. There may be evidence of increased platelet-associated immunoglobulin with reduced platelet survival. Other diseases should be excluded by appropriate investigations.

Treatment is with steroids, or sometimes with immunosuppressive drugs. Splenectomy may be necessary. Temporary remissions to allow surgery can sometimes be gained using high doses of human IgG.

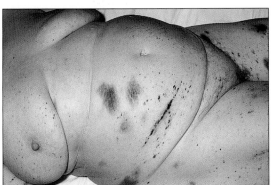

10.97 Diffuse purpuric rash with areas of sheet haemorrhage (ecchymosis) in a patient with thrombocytopenia of unknown cause.

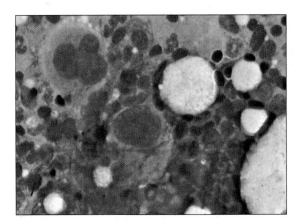

10.98 The bone marrow in idiopathic thrombocytopenic purpura shows numerous megakaryocytes, but few or no platelets are seen on the peripheral blood film.

In pregnancy the chief danger is to the fetus, which may be thrombocytopenic as a result of transplacental passage of anti-platelet IgG and thus at risk of cerebral haemorrhage at delivery.

Drug-induced immune thrombocytopenia

Many drugs may be associated with immune-mediated thrombocytopenia (**10.99**). There are probably two principal mechanisms:

- the drug may bind to the platelet to produce a neoantigen that stimulates an autoantibody

DRUGS THAT MAY CAUSE IMMUNE-MEDIATED THROMBOCYTOPENIA	
Thiazide diuretics	Quinine
Gold salts	Rifampicin
Heparin	Valproate
Carbamazepine	Sulphonamides
Phenothiazines	Penicillins

10.99 Drugs that may cause immune-mediated thrombocytopenia.

CAUSES OF VASCULAR AND NON-THROMBOCYTOPENIC PURPURA
Primary
Senile purpura
Hereditary haemorrhagic telangiectasia
Giant cavernous haemangioma (**10.112**)
Connective tissue disorders, e.g.
– Ehlers–Danlos syndrome (*see* **p. 133**)
– Marfan's syndrome (*see* **p. 134**)
Secondary
Henoch–Schönlein purpura
Metabolic
– scurvy
– Cushing's syndrome and steroid use (*see* **7.24**)
– uraemia
– liver disease
Dysproteinaemia
Purpura fulminans
Embolic purpura
Mechanical purpura

10.100 Causes of vascular and non-thrombocytopenic purpura.

- the drug binds to a plasma protein that is antigenic and the resultant antibody produces an immune complex that binds to the normal platelet Fc receptor.

Bleeding may range from mild to life-threatening. Stopping the drug usually results in the cessation of signs. Steroids may aid the return of the platelet count to normal.

When this condition is associated with the use of heparin, the bleeding may be extremely severe because of the existing state of anticoagulation of the patient. Protamine sulphate should be given to reverse the action of the heparin, along with steroids to raise the platelet count.

VASCULAR AND NONTHROMBOCYTOPENIC PURPURA

Abnormalities of the vascular endothelium may be primary or secondary (**10.100**) and, depending on their nature, extent and site, can give rise to a variety of clinical syndromes.

It is important to elicit any history of easy bruising or bleeding in the family, of epistaxis in childhood or of excessive bleeding after dental extraction, after surgery or during menstruation. Careful examination of the skin is necessary for petechiae, purpura or bruises. Tests of vascular function may be required and biopsy of lesions may give a diagnosis. Often the cause of the defect is not apparent.

PRIMARY ABNORMALITIES

Senile purpura

Senile purpura is a benign disease of the elderly, in which the characteristic lesions develop on the extensor surfaces of the hands (**10.101**), forearms and face and neck. The defect is loss

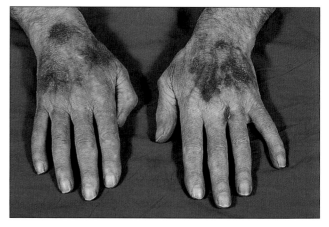

10.101   Senile purpura is a common and benign condition that results from impaired collagen production and capillary fragility in the elderly. In the absence of other signs of disease, no investigation is necessary.

of collagen support of dermal capillaries, associated with thinning of the skin. The purple spots tend to stay the same colour over many months before they fade to a brownish colour. They are often called 'age spots'. They are of no significance and are of only cosmetic importance. No treatment is available.

Hereditary haemorrhagic telangiectasia

Hereditary haemorrhagic telangiectasia (also known as HHT or the Rendu–Osler–Weber syndrome) is transmitted as an autosomal dominant trait so both sexes are equally affected. The lesions consist of dilated arterioles and capillaries that are superficial, easily traumatized and likely to ooze (**10.102**). They blanch on pressure with a glass slide. The most common site is the nasal mucosa, and epistaxis in childhood may be a presenting feature, although the disorder does not usually present until middle age. In the adult, lesions are to be found on the lips, mouth, tongue, face, hands (**10.7**), oesophagus, stomach and rectum, and more rarely in the eyes, bronchi, and reproductive and urinary tracts. Bleeding may occur from any of these sites; a common presentation is with recurrent iron-deficient anaemia associated with occult intestinal bleeding. There is an association of this disease with pulmonary arteriovenous fistulae, cirrhosis of the liver, hepatomas and splenomegaly. There may also be abnormalities of coagulation factors and platelet function that compound the bleeding tendency.

Treatment is difficult because of the diffuse nature of the lesions. If individual lesions can be identified as the source of bleeding, they may be cauterized. Oestrogens may help to prevent epistaxis.

SECONDARY ABNORMALITIES

Mechanical and factitious purpura

Sudden increase in venous pressure from coughing, vomiting, asphyxia or during an epileptic fit may cause leakage of blood even from normal capillaries (**1.117**, **10.103**). A similar situation may occur following skin suction.

Henoch–Schönlein purpura

Henoch–Schönlein purpura is an immunological disease in which the vascular endothelium is damaged by the deposition of immune complexes. It may result from reactions to drugs, food, insect bites or bacterial or viral infections. Bleeding may occur into the joints or into the bowel and there is often a generalized skin rash of a diffuse macular type which then becomes purpuric (**2.133**). Lesions may also be found in the brain and renal tract. The disorder is most common in children, and it usually resolves without complications, but about one-third of patients have associated glomerulonephritis (*see* **p. 275**) and there may be associated pleurisy, pericarditis or pneumonia.

Scurvy

Scurvy results from deficiency of vitamin C (ascorbic acid) in the diet. It is rarely seen in the developed world. Deficiency results in failure to synthesize a normal quantity and quality of collagen fibres. Bleeding occurs from the resulting capillary wall weakness.

In babies, subperiosteal bleeding is a common presentation, usually associated with anaemia. In adults, there may be gingival bleeding (**8.25**), purpura and perifollicular

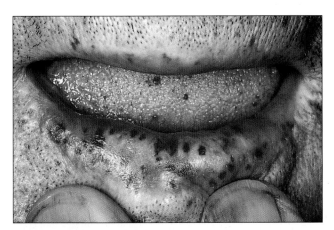

10.102 Hereditary haemorrhagic telangiectasia (HHT) is a condition in which occult blood loss in the gut may lead to severe iron deficiency anaemia. The diagnosis is usually clear from a careful clinical examination, although the telangiectases are not always as obvious as in this patient with multiple lesions on the face, lips and tongue. This patient had received multiple blood transfusions over many years because of HHT-associated gastrointestinal blood loss, and he had developed cirrhosis associated with hepatitis B antigen positivity – probably as a result of transmission of hepatitis B virus in transfused blood.

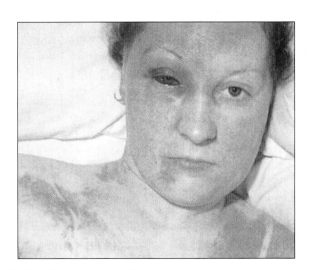

10.103 Traumatic asphyxia may produce severe petechiae and frank haemorrhage. This woman was crushed in a crowd, and on admission was unconscious as a result of cerebral petechiae and oedema. She was treated with steroids and oxygen, but retained widespread skin petechiae and a right subconjunctival haemorrhage when this photograph was taken.

haemorrhages. Severe deficiency in the adult may result in gastro-intestinal and brain haemorrhages.

Cushing's syndrome and steroid use

Excessive corticosteroids produce thin, friable, easily bruised skin that also contains purpuric spots and ecchymoses (**7.23**, **7.24**). This is a result of the loss of collagen that supports the dermal capillaries. Treatment of Cushing's syndrome or cessation of steroid therapy ultimately leads to reversal of these changes.

DISORDERS OF BLOOD COAGULATION

Blood coagulates by a complex 'cascade' that involves the sequential activation of otherwise inert factors (proenzymes) in the plasma. A platelet thrombus forms first and is the main component of primary haemostasis; this is stabilized by the fibrin clot that results from the coagulation cascade.

COAGULATION FACTOR DEFECTS

Inborn defects (quantitative or qualitative) have been described in all known coagulation factors, but the clinical presentations tend to be very similar. The most common defects result in haemophilia and Christmas disease (factor VIII and factor IX deficiency, respectively). Both are transmitted as X-linked recessive characteristics and, using gene probes, the unaffected female carriers may be identified and counselled. There is a wide range of clinical severity.

Surprisingly, there is little bleeding at birth, though excessive cord bleeding may be noted, and the signs of excessive bruising and internal bleeding usually start to manifest themselves at 6–9 months when the toddler starts to move around and fall. Bleeding may occur in every tissue of the body (**10.104**, **10.105**) but the most common bleeding site is into the joints. Acute haemarthrosis causes a sudden onset of acute pain and swelling, associated with signs that are similar to those of acute inflammation – hotness, redness, swelling and pain (**10.106**). The joint is usually held in a rigid semiflexed position and movement (and examination) is resisted by the patient. Recurrent episodes of bleeding lead to chronic degenerative joint disease which may cause chronic pain in the affected joint, with severe deformity and limitation of movement (**10.107**, **10.108**). There is usually atrophy of the surrounding muscle cuff. Compression neuropathy is also common if bleeding occurs around a nerve, for example femoral nerve compression commonly follows bleeding into the iliopsoas muscle. The most common cause of death from bleeding is cerebral haemorrhage, which produces a range of neurological deficits.

Intrarenal bleeding often produces renal pelvic or ureteric obstruction, which causes colicky abdominal pain associated with haematuria. Bleeding into the bowel wall may produce intestinal obstruction.

Investigation shows a prolongation of the APPT; this finding should be followed up by measurement of the individual factor levels.

Treatment and management of these bleeding defects is best carried out in specialized haemophilia units. The deficient plasma factors are infused intravenously until bleeding stops.

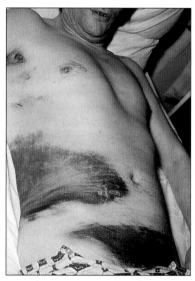

10.104 Massive haematomas in a patient with haemophilia. In the absence of major trauma, haematomas of this size always indicate a severe coagulation abnormality. Possible causes include haemophilia, Christmas disease, von Willebrand's disease and uncontrolled anticoagulant therapy. Internal bleeding is a common accompaniment, and patients require urgent investigation and treatment.

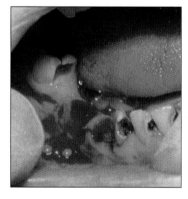

10.105 Severe haemorrhage after dental extraction is often the first clue to more minor degrees of coagulation disorder and is a common presentation in haemophilia, Christmas disease and von Willebrand's disease.

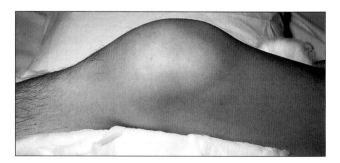

10.106 Acute haemarthrosis of the knee is a common complication of haemophilia. It may be confused with acute infection unless the patient's coagulation disorder is known, because the knee is hot, red, swollen and painful.

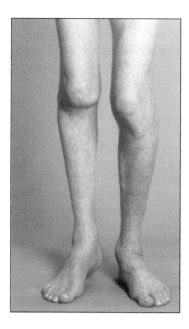

10.107 Severe chronic arthritis may occur in patients with haemophilia and Christmas disease as a result of recurrent episodes of haemorrhage into joints. The knee is the most commonly affected joint. Both knees are severely deranged in this patient. Note that he is unable to stand with both feet flat on the floor.

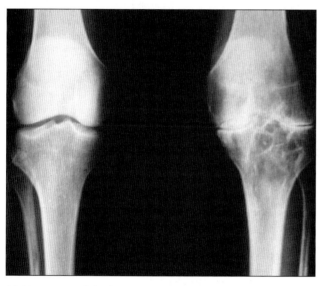

10.108 X-ray of the knees in a patient with haemophilia. The left knee joint has been severely damaged by recurrent haemarthrosis. Note the narrowing of the joint space, the presence of irregular erosions, and the evidence of cyst formation in the tibial head.

Surgery or trauma necessitate the use of appropriate plasma factor cover.

As a result of contamination of the source plasma, many patients with these disorders have been infected with HIV. This resembles HIV infection in other groups, but Kaposi's sarcoma is a rarity in the profile of HIV disorders in haemophilia. In addition, many patients have chronic active hepatitis as a result of transmitted viral hepatitis.

Von Willebrand's disease is a group of similar types of bleeding disorders to haemophilia but is wholly transmitted by an autosomal recessive route and thus affects both men and women. There is a greater range of severity from symptomless to severe. The main defect is in the synthesis of von Willebrand factor, and this produces abnormalities of platelet function and of low levels of factor VIII coagulant activity. Clinical presentation is mainly with bleeding, usually from mucosal sites, especially from the genital, renal and alimentary tracts. Severely affected patients can also bleed internally into the joints and brain, but bleeding into joints is unusual. Diagnosis is made by finding prolongation of the skin bleeding time, a platelet functional defect and a low level of factor VIII.

Minor degrees of bleeding may be controllable with tranexamic acid or vasopressin preparations, but more serious bleeding requires treatment with appropriate factor concentrates.

DEFICIENCY OF VITAMIN K

Lack of vitamin K in the diet, its malabsorption or the presence of anticoagulant drugs of the coumarin group leads to deficient hepatic synthesis of the plasma clotting factors, prothrombin, and factors VII, IX and X. Vitamin K is the cofactor necessary for the carboxylation and thus biological activation of glutamic acid. Deficiency from any of these causes can result in a bleeding tendency which may be seen in:

- haemorrhagic disease of the newborn
- intestinal malabsorption, for example Crohn's disease, coeliac disease
- hepatobiliary disease, for example hepatic failure, obstructive jaundice (**9.14**)
- dietary deficiency
- oral anticoagulant usage.

Haemorrhagic disease of the newborn

In the premature or immature infant there is defective synthesis of the vitamin K-dependent factors, which are significantly lower than those in adult life. Bleeding results on the third or fourth day of life, usually into the skin or internal organs. It is usual to give vitamin K parenterally at birth to prevent bleeding, but this policy is currently under review.

Malabsorption and dietary deficiency

These are extremely common and result from a range of disorders of the gut (*see* **p. 355**) and pancreas, and from obstructive biliary tract disease. They are usually part of a mixed clinical picture and other features often dominate. The problem is often picked up on routine screening, for example before liver biopsy, or by excessive bleeding after a minor surgical procedure. Vitamin K by injection is effective in malabsorption, but if there is serious liver cell necrosis it may not be effective.

Use of oral anticoagulants

Oral anticoagulant drugs (coumarins) such as warfarin, inhibit the action of vitamin K and result in the production of defective molecules of factors II, VII, IX and X which lack clotting activity. For normal therapeutic purposes, this depression of coagulation is maintained by testing the patient's plasma using a modification of the prothrombin time (the International Normalized Ratio, INR). It is usual to extend this to 2–3 times that of a normal control. Only when this value is exceeded is bleeding likely to occur, and this may be from or into any tissue of the body. Patients who have been stabilized on a particular dose of warfarin often bleed because other drugs have been taken that interfere with the coagulation mechanism (e.g. aspirin interferes with platelets), displace warfarin from its binding site on the albumin molecule (e.g. mefenamic acid), or decrease its metabolism (e.g. cimetidine). Bleeding often occurs early in the skin (**9.14**, **10.104**), bowel or urinary tract. Always consider the possibility of undeclared anticoagulant therapy in a bleeding patient. All patients receiving oral anticoagulant therapy require specialized care for optimal control.

Parenchymal liver disease

Necrosis of liver cells as a result of hepatitis or alcohol or other toxins results in failure of coagulation factor synthesis, and severe bruising or bleeding may result (**9.14**). The defect is usually complex and may be associated with thrombocytopenia see **p. 436**) and DIC (*see* **p. 443**). Defects of the vitamin K-dependent factors may not respond to the injection of vitamin K in this situation.

THROMBOPHILIA

A number of acquired and hereditary disorders may increase the chance of the development of arterial or venous thrombosis. These are known as thrombophilia or prethrombotic disorders.

The possibility of such a disorder should be considered in those with a family history of venous thrombosis, in all patients with recurrent venous thrombosis, in patients under the age of 40 with a first venous thrombosis, in those with venous thrombosis in an unusual site (cerebral or mesenteric veins, for example), in those with arterial thrombosis in the absence of arterial disease and in women with recurrent accidental abortions.

Factor V Leiden

This abnormality in factor V is the commonest hereditary form of thrombophilia. It occurs in 3% of individuals worldwide (5–8% of Europeans) and is found in 20–40% of patients with venous thromboembolism, especially in those with DVT at a young age. It is inherited as an autosomal dominant condition. Homozygotes have an 80-fold increased risk of DVT and heterozygotes have a seven-fold increased risk (which is increased during pregnancy or oral contraceptive treatment). The abnormality is a point mutation in which the arginine at position 506 in the factor V gene is replaced by glutamine. This eliminates the site in factor V protein which is normally cleaved by activated protein C, resulting in an extended pro-coagulant

effect in the plasma. The diagnosis can be confirmed by DNA examination. Homozygous patients should usually receive long-term anticoagulant therapy. Heterozygotes should receive thromboprohylaxis to cover surgery or trauma, but long term therapy should usually be reserved for those who have thrombotic episodes.

Protein C or S deficiency

Proteins C and S are vitamin K-dependent proteins that are synthesized in the liver, and are critical regulators of activation of blood coagulation. A range of hereditary deficiencies in the production or activity of these proteins has been described, and these are associated with an increased risk of recurrent thromboembolism, especially in younger individuals. Functional activity of protein C should be measured routinely in patients with deep vein thrombosis, especially if other family members have also been affected.

Acute skin necrosis may result when patients with protein C deficiency are given warfarin, as a result of small vessel thrombosis resulting from the warfarin-induced reduction of protective protein C. Treatment is to stop warfarin and start heparin, and skin grafting is often necessary as the slough separates.

Antithrombin deficiency

Antithrombin III (AT-III) is the most important antithrombin in the plasma and also has a major protective role against coagulation activation products at all stages in the coagulation cascade. Its activity is enhanced many hundred-fold by binding with heparin. Inherited deficiency of AT-III is found in 1 in 4000 of the population and is associated with an enhanced tendency to recurrent venous thrombosis and pulmonary embolism. Symptoms of venous thrombosis usually occur in the late teens and affect the deep veins of the legs. Antithrombin deficiency can also be acquired, following major surgery, trauma, severe proteinuria or oral contraceptive treatment. The diagnosis is made by measurement of AT levels. Patients are relatively resistant to heparin, as AT is required for its action, and treatment is usually with lifelong oral anticoagulants. In hereditary AT deficiency, an accurate family history is helpful and a determined effort should be made to measure AT-III levels in other family members.

The antiphospholipid syndrome

In the antiphospholipid syndrome, antibodies bind phospholipids and result in the inhibition of phospholipid-dependent coagulation factors. This may result in a number of thrombotic disorders, including venous thromboembolism and arterial thrombosis, which may result in abnormalities in the brain, heart, kidneys, adrenals, skin and placenta. Complications of the antiphospholipid syndrome may include recurrent abortion, strokes, chorea, epilepsy, valvular heart disease, Budd–Chiari syndrome (*see* **p. 393**) and Addison's disease (*see* **p. 302**). A minority of patients also have systemic lupus erythematosus (*see* **p. 121**). Antiphospholipid antibodies (anticardiolipin and lupus anticoagulant antibodies) can be detected by ELISA.

The management of patients with the antiphospholipid syndrome is controversial, ranging from lifelong anti-coagulation (with its potential for bleeding) to simply providing thromboprophylaxis to cover surgery, trauma or other risk periods such as pregnancy.

DISSEMINATED INTRAVASCULAR COAGULATION

DIC (also known as consumption coagulopathy) occurs when the coagulation cascade is activated by a stimulus that results in the widespread deposition of fibrin–platelet thrombi in the arterial and venous tree. This in turn stimulates secondary fibrinolysis and, as the two processes continue in parallel, the end result is depletion of platelets, consumption of clotting factors, loss of haemostasis and excessive bleeding. A large number of conditions may be the stimulus to production of acute or chronic DIC (**10.109–10.112** and *see* **10.113**).

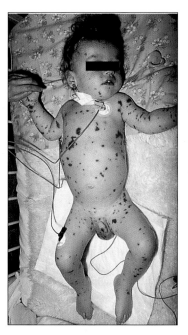

10.109 Disseminated intravascular coagulation (DIC) is often a consequence of severe infection. In this infant, meningococcal septicaemia was the underlying cause, and his widespread skin haemorrhages were accompanied by mucosal bleeding. Such devastating DIC is often fatal.

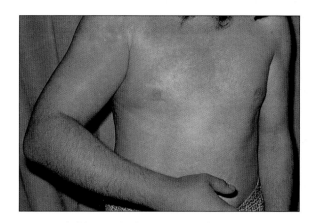

10.111 Snakebites and other venomous bites and stings are a potent cause of DIC. Adder bites in Europe rarely cause more than the severe local swelling experienced by this man, but envenomation by many other snakes and animals commonly causes DIC, and this may lead to death. Snakebite remains an important cause of death worldwide, especially in developing countries.

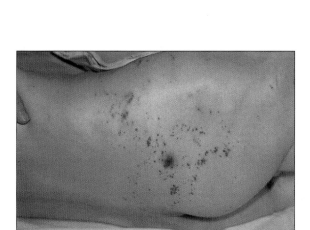

10.110 DIC resulting from staphylococcal septicaemia in a 56-year-old man. Note the characteristic skin haemorrhage ranging from small purpuric lesions to larger ecchymoses. The patient had non-insulin-dependent diabetes, and the septicaemia developed from an untreated large boil on his thigh.

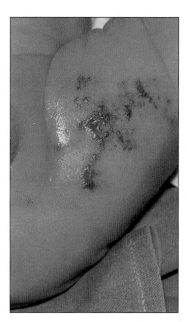

10.112 Cavernous haemangiomas may be associated with DIC (the Kasabach–Merritt syndrome). The damaged subendothelial surface of the neoplasm leads to excessive consumption of circulating platelets and clotting factors, which may result in the full clinical picture of DIC. Occasional diagnostic difficulty results from the presence of a visceral haemangioma with similar properties. Surgical excision, injection of multiple therapeutic emboli under angiographic control or radiotherapy may be successful in eliminating the lesion and the consumptive coagulopathy.

CAUSES OF DIC

Infections/infectious diseases	Haemorrhagic fevers (*see* **pp. 13, 17**), meningococcal septicaemia (*see* **p. 27**), other septicaemia Malaria (*see* **p. 48**)
Obstetric causes	Amniotic fluid embolism, pre-eclampsia, abruptio placentae, dead fetus syndrome
Malignant disease	Especially bronchus, pancreas, ovary, prostate, acute leukaemias
Shock	Traumatic, cardiac arrest, blood loss, extensive burns
Intravascular haemolysis/ massive blood transfusion	
Envenomation	
Vasculitis	e.g. haemolytic uraemic syndrome (HUS), thrombotic thrombocytopenic purpura (TTP)
Extracorporeal circulation	e.g. cardiopulmonary bypass, artificial heart, dialysis
Cavernous haemangiomas	

10.113   Causes of DIC.

Patients suffering from acute DIC present with a dramatic illness with haemorrhagic manifestations. They are usually severely ill, with fever, acidosis, and hypoxia and hypotension caused by severe blood loss. There may be extensive petechiae or frank bleeding into the skin (**1.45, 1.190, 10.109**), especially at sites of trauma, for example wounds, venepuncture sites or under a blood-pressure cuff. There may also be bleeding in the eyes (**1.90, 1.144**) and the alimentary, respiratory, genital or renal tracts. On occasions, thrombosis may dominate the initial picture, and there may be gangrene of skin and digits (**10.114**), with signs of ischaemia of heart, brain, kidneys and lungs.

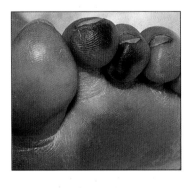

10.114   Peripheral gangrene can be a feature of DIC, as the balance between thrombosis and haemorrhage will vary from one part of the body to another and from time to time. This patient has meningococcal septicaemia, and despite his gangrenous toes he had haemorrhagic manifestations elsewhere in his body (see **1.90, 1.91, 10.109**).

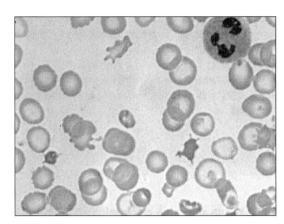

10.115   The peripheral blood film in DIC usually shows a microangiopathic haemolytic anaemia (MAHA). Abnormal red cells, including burr cells, acanthocytes with multiple sharp projections and schistocytes of irregular fragmented shape, result from physical damage to the cells caused by their passage between strands of fibrin. The platelet count is reduced. This patient presented with acute renal failure and hypertension.

A routine blood film may show fragmentation of red cells (a microangiopathic haemolytic blood picture, **10.115**) that results from cell damage by strands of fibrin thrombus. Simple screening tests for DIC include the platelet count (which is reduced), the APPT (which is prolonged) and the presence of fibrinogen–fibrin degradation products (FDPs) that have resulted from fibrin digestion. A specialist haematology laboratory can look for other evidence of coagulation consumption, fibrinolysis and platelet activation. The cause of the process (**10.113**), should be identified and treated whenever possible. The other keystones of treatment are:

* general intensive support of the patient
* restoration and maintenance of the peripheral circulation
* replacement therapy with plasma or plasma products.

Control of the thrombotic component with heparin is rarely useful, and is complicated by the effects of some heparins on platelets.

Chronic DIC occurs in some patients with chronic inflammatory or malignant disorders, and is characterized by a combination of features relating to thrombosis as well as bleeding. On investigation, fibrinogen, cryofibrinogen and FDP levels are all high.

MULTIPLE MYELOMA AND RELATED PARAPROTEINAEMIAS

The paraproteinaemias are a group of disorders in which there is proliferation of B cells leading to excessive production of immunoglobulins. Of these conditions, multiple myeloma is the most common and results from the malignant proliferation of plasma cells. It is usually a disease of the middle-aged and elderly. The clinical features result from the uncontrolled growth of plasma cells in the marrow and the production of an abnormal paraprotein – usually an IgG, but sometimes IgA or light chains and rarely IgD, IgM or other group. They include:

- lytic bone lesions resulting from local infiltration of bone, associated with hypercalcaemia (*see* **p. 139**) and painful pathological bone fractures
- bone marrow failure from infiltration, leading to anaemia, leucopenia and thrombocytopenia
- suppression of normal immunoglobulin synthesis, with resultant susceptibility to infections
- hyperviscosity syndromes caused by the physical properties of the paraprotein (M-protein); these are most common with IgG paraprotein and result in tissue ischaemia with overt arterial and venous thrombosis predominantly in the eye (**10.61**), heart, brain and kidneys
- renal impairment, which is common and is a critical factor in life-expectancy (**p. 281**); the kidney is damaged by hypercalcaemia, infection, deposition of amyloid, the deposition of light-chain fractions in the proximal tubules and hyperuricaemia
- neurological involvement, which results from ischaemia associated with hyperviscosity and from amyloid deposition.

Patients present with infections (70%), bleeding defects (10%) or renal failure (50%). Bone pain develops in all patients as the disease progresses.

Suggestive features of myeloma include a very high ESR (usually over 100 mm in the first hour), a normochromic normocytic anaemia with rouleaux formation (**10.25**), and often neutropenia and thrombocytopenia. The serum calcium levels are often elevated.

The diagnosis can be made by finding evidence of two factors out of the following three: paraproteinaemia, bone marrow plasmacytosis and lytic lesions of bones.

- paraprotein may be found in serum or urine (Bence Jones protein, **10.116**)
- bone marrow aspiration or trephine shows sheets of plasma cells (**10.117**)
- plain X-rays of the skeleton show 'punched out' areas, especially in the skull (**10.118**), ribs, pelvis and long bones (**10.119**); there may also be pathological fractures.

A range of other investigations aid prognosis.

Treatment of patients with multiple myeloma is supportive, with antibiotics for infection, analgesics for bone pain, a high fluid intake and effective management of hypercalcaemia (which may require biphosphonate treatment). Hyperviscosity and cryoglobulinaemia may be managed by plasma exchange until the tumour mass can be controlled with either melphalan or cyclophosphamide or with radiotherapy for local lesions. Hyperuricaemia should be treated with allopurinol. Stem cell autotransplants and allogenic bone marrow transplants may improve quality of life but are rarely curative.

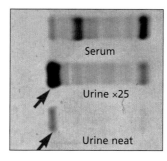

10.116 Serum and urine electrophoresis in multiple myeloma provide evidence of the presence of a paraprotein in serum and urine. In this case, the patient had IgA myeloma; the paraprotein band shows clearly in the concentrated (×25) and neat urine (arrows) and a corresponding band is present in the serum.

445

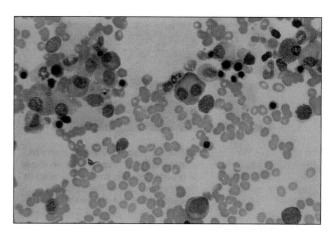

10.117 Bone marrow film in myeloma. This view is taken from the outer edge of the marrow smear to show individual cells. The marrow is generally hypercellular and contains an excess of diverse plasma cells (myeloma cells). Some are large, with immature-looking chromatin; others are small with clumping of chromatin. The cytoplasm is often pale, and Russell bodies are present in the cytoplasm, representing accumulations of IgG.

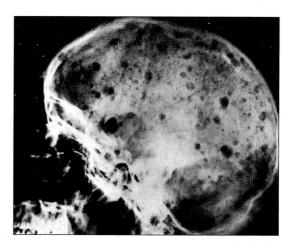

10.118 Myeloma lesions in bones show up as characteristic 'punched out' lesions without surrounding sclerosis. Secondary deposits from other tumours may occasionally give a similar appearance, but this appearance on skull X-ray is strongly suggestive of multiple myeloma.

446

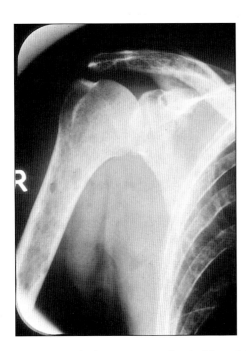

10.119   Myeloma in the humerus, scapula, clavicle and ribs. The lesions have the same 'punched out' appearance as those seen in the skull. Myeloma lesions are also commonly seen in other long bones, in the ribs and the pelvis. Pathological fractures may occur, and hypercalcaemia is common.

This is a disease of the elderly with a male preponderance of 2:1. The common presentation is with fever, anaemia, weight loss, weakness and fatigue. Qualitative platelet defects may lead to epistaxis, skin petechiae and gastrointestinal haemorrhage. Hyperviscosity features may result in strokes, myocardial infarction, loss of vision, Raynaud's phenomenon and pyoderma gangrenosum (**2.135**).

Bence–Jones protein may be found in the urine and amyloid may develop. The lymphocytic infiltrate may cause hepatomegaly and splenomegaly, but can occur in any other body tissue. Osteolytic lesions are rare.

Investigations show a normochromic normocytic anaemia with rouleaux formation on the blood film (**10.25**). There may be leucopenia but more usually there is an atypical lymphocytosis. The ESR is characteristically elevated to above 100 mm in the first hour. Bone marrow shows a generalized diffuse lympho-plasmacytoid infiltrate with excess eosinophils. Such appearances may also be found in the peripheral lymph nodes. Examination of the serum shows an abnormal M-protein, cryoglobulin, and cold-reacting antibodies.

Treatment should be aimed at the hyperviscosity that dominates the clinical picture. This may be altered by haemodilution or plasmaphaeresis. Chemotherapy with chlorambucil, cyclophosphamide or melphalan may be helpful. Supportive management is required for haemorrhage, anaemia, infections and cold-precipitation syndromes. Mean survival is 4–6 years.

The overall median survival remains about 2–3 years despite use of chemotherapy. Poor prognostic features include increasing age, anaemia, a very high ESR, low serum albumin and elevated serum creatinine at the time of diagnosis.

SOLITARY PLASMACYTOMAS

In a small number of cases of paraproteinaemia (7%) there is a localized plasma cell proliferation and the marrow elsewhere is normal. Such local plasmacytomas may arise in bone or in soft tissues and may grow to a large size before being diagnosed. Diagnosis is made by finding a solitary lytic lesion of bone, with an abnormal M-protein on electrophoresis, histological evidence of plasma cell tumour on biopsy and normal marrow at a distant site. Surgical removal or radiotherapy may produce a cure with a rapid disappearance of the M-proteins.

WALDENSTRÖM'S MACROGLOBULINAEMIA

Waldenström's macroglobulinaemia is a condition characterized by the presence of monoclonal IgM in association with excessive numbers of tissue lymphocytes and plasma cells (lymphocytic lymphoma with plasmacytoid differentiation).

MONOCLONAL GAMMOPATHY OF UNCERTAIN SIGNIFICANCE (MGUS)

A monoclonal paraprotein sometimes appears in the absence of a detectable B-cell tumour. Some patients develop this paraprotein transiently in response to an infection such as viral hepatitis or leptospirosis, in an autoimmune disease such as rheumatoid arthritis, and occasionally in non-B-cell tumours. In other (usually elderly) patients there is a stable benign paraproteinaemia that remains unchanged for many years, except in a small number who develop an overtly malignant plasma-cell myeloma.

Investigations should be directed at the underlying cause: non-B-cell malignancy, infection or autoimmune disease. Bence Jones proteins and M-band proteins are present. A level of paraprotein below 10 g/litre usually indicates a benign cause. There is no marrow infiltration or immunosuppression, and no lytic bone lesions. Patients should be followed up carefully over many years, as 10–20% develop overt myeloma. No specific treatment is necessary initially.

CRYOGLOBULINAEMIA

Malignant paraproteinaemias may be associated with the presence of circulating cryoglobulins (i.e. globulins which precipitate out when blood is cooled). They may also be found in rheumatoid arthritis, systemic lupus erythematosus, infectious mononucleosis, lymphoma, primary biliary cirrhosis and hepatitis C infection. This most commonly causes problems in the limbs and the resultant deposition on the walls of small vessels produces a generalized vasculitis, which presents with a reticular pattern of microthrombosis, and usually larger areas of gangrene, which eventually slough and require skin grafts (**10.120**). In more severe cases infarction of internal organs, especially the kidneys, may occur. There is also a high incidence of venous thrombosis, pulmonary embolism and other arterial occlusion.

Treatment is with plasmapheresis to reduce the levels of circulating cryoglobulins and also to reduce the blood viscosity due to IgG and IgM. This may allow time for appropriate chemotherapy to control the underlying pathology.

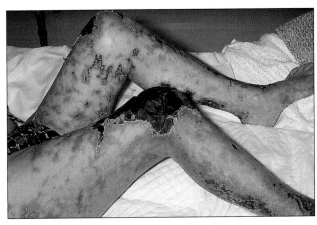

10.120 Skin infarction in cryoglobulinaemia. There is a reticulated pattern to the skin due to leakage of red cells from damaged skin capillaries. Necrosis and ulceration has occurred in peripheral sites due to vessel blockage. This patient eventually required plastic surgery.

11 Nerve and muscle

HISTORY

Consultations for neurological disorders are relatively common in general or family practice. Headache is the most common presentation, but other disorders are also seen quite frequently (**11.1**).

Important facets of the history in a patient with neurological symptoms include the following:

- Higher cerebral dysfunction – dementia, confusional states and coma are common features and are the end results of a large number of acute and chronic neurological diseases.
- Fits: a wide range of epileptic phenomena may result from neurological diseases, including generalized or partial seizures, and are often best described by family or friends rather than the patient.
- Headache, the causes of which include tension, stress, migraine and cranial arteritis. Space-occupying lesions cause headache that is often worse on waking and on coughing or bending; there may be associated vomiting. It is particularly important to define site of pain, exacerbating factors, radiation of pain and duration.
- Loss of power results from abnormalities of the upper or lower motor neuron in the brain or cord as well as disorders of the neuromuscular junction and muscle; loss of power may be of acute or gradual onset. Lower motor neuron lesions result in localized muscle atrophy; upper motor neuron lesions result in spasticity that produces a typical gait.

- Vertigo is the feeling that the surroundings are moving; it reflects disease of the labyrinth or vestibular connections. Dizziness is a common symptom – the patient usually implies unsteadiness or lightheadedness.
- Abnormal movements: a variety of tremors may suggest a diagnosis, for example the typical 'pill rolling' tremor of Parkinson's disease, or the coarse flapping tremor associated with liver, respiratory or renal failure. In contrast are the coarse movements of chorea, athetosis and hemiballismus; these are the result of extrapyramidal lesions.
- Cerebellar ataxia may produce a loss of fine control of movement that results in dysmetria, dyssynergia and a broad-based gait, with a tendency to fall to the side of the lesion if it is unilateral; there are usually other symptoms and signs of the cerebellar lesion, including diplopia, dysarthria and hypotonia. Sensory ataxia results from lesions of the sensory pathways in the peripheral nerves or spinal cord and produces a stamping gait; there is compensation from visual stimuli and when the eyes are closed the problem is exacerbated.
- Recent head injury may lead to transient or progressive neurological disorder; subdural haematomas may lead to symptoms many weeks after the original injury, which may only be recalled on close questioning.
- General medical, occupational, social and family history – all of which may point to underlying causes for neurological symptoms.

EXAMINATION

GENERAL ASSESSMENT

It is important to observe the patients and their movements. Their posture and gait may reveal abnormalities; they may show signs of personal neglect or psychiatric disorder; there may be signs of systemic disease, or of local abnormalities.

HIGHER CEREBRAL FUNCTION

Aspects of higher cerebral function often become obvious from the history, but the examination should include observations on conscious level, orientation in time and space, general level of intelligence, mental state, general attitude, speech and memory. Most of these functions can be quantified when necessary, using rating scales. Apraxia (**11.2**) and agnosia may be revealed

COMMON NEUROLOGICAL DISORDERS, AS SEEN IN A NON-SPECIALIST SETTING	
Principal presentation	**Relative frequency in family practice (%)**
Headache or migraine	37
Vertigo	25
Stroke or transient ischaemic attack	20
Epilepsy	10
Tremor or rigidity (parkinsonism)	4
Features suggesting multiple sclerosis	3
Others	1

11.1 Common neurological disorders, as seen in a non-specialist setting.

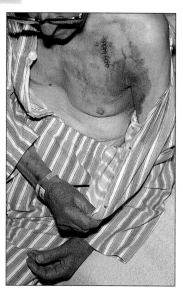

11.2 Apraxia is the inability to perform a familiar action that cannot be attributed to physical disability, incomprehension or agnosia. This patient has dressing apraxia, associated with thromboembolic stroke that followed myocardial infarction. Apraxia results from higher cerebral dysfunction. Note the recent insertion of a cardiac pacemaker – treatment for a conduction defect that followed the myocardial infarction.

FEATURES OF LOWER AND UPPER MOTOR NEURON LESIONS	
Lower motor neuron (LMN)	Upper motor neuron (UMN)
Motor weakness (root or nerve distribution)	Motor weakness (extensors in arm; flexors in leg; 'pyramidal' pattern)
Muscle wasting, fasciculation	Usually normal muscle bulk
Decreased tone	Increased tone
Decreased or absent tendon reflexes	Increased tendon reflexes, clonus
Flexor plantar response	Extensor plantar response

11.3   Features of lower and upper motor neuron lesions

by appropriate tests. Cognitive function can be rapidly screened using the mini mental state examination and other rating scales, before a more detailed assessment.

SYSTEMATIC EXAMINATION

The upper and lower limbs and trunk must be examined systematically to assess motor power, sensation, the extrapyramidal system and the cerebellum. In each muscle group, assess:

- muscle bulk, and look carefully for trophic changes and involuntary movements
- tone – spastic (clasp knife) or plastic (lead pipe)
- power
- reflexes: superficial and tendon
- coordination.

In any abnormality it must be decided whether the upper or lower motor neuron is involved (**11.3**). Patients with polyneuropathies usually present with distal weakness. Abnormal movements suggest probable extrapyramidal involvement.

Lesions of the cerebellum result in loss of tone, incoordination, altered posture, speech defects and nystagmus.

If patients have sensory symptoms, the following sensory modalities must be tested carefully. The functions to be tested include:

- tactile sensation and discrimination
- pain and deep pain
- temperature
- vibration
- proprioception

- two-point discrimination, stereognosis, and graphaesthesia if cortical lesions are suspected.

CRANIAL NERVES

I. Olfactory nerve

Chemoreceptors are present in the mucosa on the roof of the nose and pass through the cribriform plate in the ethmoid to synapse in the olfactory bulb. Secondary fibres then pass via the olfactory tract to the olfactory cortex on the anteromedial temporal lobe. Loss of smell (anosmia) may result from lesions of the:

- mucosa, for example the common cold
- cribriform plate, for example fracture
- olfactory tract, for example space-occupying lesions
- rarely, temporal lobe, for example space-occupying lesions, haematoma, or trauma.

The nerve is tested by asking the patient to smell a scent. Lesions may be unilateral or bilateral. Parosmia is a distorted sense of smell.

II. Optic nerve

From an inverted image on the light-sensitive cells of the retina, the impulses pass via the optic nerves to the optic chiasma; at the decussation, fibres from the nasal side of the retina cross to the contralateral optic tract, whereas the temporal retinal fibres remain uncrossed. The optic tracts then pass to the lateral geniculate body where they synapse. The optic radiation fibres sweep posteriorly through the temporal and parietal lobes to the occipital cortex. The left half of the field of vision is represented in the cortex of the right hemisphere and vice versa. Some fibres from the optic tract do not synapse at the lateral geniculate body but pass directly to the midbrain as the afferent limb of the pupillary light reflex.

Full examination of the second nerves should include examination of the eyes (11.4), including the retina, and an assessment of:

- visual acuity – using Jaeger or Faculty of Ophthalmologists' charts for near vision or Snellen test type for distance vision
- fields of vision by confrontation and perimetry (11.5)
- colour vision by Ishihara plates is required for individuals in many occupations
- pupillary reflexes – to light and accommodation.

The Argyll Robertson pupil (11.6) is now very rare, but is a classic feature of neurosyphilis and may also occur in diabetes. The pupil is small, irregular and reacts to accommodation but not to light directly or consensually. The abnormality is present bilaterally.

Adie's tonic pupil (11.7) is characterized by a delayed or very poor response to light but a better, though slowed, response to accommodation. The pupil appears large, is usually unilateral and may be associated with diminished or absent reflexes (Holmes-Adie syndrome). The diagnosis can be confirmed by showing there is denervation hypersensitivity of the affected pupil to weak pilocarpine drops.

Horner's syndrome (4.161, 11.8) results from paralysis of the cervical sympathetic nerve. Sympathetic supply to the pupil leaves the CNS in the lower cervical and upper thoracic portions of the cord, emerges in the first thoracic nerve root and runs via the sympathetic chain and along the internal carotid artery to the cavernous plexus and then via the ophthalmic division of the trigeminal nerve to the eye.

Any disorder that interferes with the integrity of the pathway causes Horner's syndrome, which comprises ptosis, pupillary

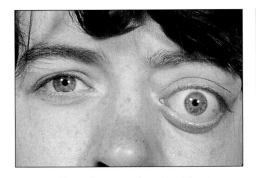

11.4 Unilateral proptosis resulted from a meningioma on the sheath of the optic nerve in this patient. A similar appearance may develop in Graves' disease (see p. 309), but exophthalmos is usually bilateral in that condition.

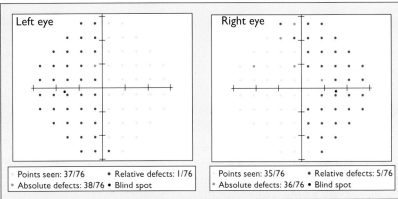

Left eye		Right eye	
Points seen: 37/76 • Relative defects: 1/76		Points seen: 35/76 • Relative defects: 5/76	
Absolute defects: 38/76 • Blind spot		Absolute defects: 36/76 • Blind spot	

11.5 Visual field testing, using the Humphrey computer-based printout. The patient had advanced acromegaly, with bitemporal hemianopia as a result of compression of the optic chiasma by an enlarging pituitary tumour. In the earlier stages of tumour enlargement, asymmetric bitemporal upper quadrantic defects are typical.

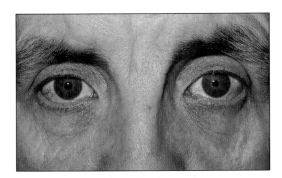

11.6 Argyll Robertson pupils are a feature of neurosyphilis. They are usually bilateral, but the abnormality was more marked in this patient's left eye. Argyll Robertson pupils are small, irregular and unresponsive to light, but they react normally on accommodation if the patient's visual acuity is adequate. They may also be found in patients with diabetes mellitus.

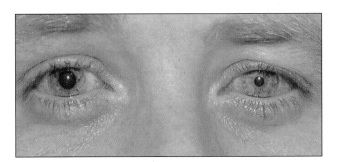

11.7 Adie's tonic pupil in the right eye of a young woman. The affected pupil is 'tonic', that is it responds slowly to light and accommodation, but on rapid testing will appear unresponsive. The site of the lesion is usually obscure, but the condition is benign. There may be associated areflexia.

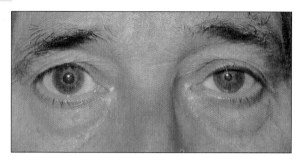

11.8   Horner's syndrome. Note the characteristic ptosis of the left eye, associated with constriction of the pupil (miosis). This patient had syringomyelia, but Horner's syndrome has many possible causes (**11.9**).

DISORDERS CAUSING HORNER'S SYNDROME

Pancoast tumour

Cervical rib

Carotid aneurysm

Carotid body tumour

Syringomyelia

Ponto-medullary CVA or tumour

Trauma

11.9   Disorders causing Horner's syndrome.

constriction (miosis), enophthalmos and loss of sweating on one-half of the face and neck (anhidrosis). The common causes of Horner's syndrome are shown in **11.9**.

III, IV and VI. Oculomotor, trochlear and abducens

The oculomotor, trochlear and abducens nerves together control the muscles of ocular movement.

Lower motor neuron lesions may lead to defective movements, squint, diplopia and pupillary abnormalities.

11.10   11.11

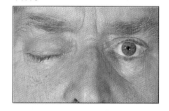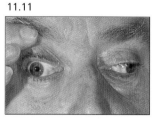

11.10 & 11.11   Third nerve palsy. Note the complete right ptosis. In the resting position, the right eye was rotated laterally and downwards, but in **11.11** the patient is looking to the left, and the right eye has rotated to the mid position, demonstrating that the trochlear (fourth) nerve is intact. This patient's third nerve palsy was the result of compression by an aneurysm of the posterior communicating artery.

- Oculomotor lesions: ptosis is present, the eyeball is rotated downwards and outwards, and the pupil is dilated and fixed (**3.76**, **11.10**, **11.11**); unilateral pupillary dilatation may be the sole manifestation of an early lesion.
- Trochlear lesions cause impaired downward movement of the adducted eye (**11.12**), giving rise to diplopia on looking down. The superior oblique muscle also in-torts the abducted eye on downgaze.
- Abducens lesions cause convergent squint with inability to move the eye outwards and diplopia on trying to look outwards (**7.83**, **11.13**).

The differential diagnosis of ptosis includes:

- third nerve palsy
- posterior communicating artery aneurysms (*see* **p. 477**)
- myasthenia gravis (*see* **p. 494**)
- Horner's syndrome (*see* **p. 451**).

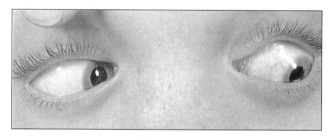

11.12   Right fourth nerve palsy. The patient is attempting to look down and to the left, but this movement is impaired in the right eye. The patient presented with diplopia, especially when reading, and difficulty in walking downstairs.

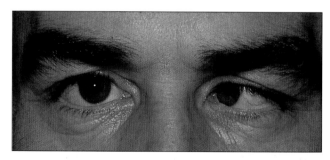

11.13   Right sixth nerve palsy. The right eye fails to abduct on lateral gaze. The lid, the pupil and other ocular movements are normal.

V. Trigeminal nerve

Lesions of the trigeminal nerve lead to loss of sensation in the skin of the face and crown of the head (**11.14**), the conjunctivae and the nasopharynx. The angle of the jaw is spared as this is supplied by the second cervical nerve. There is also diminished secretion by the lacrimal and salivary glands, which results in dry eyes and mouth, and trophic ulceration may be found in the cornea, nose and mouth. The corneal reflex is lost. The

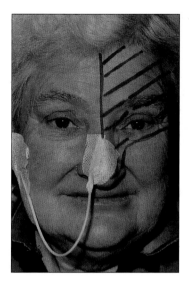

11.14 Trigeminal nerve palsy, affecting the ophthalmic division of the nerve. The distribution of sensory impairment is marked. This patient had multiple embolic phenomena from atheromatous plaques in the internal carotid artery. Note the nasogastric tube, necessary because of impairment of swallowing.

11.15

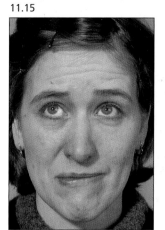

11.16

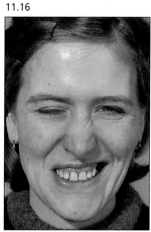

11.15 & 11.16 Lower motor neuron palsy of the right facial nerve (Bell's palsy). The face may look almost normal at rest, but this patient is unable to wrinkle her brow fully on the affected side, the right corner of her mouth droops and there is a prominent right nasolabial fold (**11.15**). When the patient is asked to close her eyes and show her teeth (**11.16**) the difference between the unaffected left side and the affected right side becomes more obvious. In upper motor neuron lesions, the weakness is less evident and the brow muscles function normally.

distribution of the first division of the fifth nerve is graphically demonstrated in ophthalmic herpes (**1.65**).

If the motor branch is involved, there is weakness and wasting of the muscles of mastication and, if this is unilateral, the jaw deviates to the affected side on opening the mouth.

Trigeminal neuralgia (tic douloureux) is a disease of unknown origin that manifests itself more commonly in women than men (usual age 50–80 years) with excruciating paroxysms of stabbing pain over the distribution of the trigeminal nerve. Paroxysms of pain are often provoked by minor touch, such as shaving, brushing teeth or chewing. The syndrome may be associated with an aberrant vascular loop and in younger patients may occasionally be an early feature of multiple sclerosis, but usually no cause is found. Severe pain usually occurs in the distribution of the maxillary or mandibular branches of the trigeminal nerve. The ophthalmic division is rarely affected. The brief, agonizing bouts are triggered by touch, chewing or cold. Carbamazepine is the drug treatment of choice although other anticonvulsants and baclofen may prove successful. If drug treatment fails, destructive lesions of the trigeminal nerve or its branches by thermocoagulation, local injection or steriotactic radiotherapy (the gamma knife) may be of value. Deccompression of the trigeminal nerve may be attempted, particularly in younger patients.

VII. Facial nerve

The facial nerve is almost entirely motor in function, supplying all the muscles of the face and scalp except for the levator palpebrae superioris. Paralysis leads to loss of facial expression and movement.

In supranuclear paralysis only the lower part of the face is involved because of the bilateral upper motor neuron innervation of the forehead. In infranuclear (lower motor neuron) paralysis both the upper and lower parts of the face are involved equally (**11.15, 11.16**).

Bell's palsy is the most common cause of infranuclear paralysis of the facial nerve. The nerve is often involved around the stylomastoid foramen, but symptoms and signs depend on the site of nerve involvement. The onset is usually acute. There is a rapid onset of unilateral paralysis of the muscles of facial expression and occasionally some pain behind the ear. Taste sensation (sweet, salt, bitter, acid) from the ipsilateral anterior two-thirds of the tongue may be lost, and there may be undue sensitivity to sounds (hyperacusis).

On the affected side, there is drooping of the corner of the mouth, with loss of skin creases and folds, particularly the nasolabial fold, and of the furrows on the forehead; the eye will often not close and attempts to close it result in it rolling upwards (Bell's phenomenon). Tears tend to run down the cheek as the lower lid sags and because of paralysis of the lip muscles, saliva dribbles from the corner of the mouth and food collects between the cheeks and gums.

The cause is possibly viral but unknown. Diagnosis is made on clinical grounds, and electromyography may be of some value in detecting interruption in the continuity of nerve fibres.

The disease is usually self-limiting and most patients recover in a few weeks. There is no specific treatment but local measures to prevent exposure keratitis are of value, and local massage and splinting may be of use. Steroids are often prescribed.

Other lesions of the facial nerve may produce similar symptoms and signs, for example mononeuritis (**7.83**), trauma and compression by tumours such as acoustic neuromas.

The Ramsay Hunt syndrome (**1.67**) results when herpes zoster affects the geniculate ganglion of the seventh nerve. Patients present with severe pain in the ear and a facial palsy on the same side. There may be a herpes rash in the external auditory meatus and in the pharynx.

VIII. Vestibulocochlear nerve

Two sets of fibres run in the vestibulocochlear nerve which serves the cochlea (for hearing) and the labyrinth and semicircular canals (for balance). Patients with lesions of the nerve may present with tinnitus, hyperacusis, deafness and dizziness.

Acoustic neurofibromas (neuromas) may develop at the cerebellopontine angle and present with insidious onset of unilateral deafness, headache, tinnitus, vertigo, ataxia, loss of sensation on the face resulting from trigeminal compression and facial weakness caused by compression of the facial nerve. Signs of a unilateral cerebellar lesion, including nystagmus develop. Further enlargement produces erosion of the petrous part of the temporal bone and pressure effects on the brainstem, with long tract symptoms and signs in the arm and leg, followed by raised intracranial pressure with papilloedema. In advanced cases hydrocephalus, long tract signs and coma may develop.

Skull X-ray with special views shows widening of the internal auditory meatus but diagnosis is best made by MRI (**11.17**, **11.120**), which clearly shows the site and extent of the lesion. Surgical removal is the aim of treatment but partial removal may be all that is possible. Early resection may allow conservation of seventh and eighth nerve function.

IX, X and XI. Glossopharyngeal, vagus and accessory

The glossopharyngeal, vagus and accessory nerves can be considered together. The glossopharyngeal nerve (IX) is predominantly sensory and supplies the posterior third of the tongue, palate, pharynx and fauces. The motor supply to this area is the vagus (X), which also supplies the oesophagus. The accessory nerve (XI) is purely motor, supplying the larynx and pharynx as well as fibres for the sternomastoid and trapezius.

Disorders of these nerves result in paralysis of the soft palate with regurgitation of fluids through the nose, difficulty in swallowing (**11.14**), change in the voice, which may become deeper and hoarse, and a diminution of coughing (bulbar palsy). Palsy of the accessory nerve leads to difficulty in flexion or extension of the neck and in shrugging the shoulders (**11.18**).

The left recurrent laryngeal nerve branch of the vagus is particularly liable to damage as it loops round the aorta and runs a long course back up to supply sensation and motor fibres to the larynx below the level of the vocal cords. Lesions of this branch result in dysphonia (**4.162**) and a 'bovine' cough.

XII. Hypoglossal

The hypoglossal nerve is wholly motor, supplying the tongue and the depressors of the hyoid bone. Lesions of the nerve result in unilateral paralysis, wasting and fasciculation of the tongue, which is pushed over to the paralysed side when protruded (**11.19**).

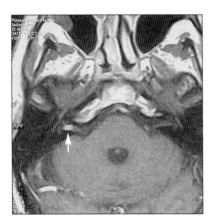

11.17 Acoustic neuroma. A gadolinium-enhanced MRI scan shows a small intracanalicular neuroma of the right eighth nerve (arrow).

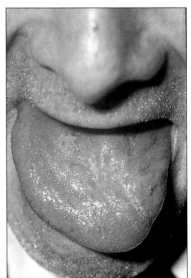

11.19 Hypoglossal nerve palsy. This patient had an isolated left lower motor neuron lesion of unknown cause, with deviation of the tongue to the affected side when it was pushed out, associated with fasciculation and fissuring caused by wasting.

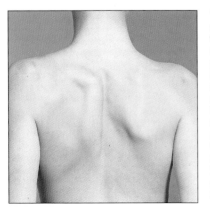

11.18 Accessory nerve palsy. The right trapezius does not contract when the patient shrugs his shoulders, and examination also revealed paralysis of the right sternomastoid muscle. The cause was avulsion of the nerve in a neck injury in an accident during a rugby football match.

INVESTIGATIONS

As in other systems, investigation of abnormalities in the CNS starts with simple investigations that lead to more specific tests to define the site and nature of the lesion and its consequences. These tests are usually more expensive, more invasive or both, and they must be selected with care.

HAEMATOLOGY

A full blood picture may show evidence of polycythaemia (in a stroke patient), anaemia and macrocytosis (in a patient with subacute combined degeneration), macrocytosis and thrombocytopenia (in alcoholism). A high ESR, C-reactive protein or plasma viscosity may suggest the possibility of vasculitis, infection or neoplasia.

BIOCHEMISTRY

Liver function abnormalities may suggest the presence of alcoholism in patients with peripheral neuropathy or coma, or of metastases or liver failure with an associated neurological syndrome. Direct measurement of levels of alcohol or narcotic drugs is of value in patients admitted in coma. Disturbances in serum potassium levels may explain episodes of paralysis; and abnormal thyroid hormone or parathyroid hormone and calcium levels are associated with peripheral and central neuron dysfunction. Calcium and glucose levels are of value in patients presenting with epileptic fits. Measurement of levels of creatine kinase is of value in patients suspected of muscular dystrophy, but it must be remembered that mild exertion or an intramuscular injection can also raise the level.

Measurement of myoglobin in the urine gives an indication of muscle necrosis, and high levels may be associated with precipitation in the renal tubules and subsequent renal failure. Under these circumstances exceptionally high levels of creatine kinase may be observed.

Optimal control of epilepsy demands monitoring of the serum levels of anticonvulsants to maintain safe and effective therapeutic levels.

SEROLOGY

Evidence of infection may be found by the presence of various antibodies, for example HIV infection, herpes simplex, neurosyphilis, neuroborreliosis (Lyme disease).

Measurement of IgG antibodies to cholinergic receptors in skeletal muscle is of value in confirming the diagnosis of myasthenia gravis.

NERVE CONDUCTION STUDIES

Motor and sensory conduction rates can be readily measured in large axons. There are differences in rates of conduction in different nerves and most laboratories apply their own standards. Demyelination greatly reduces conduction, as in the Guillain–Barré syndrome (*see* **p. 488**), nerve entrapment or diabetes mellitus, whereas in axonal degeneration, as found in drug-induced neuropathy, conduction velocity is only slightly reduced.

ELECTROMYOGRAPHY

Muscle or nerve action potentials can be recorded with needle or surface electrodes and are used in the differentiation of myopathic or neuropathic processes and in monitoring healing after nerve injury. In myopathies, damage to the motor units produces typical polyphasic responses. The specific cause of a myopathy cannot usually be diagnosed by this technique. Special tecniques may be used to investigate neuromuscular junction disorders.

EDROPHONIUM (TENSILON) TEST

This diagnostic test is used in patients with suspected myasthenia gravis (*see* **p. 494**).

ELECTROENCEPHALOGRAPH (EEG)

The EEG is a record of the spontaneous electrical signals generated within the brain. It is usually recorded from surface electrodes placed on the scalp, but in selected patients additional valuable diagnostic information may be obtained by neurosurgical implantation of sphenoidal, foramen ovale or cortical electrodes. A profile of waves is obtained from the electrodes and these wave patterns reflect the summation of electrical rhythms and are termed alpha, beta, theta and delta. The basic waveforms alter with eye closure, during sleep and with voluntary movements.

The EEG is valuable in detecting general abnormalities in physiological function such as occur in epilepsy (**11.42, 11.43**), encephalitis or encephalopathies. It can be of value in localizing a structural abnormality, but has largely been replaced by MRI and CT. Distinct patterns form the basis of classification of epilepsy. Videotelemetry is sometimes of value in diagnosing patients with 'funny turns' of unknown origin and is particularly important when localizing seizure foci before surgery.

EVOKED RESPONSES

Sensitive scalp electrodes allow the measurement on EEG of cortical responses to controlled stimuli, which may be visual, auditory or somatosensory. Delayed or abnormal waveforms may provide evidence of physiological dysfunction. Visual-evoked responses are used in the diagnosis of multiple sclerosis,

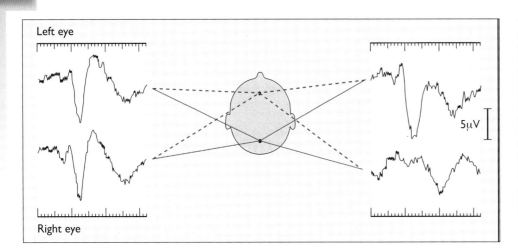

Left eye

Right eye

5μV

11.20 Visual-evoked response in optic neuritis of the right eye. Visual stimulation with a chequered pattern produces a predictable response on the EEG, and this response is delayed and deformed in this patient (bottom right trace). Optic neuritis is the most common cause of this abnormality and, as damage caused by subclinical or forgotten episodes can be detected, the test is of value; however, it is not specific (see text).

but the test is not specific and abnormalities in any part of the pathway from the eye to the occipital cortex will prolong the response time. If the patient's vision is normal, however, it is likely that the delayed response is caused by demyelination (**11.20**).

If CT or MRI is readily available, lumbar puncture is sometimes unnecessary (e.g. subarachnoid haemorrhage can often be diagnosed on CT). In all patients with altered consciousness or focal neurological signs, CT or MRI is advisable before carrying out lumbar puncture.

LUMBAR PUNCTURE

Samples of CSF are usually obtained by lumbar puncture at L3–L4 level (**11.21**). The important clinical indications are:

- probable infections of the CNS, including meningitis, encephalitis and neurosyphilis
- possible subarachnoid bleeding
- possible myelopathies or multiple sclerosis
- pressure measurement, for example in benign intracranial hypertension.

Definite contraindications to lumbar puncture are: raised intracranial pressure caused by space-occupying lesions (because of the risk of 'coning' – downward displacement of the cerebellum into the spinal canal, which is potentially fatal); cord compression; local skin sepsis; and any bleeding tendency (including anticoagulant therapy). Access to the subarachnoid space allows the pressure of CSF to be measured; it normally ranges from 80 to 180 mm of CSF and moves with respiration. Pressure on the jugular vein (Queckenstedt's test) results in a rise of up to 40 mm in CSF pressure. If the pressure does not rise, a block in the spinal canal is possible. This is usually associated with a dense yellow coloration of CSF caused by its protein content (Froin's syndrome).

CSF is collected for cell count, biochemistry and serology. If blood-staining is present initially, the CSF should be collected in three tubes to determine if the later tubes clear. Samples should be examined for pus and blood, and centrifuged to see if the supernatant is xanthochromic (**11.22**). (*See* **11.61** for changes in infection and **11.23** for changes in other conditions.)

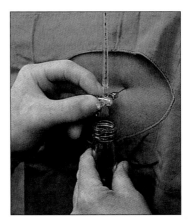

11.21 Lumbar puncture. The patient lies on his side (his head is to the left of the picture). After infiltration with local anaesthetic, the lumbar puncture needle is introduced through the third or fourth lumbar interspace. Its stylet is withdrawn, and a drop of CSF should appear. A manometer and three-way tap allows measurement of the CSF pressure and collection of fluid for examination.

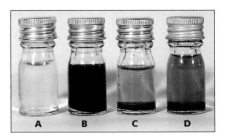

11.22 CSF examination. a) Normal crystal-clear CSF; **b)** blood in the CSF, which could result from a traumatic (bloody) tap or from subarachnoid haemorrhage – in a traumatic tap, subsequent tubes of CSF are usually less bloody; **c)** centrifuged CSF in a traumatic tap – the supernatant is nearly clear; **d)** CSF from a patient with subarachnoid haemorrhage – there is blood at the bottom of the tube and the supernatant is yellow (xanthochromic) as a result of breakdown of blood cells in the CSF before the lumbar puncture.

CEREBROSPINAL FLUID IN DISEASE STATES

	Appearance	Pressure (mm CSF)	Cells (per mm³)	Protein (mg/100 ml)	Glucose (mmol/litre)	Other
Normal	Crystal clear	80–180	0–5 (lymphocytes)	15–45	3.5–4.5	–
Traumatic tap	Bloodstained: clears	Normal	Red cells	Raised	Normal	Supernate clear
Subarachnoid haemorrhage	Bloody	Raised	Red cells	Raised	Normal	Xanthochromia
Multiple sclerosis	Clear	Normal	0–20 (lymphocytes)	Raised	Normal	Presence of oligoclonal bands
Froin's syndrome	Yellow	Low	Normal	Raised	Normal	May clot on standing
Syphilis	Clear	Normal	Up to 50 (lymphocytes)	Up to 100	Normal	Positive antibody
Viral meningitis	Clear/yellow	Raised	↑ lymphocytes	Normal	Normal	Elevated IgG index
Bacterial meningitis	Clear/yellow	Raised	↑ polymorphs	Raised	Reduced	–
TB meningitis	Clear/yellow	Raised	↑ lymphocytes	Raised	Reduced	Bacteria or Gram stain ZN stain can be negative

11.23   Cerebrospinal fluid in disease states.

BIOPSIES

Biopsy of peripheral nerves may give valuable information that can be both diagnostic and prognostic and may suggest therapy. The biopsy is best done at the wrist (superficial radial nerve) or at the ankle (distal sural nerve) and should be partial thickness to reduce the sensory loss.

Muscle biopsy may be done by needle or open biopsy under local anaesthesia. Enough material should be taken for histology, including electron microscopy, and histochemistry for muscle enzymes. Diagnostic changes are found in muscular dystrophies and inflammatory myopathies. In addition, vessel changes may indicate polyarteritis nodosa.

Brain biopsy is carried out in highly selected patients when there is a possibility that a course of therapy might be indicated, for example in suspected brain tumours or in possible herpes simplex encephalitis. It is not justified in dementia as there are currently no therapeutic possibilities, but meningeal biopsy may identify potentially treatable angiitides.

IMAGING TECHNIQUES

Straight X-rays of the skull are usually of limited value in neurological disease, unless there is a history of head injury that may be seen as a fracture (**11.24**) or a foreign body, or a disorder associated with ectopic calcification. Special views of the pituitary fossa, orbit, internal auditory canal, sinuses and spine give valuable additional information.

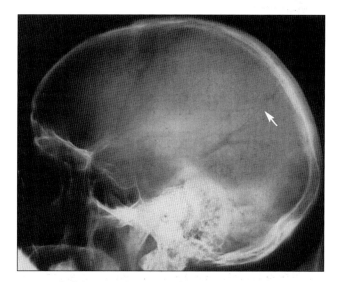

11.24   Skull fracture shown on plain X-ray. The line of the fracture (arrow) runs across the line of a meningeal artery, so the patient is at high risk of developing an extradural haematoma.

CT is extremely valuable in outlining the anatomy of the brain and skull, especially in defining cerebral haemorrhage and infarction, space-occupying lesions (**11.25**), subdural haematomas, the presence of hydrocephalus and cerebral atrophy. Structures above the tentorium are better seen than those in the posterior fossa. The spinal canal, disc spaces and cord are also well visualized. Modern techniques allow discrimination down to 5 mm. Intravenous contrast media may be given to enhance imaging.

MRI is also extremely valuable. Differences between white and grey matter are better demonstrated than with CT and the contents of the posterior fossa and the craniocervical region of the spinal canal are well visualized. Brain and spinal cord tumours, vascular abnormalities, anatomical abnormalities (syringomyelia) and demyelinating disorders are particularly well shown (**3.77**, **11.26–11.29**). MRI has largely replaced myelography in the investigation of possible pathology within

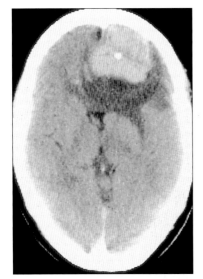

11.25   CT showing a left frontal meningioma. The contrast enhancement technique used in this scan demonstrates the classic appearance of a densely enhancing, sharply marginated tumour, tightly against the dura. The dark area posterior to the tumour represents extensive cerebral oedema. For angiograms of the same tumour see **11.31** and **11.32**.

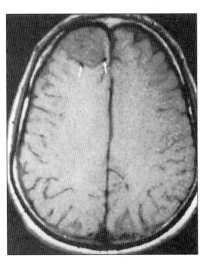

11.26   MRI picture of a right frontal meningioma. MRI shows the fissures of the brain more clearly than CT; it shows the tumour well, and parts of its vascular supply appear as hyperdense images (arrows).

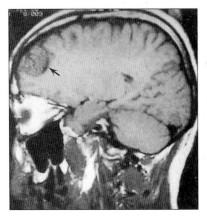

11.27   MRI sagittal view of the patient seen in 11.26. This view demonstrates the relationship of the meningioma to the dura and skull very clearly, and shows the vascular capsule posteriorly (arrow).

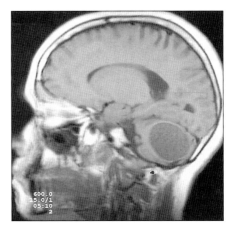

11.28   MRI sagittal view, showing a large cerebellar cyst. MRI is of particular value in demonstrating lesions in the posterior fossa.

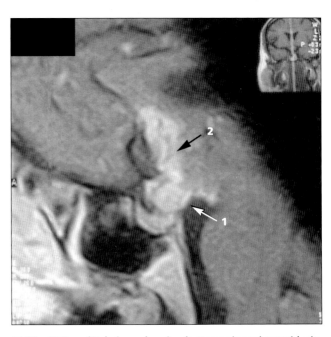

11.29   MRI sagittal view, showing leptomeningeal sarcoidosis. This gadolinium-enhanced MRI scan shows a mass around the optic chiasma (1), with extensive meningeal thickening along the adjacent brain surfaces (2).

the spinal cord or canal (**11.108**, **11.109**). As with CT, contrast medium injected intravenously may add to the yield of MRI. Dynamic MRI may provide information about blood flow.

Radionuclide scans have been largely replaced by MRI and CT for anatomical localization, but are still of value in assessing blood flow and in the detection of large ischaemic infarcts, arteriovenous malformations and subdural haematomas. A development of this technique is single photon emission computed tomography (SPECT) (**11.30**). Technetium is given attached to a carrier molecule (hexamethylene propyleneanine oxime, HMPAO) that enters the cerebral cells, and its presence is a reflection of blood flow and cell metabolism. It has a value in the investigation of patients with epilepsy because it may allow localization of foci. Another radionuclide test involves the use of isotopes of oxygen and glucose, which localize in cerebral cells and provide information on local cerebral perfusion and function – positron emission tomography (PET).

Ultrasound and the Doppler flow technique are now widely used to define the waveform, measure blood flow and define anatomical abnormalities in the carotid arteries (**11.74**). The techniques are non-invasive, cheap and readily repeatable and they have transformed the investigation of transient ischaemic attacks and permitted the screening of patients before selection for arteriography.

Cerebral angiography may be carried out by direct injection of contrast medium into the carotid or vertebral arteries, usually via a catheter inserted into the femoral artery. There is a small morbidity and mortality associated with the procedure. A series of films is taken in two planes to detect arterial and venous obstruction, aneurysms, arteriovenous malformations, tumour circulations (**11.31**, **11.32**) and arteritides. An alternative technique is digital subtraction angiography (DSA), in which the injection of contrast may be made intravenously and images of the artery are obtained by computer subtraction of images (**11.33**). MR angiography (MRA) is increasingly used to look at the cerebral circulation (**11.34**) although angiography is still preferred by many surgeons.

HEADACHE

Headache is an extremely common symptom and affects most people many times in their lives. It is rarely a symptom of serious neurological disease and usually responds rapidly to analgesics. However, more significance should be given to headache if it has any of the following features:

- dramatic onset – may suggest a subarachnoid haemorrhage (*see* **p. 477**).
- accompanied by confusion, coma or impairment of higher function.
- scalp tenderness in middle or old age – suggesting temporal arteritis (*see* **p. 128**).
- pyrexia and petechial rash may suggest meningococcal meningitis (*see* **p. 27**).
- neck stiffness suggests meningism or meningitis (*see* **p. 471**).

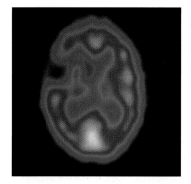

11.30 Single photon emission computed tomography (SPECT), demonstrating a right parietofrontal cerebral tumour, which proved to be a meningioma.

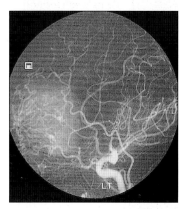

11.31 Cerebral angiogram demonstrating a left frontal meningioma. This left lateral view shows the extreme vascularity of the tumour and its penumbra (same patient as **11.25**).

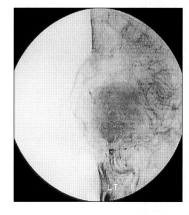

11.32 Digital subtraction angiogram of the meningioma shown in 11.25 and 11.31. This clearly demonstrates the vascularity of the tumour and its penumbra, and the encroachment of the tumour across the midline, with pressure on the right cerebral cortex.

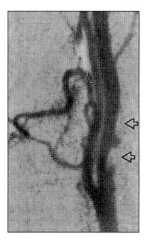

11.33 Digital subtraction angiography of the right carotid arteries. This view shows an extensive atheromatous plaque that has ulcerated in its centre and was the source of emboli in a patient with transient ischaemic attacks (TIAs).

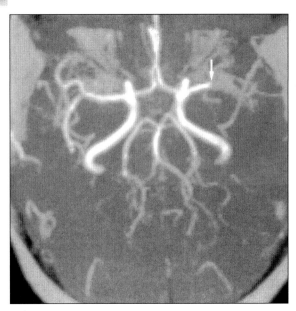

11.34   Magnetic resonance angiography (MRA), demonstrating occlusion of the left middle cerebral artery **(arrow)** non-invasively. The patient presented with a right-sided stroke, and CT suggested a thromboembolic origin.

- headache on rising in morning suggests intracranial space-occupying lesion (*see* **pp. 467, 468**).
- headache after recent head trauma suggests subdural haematoma (**p. 478**).

The most common headaches are tension headaches and migraine. These can usually be distinguished from other causes on the clinical history alone.

TENSION-TYPE HEADACHE

Tension-type headache is usually a dull, nagging pain in the frontal, occipital or temporal regions, around the head 'like a band', or pressing on the vertex. There may be tender spots in the scalp and also a throbbing sensation behind the eyes. The headaches may persist for hours, days or weeks, and are often worse at the end of the day. Many, but not all, sufferers recognize a relationship to stress. Tension-type headaches are rarely caused by visual refractive errors or hypertension, but these possibilities should be excluded. Tension-type headaches are benign in nature and respond to reassurance, avoidance of stress and simple analgesics; beta blockers may also help if there is a vascular component and some patients respond to antidepressant therapy.

MIGRAINE

Migraine is an episodic, severe headache that usually lasts between 4–72 hours. It affects 8–12% of the population and 75% of sufferers are female. It can occur at any age but is commonest in children and young adults.

There are two broad categories. The commonest is *migraine without aura (common migraine)* which should have at least two of the following features:

- pulsating pain
- unilateral
- severe intensity
- worse on activity
- nausea and/or vomiting
- photophobia or phonophobia

Patients often prefer to retire to a darkened room and sleep. Some patients describe a change in mood and appetite, and fluid retention, for a day or two before the migraine.

The second category is *migraine with aura (classic migraine)* in which the headache phase is preceded by gradually developing then receding neurological symptoms usually for 10–30 minutes. The commonest symptoms are visual disturbances such as flashing lights, zigzag lines, colours and scotomas. Other variants are hemisensory symptoms, dysphasia, hemiparesis or perceptual changes. If the aura affects the brainstem there may be vertigo, diplopia, quadriparesis, drowsiness or even coma. An ocular palsy may occasionally persist for a few days. Rarely there is a stroke, but usually only when other risk factors for stroke are also present.

There may be a familial predisposition to migraine, and a gene has been identified for familial hemiplegic migraine.

The mechanisms in migraine are poorly understood but involve both neurological and vascular events. Vasoactive peptides are released from the trigeminal nerve producing both pain and vascular changes. There are also demonstrable changes in brain function, associated with the aura, mood change and other premonitory features.

Trigger factors may include cheese, chocolate, red wine, coffee, shellfish, menstruation, minor head trauma and stress (or, paradoxically, relaxation from stress). The relationship to oral contraceptive use is variable: some women have an increase in migraine, others a decrease and some no change.

The first approach to management is to prevent migraine by identifying and eliminating trigger factors, if possible. Acute headaches may be treated with analgesics such as paracetamol or aspirin, sometimes with metoclopramide, and bed rest in a darkened room. Alternative treatments include non-steroidal analgesic drugs, the newer, more specific 5-HT_1-receptor agonists (triptans) or ergotamine. Prophylactic drugs such as pizotifen, propranolol or amitriptyline may be useful for patients with frequent, incapacitating migraines.

OTHER FORMS OF HEADACHE

Migrainous neuralgia (cluster headache)

Migrainous neuralgia occurs mainly in men as an intense, throbbing, unilateral pain, usually retro-orbital but often spreading to the upper face. It occurs in bouts or 'clusters', with one or more episodes daily, often at regular times, including wakening from sleep. Bouts last for days or weeks before clearing for weeks, months or years. There may be associated lacrimation, rhinorrhoea, and a transient Horner's syndrome, but nausea is not a feature. Acute attacks may be prevented by ergotamine, or controlled by injections of sumatriptan, or by oxygen inhalation.

Temporal arteritis

Temporal or cranial arteritis usually occurs in older patients with throbbing or persistent headache and tenderness in the temporal region (**3.98**), or more rarely in the occipital regions or the jaw on chewing. Urgent diagnosis and treatment are essential (*see* **p. 128**).

Atypical facial pain

The syndrome of 'atypical facial pain' is a nagging, protracted pain in the maxillary region, usually occurring in middle-aged depressed women. The pattern of pain does not usually conform to an anatomical distribution and there should be no abnormal signs. It may respond to amitriptyline.

Headache of increased intracranial pressure

Increased intracranial pressure (*see* **p. 467**) is suggested by early morning headache, usually in the occipital region, with exacerbation on coughing or bending. Nausea, vomiting and brief visual disturbance, often on bending, may occur. There are often additional neurological features such as papilloedema, confusion and localizing neurological signs. Sixth cranial palsy may occur as a false localizing sign.

Meningeal pain

Subarachnoid haemorrhage produces sudden severe headache and neck stiffness, usually with focal signs or coma, or both (*see* **p. 477**). Meningitis also produces headache and neck stiffness together with nausea, vomiting and photophobia (*see* **p. 471**).

Cervical spondylosis

Cervical spondylosis may cause headaches referred to the occipital region or anteriorly, which are often worse with head movement (*see* **p. 132**).

Miscellaneous other headaches

Trigeminal neuralgia causes severe, paroxysmal facial and head pain (*see* **p. 453**). Headaches may occur with cough (cough headache), and in the masticatory syndrome (Costen syndrome), in which there is pain in the maxillary regions and exacerbation with chewing. In patients with severe headache, orbital pain and visual failure, the possibility of acute glaucoma must also be considered. Exertional headaches are usually benign but occasionally foramen magnum anatomical abnormalities, vascular lesions or intermittent obstructive hydrocephalus may be responsible.

CHRONIC FATIGUE SYNDROMES

Chronic fatigue (CF) syndromes form an ill-defined group of problems that risks becoming a 'catch-all' diagnosis for many undefined disorders. The term myalgic encephalomyelitis (ME), previously applied to many of these patients, is inaccurate and should not be used. Fatigue after a whole range of illnesses is well recognized and is usually self-limiting and not recurrent. However, after some viral and bacterial illnesses it may be prolonged and recurrent.

It is important that CF should only be diagnosed after strenuous efforts have been made to exclude other recognized and treatable diseases.

CF affects all ages and all social classes and often affects people who have been extremely conscientious and highly motivated. There is usually both a physical and psychosocial element to the illness. The presenting symptoms are all nonspecific, for example mental and physical fatigue, great variation in symptoms day by day, fatigue that is worse after stress or exercise and emotional lability. There may occasionally be physical signs such as low grade fever, lymphadenopathy (cervical), recurrent tonsillitis, muscle tenderness and generalized weakness.

Extensive investigations may be required to exclude other diseases and these should include a search for evidence of recent viral infection. No diagnostic tests for CF are available.

There is no recognized treatment. Patients often require continuing psychosocial counselling. Cognitive behavioural therapy and antidepressants have been found helpful in selected patients. Complementary medical techniques are often advocated, but there is no scientific evidence of benefit.

DEMENTIA

Dementia is an acquired impairment of multiple cognitive capacities such as intellect, behaviour and personality. In the UK about 5% of people aged 65 years and over have some form of dementia and by age 85 years 20% are affected. The diagnosis requires careful assessment of short-term and long-term memory, language, calculation, behaviour, mood, and personality. A relative's history of the patient's decline is often the key to the diagnosis. Dementia differs from acute confusional states that have toxic, metabolic or infective causes. Causes of dementia include vascular, traumatic, degenerative, infectious, demyelinating, inflammatory, neoplastic, metabolic and toxic disorders.

Alzheimer's disease is the most common cause (50% of cases) of slowly progressive dementia over several years. The mental symptoms and signs precede the physical signs by several months to years. Nearly all patients are over 60 years of age, and it is estimated that 5–10% of people over 65 are affected. Pathologically, there are characteristic senile plaques, neurofibrillary tangles and amyloid angiopathy. In addition to ageing, other risk factors include a family history of the disease, head injury, low educational achievement and Down's syndrome.

The most common presentation is with a loss of recent memory, often associated with a personality change, apathy and antisocial behaviour followed by focal signs such as dysphasia, dyslexia, dyspraxia, agnosia and later loss of sphincter control. Sleep disturbance is common. Disturbance of gait reduces mobility, but in the later stages patients are inclined to wander, especially at night, and may injure themselves by falling. The end result is that patients become bed-bound and incontinent.

In addition to Alzheimer's disease, a wide range of other conditions may cause dementia (**11.35**). Some are treatable, so investigation is important in younger patients with dementia. Tests may include CT scanning (**11.36**), MRI or SPECT scanning (**11.37**), and may also involve full blood count (including serum B_{12} and folate), renal, liver and thyroid function tests, blood sugar and calcium. Serology for syphilis and HIV, chest and skull X-rays, EEG, CSF examination and heavy metal screening may be appropriate in selected cases.

Multi-infarct dementia can be difficult to distinguish clinically from Alzheimer's disease. The cause is occlusion of vessels supplying the cerebral cortex and subcortex. The clinical presentation is with features of cortical dysfunction. Sudden deteriorations in neurological status are common in this form of disorder in which there are multiple small infarcts in the brain, best shown on a CT scan (**11.38**). Clinical examination usually demonstrates physical signs that correspond to the lesions.

Dementia with Lewy bodies has been recently recognized. Features include fluctuating cognition, recurrent visual hallucinations and motor features of parkinsonism. Tremor is less common. Patients with Lewy body dementia may be very sensitive to the effects of neuroleptic medication.

Subdural haematoma may produce gradually increasing mental impairment over several weeks or months (*see* **p. 478**).

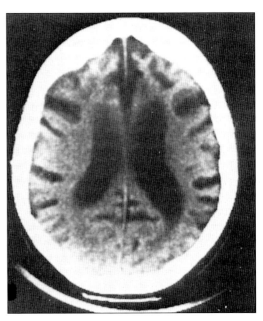

11.36 CT scan in Alzheimer's disease at ventricular body level. Note the marked dilatation of the sulci and fissures, especially frontally, the poor visual distinction between grey matter and white matter, the ventricular enlargement – greater on the patient's left (right of picture) – and the general reduction in brain size. The picture is not diagnostic of Alzheimer's disease: similar abnormalities occur in Huntington's disease and Niemann–Pick's disease.

CAUSES OF DEMENTIA

Unknown	Alzheimer's disease Dementia with Lewy bodies Multiple sclerosis Parkinson's disease
Vascular	Multiple cerebral infarcts Diffuse small vessel disease
Metabolic	Uraemia Liver failure Hypothyroidism Vitamin B_{12} deficiency Other vitamin B deficiency Hypoparathyroidism Hypoglycaemia
Physical	Space-occupying lesions (tumour, haematoma) Post-head injury, especially in subdural haematoma
Genetic	Huntington's chorea Down's syndrome
Infections	HIV infection Progressive multifocal leucoencephalopathy (PML) Tuberculosis Toxoplasmosis Syphilis Creutzfeldt–Jakob disease
Toxic	Poisoning with mercury, manganese, carbon monoxide, alcohol, copper
Other	Pseudo-dementia (depression)

11.35 Causes of dementia.

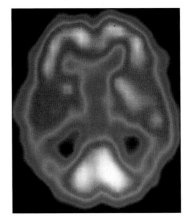

11.37 Single photon emission computed tomography (SPECT scan) in Alzheimer's disease. There is a marked symmetrical reduction in perfusion to both post-temporoparietal areas.

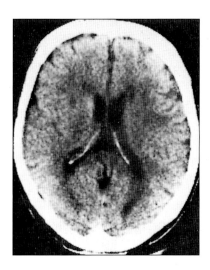

11.38 CT scan in multi-infarct dementia (cut at same level as that seen in **11.36**). The ventricles are normal in size, but there are patchy radiolucencies throughout the white matter. These indicate the presence of demyelinated patches, which result from multiple small infarcts in the brain.

The initiating head injury may have been slight and unrecognized. It is treated by surgical decompression.

In normal-pressure hydrocephalus there is dementia with gait and bladder disorder caused by marked ventricular dilatation. Meningitis, cerebral haemorrhage and trauma are predisposing factors, but it may occur without this history. The surgical creation of a shunt from ventricle to peritoneum may arrest the process.

Alcoholism is a common cause of behavioural change and dementia, and is often complicated by B-group vitamin deficiencies, especially of thiamine. Vitamin B_{12} deficiency can produce severe mental impairment, and hypothyroidism can also cause a marked slowing of mental function.

Dementia resulting from HIV infection is now increasingly common (*see* **p. 5**); whereas general paralysis of the insane from neurosyphilis (*see* **p. 61**) is very rare. Creutzfeldt–Jakob disease (CJD and vCJD) is a rare but rapidly progressive dementia now shown to be transmissible from infected human nervous tissue and thought to be caused by prions (*see* **p. 58**).

In severe brain damage from encephalitis, abscess, tumour, cerebral infarction (**11.39**), head injury, severe ischaemia or hypoglycaemia, the cause is usually clear.

Huntington's chorea is a dominantly transmitted condition that is associated with progressive dementia and chorea. The worldwide prevalence is between 1 in 10 000 and 1 in 20 000. The mutation is on the short arm of chromosome 4. The onset of symptoms is usually gradual in the middle years of life. There is usually a family history and, because of knowledge of the outcome, there is a high incidence of depression. The course is progressively downhill over a few years with increasing chorea and dementia. The diagnosis is made on clinical grounds and on the family history and DNA testing now allows presymptomatic diagnosis. Genetic counselling and appropriate support are essential.

Management of dementia involves:

- treating the disorder that is causing the cognitive problem (if possible)
- controlling the symptom or behaviour pattern
- controlling the resultant disability
- providing help for the carers at a social, nursing and medical level; this includes especially home care, day care and long-term residential care.

Recently some anticholinesterase inhibitors, such as donepezil and rivastigmine have been introduced. These may give a transient benefit in some patients with mild to moderate dementia.

EPILEPSY

Epileptic seizures are manifestations of abnormal synchronous activity in populations of neurons in the brain. The liability to recurrent seizures constitutes epilepsy. Many potential mechanisms may contribute to seizures. Some epilepsies are genetically determined, including many of those seen in childhood. Other causes include metabolic abnormalities (e.g. hypoglycaemia), drugs (e.g. alcohol withdrawal) and structural brain disease such as tumour, encephalitis, infarction or head-injury. In many patients there is a combination of mechanisms.

Seizures may be broadly classified as:

- **Partial seizures,** arising focally and giving clinical features that reflect the site of origin. They are labelled 'simple' where there is no loss of consciousness (e.g. discharges in the motor cortex leading to localized twitching, in the sensory cortex leading to focal sensory symptoms, and in the occipital region to visual symptoms). The commonest seizures arise in the temporal and frontal lobes. Patients may describe hallucinations of smell or taste, epigastric sensations, déja vu, jamais vu. Partial seizures are labelled 'complex' when the

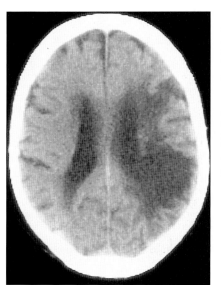

11.39 CT scan in a patient with dementia and cerebral infarction. The low-density area in the left parietal region represents a large cerebral infarct with subsequent cortical atrophy. Ventricular dilatation is also seen.

patient becomes unaware; these may be accompanied by complex behaviour called automatism, e.g. lip-smacking, fumbling, muttering or walking. Sometimes partial seizures spread to become secondarily generalised convulsions.

- **Generalized seizures,** which may be generalized convulsions, sometimes with tongue-biting (**11.40**) and/or incontinence (tonic-clonic); brief loss of awareness (petit mal); brief jerkings (myoclonus); or sudden falls (akinetic or drop attacks) (**11.41**).

- **Unclassified** when there is not enough evidence to specify the type.

Epilepsy can start at any age but the highest incidence is in the young and the elderly. About 1 in 200 persons has active epilepsy.

Making an accurate diagnosis is vital for decisions on investigation and management. The history from the patient and/or from witnesses is central to the diagnosis. The main differential diagnoses are shown in **11.42**. Differentiating these from seizures requires descriptions of the circumstances of the episodes, and of the sequence of events before, during and after the event(s). It also requires knowledge of the background medical, neurological and psychiatric history.

Investigations may include EEG (**11.43**, **11.44**) where there is diagnostic uncertainty, but a normal EEG does not exclude

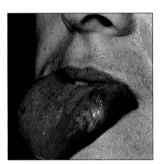

11.40 The bitten tongue as a sign of epilepsy. Damage to the tongue is a common complication of generalized seizures and may be helpful evidence where there is doubt about the diagnosis. During epileptic attacks the patient should be protected from harm if possible; but forcible attempts to open the mouth or restrain the patient often do more harm than good.

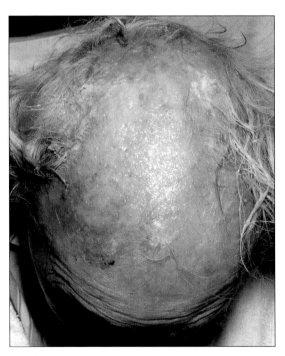

11.41 Serious injury may occur during generalized seizures in epilepsy. This patient has a large full-thickness burn, sustained when he fell in a fire during a fit.

THE DIFFERENTIAL DIAGNOSIS OF SEIZURES

Commonest

Epilepsy

Syncope (including convulsive syncope)

Non-epileptic attacks (previously known as pseudoseizures)

Cardiac arrhythmias

Less common

Hypoglycaemia

Parasomnias (sleep paralysis, sleepwalking)

Transient ischaemic attacks

Migraine

Cataplexy or narcolepsy

11.42 Differential diagnosis of seizures.

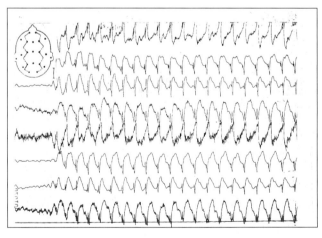

11.43 EEG in a patient with generalized seizures. This shows the typical spike and wave discharge of epilepsy. If the EEG is taken during an attack, this appearance may be diagnostic of epilepsy, but gives no indication of the cause; if spike and wave activity is observed between attacks, the appearance does not prove that an episode was epileptic, but the findings support the diagnosis. Ambulatory monitoring of the EEG provides a much more valuable assessment of the relationship of EEG abnormalities to symptoms.

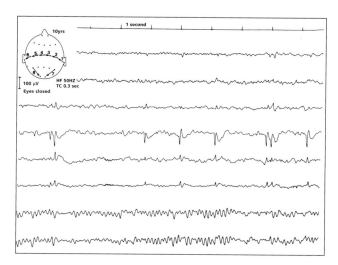

11.44 EEG in a patient with partial seizures. Focal sharp waves are seen in the left temporoparietal region.

epilepsy. Imaging the brain is important, particularly with partial seizures. MRI is the investigation of choice because it shows structural lesions much more clearly than CT, including mesial temporal damage (hippocampal sclerosis) (**11.45**) and developmental disorders. CT is also useful, however, particularly in older patients where major brain lesions such as stroke, or brain tumour may be shown.

Treatment with anti-epileptic drugs is required in all patients except those with seizures that can be avoided (e.g. photogenic or alcohol withdrawal seizures), or where the seizures are very slight or infrequent and the patient declines

medication. There is debate on whether to start after one untriggered tonic-clonic seizure or to withhold treatment unless there is another. The commonest drug for partial seizures is carbamazepine although phenytoin and sodium valproate are alternatives. Sodium valproate is the treatment of choice for generalized seizures with lamotrigine an increasing contender. A number of newer anti-epileptic drugs (gabapentin, levetiracetam, tiagabine, topiramate) are second choice for the 20–40% who fail on the initial treatment.

All patients should have a full discussion about their epilepsy, tailored to their needs, but including the cause of their epilepsy, the possible prognosis, first aid for seizures and the treatment choices. Further topics may include the impact on driving, work and leisure, and coping with stigma. There are other important issues for women: the use of oral contraceptives, the teratogenic effects of anti-epileptic drugs, genetic risks of epilepsy and coping with epilepsy in pregnancy.

Withdrawal of anti-epileptic drugs may be considered after 2 years free of seizures but the decision should be carefully discussed, weighing up the risks of recurrence and the impact of having further seizures after withdrawal on work, driving and social life.

A small proportion of patients with refractory partial seizures may be offered surgery. The best results are for temporal lobe epilepsy (**11.45**). Resection of the anterior part of the temporal lobe abolishes seizures in about 60% and markedly reduces them in another 20-25% of patients.

COMA

Coma is defined as a state of unrousable unresponsiveness (**1.143**, **11.46**), and for practical clinical purposes this may be refined into a spectrum of symptoms and signs by use of a coma scale such as the Glasgow Coma Scale (**11.47**).

Coma has many possible causes (**11.48**), and the management of patients in coma always involves the investigation of underlying cause together with appropriate supportive and specific treatment. Immediate maintenance of airway patency is essential (**11.46**) and further treatment is dependent on the underlying cause and duration of the coma.

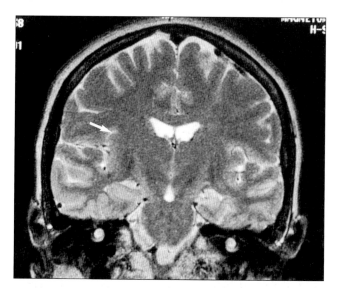

11.45 Hippocampal atrophy in a patient with refractory temporal lobe epilepsy, demonstrated by MRI in this coronal section (arrow). Anterior temporal lobectomy abolished the patient's seizures.

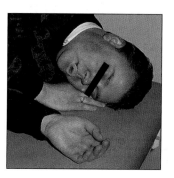

11.46 The correct position for the unconscious patient. The patient should be placed in the semiprone position, and a simple airway should be placed in the mouth. Exactly the same management should be applied to any unconscious patient who does not require cardiac or respiratory support.

							Date	
							Time	

OBSERVATION CHART (COMA)

Ward/Clinic/.. Cons. ....
Hosp .... D D M M Y Y .... C.H.I No.
Surname ....
First name .... M. state
Address .... Sex

COMA SCALE

Eyes open — Spontaneously / To speech / To pain / None — Eyes closed by swelling = C

Best verbal response — Oriented / Confused / Inappropriate words / Incomprehensible sounds / None — Endotracheal tube or tracheostomy = T

Best motor response — Obey commands / Localise pain / Flexion to pain / Extension to pain / None — Usually record the best arm response

Pupil scale (mm): 1, 2, 3, 4, 5, 6, 7, 8

Blood pressure and pulse rate — 240 230 220 210 200 190 180 170 160 150 140 130 120 110 100 90 80 70 60 50 40

Temperature °C — 40 39 38 37 36 35 34 33 32 31 30

RESPIRATION — Rate/min — Regular/irregular

PUPILS — + reacts / – no reaction / c eye closed — right — Size Reaction / left — Size Reaction

PATTERN OF LIMB MOVEMENTS — Score 1 – 5 as below — right — Arm Leg / left — Arm Leg

1, 2, 3 record differences in strength between limbs with movements better than types 4 and 5
1 – normal strength 2 – weakness When L and R limbs are both weak but to different degrees, then
3 – weakest side 4 – spastic/abnormal flexion 5 – extension

11.47 Glasgow Coma Scale. This widely used scoring system can be employed to monitor progression of coma and to predict outcome in some cases. Points are allocated for cortical and brainstem functions, including eyes open, best verbal response, best motor response. To these may be added pupil size, blood pressure, pulse, temperature, respiration, pupillary reaction to light and patterns of limb movement.

CAUSES OF COMA RANKED IN APPROXIMATE ORDER OF INCIDENCE

Head injury

Drug overdose
Attempted suicide or parasuicide
Drug misuse
Alcohol misuse
Therapeutic error

Diabetes mellitus
Hypoglycaemia (common)
Hyperglycaemia (rare)

Stroke or transient ischaemic attack

Epileptic seizure

Infection
Meningitis
Encephalitis
Cerebral malaria
African trypanosomiasis
Other

Metabolic
Renal, hepatic or respiratory failure, myxoedema, chemical toxins, non-diabetic hypoglycaemia

Cardiorespiratory arrest

Psychiatric causes

11.48 Causes of coma ranked in approximate order of incidence.

RAISED INTRACRANIAL PRESSURE

A rise in the pressure of CSF above 250 mm is usually a reflection of serious neurological disease, caused by a space-occupying lesion, obstruction to the outflow of CSF, obstruction of the venous return or intracranial infection.

It is possible to measure CSF pressure by lumbar puncture, but this is potentially hazardous and may not accurately reflect pressure in the brain, for example if there is obstruction by spinal tumours or herniation of brain through the foramen magnum.

A rise in intracranial pressure is usually associated with headache, especially in the morning, nausea, vomiting and loss of vision and balance. There may be false localizing signs, for example sixth nerve palsies. The most reliable sign is the appearance of papilloedema (**11.49**, **11.50**), but only 50% of adults with space-occupying lesions show disc swelling.

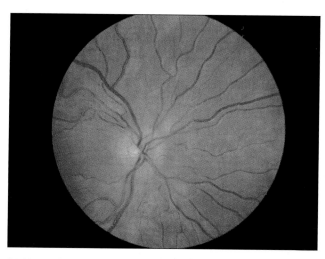

11.49 Early papilloedema in a patient with a cerebral tumour. There is hyperaemia of the optic disc, with blurring of the inferonasal margin.

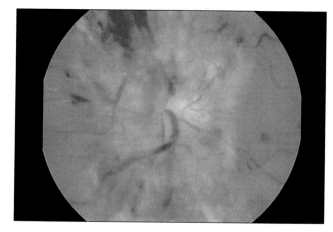

11.50 Chronic papilloedema in the right eye of a middle-aged woman with benign intracranial hypertension. The disc margins are completely blurred, and there are widespread haemorrhages and ischaemic areas in the retina. The appearance of chronic papilloedema should be compared with the less-marked changes seen in early papilloedema (**7.10**).

Urgent action to reduce pressure is needed in patients with impending herniation of brain through the foramen magnum. This should usually include high doses of dexamethasone and intravenous mannitol. The airway must be maintained and hyperventilation to reduce the $PaCO_2$ may be of transient value. After stabilization, imaging procedures should be used to establish the underlying diagnosis, which should be treated appropriately.

Benign intracranial hypertension (pseudotumour cerebri) is usually an unexplained disorder, most commonly occurring in overweight young women. There are other causes including drugs and the oral contraceptive pill. It is always important to exclude a cerebral venous thrombosis. Patients may present with a headache, visual upset and papilloedema. The process

may not be benign as patients can lose vision and go blind with eventual optic atrophy. The diagnosis is by exclusion of a mass lesion or sinus thrombosis by MRI or CT. The raised pressure is confirmed by lumbar puncture: the CSF should be normal. Treatment includes weight reduction, diuretics and occasionally a shunt or optic nerve decompression.

HYDROCEPHALUS

Hydrocephalus is the enlargement of the cerebral ventricles that is associated with the accumulation of CSF. This may result from a variety of causes including:

Communicating hydrocephalus
* excess production of CSF – choroid plexus papilloma
* impaired CSF absorption – in meningitis
* cerebral dysgenesis or atrophy.

Noncommunicating hydrocephalus
* obstruction to the flow of CSF – intracerebral tumours, aqueduct or foramen stenosis, by blood in subarachnoid haemorrhage.

The clinical features depend on whether the disease process is acute or chronic and whether the process produces complete or partial obstruction. The acute presentation is usually accompanied by severe headache, nausea and vomiting. There are usually no localizing symptoms or signs, but there is papilloedema (**11.49. 11.50**) and there may be a sixth nerve lesion. Neurological signs usually suggest a bilateral upper motor neuron disorder (i.e. bilateral extensor plantar signs and brisk reflexes). There is progressive impairment of higher cerebral functions with loss of memory, impairment of mobility and loss of sphincter control.

CT and MRI show the abnormality of the ventricles (**11.51**) and may suggest the site of the block (**11.122**).

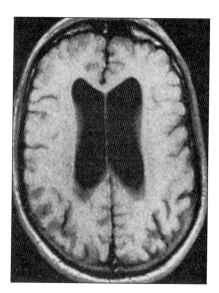

11.51 Hydrocephalus in a 69-year-old man. This axial MRI at the level of the ventricular bodies shows severe ventricular enlargement, but the sulci of the brain are normal.

Lumbar puncture may be of little value as the pressure is often normal.

If the primary lesion is not amenable to treatment, drainage of the affected ventricles is of value. This involves the surgical creation of a shunt with a valve that allows the one-way drainage of CSF from the ventricles to the peritoneal cavity.

INFANTILE HYDROCEPHALUS

A variety of congenital abnormalities may lead to hydrocephalus which may be present before birth (and hence produce difficulties at birth) or develop during childhood or adult life.

Progressive enlargement of the head is usually obvious, with failure of closure of the fontanelles (**1.141**, **11.52**). Milestones of development are delayed and the end result may be mental retardation complicated by epilepsy and motor impairment. CT (**11.53**) or MRI may show the abnormality and sometimes the

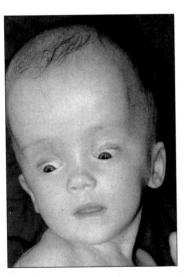

11.52 Infantile hydrocephalus. The head is obviously enlarged and prominent subcutaneous scalp veins are visible. In neglected cases the eyes are displaced downwards (the 'setting sun' sign) so that the upper sclerae are visible. The cranial sutures are widely splayed. This appearance may result from 'internal' (obstructive) or 'external' (communicating) hydrocephalus.

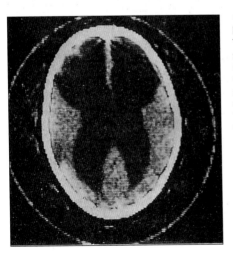

11.53 Severe hydrocephalus. This CT scan shows gross dilatation of the ventricular system and compression of the remaining cortical tissue.

cause, and the early implantation of a shunt may arrest the physical and mental deterioration that would otherwise occur.

INTRACRANIAL TUMOURS

Intracranial tumours can arise from any cell type within the cranial vault. Those that arise from within the brain are called 'intrinsic' brain tumours and those that arise from the skull base, vault or meninges are called 'extrinsic' brain tumours. This is an important distinction as extrinsic brain tumours manifest by exerting pressure on the nearby brain and their main treatment is surgical excision with a good chance of full recovery.

The incidence of primary intrinsic brain tumours is 9.5 cases per 100 000 population and recent data suggests that this incidence is rising. In children, brain tumours represent 20% of all childhood malignancies and are the number two cause of cancer death in this age group.

Primary intrinsic brain tumours are slightly commoner in males and more than two-thirds are high grade. Less than 5% of glioma patients have a family history. Known risk factors include: tuberous sclerosis, neurofibromatosis type I, previous cranial irradiation, severe head trauma, chronic exposure to petrochemicals and employment in the aerospace industry.

The most common primary intrinsic brain tumours are gliomas, which account for 60% of all brain tumours, meningiomas (20%), pituitary adenomas (10%), acoustic neuromas (8%) and other tumour types (each about 1–2%). Secondary tumours in the brain are up to eight times more common than primary tumours.

The usual clinical presentations include:

- headache, vomiting and papilloedema (**11.49**, **11.50**), i.e symptoms and signs of raised intracranial pressure
- epileptiform seizures
- pressure effects on adjacent structures, which produce focal neurological defects
- endocrine changes in some pituitary lesions.

These symptoms are also found with other space-occupying lesions, such as intracerebral haematomas, abscesses and subdural haematomas.

CT and MRI are the preferred methods of investigation, and MRI usually provides better information when tumours are in the posterior fossa or at the base of the skull. Radionuclide imaging and SPECT (**11.30**), where available, may also add diagnostic information on occasions. Biopsy for histology is an essential prelude to treatment. Lumbar puncture should be avoided because of the risk of 'coning' (*see* **p. 456**).

GLIOMA

Gliomas arise from neuroglial cells – usually in the cerebral hemispheres and rarely in the cerebellum. The most common type is the astrocytoma, which originates in astrocytes and has a range of degrees of malignancy: grade I has a long survival (up to 25 years) and grade IV has a survival of only several months (this rapidly invasive tumour is also known as glioblastoma multiforme). Such tumours rarely metastasize beyond the brain, tending to invade locally in one hemisphere or, less commonly, across the corpus callosum ('butterfly glioma'). In children, the most common sites are the hypothalamus, optic nerve and cerebellum (where they may be cystic and benign). Diagnosis of the space-occupying lesion is by CT (**11.54**) or MRI (**11.55**), followed by stereotactic biopsy. Solitary low-grade malignant lesions may be amenable to surgery and the more malignant lesions may respond to radiotherapy.

Oligodendrogliomas arise from oligodendroglia and grow extremely slowly (5-year survival 30–50%). They may sometimes be recognized on a straight skull X-ray by the presence of calcium.

Ependymomas arise from the lining cells of the lateral and fourth ventricles. They tend to occur in the young and are associated with a short survival. They disseminate locally and via the CSF. They may occasionally respond to radiotherapy.

MENINGIOMA

Meningiomas are slowly growing benign tumours that arise from the arachnoid and produce symptoms by compression of adjacent structures. They may arise at any site, even in the spinal canal, but most commonly over the hemispheres. Women over 40 years of age are most commonly affected, and because the tumours are slow growing they may reach a large size before patients present with partial seizures, features of raised intracranial pressure or localized neurological deficits. The tumours have a rich blood supply, may erode bone locally and may calcify. The diagnosis is usually suggested by CT (**11.25**) or MRI (**11.26, 11.27, 11.56, 11.120**) and occasionally localized calcification is seen on the plain X-ray of the skull. Surgery may be curative with early lesions, but local erosion of other structures may make resection extremely difficult, for example sphenoidal ridge tumours may envelop the carotid artery and other parapituitary structures. If incompletely removed, meningiomas tend to regrow. Malignant change is rare. If situated in the spinal canal, they are most likely to occur

469

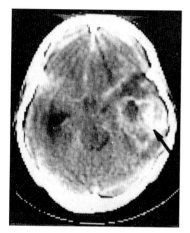

11.54 Glioma involving most of the left parietal lobe – seen to the right on this axial CT scan (arrow). The appearance is of a cystic tumour, but biopsy and histological confirmation are necessary to be certain of its nature.

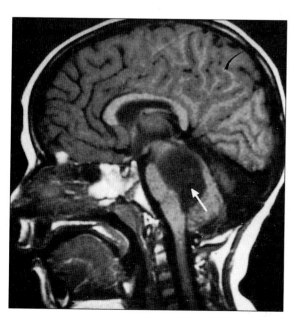

11.55 Cystic glioblastoma of the brainstem (arrowed), clearly demonstrated by MRI. The sagittal section shows that the tumour involves the posterior part of the brainstem and extends into the cerebellum.

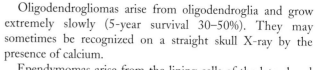
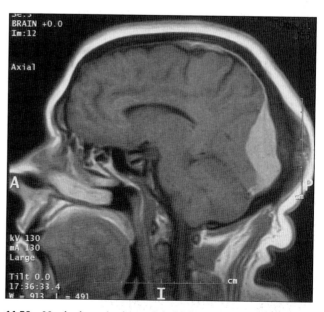

11.56 Meningioma in the occipital lobe, as revealed on gadolinium-enhanced MRI. The patient presented with a contralateral homonymous hemianopia. Note also the reactive hyperostosis of the skull in the region of the meningioma.

in the thoracic region where they manifest themselves with the gradual onset of paraparesis; surgery carries a good prognosis because of the earlier presentation.

PITUITARY TUMOURS

Pituitary tumours are classified into non-functioning (25%) and functioning adenomas. The functioning group (*see* **p. 294**) encompasses prolactinoma (40%), growth hormone secreting adenoma (20%) and ACTH secreting adenoma (15%). Hypersecretion may lead to Cushing's disease (ACTH), acromegaly (GH) or galactorrhoea and amenorrhoea (prolactin). These tumours may also present with symptoms and signs of pressure or invasion of the surrounding structures. Bitemporal hemianopia (**11.5**) occurs as a result of pressure on the optic chiasma (**7.4–7.7**); oculomotor palsy and opthalmoplegia may occur due to invasion of the cavernous sinus; and epilepsy rarely occurs due to invasion of the temporal lobe. Rarely, pituitary adenomas present with sudden onset of headache or collapse (pituitary apoplexy, *see* **p. 296**).

The adenoma appears on skull X-ray (**7.4**) and MRI (**7.5–7.7**, **2.26**) as a mass arising from the sella turcica and the sella may be enlarged and eroded (**7.4**, **7.6**). The tumour may extend into the suprasellar region (**7.5–7.7**).

The differential diagnosis is suprasellar meningioma, metastases, craniopharyngioma and chordoma. Surgical treatment is indicated to relieve chiasmatic pressure, for Cushing's syndrome, acromegaly and failed medical treatment in prolactinoma. Medical treatment is indicated in prolactinoma (*see* **p. 298**) and is used to supplement surgery to control the symptoms of Cushing's syndrome (*see* **p. 299**) and acromegaly (*see* **p. 297**). Adjuvant radiotherapy is also used in the treatment of pituitary tumours.

NEUROMA

Neuromas are benign tumours that arise from the Schwann cells of the cranial nerves and spinal roots. The most common intracranial site is on the acoustic nerve at the cerebellopontine angle. (*see* **p. 454**).

METASTASES

Metastases account for about one-quarter of all cerebral tumours and most frequently arise from lung, breast, kidney, colon, skin and reticulosis. Metastatic lesions may develop in any part of the brain, including the cerebellum. Many lesions are found by chance at autopsy and they tend to be multiple. The diagnosis may be suggested by the development of neurological deficits in patients who have a known malignancy. The clinical course is variable: many patients present with slowly progressive symptoms, whereas in others an acute

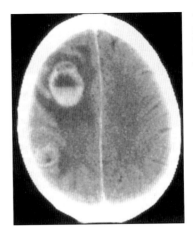

11.57 Multiple cerebral metastases in a patient with carcinoma of the bronchus, demonstrated on CT scan. 'Cuts' at other levels in the brain demonstrated further lesions.

presentation may result from haemorrhage within the mass. Diagnosis is most easily made by CT (**4.165**, **11.57**) or MRI. Solitary lesions may be amenable to surgical removal with occasional good long-term results. Corticosteroids are of interim value in reducing oedema and temporarily improving clinical status to allow chemotherapy or radiotherapy to be of value.

INFECTIONS OF THE NERVOUS SYSTEM

Many infections involve the CNS. Meningitis, encephalitis and cerebral abscess are considered here, and many other infections that may involve the CNS are reviewed in Chapter 1. CNS infections are a major problem in immunocompromised patients, including those with AIDS. The Guillain–Barré syndrome (*see* **p. 488**) is probably of infective origin, and infection may prove to have a causative role in some patients with dementia and other degenerative diseases of the nervous system.

MENINGITIS

Meningitis is defined as inflammation of the pia and arachnoid mater and is usually caused by bacteria (*see also* **p. 27** and **38**) or viruses (**11.58**); it may also be caused by fungi, malignant infiltration, blood (subarachnoid haemorrhage) or chemicals (drugs or contrast medium).

Viruses are the most common cause of meningitis. They produce a lymphocytic reaction in the CSF and there may be associated encephalitis. Bacteria are the second most common cause of acute meningitis and they usually provoke a polymorphonuclear leucocytosis in the CSF. A chronic reaction is found in tuberculosis. Fungal infection is uncommon, except in immunocompromised patients (e.g. those with HIV), and it may run a chronic or subacute course.

The clinical presentation may be with acute or gradual onset of fever, vomiting, headache, lethargy, impaired consciousness

INFECTIVE CAUSES OF MENINGITIS

Bacteria

Streptococcus pneumoniae

Neisseria meningitidis

Haemophilus influenzae

Streptococci

Staphylococci

Listeria monocytogenes

Gram-negative bacilli

Leptospirosis

Mycobacterium tuberculosis

Viruses

Echo

Coxsackie

Epstein–Barr

Poliomyelitis

Mumps

Herpes simplex

Fungi

Cryptococcus

Histoplasma

Coccidoides

Blastomyces

11.58   Infective causes of meningitis.

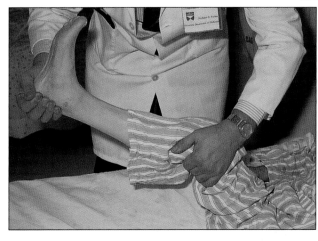

11.59   Kernig's sign. The hip is flexed to 90° degrees with the knee bent; pain is felt on attempting to straighten the patient's leg. A positive response suggests menigeal irritation.

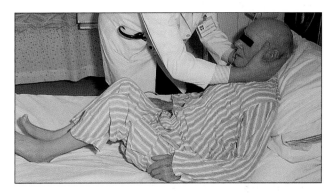

11.60   Brudzinski's sign. Flexion of the neck causes the legs to be drawn up. A positive response suggests meningeal irritation.

or seizures; signs include a stiff neck, focal signs such as cranial nerve abnormalities (third, fourth, sixth and seventh), hemiparesis, dysphasia, visual field defects and papilloedema. A rash may be present in viral and meningococcal infections. A non-blanching rash is an important clinical sign in meningococcal disease (**1.90**, **1.91**), but often only a few petechiae are seen so examination of the whole skin surface is important. Two important clinical signs of meningitis are dependent on traction of spinal nerves causing pain in the inflamed meninges. These are present in about 50% of cases.

- Kernig's sign (**11.59**)
- Brudzinski's sign (**11.60**).

A search must also be made for associated diseases, for example mastoiditis, pulmonary tuberculosis or malignancy. Laboratory diagnosis depends on lumbar puncture, which may show a rise in CSF pressure and perhaps a turbid fluid that should be sent for microbiology, microscopy and biochemistry. These results (**11.61**) will define the infection. If a space-occupying lesion (e.g. abscess) is suspected, then CT or MRI is essential before undertaking lumbar puncture.

Molecular polymerase chain reaction (PCR) techniques are now available for the raid diagnosis of some infections including meningococcal infection. Acute bacterial meningitis is a life-threatening emergency. Delay in starting treatment increases the mortality and mobidity. Antiobiotics are given intravenously, the type being dictated by the organism found, although empirical treatment will usually have been started before culture results are available (*see* **p. 27** for meningococal meningitis). Intrathecal antibiotic injection is now rarely used.

Viral meningitis is usually a benign, self-limiting condition.

ENCEPHALITIS

Encephalitis is a generalized non-suppurative inflammation of the brain that is usually caused by infection by a virus but is also found in a variety of bacterial infections. Such infections may also involve the spinal cord, cranial nerves and nerve roots. In Europe, encephalitis may follow infection with measles,

CEREBROSPINAL FLUID (CSF) FINDINGS IN MENINGITIS					
	Cells		**Biochemistry**		
	Number (per mm³)	**Type**	**Protein (mg/100 ml)**	**Glucose (mmol/litre)**	**Others**
Normal	0–5	Lymphocytes	15–45	3.3–4.5	
Viral infection	5–500	Lymphocytes	40–90	Normal range	No bacteria on Gram stain
Acute bacterial infection	5–10 000	Polymorphs	Elevated	Reduced	Bacteria present on Gram stain or culture
Tuberculosis	5–1000	Lymphocytes	Markedly elevated (often >100)	Reduced	Fibrin clot forms on standing; AFBs on ZN staining or culture

11.61   Cerebrospinal fluid (CSF) findings in meningitis.

rubella, chickenpox, influenza virus, herpes simplex and HIV. In the Far East and other parts of the world, epidemic viral encephalitis carries a high morbidity and mortality (*see* **p. 14**).

The usual clinical features include fever, nausea and vomiting, headache, impairment of the conscious level (**1.46**), the development of focal neurological signs, meningism and features of raised intracranial pressure. Seizures are common. The disease is often followed by complete recovery after a period of weeks.

The EEG may show diffuse or focal abnormalities. CT or MRI often show abnormalities (**11.62**). Serology may show a changing level of viral antibody. Lumbar puncture may show a rise in CSF pressure with lymphocytosis, elevated protein content and a normal glucose level.

Treatment consists of nursing and supportive care. Aciclovir should be given in all cases of suspected encephalitis because the consequences of untreated herpes simplex encephalopathy in the minority are considerable. In patients who are immunocompromised cytomegalovirus should also be considered and this responds to ganciclovir.

Acute demyelinating encephalomyelitis is an allergic demyelination disease which follows some types of vaccination and may follow measles or chickenpox infection after several weeks. Its presentation is similar to that of encephalitis.

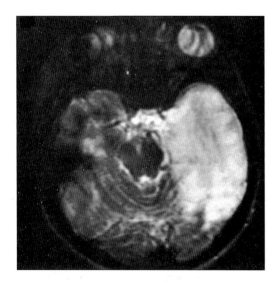

11.62   Herpes simplex encephalitis. This MRI view shows abnormally increased signal in the left temporal lobe (right of picture). MRI and CT appearances in encephalitis vary; often diffuse or scattered abnormalities are seen.

BRAIN ABSCESS

Brain abscess is a localized collection of pus in the brain. The infection may be bloodborne from a distant site, be introduced by a penetrating head injury, or extend from local infections in the head (mastoiditis or sinusitis). Anaerobic bacteria are particularly commonly found in brain abscesses.

The clinical symptoms are those of infection and of the development of a space-occupying lesion in the brain. There is usually fever, headache, nausea, vomiting, clouding of the conscious level, focal signs and fits. There may be signs of a focus of infection, of an increase in intracranial pressure and of papilloedema. Additional focal signs may occur depending on the anatomical site of the abscess.

The white cell count and ESR are usually elevated, but not always so. Blood cultures should always be set up. The lesion can be identified on an enhanced CT (**1.26**, **11.63**. **11.64**) or MRI as a ring-enhancing lesion with surrounding oedema. If there is doubt about the diagnosis, it can be confirmed by stereotactic biopsy. Lumbar puncture may be dangerous.

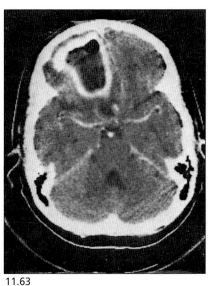

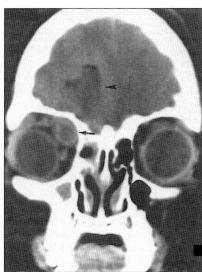

11.63 & 11.64 Cerebral abscess secondary to sinusitis. 11.63 shows an enhanced axial CT scan. A right frontal abscess (left of picture) is seen, and it contains some gas in the anterior region. The coronal CT scan demonstrates the frontal abscess (arrowhead) and also an abscess in the orbit (arrow); both followed infection of the ethmoidal sinuses. Note the soft-tissue density in the ethmoids on this side (below the arrow).

11.63   11.64

473

Treatment is with appropriate antibiotic combinations, corticosteroids to reduce swelling and, in selected patients, neurosurgery, to drain the abscess. If a predisposing cause has been identified, this also requires treatment.

Infections may also localize in the subdural or extradural spaces of both brain and spinal cord. Patients with spinal epidural abscesses present with severe back pain and paraparesis.

CEREBROVASCULAR DISEASE

STROKE

Completed stroke is defined as a focal loss of neurological function of presumed vascular origin, which causes death or lasts for over 24 hours. This timescale differentiates it from a transient ischaemic attack (see below). In addition, some clinicians describe a reversible ischaemic neurological deficit (RIND) in which the neurological deficit lasts more than 24 hours and reverses within 3 weeks. Stroke-in-evolution is a condition in which the symptoms and signs suggest a focal lesion within the distribution of a major artery and this gradually extends over a period of days or weeks to involve an adjacent motor or sensory site.

Around 90% of strokes result from thrombosis or embolism in a major cerebral artery, and 10% result from haemorrhage.

Stroke remains one of the most common causes of death (10–15%) and disability in the developed world with an incidence of 2–5 per 1000. It is especially important because of the high mortality (20–30% in the first month) and the high dependency (60%) of the survivors. Most countries also have an ageing population and it is predicted that the incidence of strokes will rise by up to 40% in the next 10 years.

The clinical presentations of strokes caused by cerebral thrombosis, embolism and haemorrhage are similar. They involve a combination of features that may include hemiparesis, hemianaesthesia, loss of speech if the dominant hemisphere is involved and loss of vision. Lesions affecting the non-dominant hemisphere are more likely to be associated with neglect. The clinical onset is often rapid and reaches a maximum within a few hours. The limbs are flaccid and reflexes are initially absent. The patient may have an impaired conscious level because of cerebral oedema, and there may also be papilloedema. Over the next 24-hour period tone increases, some power may return, the tendon reflexes are exaggerated and the plantar response is extensor.

Lacunar infarcts are small lesions around the basal ganglia, thalamus and pons that result in localized motor or sensory deficits. Brainstem infarcts produce complex neurological syndromes, as they involve the long tracts, the cranial nerve nuclei and cerebellar connections.

The signs of acute stroke are usually obvious, but careful examination is necessary to localize the site of damage and the artery involved. CT scanning is useful in detecting a haemorrhagic lesion in the first 48 hours; however, some infarcts may be missed (**11.65–11.67**). Exclusion of haemorrhage is important if any form of antithrombotic therapy is contemplated. MRI may be used to detect cerebrovascular lesions, particularly those in the posterior fossa (**11.68**), and MR angiography has a developing role in the investigation of stroke (**11.34**).

Immediate examination and investigation should focus on the possibility of a treatable cause of stroke, such as temporal arteritis (see **p. 128**), embolism from the heart (**5.85**, **5.94**) or the large arteries, or, occasionally, a surgically treatable haemorrhage. No specific treatment is available for most patients with stroke, so their immediate management is

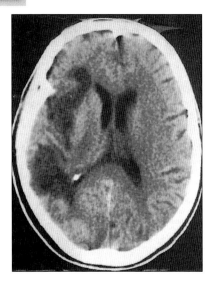

11.65 Extensive right-sided cerebral infarction (left side of picture) demonstrated by unenhanced CT scan, performed 4 days after the onset of stroke. There is no evidence of haemorrhage (cf. **11.66**). High-quality CT scanners usually allow the diagnosis of cerebral infarction within 6–8 hours of onset.

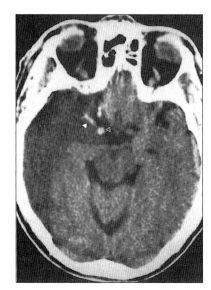

11.67 Cerebral embolism in a patient after cardiac surgery, demonstrated by unenhanced CT scan. The open arrowhead points to a high-density embolus within the distal right internal carotid artery; the filled arrowhead points to a similar embolus in the right middle cerebral artery. There is extensive hypodensity in the right middle cerebral artery distribution, reflecting an extensive area of infarction.

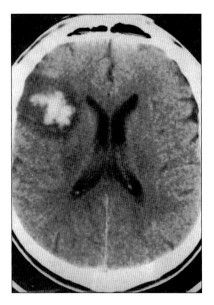

11.66 Haemorrhagic cerebral infarction demonstrated by unenhanced CT scan 1 day after the onset of stroke. Note the high-density haemorrhage within the low density of the oedematous, infarcted region in the right hemisphere. Haemorrhage is evident from its onset on CT scanning.

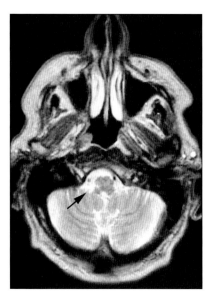

11.68 Small medullary infarct revealed by MRI. CT is most helpful in cerebral vascular lesions, but MRI is valuable in posterior fossa and brainstem lesions. Here, a small medullary infarct is revealed by the high signal area on the right (arrow).

supportive. Skilled nursing care prevents the development of pressure sores (**11.69**) and allows adequate nutrition and hydration.

Most recovery from stroke occurs during the first 6 months. Permanent disability is a common consequence of stroke (**11.70–11.71**). Long-term rehabilitation, with intensive physiotherapy (**11.72**), speech therapy and occupational therapy, should be carefully planned and allows about 25% of stroke patients to return to work or normal retirement. Mortality during the first month is about 40–50% because of extension of the cerebral damage, aspiration pneumonia and deep vein thrombosis with pulmonary embolism.

An intracerebral haemorrhage (apoplectic stroke) usually results from the rupture of a vessel or microaneurysm. Commonly these arise in hypertensive patients, occasionally in

those with bleeding disorders or on anticoagulants. The intracerebral haematoma often resolves over 2–3 weeks. Acute cerebellar haemorhages may require surgical evacuation, which can be life-saving.

Secondary prevention of stroke by control of cardiovascular risk factors (*see* **pp. 212–219**) is as important after stroke as in coronary heart disease. Hypertension must be controlled, and long-term antiplatelet therapy is usually indicated unless the stroke was haemorrhagic. Patients with atrial fibrillation should have cardiac ultrasound to determine whether thrombus is present in the fibrillating atrium. All patients with atrial fibrillation should be considered for oral anticoagulation or, if there is a major contraindication, should receive antiplatelet agents.

Primary prevention of stroke should be directed towards:

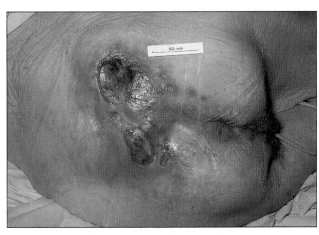

11.69   Severe sacral pressure sore – one of the serious but preventable complications of immobility following stroke. Note also the presence of a urinary catheter, commonly associated with recurrent urinary infections.

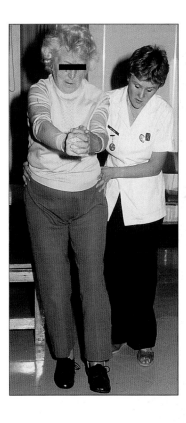

11.72   Skilled assistance can greatly aid rehabilitation from stroke. This patient with hemiplegia is being taught to walk without the use of mechanical aids; however, a walking frame can be an important aid in the early stages of rehabilitation.

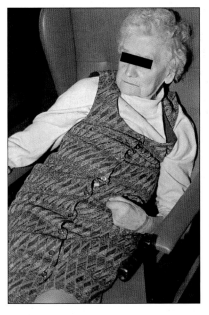

11.70   Loss of postural stability is common after stroke. When the non-dominant hemisphere is involved, walking apraxia and loss of postural control are usually apparent. The patient is unable to sit upright and tends to fall sideways. Appropriate support with pillows or cushions should be provided.

- control of blood pressure
- diagnosis and surgical treatment of carotid atheroma
- lowering lipid levels
- antithrombotic treatment in atrial fibrillation
- stopping smoking
- control of diabetes mellitus
- reducing haemoglobin in primary proliferative polycythaemia.

TRANSIENT ISCHAEMIC ATTACKS

A transient ischaemic attack (TIA) is defined as sudden focal loss of neurological function, presumed to be caused by a vascular lesion, which lasts less than 24 hours and leaves no residual signs. TIAs become more frequent with advancing years and there is an annual incidence of 0.5 cases per 1000 of the population. Two distinct clinical varieties are described – those in which the damage occurs in the territory supplied by the carotid artery and those in which the territory of the vertebral arteries is affected. The diagnosis of the attack is made on clinical grounds, but often the actual cause is unknown. Most are assumed to be embolic in origin and the source of these emboli is most commonly a plaque of atheroma, which ulcerates and allows formation of small amounts of platelet–fibrin thrombus that, in turn, break off and produce multiple small emboli. Emboli may be seen in the retina (**11.73**). Sites of thrombus formation include the internal and

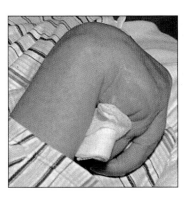

11.71   Permanent flexion contracture of the right hand has occurred in this patient several months after the onset of a dense hemiplegia. This type of disability can be prevented by early and continuing physiotherapy.

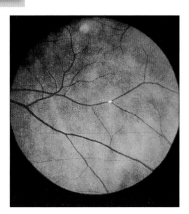

11.73 Retinal embolus in a patient with transient ischaemic attacks. Emboli may sometimes be seen in the retina in patients who have symptoms suggesting a TIA. Larger emboli from the carotid territory may even cause transient monocular blindness (amaurosis fugax).

common carotid artery, the mitral and aortic valves, the left ventricular wall after acute infarction (*see* **p. 217**), a dilated fibrillating left atrium, especially when there is mitral stenosis (*see* **p. 220**), and rarely an atrial myxoma (*see* **p. 235**). In addition to emboli, a search must be made for cardiac arrhythmias, hypertension, bacterial endocarditis, polycythaemia or myeloma – all of which may predispose to TIA.

Patients with carotid territory TIAs (anterior circulation TIAs) present with transient monocular blindness (amaurosis fugax), loss of power or sensation, or loss of speech. Those with vertebrobasilar TIAs (posterior circulation TIAs) present with loss of balance, staggering, and sensory impairment.

Investigation may include 24-hour monitoring for abnormalities of heart rhythm, echocardiography for thrombus on the left ventricular wall or in the left atrium, for mitral valve lesions or for vegetations, and routine chest X-ray. A full blood count, ESR, blood sugar and serology for syphilis are also necessary. Colour-flow Doppler (**11.74**) has revolutionized the imaging of carotid arteries. This technique is of great value for screening as it is non-invasive, easily repeatable and relatively cheap. It is now of such specificity that surgeons may use it to define the extent of proposed surgery without resorting to angiography (**11.33**), which carries a 1–2% risk of producing acute stroke. Treatment of patients with TIA is required to reduce the risk of completed stroke, which occurs at a rate of

5% per year. TIA is also a marker for subsequent myocardial infarction, which is a frequent cause of later death. Antiplatelet agents such as aspirin and dipyridamole are helpful, as are conventional anticoagulants. Carotid artery surgery is useful for severe carotid artery atheroma; it is most likely to be beneficial if the arterial lumen is narrowed by 70% or more. Angioplasty and stenting is a developing alternative.

VERTEBROBASILAR INSUFFICIENCY

Vertebrobasilar insufficiency (VBI) produces intermittent ischaemia in the brainstem and sometimes in the labyrinth. Symptoms, often in the elderly, include episodic dizziness, sometimes linked with head movement (**11.75**), visual disturbances, double vision, drop attacks, slurred speech and ataxia. Occasionally there may be alternating hemipareses or sensory disturbances. Vertigo is usually of abrupt onset lasting only minutes but may be associated with nausea and vomiting. Other causes of vertigo must be considered, including postural hypotension, Stokes-Adams attacks, transient changes of heart rhythm, epilepsy with a vertiginous aura and even benign positional vertigo. There may be a link with cervical spondylosis and some VBI attacks may arise from altered blood flow provoked by compression of the vertebral arteries by osteophytes. The diagnosis of VBI should not be made on dizziness alone.

In most instances the diagnosis is clinical. Plain neck X-rays usually show some spondylotic changes, often as an age change. Doppler ultrasound scans may assess the patency of the carotid arteries and the origins of the vertebral arteries. The vertebral vessels can only be shown in full by MRA or angiography. However, it is rare for any surgical intervention to be made on such a vessel. Most treatment of VBI ischaemic attacks includes

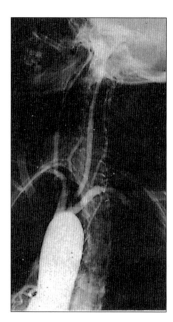

11.75 Aortogram in a patient with vertebrobasilar insufficiency, who presented with intermittent syncope. The carotid arteries are normal, but on turning her head to the left, the flow of contrast medium through the patient's left vertebral artery is interrupted. This anomaly may also be found in asymptomatic normal individuals.

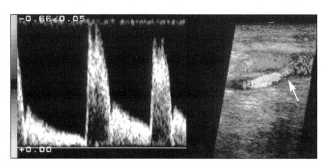

11.74 Stenosis of the internal carotid artery (arrow) shown by extracranial colour duplex scanning and conventional Doppler sonography.

controlling the vascular risk factors (diabetes, hypertension, hyperlipidaemia), with the addition of antiplatelet drugs such as aspirin and dipyridamole, and sometimes splinting the neck with a collar.

SUBARACHNOID HAEMORRHAGE

Subarachnoid haemorrhage (SAH) has an incidence of 10–15/100 000/year. It usually results from rupture of an arterial berry aneurysm (70–80%), or leakage from an arteriovenous malformation (5–10%); in 10–20% of cases, no source for the bleeding is found. Berry aneurysms develop at the bifurcations of the intracerebral arteries, probably as a result of an inherited weakness in the vessel wall. They are multiple in about 20% of patients. The common sites are on the anterior cerebral artery or anterior communicating artery (30%), the internal carotid and posterior communicating artery (25%), the middle cerebral bifurcation (13%), at branches from the internal carotid artery (15%) and on the vertebrobasilar system (5%). Most aneurysms are in the subarachnoid space, so their rupture produces SAH. Aneurysms of the internal carotid artery, when this runs in the cavernous sinus, produce pressure on the adjacent cranial nerves.

The clinical presentation is often dramatic with sudden onset of severe headache, often associated with nausea, vomiting and neck pain. The patient may become unconscious. Focal signs are usually absent. Rarely, an aneurysm may present before rupture, with signs of direct pressure on an adjacent nerve (**11.10**, **11.11**). Examination demonstrates neck stiffness and a positive straight-leg raising test. Fundal examination may show papilloedema and occasionally a subhyaloid haemorrhage.

The investigation of choice is CT which within 48 hours of onset will show the presence of blood in some 95% of patients (**11.76**). However, if the scan is delayed for 5 days, only 50% of

bleeds will show blood. The other investigation is a CSF examination with special attention given to the presence of xanthochromia in the spun supernatant. MRI (**11.77**) and MRA may be useful in showing aneurysms (> 3 mm size), AVMs and clots, but the most specific investigation is four-vessel angiography (**11.78**). This should only be undertaken in possible candidates for surgery who are fit enough for such intervention. Neuroradiologists may now be able to obliterate selected aneurysms by inserting fine platinum coils within the aneurysm sac, which cause thrombosis of the lesion.

The important of treating such aneurysms lies in the high mortality associated with re-bleeding: some 33% of patients

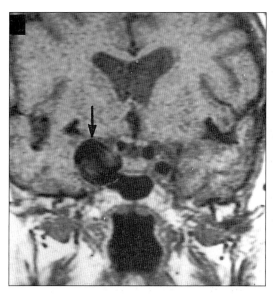

11.77 Right cavernous carotid aneurysm (arrowed), shown on coronal MRI. The signal void at the periphery of the aneurysm represents flowing blood, whereas the intensity in the central portion may represent either a clot or slowly flowing blood. MRI may demonstrate aneurysms clearly, but is much less successful than CT at demonstrating the presence or absence of blood in the subarachnoid space.

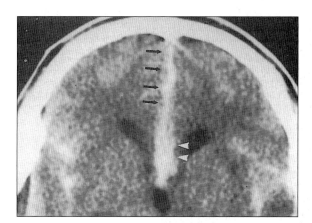

11.76 Subarachnoid haemorrhage from an anterior communicating artery aneurysm. This uncontrasted CT scan shows areas of increased density representing blood in the interhemispheric fissure (arrows) and the septum pellucidum (arrowheads). A lesser amount of blood is present in the sylvian fissures and the perimesencephalic cistern.

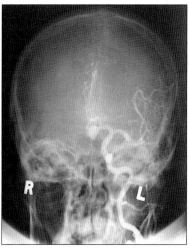

11.78 Berry aneurysm on the anterior communicating artery. The patient presented with a subarachnoid haemorrhage.

rebleed in the first 4 weeks. Progressive drowsiness in patients who have had a SAH may reflect acute hydrocephalus, cerebral oedema or rebleeding. Shunting may relieve the first.

The only other treatment of proven value once a diagnosis has been made is the use of calcium blockers, which relieve the spasm in adjacent arteries and hence reduce ischaemia in the surrounding brain.

Bleeding from an arteriovenous malformation (**11.79**) tends to be less severe and such patients present less acutely. There is also a significant incidence of previous epilepsy (*see* **p. 463**). Arteriovenous malformations may also be found in the spinal cord and may be difficult to remove safely. Some are amenable to interventional radiology (embolization procedures) and stereotactic radiotherapy, but both methods may damage the function of adjacent brain.

As this is a disease of young and otherwise fit people and the mortality is so high (60% if untreated; 35% if treated), consideration should be given to the question of organ donation in those who die.

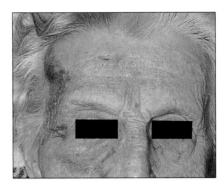

11.80 Subdural haematoma often follows a fall in an elderly patient, as in this woman who developed suggestive symptoms within a few days of a fall, despite the absence of skull fracture. The diagnosis is often missed because of the slow development of symptoms.

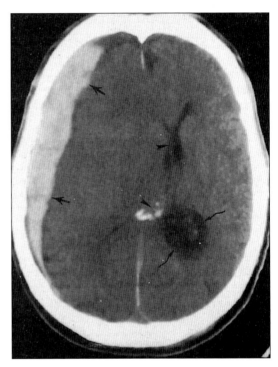

11.81 Large acute subdural haemorrhage (arrows) revealed by CT scan at the level of the lateral ventricles. The haemorrhage has resulted in midline shift, with marked compression and displacement of the right lateral ventricle (arrowheads). Because of the brain distortion and obstruction of CSF outflow, the left lateral ventricle is dilated (wavy arrows).

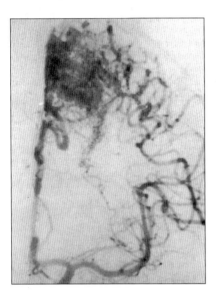

11.79 Left parietal arteriovenous malformation, shown in an anteroposterior view of an internal carotid angiogram. Bleeding from arteriovenous malformations is usually less severe than that from aneurysms, but their size may lead to other symptoms, including epilepsy.

SUBDURAL AND EXTRADURAL HAEMATOMAS

Subdural haematoma is the accumulation of blood in the potential subdural space (i.e. the dura–arachnoid interspace). It often results from a deceleration head injury, as in a fall (**11.80**) or a road traffic accident, but may also occur spontaneously, especially in the elderly. About 40% of patients also have a skull fracture. The diagnosis is often missed because of the slow development of symptoms. These include headache, intermittent fluctuation of conscious level, confusion and coma. There are often no immediate focal signs, but pupillary size may be asymmetrical. CT (**11.81**) or MRI (**11.82**) confirm

the diagnosis. Later, hemiparesis and hemisensory loss may occur.

A chronic subdural haematoma is one that has been present for over 3 weeks. These occur particularly in the aged, often after a trivial injury, so insignificant that it is not remembered. About 20% are bilateral. In only a few cases (about 5%) is there X-ray evidence of a fractured skull. In the long term, if untreated, these chronic subdural haematomas may calcify

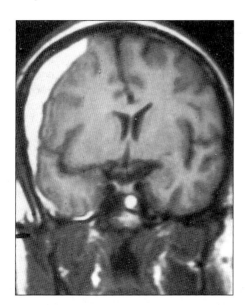

11.82   Right subdural haemorrhage revealed by MRI. The high intensity (white) haemorrhage has dissected under the temporal lobe, and the midline has been displaced to the left.

(**11.83**). CT and MRI appearances reflect the location, extent and age of the haemorrhage.

Extradural haematoma is often caused by rupture of the middle meningeal artery, associated with skull fracture resulting from direct injury. A haematoma forms and expands between the dura mater and the calvarium. The patient may have a lucid interval after awakening from the unconscious state after

trauma. The rapidly accumulating haematoma compresses the hemisphere and produces coma and death. For extracerebral clots, a deteriorating conscious level is often the first sign. An abnormal pupillary response may be the only focal sign early in the disease. Regular monitoring using the Glasgow Coma Scale (**11.47**) is essential. Confirmation of a haematoma is made by CT (**11.84**) and the clot may be removed surgically.

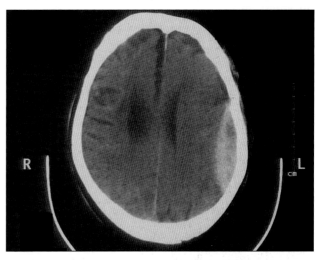

11.84 Extradural haematoma. A well defined biconvex collection of blood compresses the left cerebral hemisphere. There is inward displacement of the grey–white junction and slight rightward displacement of the left lateral ventricle.

11.83   Chronic bilateral subdural haematoma. This skull X-ray shows areas of calcification adjacent to the inner table of both parietal bones (arrows). The diagnosis was confirmed by CT.

CEREBRAL VENOUS THROMBOSIS

Thrombosis in the large dural venous sinuses or cortical veins is almost always associated with spread of infection from an adjacent focus, with obstruction caused by focal malignancy or with thrombophilia (*see* **p. 442**) which may have been exacerbated by dehydration, post-partum, the oral contraceptive ill, or sickle cell disease. The lateral sinus, cavernous sinus, superior sagittal sinus and cortical veins may be involved. The common sites of initial infection are the middle ear, the maxillary sinus, the nose (**2.50**) and the periorbital region. Infection of the sagittal venous sinus may result from extension of thrombophlebitis from other dural veins or venous sinuses.

The presenting features are often acute, with abrupt onset of fever, rigors, headache, coma or paresis. Cavernous sinus thrombosis may cause severe eye manifestations (**11.85**) and there may be papilloedema with visual loss. Occasionally the adjacent cranial nerves may be involved (fifth, sixth).

The diagnosis may be made by MRI (**11.86**), MR venography or CT scan.

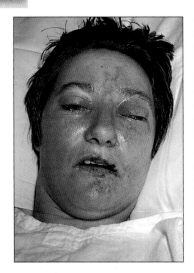

11.85 Cavernous sinus thrombosis occurred as a complication of sinusitis in this patient who presented with fever, rigors, headache and painful swelling around the left eye. The eye was difficult to examine, but she had papilloedema. The underlying infection was with *Staphylococcus aureus*, and she responded to appropriate antimicrobial therapy, making a full recovery.

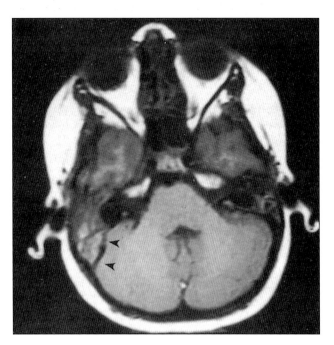

11.86 Acute right sigmoid sinus thrombosis (arrows) demonstrated by MRI.

Treatment is with antibiotics and anticoagulants to stop the spread of thrombosis even if haemorrhagic lesions are present. Repeated imaging may be necessary to monitor progress and treatment.

CEREBRAL PALSY

Cerebral palsy is the end result of brain damage caused by a range of disorders which may have been present in the growing fetus, at birth or in early infancy. The most common factors are hypoxia, intracerebral bleeding, trauma, kernicterus, hypoglycaemia and cerebral infection.

The result is a degree of cognitive impairment, motor and sensory impairment and epileptic fits, all of which produce social and behavioural problems as the child grows. The most common defects are motor: spastic hemiplegias and paraplegia are often compounded by choreo-athetosis and dystonia (**11.87**, **11.88**). There is a wide range of other possible neurological defects. Such children need careful assessment so that they may be given the opportunity to develop their residual mental and physical skills. Special schooling is often required. These children are now encouraged to lead independent and productive lives, and control of fits and surgical correction of muscle and joint abnormalities are important.

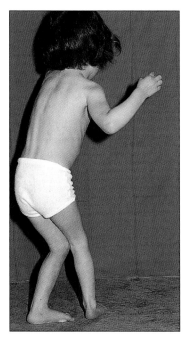

11.87 Spastic quadriplegia in cerebral palsy. Note the asymmetrical spasticity, with flexion contractures of the right arm and both knees, and internal rotation of the left lower limb. The spasticity was complicated by uncontrollable choreo-athetoid movements.

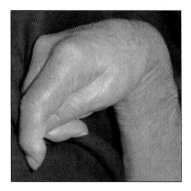

11.88 The spastic hand in cerebral palsy. This common deformity includes pronation of the forearm, flexion of the wrist, the 'thumb in palm' position and flexion of the metacarpophalangeal joints.

MOVEMENT DISORDERS

PARKINSON'S DISEASE

Parkinson's disease is a progressive degenerative disease of the extrapyramidal system that results from loss of the functional dopaminergic neurons that radiate from the substantia nigra to the caudate nucleus and putamen. This loss results in bradykinesia or akinesia, a resting tremor, restricted mobility resulting from muscular rigidity (cogwheel rigidity) and postural instability. The cumulative lifetime risk of developing parkinsonism is about 1 in 40. Symptoms usually first appear over the age of 50 years. A slow tremor of the hands, often unilateral, is the most common initial sign. This is typically 'pill rolling' in form and it diminishes on voluntary movement. It usually becomes bilateral, and may involve the upper and lower limbs and the jaw. Slowness of movements is often noticed first by the family rather than the patient. Rigidity compounds this slowness and leads to abnormalities in posture, which is typically stooped (**11.89**) and to gait abnormalities (a 'shuffling' or 'festinant' gait). The patient often has a mask-like face (**11.90**) with a reduced blinking rate, dribbles saliva because of difficulty in swallowing, and has monotonous speech, caused by dysarthria and dysphonia; writing is also impaired, often with micrographia. Parkinson's disease is a major cause of disability and increased mortality results from aspiration pneumonia, bed sores and urinary tract infections.

Diagnosis is made on the clinical picture, which is usually characteristic, but a careful history and examination are required to exclude identifiable causes of parkinsonism (**11.91**).

The mainstay of treatment is levodopa, which dramatically improves the symptoms of Parkinson's disease, especially akinesia, but not survival. Small doses are now used to minimize side-effects, often with concomitant therapy with a decarboxylase inhibitor or with an anticholinergic agent for tremor. After treatment for some years a number of disabling problems may develop. Levodopa effects may become shorter-lasting with deterioration at the end of each dose period. Increasing periods of rapid dyskinetic movements or longer-

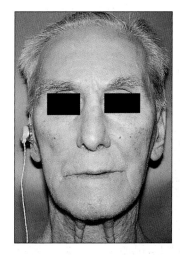

11.90 Parkinson's disease is characteristically associated with a mask-like face, devoid of emotion despite changes in circumstance. The patient often dribbles saliva, and commonly has monotonous speech.

481

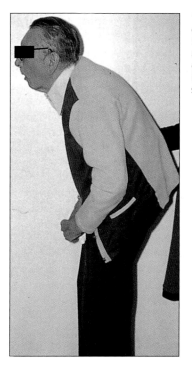

11.89 Parkinson's disease – typical posture. Note the stooped posture and the typical position of his arms, which are held slightly flexed at the sides.

IDENTIFIED CAUSES OF PARKINSONISM

Secondary causes:

Drugs:	phenothiazines, reserpine, methyldopa
Infections:	post-encephalitis lethargica
Toxins:	carbon monoxide, manganese and MPTP (1-methyl-4-phenyl-1,2,3,6-tetrahydropyridine) – a synthetic opiate byproduct

Hypoparathyroidism

Vascular:	cerebrovascular disease
Trauma:	e.g. in boxers (pugilist's encephalopathy)

Space-occupying lesions

Parkinsonisn in combination with:

Progressive supranuclear palsy (Steele–Richardson)

Alzheimer's disease

Shy–Drager syndrome (primary autonomic failure)

Normal pressure hydrocephalus

Huntington's chorea

Hepato-lenticular degeneration (Wilson's disease)

Athetoid cerebral palsy

11.91 Identified causes of parkinsonism.

maintained dystonias may occur with a variable relationship to the doses of levodopa. Periods of unpredictable immobility, the 'on–off' phenomenon, may occur many times a day. These complications are best treated with small, frequent levodopa doses, dopamine receptor agonists (bromocriptine, lisuride) and, occasionally, selegiline.

The use of dopamine agonists (pergolide, pramipexole or ropinirole) to initiate treatment has proved helpful in reducing the long term side effects from combined dopa treatment. In selected disabled patients there has recently been a return to stereotactic surgical lesions, such as pallidotomy, and/or deep brain stimulation of the subthalamic nuclei.

INVOLUNTARY DISORDERS OF MOVEMENT

A number of involuntary disorders of movement may occur.

Physiological tremor at about 8–13 Hz is normal, but increases to a noticeable level in anxiety, panic attacks, thyrotoxicosis, hypoglycaemia, after excessive intake of coffee or tea and with some drug use or misuse.

Postural tremor, usually at about 6–7 Hz, may occur spontaneously as an essential tremor or in families as a familial tremor. This is seen in the outstretched hands and during

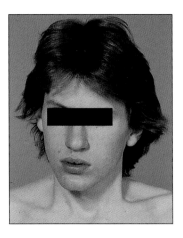

11.92 Spasmodic torticollis. In this condition, the head turns spasmodically as a result of asymmetrical contraction of the neck muscles. The condition is not usually associated with any other pathology.

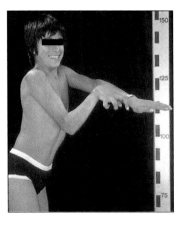

11.93 Torsion dystonia. This congenital condition is associated with severe fixed posturing of the hands, arms, neck and trunk. It is difficult or impossible to treat.

movement. Stress increases it and alcohol inhibits it. Beta blockade with propranolol is the treatment of choice.

Chorea is a rapid, semipurposeful movement seen in levodopa toxicity (dyskinesia), and also in Huntington's disease (*see* **p. 463**), and other disorders such as Sydenham's chorea (*see* **p. 220**), pregnancy chorea, systemic lupus erythematosus and drug-induced chorea (e.g oral contracteptives).

Hemiballismus is a unilateral disorder with dramatic, wild flailing of the limbs. It is attributed to a lesion, usually vascular, in the subthalamic nucleus.

Dystonias are a group of disorders in which spasm may be restricted to one area, for example in the neck (spasmodic torticollis, **11.92**), in the facial muscles around the eyes (blepharospasm) or in the hand (writer's cramp). Dystonias may rarely be widespread as a grossly disabling disorder that includes the trunk (torsion dystonia, **11.93**). Muscle spasm is amenable to local treatment with injected botulinum toxin type A, which causes irreversible neuromuscular blockade over a period of 3 months and may produce dramatic improvements in selected patients. A small number of dystonic patients have dopa-responsive dystonia: this should always be excluded by a therapeutic trial.

Tardive dyskinesias are involuntary movements of the face and tongue (orofacial dyskinesias), and of the limbs, caused by treatment with phenothiazines and butyrophenones. They are common in treated patients with chronic schizophrenia.

MULTIPLE SCLEROSIS

Multiple sclerosis is the most common disorder of myelin affecting the CNS, but there are many other acquired and inherited leucodystrophies.

It is a disease of unknown cause in which there is patchy demyelination in brain and spinal cord. The acute lesions are infiltrated by lymphocyte and plasma cells and may have an immunological basis. The end result of recurrent acute lesions is a chronic disease with relapses and remissions, but with the development of progressive neurological deficit. The disease has a definite geographical predilection, being rare in equatorial countries and increasing in incidence further away from the equator. In the UK, there is a higher incidence in the northern Isles of Orkney and Shetland compared with the south of England. It affects mainly young adults and is the most common neurological disorder of early adult life (mean age at onset in the UK is 34 years). The clinical features take many forms (**11.94**).

Optic neuritis is one of the most common early presentations of multiple sclerosis, but is not always followed by further features of progressive disease. It is usually unilateral, and is associated with loss of visual acuity, loss of colour vision and, sometimes, pain in the eye. These symptoms may come on suddenly and progress rapidly to a central scotoma. Examination shows the extent of visual loss and the presence and size of a scotoma. There is a defective pupillary response

CLINICAL FEATURES OF MULTIPLE SCLEROSIS

Site	Features
Optic neuritis (retrobulbar neuritis)	Pain on ocular movement, loss of central vision, sometimes papillitis
Brainstem lesions, III, IV, VI nerves	Diplopia
Cerebellum and its brainstem connections	Ataxia, dysarthria, oscillopsia
Subcortex, brainstem, spinal cord	Paraesthesiae, numbness, impaired position sense, trigeminal or other acute pain syndromes
Pyramidal tract	Limb or bulbar weakness, spasticity, clonus, brisk tendon reflexes, extensor plantar responses, urgency, frequency, urinary retention
Subcortical demyelination	Dementia, euphoria, depression

11.94 Clinical features of multiple sclerosis.

motor, sensory, and bladder function abnormalities. Brisk reflexes are usual with an extensor plantar response.

Brainstem involvement may present as sixth nerve palsy (**11.13**), as internuclear ophthalmoplegia (**11.97**) or with nystagmus. Involvement of the cerebellum results in ataxia and dysarthria. Subcortical involvement results in dementia and euphoria. Depression is also a common feature at all stages of the disorder.

There is no definitive diagnostic test, and sometimes the diagnosis only becomes clear clinically over the course of years because of the relapsing nature of the neurological findings. Evoked responses – visual (**11.20**), auditory or somatosensory – may be of value; they depend on the demonstration of delayed nerve conduction. Lumbar puncture may show a mild lymphocytic pleocytosis or a modest rise in the CSF protein. Oligoclonal bands of IgG in the CSF protein (but not in the serum), indicating the local synthesis of immune globulins, are present in 90% of patients. MRI of the brain (**11.98**) and spinal cord are now the most useful diagnostic tests confirming anatomical dissemination and excluding other pathology.

(afferent pupillary defect). The retina may show papilloedema (or papillitis; **11.95**) in the early stages. Most patients show rapid resolution of the acute symptoms but residual signs often remain. The patient may have visual impairment, and the optic disc may show swelling (papillitis, **11.95**), appear pale (optic atrophy, **11.96**) or remain normal.

Sensory impairment is also common at onset with numbness and paraesthesiae. Involvement of the pyramidal tracts usually occurs later. It is usually bilateral, and the patient presents with

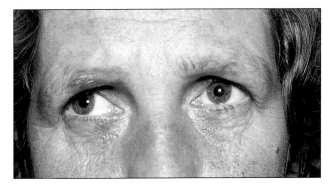

11.97 Internuclear ophthalmoplegia may be a presenting feature of brainstem involvement in multiple sclerosis. On lateral gaze to the right, adduction of the left eye is incomplete. On convergence, eye movement was normal. The lesion is in the left medial longitudinal bundle – between the nucleus in the pons and the third nerve nucleus on the opposite side.

11.95

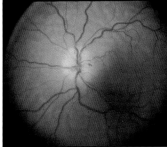

11.95, 11.96 Optic neuritis is a common initial presentation of multiple sclerosis. In the early stages the disc may appear normal, or may develop papillitis with blurred margins and occasional haemorrhages (**11.95**). Later, the patient may develop the complete pallor of optic atrophy (**11.96**); alternatively the disc may return to a normal appearance.

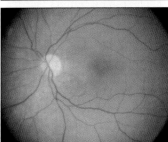

11.96

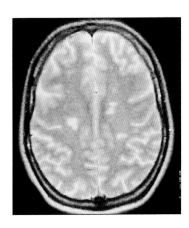

11.98 Multiple sclerosis. This MRI picture shows multiple 'high signal' lesions in the white matter of both hemispheres. These represent multiple areas of demyelination.

There is no specific treatment but high-dose intravenous steroids have a place in the acute episode. Dietary manipulation and hyperbaric oxygen have been used, but there is little evidence of their efficacy. Physiotherapy, psychotherapy and family counselling and support are mandatory. Depression should be actively treated and spasticity may respond to baclofen. Pain and troublesome paraesthesiae may respond to carbamazepine. Urinary retention and incontinence are treated symptomatically and care must be taken to avoid pressure sores (**11.69**) as the patient becomes immobile.

Recently beta-interferons have been show to reduce the frequency and severity of relapses and to slow progression of the disease. Such treatments require regular injections and are very costly.

MOTOR NEURON DISEASE

Motor neuron disease is found in 1 in 12 000 of the population (in the UK), with a male:female ratio of 3:2 and a peak incidence at the age of 70 years. It is a rare, progressive degenerative disease of the upper and lower motor neurons that causes severe disability; patients have a 5-year survival of about 40%. There is no impairment of intellect, sensation, sexual, bowel or bladder function or balance. Frontal lobe dementia may occur. No cause has been found, although there is a family history with dominant inheritance in 10% of cases. Clinical presentation may be in one of three patterns:

- Progressive muscular atrophy (PMA) patients present with wasting of the small muscles in one hand (**11.99**), which is rapidly followed by wasting in the other and proximal spread to involve the arms; the feet may be similarly involved. Symptoms usually include weakness, easy fatigability, muscle cramps and lack of muscle strength. The main signs are muscle wasting with loss of power and fasciculation. Tendon reflexes may be absent.

- Amyotrophic lateral sclerosis (ALS) patients present with features of degeneration of the upper motor neuron and the lateral corticospinal tracts. There is usually an associated progressive muscular atrophy, so that the clinical picture is of combined upper and lower motor neuron degeneration.

- Progressive bulbar palsy mainly affects women. Patients have involvement of the cranial nerves with upper and lower motor neuron lesions. The dominant and distressing features are dysarthria and dysphonia, difficulties in chewing and swallowing, and regurgitation of food and fluids via the nose because of palatal palsy. The tongue may be wasted (**11.100**) and fasciculation is obvious. Paralysis of the respiratory muscles is also apparent. Aspiration pneumonia is a common complication and, with hypoventilation, causes death.

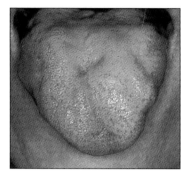

11.100 Motor neuron disease. This patient had progressive bulbar palsy. An early feature was fasciculation of the tongue, followed by progressive wasting, with furrowing of the surface. Progressive difficulties in chewing, swallowing and respiration accompanied this sign.

The diagnosis may be made on clinical grounds alone but electromyography may provide evidence of widespread denervation and exclude a neuropathy, particularly multifocal motor neuropathy with conduction block. The CSF is normal. Cervical and lumbar spondylosis and motor neuropathies must be excluded, as they also cause amyotrophy (**7.84**). There is no specific treatment, although riluzole may slightly slow progression. Severe bulbar weakness may require feeding by PEG (*see* **p. 331**). Patients and their families may need physical and psychosocial support.

DISORDERS OF THE SPINAL CORD

SYRINGOMYELIA

Syringomyelia results from the formation of a 'syrinx' in the spinal cord. This is a cavity filled with CSF that probably arises during development, when it may be associated with an Arnold–Chiari malformation. Less commonly it occurs after trauma. The syrinx may extend all the way down the central canal of the cord, but is usually most prominent in the upper cervical cord and in the brainstem (syringobulbia). As the cavity enlarges there is progressive neurological impairment,

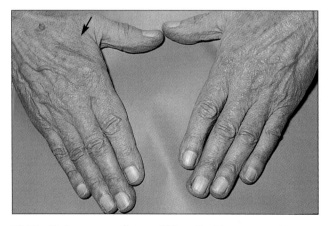

11.99 Motor neuron disease. This patient has progressive muscular atrophy and presented with fasciculation and wasting of the muscles between the thumb and index finger on the dorsal (arrow) and palmar surfaces. Wasting in the right hand was followed by the development of similar wasting in the left hand, and subsequently by progressive wasting and fasciculation elsewhere.

starting with the decussating fibres of the spinothalamic tract, which carry pain and temperature, and resulting in disassociation sensory impairment of the trunk and upper limbs. This impairment results in the development of painless ulcers of the hands from unrecognized trauma and burns (**11.101**) and later to Charcot's joints in the upper limb (**11.102**). Later, the anterior horn cells are affected, leading to

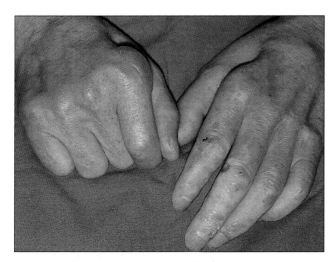

11.101   Syringomyelia. The patient has severe wasting of the small muscles of both hands. He has also sustained a painless burn at the base of the right index finger – a result of the sensory loss associated with the condition.

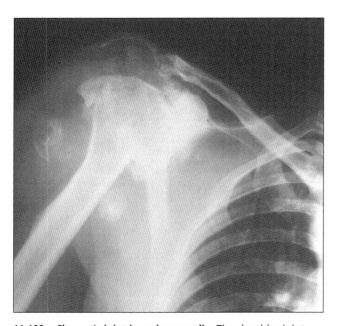

11.102   Charcot's joint in syringomyelia. The shoulder joint has been destroyed, and the radiological appearance is complicated by new bone formation. This painless joint destruction is the result of sensory loss. In syringomyelia it is usually confined to the upper limbs, but similar changes may occur in the upper or lower limbs in diabetes, leprosy and tertiary syphilis (*see* **1.193**, **1.194**).

wasting of the small muscles of the hand (**11.101**) and arms with absent reflexes. Extension to the corticospinal tracts produces a spastic paraplegia. A syrinx in the brainstem (syringobulbia) results in loss of cranial nerve motor function with dysphagia and dysarthria, hemiatrophy of the tongue, weakness and wasting of the sternomastoid, impairment of hearing and loss of fifth nerve sensation or a Horner's syndrome (**11.8**).

The diagnosis is made by demonstrating the presence of a cavity on MRI (**11.103**).

Treatment is surgical by posterior decompression of the foramen magnum, which may arrest or slow progression.

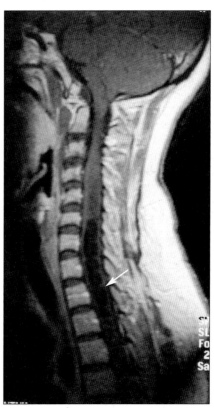

11.103 Syringomyelia. This T1-weighted gadolinium-enhanced MRI shows an extensive fluid-containing cavity in the lower cervical and upper thoracic region (arrow). There were also congenital anomalies of the upper cervical vertebrae.

FRIEDREICH'S ATAXIA

Friedreich's ataxia is an autosomally transmitted (usually recessive) form of spinocerebellar degeneration. Patients with the disease usually present between the ages of 5 and 10 years, with clumsiness in walking. This progresses inexorably and is associated with loss of proprioception and vibration sense, which produces lower limb atrophy and loss of tone. Tendon reflexes are lost and the plantar responses are extensor. The degenerative process moves upwards with time, to affect speech and eye movements.

In addition to the neurological defects, there are skeletal abnormalities, notably a scoliosis and pes cavus (**11.104**).

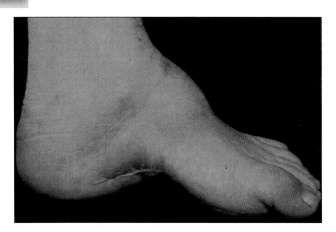

11.104   Pes cavus is a characteristic finding in Friedreich's ataxia. Both feet are usually more or less symmetrically high-arched and stubby. This patient has undergone surgery in a previous attempt to correct the deformity.

There may be a cardiomyopathy in some 75% leading to conduction defects and heart failure. Rare associated nerve defects include retinal degeneration, optic atrophy, deafness, mental retardation and LMN degeneration.

Diagnosis is made on clinical finding and family history. Genetic counselling is important. Treatment is purely supportive.

SPINA BIFIDA

Spina bifida results from defective fusion of the vertebral arches. The most common site is in the lumbar region. Spina bifida occulta may be found in asymptomatic people who are X-rayed for some other reason (**11.105**). In some patients,

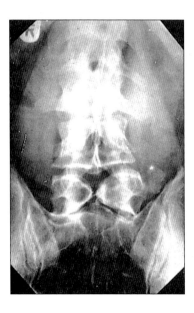

11.105   Occult spina bifida, discovered by chance on X-ray. The fifth lumbar and first sacral vertebrae have failed to fuse posteriorly in the midline, but the patient had no symptoms.

there may be an associated tuft of hair over the lower back (**11.106**) or tethering of the cord with a 'dimple' in the skin. Spina bifida occulta is often a benign complaint that requires no treatment, but occasionally may lead to progressive motor and sensory deficits.

Diastematomyelia is a congenital anomaly in which the spinal cord is split in two by a long, cartilaginous or fibrous band arising from the posterior surface of a vertebral body in the thoracic or lumbar spine.

In spina bifida, there is often a progressive lower motor neuron deficit involving bowel, bladder and lower limbs. The common cutaneous sign is a tuft of hair over the lower back (**11.106**) or a dimple, haemangioma, lipoma, sinus or skin tag. Symptoms start when the child starts to walk and gait may be abnormal due to weakness or pain. Neuropathic changes may subsequently appear in the feet.

In the severe form of spina bifida, the meninges may protrude through the bony defect (meningocele) and may include neural elements (meningomyelocele). These abnormalities are often associated with hydrocephalus and usually there is impairment of leg and bladder function. Surgery is required to cover the defect and shunting is necessary for hydrocephalus.

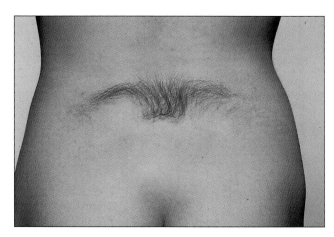

11.106   Occult spina bifida may be suggested by the presence of a tuft of hair over the base of the spine. This is usually a harmless anomaly, but may be associated with diastematomyelia.

PARAPLEGIA

Paraplegia is paralysis of both lower limbs and may be acute or chronic. The limbs are flaccid in the acute phase and become spastic later. There is loss of bladder control. A large number of diseases may produce similar clinical features (**11.107**).

Investigations should include a full blood count, ESR, serum B_{12} level, and an MRI (**11.108**). Plain spinal X-rays may show collapse, malalignment or vertebral pathology. CT with contrast and/or myelography may be used in selected patients.

CAUSES OF PARAPLEGIA

Skeletal diseases	Disc prolapse (above L1)
	Spondylosis
	Metastatic carcinoma
	Paget's disease
	Rheumatoid arthritis
Spinal tumours	Neurofibromas
	Meningiomas
	Secondary carcinoma/lymphoma
	Ependymoma
Infections	Abscess (pyogenic)
	Tuberculosis (Pott's spine)
	Myelitis
	HIV
	Syphilis
Demyelination	Multiple sclerosis
Blood disorders (spinal haematoma)	Bleeding disorders Anticoagulants
Vascular occlusion	Emboli
	Thrombosis
Trauma	Falls, road traffic accidents
Metabolic	Vitamin B_{12} deficiency

11.107 Causes of paraplegia.

NEOPLASMS OF THE SPINAL CORD

Primary neoplasia causing nerve root or cord compression may arise from any of the tissues in the area, and metastases from distant organs may also involve the spinal cord, nerve plexi or surrounding structures. The lesions may therefore be paravertebral, extradural, intradural or intramedullary. Symptoms may be produced by direct invasion, by compression or, more rarely, by ischaemia resulting from invasion of the nutrient arteries. The process is usually insidious, with local pain that may radiate along a dermatome and may produce motor signs such as muscle wasting (**4.160**), sensory signs and occasionally autonomic changes (anhidrosis, hyperhidrosis or Horner's syndrome, **4.161**, **11.8**). Cord compression may result in lower motor neuron features at the level of the lesion, coupled with sensory loss and progressive features of upper motor signs below this level. Pain may be local or referred. Dysfunction of the bowel and bladder may be prominent early features. Occasionally, patients may present acutely with paraplegia.

MRI will establish the diagnosis in most instances (**11.109**). There is seldom a need for myelography, CT or CSF examination except in selected patients where either there are diagnostic difficulties or technical reasons why MRI is not possible (e.g. pacemaker).

Treatment is dependent on the diagnosis. If the patient has suffered from previous malignancy, especially of lung or breast or a lymphoma, treatment may be possible with radiotherapy or appropriate chemotherapy, or both. Biopsy may be necessary to establish a diagnosis and surgical resection to relieve cord or nerve root compression.

487

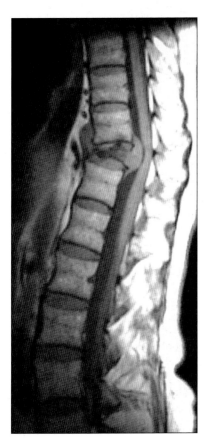

11.108 Compression of the spinal cord leading to paraplegia, revealed by MRI scan. A secondary deposit from carcinoma of the breast led to complete collapse and fracture of a vertebra with consequent cord compression.

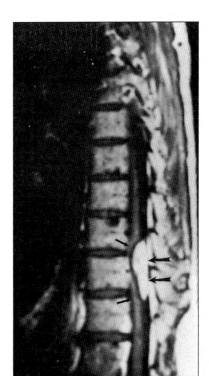

11.109 Subdural lipoma demonstrated by MRI in sagittal section. The lipoma (large arrows) is severely compressing the spinal cord (small arrows).

DISORDERS OF PERIPHERAL NERVES (NEUROPATHIES)

Many disease processes produce peripheral neuropathy (11.110). Most patients present with features of lower motor neuron involvement and sensory changes, but sometimes also or predominantly with motor changes. The cranial nerves may be affected by the same processes (see p. 450). The condition may be symmetrical or localized to one side. There are great variations in the degree of defects and their distribution. Motor involvement is associated with wasting and loss of power (7.90, 11.111, 11.112). Sensory features include numbness, paraesthesiae or hyperaesthesiae, pain and impaired temperature sensation. There may be associated skin ulceration and loss of skin hair. The tendon reflexes are absent.

Patients with autonomic neuropathy typically present with orthostatism and may have associated dysphagia, gastric atony with vomiting, diarrhoea and gustatory sweating (7.91). There is usually retention of urine with overflow incontinence and failure of erection. Hypotension may occur on standing (postural hypotension).

CAUSES OF PERIPHERAL POLYNEUROPATHIES	
Metabolic	Endocrine: diabetes (see also **p. 319**), hypothyroidism, acromegaly Renal failure Chronic liver failure Vitamin deficiency – B_1, B_6, nicotinic acid, B_{12}, vitamin E Amyloid Acute intermittent porphyria
Infections	Diphtheria exotoxin Leprosy Herpes zoster HIV
Toxic	Alcohol Drugs, e.g. lithium, isoniazid, gold, phenytoin, vincristine, chlorambucil, cisplatin, taxol, metronidazole, dapsone Heavy metals: lead, arsenic, thallium, mercury Organic solvents: trichlorethylene, ethylene oxide, organophosphates, n-hexane, tri-orthocresyl phosphate
Autoimmune disorders	Systemic lupus erythematosus
Neoplasia	Tumours, especially carcinoma of bronchus and myeloma
Hereditary disorders	Fabry's disease, Refsum's disease Charcot–Marie–Tooth disease (HMSN types I and II)
Idiopathic	Guillain–Barré syndrome

11.110 Causes of peripheral polyneuropathies.

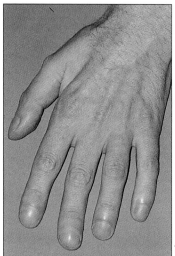

11.111 & 11.112
Wasting of the hand as a consequence of ulnar neuropathy. Note the marked wasting of the interosseous muscles, especially the first dorsal interosseous. This patient also had early finger clubbing, and he proved to have a bronchial carcinoma.

11.111

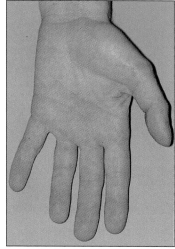

11.112

It is always important to exclude potentially treatable causes of a peripheral neuropathy such as diabetes, B_{12} deficiency, dysproteinaemias, drugs, alcohol and connective tissue disorders. Genetic testing is now possible for some of the more common inherited neuropathies, such as Charcot–Marie–Tooth disease, hereditary motor and sensory neuropathy (HMSN) type 1.

IMMUNE POLYNEUROPATHY

Guillain–Barré syndrome (acute infectious polyneuropathy, AIP) is thought to be an immune polyneuropathy as it appears 2–3 weeks after an infection of the upper respiratory or gastrointestinal tract, or following recent immunization. It may affect all ages, but is most commonly found in the middle years of life. There may be a range of prodromal symptoms, including pyrexia, headache, nausea and vomiting; these are followed by back and limb pain, with a gradual onset of ascending motor neuropathy (LMN type) starting in the limbs, then involving the truncal muscles, cranial nerves and muscles of respiration. Sensory changes may be present early in the disease and dysaesthesia may be severe. Autonomic involvement may also be present and associated with postural hypotension and arrhythmias. Death may occur from respiratory impairment or from arrhythmias.

The diagnosis is made on the clinical picture, and it may be substantiated by finding a normal cell count in the CSF, with normal pressure but a high protein level, which may give a deep yellow colour to the CSF. There may be evidence of delayed nerve conduction velocities.

The natural history of the disease is of a progressive neuropathy over several days, a period of stable neuropathy and then gradual recovery of normal function in the majority of cases. Intensive respiratory support may be required at any stage if the respiratory muscles are involved. In the early stages of the disease intravenous immune globulin and plasmaphaeresis have been used with benefit. Steroids may be of value in chronic inflammatory demyelinating polyneuropathy. Thrombo-prophylaxis may reduce the risk of DVT and PE associated with immobility.

DIRECT INJURY AND COMPRESSION NEUROPATHY

Acute

Acute damage to peripheral nerves can result from direct penetrating or non-penetrating trauma and may involve any nerve or plexus. The result is loss of motor and sensory function, and atrophy of muscle and skin in the areas supplied. The most common types of injury include acute stretching resulting from difficult delivery (11.113) or from trauma in later life (especially road traffic accidents), and compression from coma resulting from alcohol, drugs, during general anaesthesia or simply from lying or sitting in a cramped position for a prolonged period. Penetrating injuries include bullet or knife wounds and ill-placed intramuscular injections. The most common such lesion is that involving the radial nerve, which is usually injured as it winds round the back of the humerus (Saturday night palsy – as a result of alcoholic coma – 11.114). Other examples are the peroneal nerve which may be compressed as it passes over the head of the fibula and the ulnar nerve at the elbow (producing signs similar to those in 7.90).

Chronic

Carpal tunnel syndrome is more common in women (3 per 1000 patients per year) than in men (1 per 1000 patients per year) and is most common in middle-aged women. It results from compression of the median nerve as it passes through the carpal tunnel deep to the flexor retinaculum. The cause is often unclear, but sometimes a predisposing disorder is present (11.115). The main complaints are of pain, numbness and paraesthesiae in the fingers supplied by the median nerve. The symptoms are often worse on awakening. Pain may radiate up

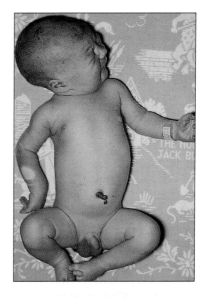

11.113 Right upper brachial plexus birth injury leading to a right-sided Erb's palsy. There is paralysis of shoulder abduction, external rotation of the arm and paralysis of forearm supination, leading to a characteristic 'porter's tip' position of the right hand. Difficult delivery is a common cause of acute injury to peripheral nerves.

489

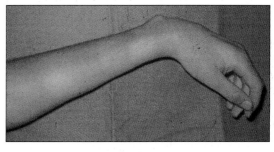

11.114 Radial nerve palsy. The patient is unable to extend the wrist and the metacarpophalangeal joints of the fingers or thumb – he has 'wrist drop'. Compression is a common cause of this injury; laceration of the nerve is another possible cause, usually after a closed midshaft humeral fracture. Electromyograms will show the first evidence of reinnervation of muscles.

CAUSES OF THE CARPAL TUNNEL SYNDROME
Idiopathic
Pregnancy
Hypothyroidism
Diabetes mellitus
Acromegaly
Rheumatoid arthritis
Trauma to wrist

11.115 Causes of the carpal tunnel syndrome.

the arm to the elbow, and it may be relieved by elevation of the hand or by gentle shaking of the hand in the air (flick test). Use of the hand leads to loss of the symptoms. Examination shows sensory loss over the distribution of the median nerve – usually the thumb, index and middle fingers and one half of the ring finger (**11.116, 11.117**). There may be power loss in the thumb, both in abduction and adduction (i.e. abductor pollicis brevis, flexor pollicis brevis and opponens) and there may be wasting of the thenar eminence.

Additional tests include:

- Tinel's sign which is elicited by tapping with a finger over the carpal tunnel – this produces paraesthesiae in the hand and travelling up the arm
- Phalen's test is similar to the above, but the stimulus is flexion of the wrist for 60 seconds; a positive test is the production of paraesthesiae
- tourniquet test is the testing of sensation deficit resulting from application of an upper arm tourniquet

Nerve conduction studies are also of value in early diagnosis.

Management depends on the cause. If this is temporary (e.g. pregnancy), then simple measures such as splints or diuretics may buy enough time for spontaneous resolution to occur after delivery. Steroid injection into the carpal tunnel gives symptomatic relief and is sometimes curative. Otherwise, surgical decompression is required; this leads to return of motor function and usually to some sensory recovery.

In the thoracic outlet syndrome there is compression of the lower trunks of the brachial plexus as they pass over an abnormal cervical rib (**5.185**) or fibrous band, or over the normal first rib and muscle. Damage is usually confined to the C8, T1 fibres. Patients present with paraesthesiae, weakness, numbness of the ulnar fingers and wasting of the small muscles of the hand, especially the thenar muscles. There may be coincidental obstruction of the arterial supply of the limb (*see* **p. 249**). Symptoms are usually more apparent when the arm is abducted. Treatment is by removal of the fibrous band or rib.

Ulnar nerve damage (entrapment) is usually caused by recurrent trauma to the nerve in its shallow groove at the back of the medial condyle of the humerus. It can also occur after fracture of the condyle and subsequent healing. There is usually weakness and atrophy of the interossei with clawing of the fingers and difficulty with fine movements. Sensory loss may be detected in the small finger and the adjacent half of the ring finger and it may be possible to elicit sensory complaints by compressing the nerve at the elbow.

Compression of the lateral cutaneous nerve of the thigh may occur as it passes under the inguinal ligament, especially in grossly obese individuals wearing a tight belt or corset. Paraesthesiae occur in the nerve distribution, that is the lateral surface of the thigh as far down as the knee. Symptoms may be brought on by change in posture, especially by sitting. Resolution of symptoms can be produced by advice about clothing and by weight control and some patients require surgical decompression.

NEUROCUTANEOUS SYNDROMES

STURGE–WEBER SYNDROME

Sturge–Weber syndrome, a congenital condition with a diffuse capillary haemangioma of the face, forehead and anterior crown, in the distribution of the ophthalmic division of the trigeminal nerve (**11.118**), is associated with similar ipsilateral angiomas of the pia mater and underlying cortex, typically in

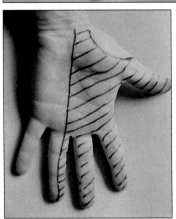

11.116 & 11.117 Carpal tunnel syndrome. The common areas of sensory impairment are marked in this patient. Note that they usually extend round the fingertips on to the nail area in the affected fingers and even further over the extensor surface on the thumb. Wasting of the thenar eminence is also seen.

11.116

11.117

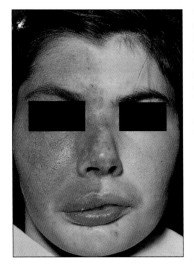

11.118 Sturge–Weber syndrome. This patient has a classic diffuse capillary haemangioma in the distribution of the ophthalmic, nasociliary and maxillary branches of the trigeminal nerve. The lesion extends backwards over the anterior two-thirds of the crown of the head.

the parieto-occipital region. This combination is associated with the development of epilepsy – usually generalized seizures – with associated mental retardation or hemiparesis, or both. Straight X-ray of the skull or CT scan (**11.119**) show calcification in the deep layers of the cortex.

Treatment is by drug control of epilepsy and cosmetic covering of the facial lesions.

- **Type II** (abnormality on chromosome 22) is generally associated with central lesions – bilateral acoustic neurofibromas, multiple intracranial meningiomas (**11.120**), schwannomas of cranial nerves and a few cutaneous lesions.

Diagnosis is readily confirmed by biopsy. Excision of peripheral lesions that rapidly change in size is important, because sarcomatous change may occur. Gene markers are of value in antenatal diagnosis and subsequent counselling is required.

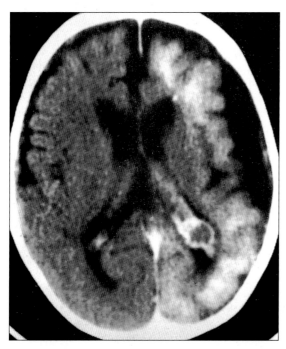

11.119   Sturge–Weber syndrome. This enhanced CT scan shows increased density throughout the atrophic left cerebral hemisphere, probably representing a combination of calcification and enhancement of the pial angiomas. There is enhancement of an enlarged left ventricular choroid plexus, which is again angiomatous. The right frontal lobe also shows some atrophy, and this patient may have bilateral involvement.

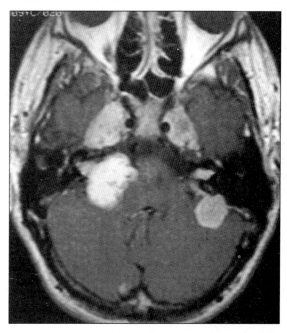

11.120   Neurofibromatosis (type II). This patient has multiple cerebral tumours, as demonstrated by gadolinium-enhanced MRI. This scan shows bilateral eighth nerve tumours, a meningioma along the left petrous bone and bilateral parasellar meningiomas.

NEUROFIBROMATOSIS

Neurofibromatosis (von Recklinghausen's disease) is a rare disease with an autosomal dominant transmission, in which multiple neurofibromas develop in peripheral and cranial nerves, and in which CNS tumours also appear (gliomas and meningiomas). There is also a rare association with the development of phaeochromocytomas (*see* **p. 304**). Two distinct types are now recognized.

- **Type I** (abnormality on chromosome 17) is generally associated with peripheral lesions – papillomas of skin, multiple cutaneous neurofibromas (**2.86**), café-au-lait spots, pigmented hamartomas of iris (Lisch nodules), axillary freckling, spinal and autonomic neurofibromas, phaeo-chromocytomas and optic gliomas.

Tuberous sclerosis (epiloia)

Tuberous sclerosis (epiloia) is inherited as an autosomal dominant trait (prevalence 3–9/100 000) and those affected present in childhood with mental retardation (50%), epilepsy (75%) and typical facial lesions (adenoma sebaceum, **11.121**). These lesions are angiofibromas. They are rarely seen before the age of 2 years, and may not appear until middle age, but are present in 85% of all cases. The diagnosis is usually clinically obvious. There may also be nodules in the retina (phakomas). Skin changes in addition to those on the face include white oval patches on the thorax (ash leaf patches – found in 80% of all cases), fibromas under the nails and naevi at the base of the spine (shagreen patches). There is a rare association with intracranial gliomas, multiple angiomyolipomas of the kidney and cardiac rhabdomyomas. X-ray of the skull or CT scan may show calcification in the walls of the lateral ventricles (**11.122**).

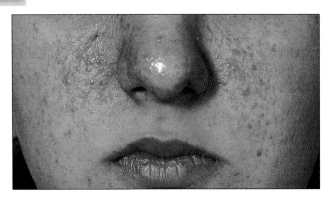

11.121 Adenoma sebaceum of the face – a marker of tuberous sclerosis (epiloia). The lesions are angiofibromas and in tuberous sclerosis they are associated with mental retardation, epilepsy and other skin changes.

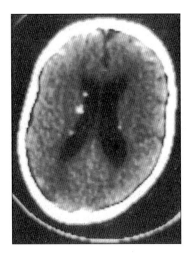

11.122 Tuberous sclerosis. This CT scan shows calcified periventricular lesions. These are hamartomatous tubers, containing both neurons and astrocytes. The patient also shows bilateral ventricular enlargement (hydrocephalus) that probably results from the presence of tubers near the foramen of Munro, causing CSF obstruction.

Treatment involves control of epilepsy. Genetic counselling is important.

DISORDERS OF MUSCLE

MUSCULAR DYSTROPHIES

Muscular dystrophies are a large group of poorly understood genetic disorders in which there is progressive degeneration of selected muscle groups. Those affected usually present with progressive muscle weakness in the early years of life.

One of the most common is **Duchenne muscular dystrophy** (DMD), which is transmitted as an X-linked recessive disorder and affects males. DMD affects 1 in 3500 live male births and about one-third of cases arise in previously unaffected families. The syndrome is caused by deletion of the dystrophin gene on the X chromosome. This results in failure to produce dystrophin, which is located on the muscle fibre surface membrane and is necessary for optimum muscle function.

Blood tests are now available to detect the faulty gene and its presence in carriers. Symptoms and signs become obvious at the age of about 2 years, with weakness of the pelvic and shoulder girdle muscles, and the first signs are commonly difficulty in walking, abnormal gait, frequent falling and difficulty in climbing steps and in getting off the floor (**11.123**, **11.124**). Some muscle groups – especially in the calf – become hypertrophied. The course is inexorably downhill and by adolescence the boy is often deformed and invariably in a wheelchair (**11.125**, **11.126**). The most common cause of death is hypostatic pneumonia associated with failure of the muscles of respiration and associated cardiac failure.

The diagnosis is usually obvious clinically and from the family history. There is usually massive elevation of the serum creatine kinase. Muscle biopsy shows necrosis of short segments of muscle fibres in focal groups with some attemps at fibre regeneration. Eventually, the fibres become progressively distorted, replaced by dense collagenous bands infiltrated with fatty tissue. Immune staining shows the absence of dystrophin in muscle biopsies from Duchenne patients.

No treatment will alter the course of the disease. Genetic counselling for the family and psychosocial support are important.

A number of less common dystrophies include:

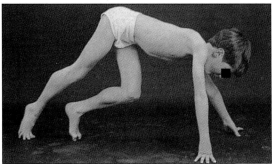

11.123

11.123 & 11.124 Duchenne muscular dystrophy leads to great difficulty in getting up from a prone position. To reach the stage shown in **11.123**, this boy rolled over and 'walked' his hands and feet towards each other. He then walked his hands to his feet and up the front of his legs to reach the position shown in **11.124**. From here, he reaches an upright position by releasing his grip on his knees and swinging his arms and trunk sideways and upwards. This manoeuvre is known as Gowers' sign. Note the prominence of the calf muscles, especially in **11.123**. This boy was 10 years old, but many patients have lost the ability to get up from the floor by this age.

11.124

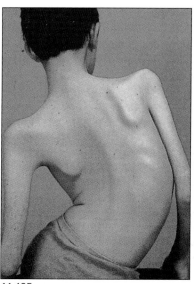

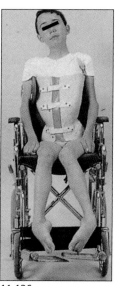

11.125   11.126

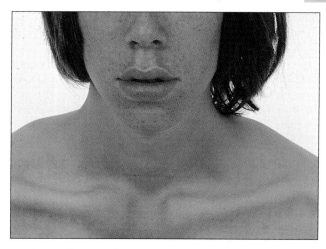

11.128   **Facioscapulohumeral dystrophy** in a 15-year-old boy. This view shows wasting of the muscles of the face, neck and shoulder girdle.

11.125 & 11.126   Duchenne muscular dystrophy. This 15-year-old boy has severe scoliosis and an equinovarus deformity of the feet. A fair degree of improvement in the scoliosis, which was still relatively mobile, was achieved with a spinal brace. By this stage in the disease, patients are invariably confined to a wheelchair.

- **Becker muscular dystrophy,** an X-linked disease, milder than DMD, in which the patients live well into adult life.
- **Limb-girdle dystrophy** is an autosomal recessive disorder that affects the pelvic and shoulder girdle of boys and girls and is progressive in symptomatology (**11.127**).
- **Facioscapulohumeral dystrophy** is an autosomal dominant disease that affects the muscles of the face, neck and shoulders; these atrophy to give characteristic winging of the scapulae and atrophy of the deltoids and pectoralis major (**11.128**). Scoliosis occurs because of loss of support from weak truncal muscles. The pelvic girdle muscles may be similarly affected. The history is of progressive muscle weakness and atrophy.

MYOTONIC DYSTROPHY

Myotonia is increased spasm of muscle fibres that results from abnormalities of the muscle membrane producing a delay in relaxation. Myotonic dystrophy (dystrophia myotonica) is an uncommon disorder (prevalence 5–50 per 100 000 of the population). It is transmitted as an autosomal dominant disorder with the recognition of a trinucleotide repeat (CTG) in a gene on chromosome 19, so there is now a blood test to confirm the diagnosis. It usually presents in the age range 20–30 years with weakness of the limb muscles associated with myotonia. This becomes apparent as failure to relax a grip. There is also cranial muscle involvement, often with ptosis, difficulty in whistling and dysarthria. There is associated wasting of the temporalis, masseter and sternomastoid muscles. A variety of other signs may occur, including the development of cataracts, frontal baldness (in men) and testicular or ovarian atrophy. The facies is very typical (**11.129**). There may be

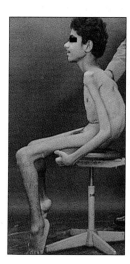

11.127   Limb-girdle dystrophy. This 18-year-old boy showed severe signs, with extreme proximal muscle wasting and weakness, and a prominent kyphosis.

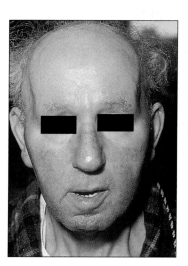

11.129   Myotonic dystrophy in a 50-year-old man. His appearance is typical, with facial weakness, atrophy of the temporal muscles and sternomastoids and frontal baldness, which produces a 'monk-like' appearance.

associated cardiomyopathy with arrhythmias, especially atrial flutter; and there may occasionally be mental retardation.

The diagnosis is made on clinical grounds. Treatment is generally unsatisfactory and is directed at the myotonia (e.g. procainamide). General anaesthetics may be hazardous in some patients. Genetic counselling is important.

Myotonia congenita (Thomsen's disease) is a rare myotonic disorder, which may be dominant or recessive and is characterized by muscle hypertrophy and a milder degree of myotonia that is provoked by cold weather and improves with exercise.

MYOPATHIES

Myopathy occurs in a number of systemic disorders, including dermatomyositis, polymyalgia rheumatica and a number of endocrine disorders such as Cushing's syndrome and thyrotoxicosis; it may occur as a remote effect of malignant tumours. A number of other rare forms of myopathy also occur.

It is important to diagnose polymyositis (characterized by high creatinine kinase levels, abnormal EMG, positive muscle biopsy) as this is responsive to treatment with steroids and/or immunosuppresives. It may present with proximal muscle weakness or even as a bulbar palsy.

CHANNELOPATHIES

Rare muscle disorders characterized by a very low or high serum potassium levels, such as the periodic paralyses, have been shown to be due to mutations on genes encoding calcium, chloride or sodium channels in skeletal muscle. These disorders are usually dominantly inherited. Commonly the presentation is with repeated attacks of generalized muscle weakness or myotonia. Symptoms usually start in adolescence and may be provoked by vigorous exercise. The limb muscles are usually affected and the weakness may last for hours. Recognition of these disorders has resulted in specific treatments: hypokalaemic attacks may respond to carbonic anhydrase inhibitors such as acetazolamide, and sodium channel disorders (paramyotonia congenita) to mexilitine. In the acute attack of hypokalaemic paralysis, added potassium supplements may give symptomatic relief.

MYASTHENIA GRAVIS

Myasthenia gravis is a disease in which a reduction in the available functional nicotinic receptors at the neuromuscular junction is associated with increased fatigability and weakness of striated muscles. It may appear at any time of life and affects women more commonly than men.

The cause is not known, but it is an autoimmune condition with evidence of IgG antibodies to acetylcholine receptor protein in 90% of patients. There is an increased incidence of other autoimmune disorders, such as rheumatoid arthritis, pernicious anaemia and systemic lupus erythematosus in patients with myasthenia gravis. Some patients have a thymoma.

The usual presentation is with muscle weakness and fatigability. This commonly involves the ocular muscles but any group may be affected. Ptosis and diplopia are frequent manifestations and get worse during the course of the day. Similarly affected are the muscles of mastication, swallowing and speech. Muscle bulk is usually maintained until late in the disease.

The pharmacological diagnostic test is edrophonium (Tensilon) given by slow intravenous injection (**11.130, 11.131**). Antibodies to the acetylcholine receptor have now been shown to be present in some 90% of patients with generalized myasthenia. Electromyography with repetitive stimulation and single fibre studies may show neuromuscular defects. A search for a thymoma should be made by X-ray (**11.132**) or thoracic CT scanning.

Drug treatment is with a long-acting anticholinesterase, which is usually symptomatically effective. Thymectomy may also result in long-term improvement, and immunosuppression with prednisolone and azathioprine may be beneficial, as is plasma exchange in severe cases. Steroid treatment can result in a temporary deterioration in myasthenic weakness so that this is best started as an in-patient in hospital.

11.130

11.131

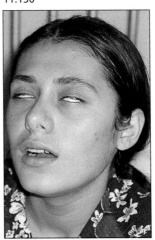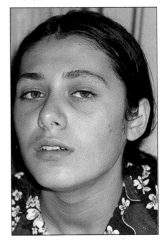

11.130 & 11.131 Myasthenia gravis. The edrophonium (Tensilon) test can be used to confirm the diagnosis. Facial weakness is provoked by repeated facial movements (**11.130**). Edrophonium chloride, a short-acting anticholinesterase, is then given by slow intravenous injection. In myasthenia gravis the facial weakness is rapidly relieved by this test (**11.131**). Objective testing of muscular power elsewhere in the body will reveal similar responses. This test should be always undertaken in hospital where there are resuscitation facilities and with a drawn up syringe of atropine present.

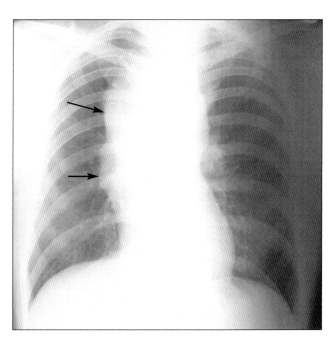

11.132 Thymoma (arrows) in a patient with myasthenia gravis. A lateral film confirmed that this mass was in the anterior mediastinum. Thymectomy may result in cure or great improvement in the myasthenia.

The course of the disease is variable but progressive, and death may result from aspiration pneumonia.

EATON–LAMBERT SYNDROME

Eaton–Lambert syndrome (myasthenic syndrome) is a rare disorder of neuromuscular transmission that is found in patients with small cell (oat cell) carcinoma of the bronchus. It is associated with antibodies to presynaptic calcium channels, and patients present with proximal muscle weakness of the limbs, which worsens with exertion. There may also be sensory features, particularly paraesthesiae. Tendon reflexes are usually absent and cranial nerves are rarely affected.

The diagnosis is made by the presence of voltage gated antibodies to the calcium channel of skeletal muscle and by the results of electromyography using repetitive stimulation. As the neurological symptoms usually precede the overt appearance of the lung lesion an intensive search should be made of the lungs (*see* **p. 194**). Plasmapheresis may be of some value in treating the Eaton–Lambert myasthenic syndrome and some patients respond to 3-4 diaminopyridine.

Index

Note: Numbers in normal type refer to page numbers; numbers in *italics* denote figures. Where both figures and text occur on the same page, only the figure number is given, except where text entry is of major importance.

The use of *versus* refers to differential diagnosis or comparisons.

This index is in letter-by-letter order, whereby hyphens, en-rules and spaces are hidden from the alphabetization.

Common abbreviations used in subentries include: COPD chronic obstructive pulmonary disease; CT computed tomography; DIC disseminated intravascular coagulation; ECG electrocardiogram; MRI magentic resonance imaging; SLE systemic lupus erythematosus

498

myxoedema 312–313
  subdural haematoma 479
  definition 465
  Glasgow Coma Scale 465, *466*, 479
  positioning the unconscious patient
    465, *465*
Common bile duct
  obstruction
    cholangiocarcinoma *381*
    gallstones 398, *398*
    see also Biliary obstruction
  stricture 402
Common cold (coryza) 10–11, *11*
Common hepatic duct, stricture *396*
Compartment syndrome 242–243
Complement, C3 deposition 272
Compression neuropathy 440, *489*,
  489–490, *490*
Computed tomography (CT)
  acute pancreatitis *400*
  cardiovascular disease
    aortic aneurysms 246, *247*
    aortic dissection *248*
  cervical spondylosis *132*
  endocrine disease
    adrenal tumour *301*
    aldosteronism *304*
    Cushing's syndrome *301*
  gastrointestinal disorders 342
    abdominal tumour *343*
    cysticercosis *370*
  Hodgkin's disease *434*
  infectious disease
    aspergillomas *157*
    hydatid cyst 56, *56*
    subphrenic abscess *5*
    tuberculosis 178, *179*
  liver disease 381, *382*
    abscess *388*
    hepatocellular carcinoma *396*
  neurological investigations 458
    brain abscess 472, *473*
    dementias 462, *462*, *463*
    gliomas 469, *469*
    hydrocephalus *468*
    meningioma *458*
    metastatic tumour *193*, *470*
    stroke 473, *474*
    Sturge–Weber syndrome *491*
    subarachnoid haemorrhage 477,
      477
    subdural haematoma *478*
  percutaneous drainage *5*
  renal disease 261, *262*
    carcinoma *289*
  respiratory disease 155
    asbestosis *189*
    bronchial carcinoma *158*, *192*,
      193
    bronchiectasis *174*
    cryptogenic fibrosing alveolitis 185,
      186
    emphysema *170*
Congenital anomalies 225
  lung 'blebs' 195, *196*
Congenital disorders
  endocrine 312
    adrenal hyperplasia 302–304, 307,
      307
    growth 305–308
    hypothyroidism 312
    multiple endocrine neoplasia
      syndromes (MEN) 304
  heart *see* Congenital heart disease
  infections
    cytomegalovirus 21, *21*
    rubella *2*, 12, *13*
    syphilis 62, *62*
    toxoplasmosis *48*
    pigmentation 87, 93, *94*
Congenital heart disease 225–230
  aetiology 225
  coarctation of aorta 228–229, *229*
  common types 226, *226*

cyanosis *225*, 229
Down's syndrome *227*, 336, *336*
Fallot's tetralogy *see* Fallot's tetralogy
  great artery transposition 230
  patent ductus arteriosus 228, *228*
  presentation 226
    'blue baby' *225*
  septal defects 226, 226–227, *227*, *228*,
    230
  squatting *226*
  Wolff–Parkinson–White (WPE)
    syndrome *208*
  see also Cardiovascular abnormalities
Congo Red stains *278*
Coning 456
Conjunctiva
  haemorrhage *231*
  Loa loa in 52, *52*
  pallor *339*
  sparganosis 56, *57*
  suffusion (leptospirosis) 42, *42*
  see also Conjunctivitis
Conjunctivitis
  kawasaki disease 57, *57*
  purulent 59, *60*
  Reiter's syndrome 116
  rheumatoid disorders *104*
  see also Conjunctiva
Connective tissue diseases 121–127
  autoimmune 96–98
  cardiac complications 220
  features 121
  overlap syndromes (MCTD) 127
  pigmentation changes 88
  pulmonary complications 183, *183*
  see also specific diseases
Conn's syndrome 303
Constrictive pericarditis 237
Consumption coagulation *see*
    Disseminated intravascular
    coagulation (DIC)
Contact blepharitis *73*
Contact dermatitis 73
  nickel *73*
  topical steroids 68
Continuous ambulatory peritoneal
    dialysis (CAPD) 266, 267, *267*,
    279
Continuous positive airway pressure
    (CPAP) 173
Cooley's anaemia (β-thalassaemia)
    421–422
Coomb's test 417, 422
COPD *see* Chronic obstructive
    pulmonary disease (COPD)
Copper
  deficiency 331
  excess 394
Core temperature 245
Cornea
  cystinosis *335*
  ectopic calcification *140*
  scarring (trachoma) *42*
  ulceration (herpetic) *20*
  see also Eye
Corneal arcus (arcus corneus) *268*
  hyperlipidaemia *324*, *325*
Cornelia de Lange syndrome *305*
Coronary angiography 205, *205*
  angina 212, *214*
Coronary angioplasty 205, *213*
  angina 212, 214
Coronary artery
  disease (CAD) 212
    see also Ischaemic heart disease
      (IHD)
  occlusion 214
  surgery 214, *214*
Coronary heart disease *see* Ischaemic
    heart disease (IHD)
Cor pulmonale *171*
Corticosteroids
  adverse effects
    Cushing's syndrome *75*, 269

    steroid-induced osteoporosis 128
    topical corticosteroid-induced striae
      75
  dermatitis/eczema management 74
  intra-articular injection 111, *111*
  nephrotic syndrome 269, *269*
  rheumatoid arthritis 112
  temporal arteritis 128
  see also Steroids
Cortisol 300, 301
Corynebacterium diphtheriae 30–31
Coryza (common cold) 10–11, *11*
Cough
  bovine 191
  'brassy' 246
  bronchial carcinoma 190–191
  headache 461
  see also Sputum
Courvoisier's sign 402
Coxiella burnetii 44
Coxsackieviruses 11–12
  pericarditis 235
Cradle cap 73
Cranial (temporal) arteritis 128–129,
    129, 461
Cranial nerves 450–454
  see also individual nerves
Craniopharyngioma 297
C-reactive protein (CRP) 105
Creatine kinase (CK) 216, *217*
Creatinine
  clearance 260
  serum 265
CREST (CRST) syndrome 123
Cretinism 312
Creutzfeldt–Jakob disease (CJD) 58, 463
CRH test 301
Cricothyrotomy 161, *161*
Crohn's disease 331, *331*, *359*, 359–361,
    360, 441
  childhood 359
  cirrhosis 395
  'cobblestone' appearance *343*, *359*
  colitis 359
  epidemiology 359
  extra-intestinal features 360
  fibrosis 359, *359*
  fistulae 359, *360*
  management 360–361
  proctitis *359*
  skip lesions 359, *360*
  small bowel meal *343*
  small intestine tumours 357
CRST (CREST) syndrome 123
Cryoglobulinaemia 445, 446–447
  skin infarction in *447*
Cryptococcosis 46
Cryptococcus neoformans 46
Cryptogenic fibrosing alveolitis (CFA)
    185, 185–186, *186*
  'honeycomb' appearance 185, *186*
Cryptosporidium parvum 368
  HIV-associated 9
Crystal arthropathies 120, 120–121, *121*,
    393
  see also Gout
CT scans *see* Computed tomography
    (CT)
Cullen's sign 399
Cushingoid features *269*
Cushing's disease 299
Cushing's syndrome 299–302, *300*, 302,
    305
  buffalo hump *301*
  CT scan *301*
  diabetes mellitus 316
  diagnosis 301
  ectopic ACTH secretion *193*
  facial features *301*
  Nelson's syndrome 300–302
  proximal muscle wasting *300*
  steroid use *269*, 440
  treatment 302
Cutaneous filariasis 53

Cutaneous larva migrans 54, *54*
Cyanosis
  'blue bloaters' *171*
  cardiovascular disease 200
    congenital heart disease 225, 229
  central *148*, 225, 344
    blood gases 153
  limb *221*
  respiratory disease 147
  tongue *148*
Cyst
  amoebic 47
  baker's 108, *109*
  bone *140*
  cerebellar *458*
  gas-filled (pneumatosis coli) 364–365,
    365
  hydatid 56, *56*
  liver 395, *395*
  ovary 308, *308*
  renal 283
  subarticular *119*
Cystadenoma 396
Cystic duct, gallstone impaction 397
Cysticercosis 370, *370*
Cystic fibrosis 175
  adolescent presentation *175*
  bronchiectasis *174*
  malabsorption 175, *175*
  neonatal presentation *175*
Cystic glioblastoma 469, *469*
Cystinosis 335
  cornea *335*
Cystography, micturating *262*, 285,
    285–286
Cystoscopy *263*
Cytomegalovirus (CMV) 21–22
  congenital infection 21, *21*
  hepatosplenomegaly 21, *21*
  HIV-associated retinitis 9, *9*
  infective oesophagitis 348
  pneumonia (pneumonitis) 21, *21*

D

Dactylitis
  psoriatic arthropathy *116*
  sarcoidosis *182*
  sickle-cell disease *419*
Darier's disease 89
D Dimer test (fibrin degeneration
    products) 410
Deafness, nerve (Alport's syndrome) *284*
Deep vein thrombosis (DVT) 250–252
  differential diagnosis 250
  following myocardial infarction 218
  leg oedema 250, *251*
  post-phlebetic syndrome 252
  risk factors 249, *250*
  symptoms/signs 250, *251*
  thrombophilia 252
  treatment 250, *252*
Defibrillation *216*
Dementia 461–463
  alcoholic 463
  Alzheimer's disease 461–462, *462*
  causes 461, *462*
  cerebral infarction 463, *463*
  clinical features 462
  Creutzfeldt–Jakob disease (CJD) 463
  epidemiology 461
  Huntington's chorea 463
  investigation 462
  Lewy body 462
  management 463
  multi-infarct 462, *463*
  normal-pressure hydrocephalus 463
  risk factors 461–462
Demodex folliculorum 85
Demyelinating disease 472
  see also Multiple sclerosis
Dendritic ulcer 18, *19*
Dengue haemorrhagic fever 13, *13*

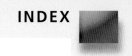

503

505

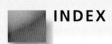

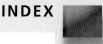
509

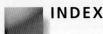

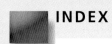

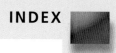

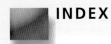

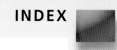

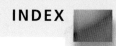